# Emerging Diseases/Viruses Prevention: Control, Surveillance, and One Health

# Emerging Diseases/Viruses Prevention: Control, Surveillance, and One Health

Editor

**Yannick Simonin**

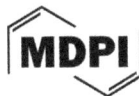

Basel • Beijing • Wuhan • Barcelona • Belgrade • Novi Sad • Cluj • Manchester

*Editor*
Yannick Simonin
University of Montpellier
Montpellier, France

*Editorial Office*
MDPI
St. Alban-Anlage 66
4052 Basel, Switzerland

This is a reprint of articles from the Special Issue published online in the open access journal *Tropical Medicine and Infectious Disease* (ISSN 2414-6366) (available at: https://www.mdpi.com/journal/tropicalmed/special_issues/Emerging_Viruses_Prevention).

For citation purposes, cite each article independently as indicated on the article page online and as indicated below:

Lastname, A.A.; Lastname, B.B. Article Title. *Journal Name* **Year**, *Volume Number*, Page Range.

ISBN 978-3-0365-8856-8 (Hbk)
ISBN 978-3-0365-8857-5 (PDF)
doi.org/10.3390/books978-3-0365-8857-5

© 2023 by the authors. Articles in this book are Open Access and distributed under the Creative Commons Attribution (CC BY) license. The book as a whole is distributed by MDPI under the terms and conditions of the Creative Commons Attribution-NonCommercial-NoDerivs (CC BY-NC-ND) license.

# Contents

**Yannick Simonin**
Emerging Diseases/Viruses Prevention, Control, Surveillance, and One Health
Reprinted from: *Trop. Med. Infect. Dis.* 2023, 8, 257, doi:10.3390/tropicalmed8050257 . . . . . . . 1

**Yannick Simonin**
Special Issue "Emerging Diseases/Viruses: Prevention, Control, Surveillance, and One Health"
Reprinted from: *Trop. Med. Infect. Dis.* 2022, 7, 301, doi:10.3390/tropicalmed7100301 . . . . . . . 5

**Bona S. H. Hutahaean, Sarah E. Stutterheim and Kai J. Jonas**
Barriers and Facilitators to HIV Treatment Adherence in Indonesia: Perspectives of People Living with HIV and HIV Service Providers
Reprinted from: *Trop. Med. Infect. Dis.* 2023, 8, 138, doi:10.3390/tropicalmed8030138 . . . . . . . 7

**Ning Li, Haidong Li, Zhengji Chen, Huan Xiong, Zhibo Li, Tao Wei, et al.**
Estimating Dengue Transmission Intensity in China Using Catalytic Models Based on Serological Data
Reprinted from: *Trop. Med. Infect. Dis.* 2023, 8, 116, doi:10.3390/tropicalmed8020116 . . . . . . . 31

**Debjit Chakraborty, Falguni Debnath, Suman Kanungo, Sandip Mukhopadhyay, Nabanita Chakraborty, Rivu Basu, et al.**
Rationality of Prescriptions by Rational Use of Medicine Consensus Approach in Common Respiratory and Gastrointestinal Infections: An Outpatient Department Based Cross-Sectional Study from India
Reprinted from: *Trop. Med. Infect. Dis.* 2023, 8, 88, doi:10.3390/tropicalmed8020088 . . . . . . . . 51

**Moufid Mhamadi, Aminata Badji, Mamadou Aliou Barry, El Hadji Ndiaye, Alioune Gaye, Mignane Ndiaye, et al.**
Human and Livestock Surveillance Revealed the Circulation of Rift Valley Fever Virus in Agnam, Northern Senegal, 2021
Reprinted from: *Trop. Med. Infect. Dis.* 2023, 8, 87, doi:10.3390/tropicalmed8020087 . . . . . . . . 63

**Victor Diogho Heuer de Carvalho, Thyago Celso Cavalcante Nepomuceno, Thiago Poleto and Ana Paula Cabral Seixas Costa**
The COVID-19 Infodemic on Twitter: A Space and Time Topic Analysis of the Brazilian Immunization Program and Public Trust
Reprinted from: *Trop. Med. Infect. Dis.* 2022, 7, 425, doi:10.3390/ tropicalmed7120425 . . . . . . . 75

**Wenbo Zeng, Zhongqiu Li, Tiange Jiang, Donghui Cheng, Limin Yang, Tian Hang, et al.**
Identification of Bacterial Communities and Tick-Borne Pathogens in *Haemaphysalis* spp. Collected from Shanghai, China
Reprinted from: *Trop. Med. Infect. Dis.* 2022, 7, 413, doi:10.3390/tropicalmed7120413 . . . . . . . 101

**Nuning Nuraini, Ilham Saiful Fauzi, Bony Wiem Lestari and Sila Rizqina**
The Impact of COVID-19 Quarantine on Tuberculosis and Diabetes Mellitus Cases: A Modelling Study
Reprinted from: *Trop. Med. Infect. Dis.* 2022, 7, 407, doi:10.3390/tropicalmed7120407 . . . . . . . 125

**Ruba Chakma, Pimolpachr Sriburin, Pichamon Sittikul, Jittraporn Rattanamahaphoom, Warisa Nuprasert, Nipa Thammasonthijarern, et al.**
Arbovirus Seroprevalence Study in Bangphae District, Ratchaburi Province, Thailand: Comparison between ELISA and a Multiplex Rapid Diagnostic Test (Chembio DPP® ZCD IgG)
Reprinted from: *Trop. Med. Infect. Dis.* 2022, 7, 378, doi:10.3390/tropicalmed7110378 . . . . . . . 145

**Min-Ju Kim, Ki-Back Chu, Su-Hwa Lee, Hae-Ji Kang, Keon-Woong Yoon, Md Atique Ahmed and Fu-Shi Quan**
Recombinant Vaccinia Virus Expressing *Plasmodium berghei* Apical Membrane Antigen 1 or Microneme Protein Enhances Protection against *P. berghei* Infection in Mice
Reprinted from: *Trop. Med. Infect. Dis.* **2022**, *7*, 350, doi:10.3390/tropicalmed7110350 . . . . . . . **159**

**Vladimir Stevanovic, Tatjana Vilibic-Cavlek, Vladimir Savic, Ana Klobucar, Snjezana Kovac, Marcela Curman Posavec, et al.**
Surveillance of Tahyna Orthobunyavirus in Urban Areas in Croatia—The "One Health" Approach
Reprinted from: *Trop. Med. Infect. Dis.* **2022**, *7*, 320, doi:10.3390/tropicalmed7100320 . . . . . . . **173**

**Coceka N. Mnyani, Andomei Smit and Gayle G. Sherman**
Infant HIV Testing Amid the COVID-19 Pandemic and Evolving PMTCT Guidelines in Johannesburg, South Africa
Reprinted from: *Trop. Med. Infect. Dis.* **2022**, *7*, 302, doi:10.3390/tropicalmed7100302 . . . . . . . **185**

**Valliammai Jayanthi Thirunavuk Arasoo, Mariyammah Masalamani, Amutha Ramadas, Nisha Angela Dominic, Darien Daojuin Liew, Robin Wai Jen Sia, et al.**
Association between Chlamydial Infection with Ectopic and Full-Term Pregnancies: A Case-Control Study
Reprinted from: *Trop. Med. Infect. Dis.* **2022**, *7*, 285, doi:10.3390/tropicalmed7100285 . . . . . . . **193**

**Pichamon Sittikul, Pimolpachr Sriburin, Jittraporn Rattanamahaphoom, Kriengsak Limkittikul, Chukiat Sirivichayakul and Supawat Chatchen**
Combining Immunoassays to Identify Zika Virus Infection in Dengue-Endemic Areas
Reprinted from: *Trop. Med. Infect. Dis.* **2022**, *7*, 254, doi:10.3390/tropicalmed7100254 . . . . . . . **203**

**Xu-Sheng Zhang, Huan Xiong, Zhengji Chen and Wei Liu**
Importation, Local Transmission, and Model Selection in Estimating the Transmissibility of COVID-19: The Outbreak in Shaanxi Province of China as a Case Study
Reprinted from: *Trop. Med. Infect. Dis.* **2022**, *7*, 227, doi:10.3390/tropicalmed7090227 . . . . . . . **211**

**Yi-Ming Zhong, Xiao-He Zhang, Zheng Ma and Wen-En Liu**
Prevalence of *Escherichia coli* ST1193 Causing Intracranial Infection in Changsha, China
Reprinted from: *Trop. Med. Infect. Dis.* **2022**, *7*, 217, doi:10.3390/tropicalmed7090217 . . . . . . . **229**

**Maxim Van Herreweghe, Annelies Breynaert, Tess De Bruyne, Corneliu Petru Popescu, Simin-Aysel Florescu, Yaniv Lustig, et al.**
Can Biomarkers of Oxidative Stress in Serum Predict Disease Severity in West Nile Virus Infection? A Pilot Study
Reprinted from: *Trop. Med. Infect. Dis.* **2022**, *7*, 207, doi:10.3390/tropicalmed7090207 . . . . . . . **237**

**Michal Solomon, Inbal Fuchs, Yael Glazer and Eli Schwartz**
Gender and Cutaneous Leishmaniasis in Israel
Reprinted from: *Trop. Med. Infect. Dis.* **2022**, *7*, 179, doi:10.3390/tropicalmed7080179 . . . . . . . **243**

**Zhongqiu Li, Wenbo Zeng, Yufeng Yang, Peijun Zhang, Zhengbing Zhou, Yuanyuan Li, et al.**
Expression Profile Analysis of Circular RNAs in Leishmaniasis
Reprinted from: *Trop. Med. Infect. Dis.* **2022**, *7*, 176, doi:10.3390/tropicalmed7080176 . . . . . . . **251**

**Giulia Mencattelli, Federica Iapaolo, Andrea Polci, Maurilia Marcacci, Annapia Di Gennaro, Liana Teodori, et al.**
West Nile Virus Lineage 2 Overwintering in Italy
Reprinted from: *Trop. Med. Infect. Dis.* **2022**, *7*, 160, doi:10.3390/tropicalmed7080160 . . . . . . . **263**

**Vanessa Chong, Jennifer Zi Ling Tan and Valliammai Jayanthi Thirunavuk Arasoo**
Dengue in Pregnancy: A Southeast Asian Perspective
Reprinted from: *Trop. Med. Infect. Dis.* 2023, *8*, 86, doi:10.3390/tropicalmed8020086 . . . . . . . . 273

**Allan Mayaba Mwiinde, Enock Siankwilimba, Masauso Sakala, Faustin Banda and Charles Michelo**
Climatic and Environmental Factors Influencing COVID-19 Transmission—An African Perspective
Reprinted from: *Trop. Med. Infect. Dis.* 2022, *7*, 433, doi:10.3390/tropicalmed7100320 . . . . . . . 297

**Rafaella de Carvalho Cardoso, Bismarck Rezende, Allan Kardec Nogueira Alencar, Fabrícia Lima Fontes-Dantas and Guilherme Carneiro Montes**
Role of Arbovirus Infection in Arthritogenic Pain Manifestation—A Systematic Review
Reprinted from: *Trop. Med. Infect. Dis.* 2022, *7*, 390, doi:10.3390/tropicalmed7110390 . . . . . . . 321

**Amira Wahida Mohamad Safiee, Mohammad Ridhuan Mohd Ali, Muhammad Zarul Hanifah Md Zoqratt, Tan Hock Siew, Chua Wei Chuan, Lee Lih Huey, et al.**
Putative Pathogenic Genes of *Leptospira interrogans* and *Leptospira weilii* Isolated from Patients with Acute Febrile Illness
Reprinted from: *Trop. Med. Infect. Dis.* 2022, *7*, 284, doi:10.3390/tropicalmed7100284 . . . . . . . 331

**Nadia A. Fernández-Santos, Gabriel L. Hamer, Edith G. Garrido-Lozada and Mario A. Rodríguez-Pérez**
SARS-CoV-2 Infections in a High-Risk Migratory Population Arriving to a Migrant House along the US-Mexico Border
Reprinted from: *Trop. Med. Infect. Dis.* 2022, *7*, 262, doi:10.3390/tropicalmed7100262 . . . . . . . 343

**Polrat Wilairatana, Wanida Mala, Kwuntida Uthaisar Kotepui and Manas Kotepui**
Prevalence and Characteristics of Malaria and Influenza Co-Infection in Febrile Patients: A Systematic Review and Meta-Analysis
Reprinted from: *Trop. Med. Infect. Dis.* 2022, *7*, 168, doi:10.3390/tropicalmed7080168 . . . . . . . 351

**Deborah N. Melo, Giovanna R. P. Lima, Carolina G. Fernandes, André C. Teixeira, Joel B. Filho, Fernanda M. C. Araújo, et al.**
Post-Mortem Diagnosis of Pediatric Dengue Using Minimally Invasive Autopsy during the COVID-19 Pandemic in Brazil
Reprinted from: *Trop. Med. Infect. Dis.* 2022, *7*, 123, doi:10.3390/tropicalmed7070123 . . . . . . . 367

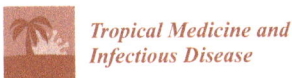 Tropical Medicine and Infectious Disease

*Editorial*

# Emerging Diseases/Viruses Prevention, Control, Surveillance, and One Health

Yannick Simonin

Pathogenesis and Control of Chronic and Emerging Infections, University of Montpellier, INSERM, Etablissement Français du San, 34394 Montpellier, France; yannick.simonin@umontpellier.fr

**Citation:** Simonin, Y. Emerging Diseases/Viruses Prevention, Control, Surveillance, and One Health. *Trop. Med. Infect. Dis.* **2023**, *8*, 257. https://doi.org/10.3390/tropicalmed8050257

Received: 23 April 2023
Accepted: 24 April 2023
Published: 29 April 2023

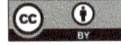

**Copyright:** © 2023 by the author. Licensee MDPI, Basel, Switzerland. This article is an open access article distributed under the terms and conditions of the Creative Commons Attribution (CC BY) license (https://creativecommons.org/licenses/by/4.0/).

Emerging diseases have posed a constant threat and major challenge to human health throughout our history. From the Black Death in the Middle Ages to the COVID-19 pandemic, these diseases have generated significant human suffering and economic disruption. The emergence of new pathogens, such as Ebola, Zika, SARS-CoV-2 or mpox, has illustrated the potential for these diseases to spread extraordinarily rapidly. Far from dissipating despite remarkable advances in medical science and public health in recent decades, emerging diseases continue to appear and proliferate at an alarming rate. Changes in our environment, produced primarily by human activity and the evolution of human/animal interactions, are likely to be responsible for novel health crises in the future.

Therefore, prioritizing the prevention of emerging diseases is essential in order to prepare for these future health crises. Preventive measures for emerging diseases involve early detection and rapid responses, but also the development of effective vaccines and treatments. Strengthening surveillance systems and enhancing diagnostic capacities are essential in order to detect and respond rapidly to epidemics. In addition, it is vital to boost investment in public health infrastructure, particularly with regard to sanitation and hygiene in general, in order to mitigate the risk of disease transmission. In order to achieve this, public health systems must be equipped with the necessary resources and trained personnel to detect and respond rapidly to epidemics, which both require significant investment. In addition to preventive measures, control measures are required in order to contain emerging diseases. The SARS-CoV-2 pandemic has revealed to us that the contact tracing of patients and the isolation and quarantine of infected people, all coupled with extensive vaccination campaigns, are productive control measures. In addition, effective communication strategies are required in order to prevent emerging diseases and must be designed to reach all factions of the population, including isolated groups and those with limited access to health care, particularly those who live on the streets.

Prevention measures for emerging diseases must often be implemented on a global scale. This requires international cooperation and coordination to quickly detect and respond to outbreaks. A fundamental approach to strengthening surveillance systems is the One Health concept. This concept recognizes that human health, animal health and environmental health are interdependent. Zoonoses represent at least 60% of infectious diseases and no less than two-thirds of novel emerging diseases. Therefore, monitoring and containing animal populations can greatly aid in the prevention of novel pathogens emerging. Furthermore, monitoring environmental factors, such as temperature and humidity, may help anticipate the emergence of novel pathogens, including vector-borne diseases.

Amongst the pathogens that possess a significant potential for emergence are arboviruses, whose distribution is constantly expanding in correlation with their vectors, particularly mosquitoes. Indeed, climate change, urbanization and land use all affect the dynamics of vectors, as well as reservoir host populations and the transmission of vector-borne pathogens. In this context, the geographical distribution of arboviruses is expanding; it now affects all five continents and has become a major public health concern. Among the 26 articles collected in this SI, 10 articles attend to arboviruses. Dengue (DENV) is the most diffuse arbovirosis in the world, and DENV cases have been surging in recent years. Li et al. review the literature and reveal studies that have collected age-specific DENV serological data in China; they discover that the transmission intensity varies depending on age in most of the study populations, and the attenuation of antibody protection was identified in some study populations [1]. Melo et al. report the first pediatric disease in which the use of minimally invasive autopsy has confirmed severe dengue as the cause of death [2]. Chong et al., in a narrative review, detail the impact of DENV on pregnancy in Southeast Asia, revealing, in particular, the specific physiological effects of dengue during the trimesters of pregnancy [3]. Another study uses the combination of a DENV and zika virus (ZIKV) nonstructural protein 1 IgG enzyme-linked immunosorbent assay and a ZIKV NS1 blockade-of-binding ELISA in order to test the convalescent sera of non-flavivirus, primary DENV, secondary DENV, and ZIKV infections. The authors discover that primary testing via a ZIKV NS1 IgG ELISA is the prime option for large-scale ZIKV serosurvey studies and provides relatively high sensitivity [4]. Regarding WNV, one article of this SI details the detection of WNV lineage 2 infection in birds from the Umbria region during the cold season; it confirms that the L2 strains of WNV that circulate in Italy are genetically stable and provides evidence of a continuous circulation of WNV in Italy throughout the year [5]. Another study foregrounds the correlation between oxidation and severe disease in WNV-infected patients [6]. Mhamadi et al. illustrate the circulation of Rift Valley fever virus in northern Senegal through human and livestock surveillance [7], while Stevanovic et al. demonstrate the rather high seroprevalence of Tahyna orthobunyavirus, a neglected mosquito-borne bunyavirus, in human and animal (horses and pets) serum in a One Health approach; this evidences the criticality of studying this neglected arbovirus [8]. Another report studies the seroprevalence of DENV, ZIKV, or CHIKV in Bangphae District, Ratchaburi Province, Thailand, via enzyme-linked immunosorbent assays and rapid diagnostic tests [9]. Furthermore, one review details the role of CHIKV infection in arthritogenic pain, which appears to be comparable to rheumatoid arthritis as both diseases share common symptoms [10].

Five articles in this SI attend to the COVID-19 pandemic from various perspectives. De Carvalho et al. summarize the COVID-19 infodemic on Twitter in Brazil via a study that applies a thematic analysis across space and time with respect to public opinion regarding the Brazilian COVID-19 immunization program [11]. Another study highlights the influence of climatic and environmental elements on the proliferation of COVID-19 in Africa [12]. The research article by Zhang et al. proposes five models through which to study the early COVID-19 outbreak in Shaanxi, China. They demonstrate that the renewal equation model provides the optimum modelling and significantly enhances the estimate of transmissibility [13]. In a brief report, Fernández-Santos et al. suggest that vulnerable populations traveling from Latin American countries and seeking residence in the United States are at a high risk of exposure to SARS-CoV-2 [14]. Another study reveals that quarantine effectively diminishes the number of COVID-19 cases but induces an escalating number people suffering from tuberculosis and diabetes; this emphasizes the criticality of promoting a healthy lifestyle when implementing quarantine [15].

Two further articles attend to HIV; the first studies the barriers to and facilitators of adherence to antiretroviral therapy in Indonesia by employing a socioecological approach [16]. The second evaluates the impact of COVID-19 on receiving an HIV diagnosis in children, particularly regarding the prevention of the mother-to-child transmission of HIV in Johannesburg, South Africa [17].

This SI also includes four articles that focus on parasite-related issues and in particular, two articles on leishmaniasis. The first, from Israel, reveals that there is no tangible variation regarding sex difference in leishmanial infection in humans [18]. The second article provides novel evidence for the modification of differentially expressed circRNAs and their potential function in leishmaniasis [19]. Kim et al. compare the efficacies of the recombinant vaccinia viruses that express either the AMA1 or microneme protein (MIC) of *Plasmodium berghei* in mice. Their results indicate that the recombinant vaccinia viruses that express MIC could be an advantageous candidate vaccine- antigen [20]. Another study aims to analyze the prevalence and characteristics of malaria and influenza co-infection in febrile patients. The prevalence of this co-infection among these patients is revealed to be heterogeneous by country, the characteristics of the febrile participants, and the diagnostic tests for influenza virus [21].

Four further articles attend to bacterial infections. An article from Zhong et al. reveal that *Escherichia coli* ST1193 isolates have emerged as the predominant type of *E. coli* strain that causes intracranial infections in Changsha, China [22]. A case report by Safiee et al. indicates that the various infecting *Leptospira* species and the presence of a range of virulence factors result in a modest variation in the clinical manifestations and laboratory findings of leptospirosis [23]. Another study conducted in Malaysia demonstrates that women who experience an ectopic pregnancy are more likely to have tested positive for chlamydia than those who give birth at term [24]. Zheng et al. from Shanghai, China, investigate the bacterial communities and the prevalence of some primary pathogens in *Haemaphysalis* spp., the dominant species of ticks in Shanghai [25]. Chakraborty et al. analyze the prescriptions of patients suffering from diarrhea or acute respiratory infection in order to understand the prescription pattern among various categories of prescribers in two tertiary care centers in West Bengal, India. They reveal that irrational prescribing patterns prevail in tertiary care centers [26].

Cumulatively, the 26 articles collected in this issue provide readers with a broad overview of emerging diseases and foreground the advances made in our understanding of several domains related to the knowledge, surveillance and control of zoonotic diseases. We sincerely thank the authors, reviewers and the editorial staff members for their contributions to this Special Issue.

**Acknowledgments:** Author thanks all authors for contributing their work to this Special Issue.

**Conflicts of Interest:** The author declare no conflict of interest.

# References

1. Li, N.; Li, H.; Chen, Z.; Xiong, H.; Li, Z.; Wei, T.; Liu, W.; Zhang, X.S. Estimating Dengue Transmission Intensity in China Using Catalytic Models Based on Serological Data. *Trop. Med. Infect. Dis.* **2023**, *8*, 20116. [CrossRef]
2. Melo, D.N.; Lima, G.R.P.; Fernandes, C.G.; Teixeira, A.C.; Filho, J.B.; Araújo, F.M.C.; Araújo, L.C.; Siqueira, A.M.; Farias, L.A.B.G.; Monteiro, R.A.A.; et al. Post-Mortem Diagnosis of Pediatric Dengue Using Minimally Invasive Autopsy during the COVID-19 Pandemic in Brazil. *Trop. Med. Infect. Dis.* **2022**, *7*, 123. [CrossRef] [PubMed]
3. Chong, V.; Tan, J.Z.L.; Arasoo, V.J.T. Dengue in Pregnancy: A Southeast Asian Perspective. *Trop. Med. Infect. Dis.* **2023**, *8*, 86. [CrossRef] [PubMed]
4. Sittikul, P.; Sriburin, P.; Rattanamahaphoom, J.; Limkittikul, K.; Sirivichayakul, C.; Chatchen, S. Combining Immunoassays to Identify Zika Virus Infection in Dengue-Endemic Areas. *Trop. Med. Infect. Dis.* **2022**, *7*, 254. [CrossRef] [PubMed]
5. Mencattelli, G.; Iapaolo, F.; Polci, A.; Marcacci, M.; Di Gennaro, A.; Teodori, L.; Curini, V.; Di Lollo, V.; Secondini, B.; Scialabba, S.; et al. West Nile Virus Lineage 2 Overwintering in Italy. *Trop. Med. Infect. Dis.* **2022**, *7*, 160. [CrossRef] [PubMed]
6. Van Herreweghe, M.; Breynaert, A.; De Bruyne, T.; Popescu, C.P.; Florescu, S.A.; Lustig, Y.; Schwartz, E.; Gobbi, F.G.; Hermans, N.; Huits, R. Can Biomarkers of Oxidative Stress in Serum Predict Disease Severity in West Nile Virus Infection? A Pilot Study. *Trop. Med. Infect. Dis.* **2022**, *7*, 207. [CrossRef]
7. Mhamadi, M.; Badji, A.; Barry, M.A.; Ndiaye, E.H.; Gaye, A.; Ndiaye, M.; Mhamadi, M.; Touré, C.T.; Ndiaye, O.; Faye, B.; et al. Human and Livestock Surveillance Revealed the Circulation of Rift Valley Fever Virus in Agnam, Northern Senegal, 2021. *Trop. Med. Infect. Dis.* **2023**, *8*, 87. [CrossRef]
8. Stevanovic, V.; Vilibic-Cavlek, T.; Savic, V.; Klobucar, A.; Kovac, S.; Curman Posavec, M.; Petrinic, S.; Bogdanic, M.; Santini, M.; Tesic, V.; et al. Surveillance of Tahyna Orthobunyavirus in Urban Areas in Croatia-The "One Health" Approach. *Trop. Med. Infect. Dis.* **2022**, *7*, 320. [CrossRef]
9. Chakma, R.; Sriburin, P.; Sittikul, P.; Rattanamahaphoom, J.; Nuprasert, W.; Thammasonthijarern, N.; Maneekan, P.; Thaipadungpanit, J.; Arunsodsai, W.; Sirivichayakul, C.; et al. Arbovirus Seroprevalence Study in Bangphae District, Ratchaburi Province, Thailand: Comparison between ELISA and a Multiplex Rapid Diagnostic Test (Chembio DPP® ZCD IgG). *Trop. Med. Infect. Dis.* **2022**, *7*, 378. [CrossRef]
10. de Carvalho Cardoso, R.; Rezende, B.; Alencar, A.K.N.; Fontes-Dantas, F.L.; Montes, G.C. Role of Arbovirus Infection in Arthritogenic Pain Manifestation-A Systematic Review. *Trop. Med. Infect. Dis.* **2022**, *7*, 390. [CrossRef]

11. de Carvalho, V.D.H.; Nepomuceno, T.C.C.; Poleto, T.; Costa, A.P.C.S. The COVID-19 Infodemic on Twitter: A Space and Time Topic Analysis of the Brazilian Immunization Program and Public Trust. *Trop. Med. Infect. Dis.* **2022**, *7*, 425. [CrossRef]
12. Mwiinde, A.M.; Siankwilimba, E.; Sakala, M.; Banda, F.; Michelo, C. Climatic and Environmental Factors Influencing COVID-19 Transmission-An African Perspective. *Trop. Med. Infect. Dis.* **2022**, *7*, 433. [CrossRef] [PubMed]
13. Zhang, X.S.; Xiong, H.; Chen, Z.; Liu, W. Importation, Local Transmission, and Model Selection in Estimating the Transmissibility of COVID-19: The Outbreak in Shaanxi Province of China as a Case Study. *Trop. Med. Infect. Dis.* **2022**, *7*, 227. [CrossRef] [PubMed]
14. Fernández-Santos, N.A.; Hamer, G.L.; Garrido-Lozada, E.G.; Rodríguez-Pérez, M.A. SARS-CoV-2 Infections in a High-Risk Migratory Population Arriving to a Migrant House along the US-Mexico Border. *Trop. Med. Infect. Dis.* **2022**, *7*, 262. [CrossRef] [PubMed]
15. Nuraini, N.; Fauzi, I.S.; Lestari, B.W.; Rizqina, S. The Impact of COVID-19 Quarantine on Tuberculosis and Diabetes Mellitus Cases: A Modelling Study. *Trop. Med. Infect. Dis.* **2022**, *7*, 407. [CrossRef]
16. Hutahaean, B.S.H.; Stutterheim, S.E.; Jonas, K.J. Barriers and Facilitators to HIV Treatment Adherence in Indonesia: Perspectives of People Living with HIV and HIV Service Providers. *Trop. Med. Infect. Dis.* **2023**, *8*, 138. [CrossRef] [PubMed]
17. Mnyani, C.N.; Smit, A.; Sherman, G.G. Infant HIV Testing Amid the COVID-19 Pandemic and Evolving PMTCT Guidelines in Johannesburg, South Africa. *Trop. Med. Infect. Dis.* **2022**, *7*, 302. [CrossRef] [PubMed]
18. Solomon, M.; Fuchs, I.; Glazer, Y.; Schwartz, E. Gender and Cutaneous Leishmaniasis in Israel. *Trop. Med. Infect. Dis.* **2022**, *7*, 179. [CrossRef]
19. Li, Z.; Zeng, W.; Yang, Y.; Zhang, P.; Zhou, Z.; Li, Y.; Guo, Y.; Zhang, Y. Expression Profile Analysis of Circular RNAs in Leishmaniasis. *Trop. Med. Infect. Dis.* **2022**, *7*, 176. [CrossRef]
20. Kim, M.-J.; Chu, K.-B.; Lee, S.-H.; Kang, H.-J.; Yoon, K.-W.; Ahmed, M.A.; Quan, F.-S. Recombinant Vaccinia Virus Expressing Plasmodium berghei Apical Membrane Antigen 1 or Microneme Protein Enhances Protection against *P. berghei* Infection in Mice. *Trop. Med. Infect. Dis.* **2022**, *7*, 350. [CrossRef]
21. Wilairatana, P.; Mala, W.; Kotepui, K.U.; Kotepui, M. Prevalence and Characteristics of Malaria and Influenza Co-Infection in Febrile Patients: A Systematic Review and Meta-Analysis. *Trop. Med. Infect. Dis.* **2022**, *7*, 168. [CrossRef] [PubMed]
22. Zhong, Y.M.; Zhang, X.H.; Ma, Z.; Liu, W.E. Prevalence of Escherichia coli ST1193 Causing Intracranial Infection in Changsha, China. *Trop. Med. Infect. Dis.* **2022**, *7*, 217. [CrossRef]
23. Safiee, A.W.M.; Mohd, A.M.R.; Zoqratt, M.Z.H.M.; Siew, T.H.; Chuan, C.W.; Huey, L.L.; Fauzi, M.H.; Besari, A.M.; Yean, Y.C.; Ismail, N. Putative Pathogenic Genes of Leptospira interrogans and *Leptospira weilii* Isolated from Patients with Acute Febrile Illness. *Trop. Med. Infect. Dis.* **2022**, *7*, 284. [CrossRef]
24. Thirunavuk, A.V.J.; Masalamani, M.; Ramadas, A.; Dominic, N.A.; Liew, D.D.; Sia, R.W.J.; Wanigaratne, A.; Weerawarna, K.; Wong, W.L.L.; Jeganathan, R. Association between Chlamydial Infection with Ectopic and Full-Term Pregnancies: A Case-Control Study. *Trop. Med. Infect. Dis.* **2022**, *7*, 285. [CrossRef] [PubMed]
25. Zeng, W.; Li, Z.; Jiang, T.; Cheng, D.; Yang, L.; Hang, T.; Duan, L.; Zhu, D.; Fang, Y.; Zhang, Y. Identification of Bacterial Communities and Tick-Borne Pathogens in Haemaphysalis spp. Collected from Shanghai, China. *Trop. Med. Infect. Dis.* **2022**, *7*, 413. [CrossRef] [PubMed]
26. Chakraborty, D.; Debnath, F.; Kanungo, S.; Mukhopadhyay, S.; Chakraborty, N.; Basu, R.; Das, P.; Datta, K.; Ganguly, S.; Banerjee, P.; et al. Rationality of Prescriptions by Rational Use of Medicine Consensus Approach in Common Respiratory and Gastrointestinal Infections: An Outpatient Department Based Cross-Sectional Study from India. *Trop. Med. Infect. Dis.* **2023**, *8*, 88. [CrossRef] [PubMed]

**Disclaimer/Publisher's Note:** The statements, opinions and data contained in all publications are solely those of the individual author(s) and contributor(s) and not of MDPI and/or the editor(s). MDPI and/or the editor(s) disclaim responsibility for any injury to people or property resulting from any ideas, methods, instructions or products referred to in the content.

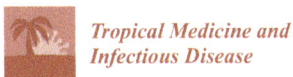 *Tropical Medicine and Infectious Disease*

*Editorial*

# Special Issue "Emerging Diseases/Viruses: Prevention, Control, Surveillance, and One Health"

Yannick Simonin

Pathogenesis and Control of Chronic and Emerging Infections, University of Montpellier, INSERM, Etablissemnt Français du Sang, 34000 Montpellier, France; yannick.simonin@umontpellier.fr

**Citation:** Simonin, Y. Special Issue "Emerging Diseases/Viruses: Prevention, Control, Surveillance, and One Health". *Trop. Med. Infect. Dis.* **2022**, *7*, 301. https://doi.org/10.3390/tropicalmed7100301

Received: 8 October 2022
Accepted: 10 October 2022
Published: 15 October 2022

**Publisher's Note:** MDPI stays neutral with regard to jurisdictional claims in published maps and institutional affiliations.

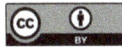

**Copyright:** © 2022 by the author. Licensee MDPI, Basel, Switzerland. This article is an open access article distributed under the terms and conditions of the Creative Commons Attribution (CC BY) license (https://creativecommons.org/licenses/by/4.0/).

Zoonotic diseases account for at least 60% of all infectious diseases and no less than two-thirds of new emerging ones, which underlines the importance of monitoring them as early as possible. Understanding the nature of the animal-to-human transmission of zoonotic diseases is a fundamental requirement for their effective anticipation and control. The SARS-CoV-2 pandemic, and more recently, the monkeypox epidemic, have revealed our limited preparedness against a diversity of emerging and re-emerging pathogens. There are different modes of transmission of zoonotic diseases: direct or indirect contacts, vector-borne, or environmental (water, soil, food, etc.), making their monitoring more complex. Effective control of zoonotic diseases requires early detection of the source of the disease and the factors that contribute to its spread. Combining wildlife, farm animal, and domestic animal health monitoring with human health monitoring can greatly reduce the risk of major epidemics or pandemics of zoonotic origin.

The changes in our environment caused mainly by human activity and the evolution of human–animal interactions are and will undoubtedly be responsible for several new health crises. These crises will be manifested in particular by an increase in the frequency and intensity of epidemics and epizootics. Numerous factors favor the increase in interactions between humans, animals, and their environment, such as the increase in animal and human population movements, or the demographic increase in the human population and its expansion into new geographical areas (ultimately increasing human/wildlife interactions). Over half of known human pathogenic diseases can be aggravated by climate change, including warming, precipitation, and floods [1]. These profound changes can have major consequences for human health. Consequently, the need to understand the emergence of a disease in humans through an approach that integrates a large number of environmental parameters, described as global, has been reinforced.

The links and analogies between animal health and human health have been known since Antiquity, particularly with the transposition of anatomical knowledge from animals (particularly from dissections) to humans. This notion was expressed more concretely in the mid-1800s by a Prussian pathologist, Rudolf Virchow, who emphasized the lack of distinction between animal and human medicine. The "One Health" concept has since developed by basing the study of these issues on multidisciplinary and multisectoral approaches [2]. Its general principle is to study the interactions between animals, humans, and their various environments. Despite its rich content and the fact that the concept has been around for a long time, its practical application remains very limited and is confronted with organizational difficulties. It is in the fight against zoonoses, which are responsible for emerging diseases that tend to become epidemic or even endemic, that the One Health concept was applied the earliest and most effectively. Indeed, awareness of the importance of this concept became more prevalent during health crises initially involving animal health, particularly in Africa. There are many examples of surveillance of zoonotic diseases using integrated approaches, particularly in areas of the world where humans, domestic animals, and wildlife live in close contact. Examples include brucellosis in many countries, including the Middle East; bovine tuberculosis in sub-Saharan Africa; leptospirosis in Fiji; and Ebola in West Africa. These examples underline the need for integrated approaches to the efficient management of complex health problems. The COVID-19 crisis has demonstrated the need to better implement integrated approaches to health and has prompted us to look ahead to the post-crisis period and to anticipate the management of future crises. Historically focused on zoonotic issues, the One Health concept has evolved into a broader disciplinary field, including food safety, water safety, biodiversity, and climate change adaptation. This evolution is due to the awareness that the factors at the origin of health problems are multiple and complex and are not limited to the study of the direct or indirect interactions between animals and humans.

In this Special Issue, we invite colleagues to submit original research articles and scientific reviews to assemble a collection of papers highlighting the progress in our understanding of all aspects related to surveillance and control of zoonotic diseases, including (1) the development of new diagnostic tools, (2) outbreak investigation and surveillance programs of emerging pathogens (including One Health approaches), and (3) understanding the mechanisms of pathogen emergence. The first 10 papers published in this Special Issue address topics related to viruses (SARS-CoV-2, influenza, DENV, WNV, ZIKV), bacteria (*Escherichia coli*), and parasites (Leishmania, Plasmodium) [3–10].

**Funding:** This research received no external funding.

**Acknowledgments:** We thank all authors for contributing their work to this special issue.

**Conflicts of Interest:** The author declares no conflict of interest.

## References

1. Mora, C.; McKenzie, T.; Gaw, I.M.; Dean, J.M.; von Hammerstein, H.; Knudson, T.A.; Setter, R.O.; Smith, C.Z.; Webster, K.M.; Patz, J.A.; et al. Over half of known human pathogenic diseases can be aggravated by climate change. *Nat. Clim. Change* **2022**, *12*, 869–875. [CrossRef] [PubMed]
2. Lerner, H.; Berg, C. The concept of health in One Health and some practical implications for research and education: What is One Health? *Infect. Ecol. Epidemiol.* **2015**, *5*, 25300. [CrossRef] [PubMed]
3. Melo, D.N.; Lima, G.R.P.; Fernandes, C.G.; Teixeira, A.C.; Filho, J.B.; Araújo, F.M.C.; Araújo, L.C.; Siqueira, A.M.; Farias, L.A.B.G.; Monteiro, R.A.A.; et al. Post-Mortem Diagnosis of Pediatric Dengue Using Minimally Invasive Autopsy during the COVID-19 Pandemic in Brazil. *Trop. Med. Infect. Dis.* **2022**, *7*, 123. [CrossRef] [PubMed]
4. Wilairatana, P.; Mala, W.; Kotepui, K.U.; Kotepui, M. Prevalence and Characteristics of Malaria and Influenza Co-Infection in Febrile Patients: A Systematic Review and Meta-Analysis. *Trop. Med. Infect. Dis.* **2022**, *7*, 168. [CrossRef] [PubMed]
5. Mencattelli, G.; Iapaolo, F.; Polci, A.; Marcacci, M.; Di Gennaro, A.; Teodori, L.; Curini, V.; Di Lollo, V.; Secondini, B.; Scialabba, S.; et al. West Nile Virus Lineage 2 Overwintering in Italy. *Trop. Med. Infect. Dis.* **2022**, *7*, 160. [CrossRef] [PubMed]
6. Li, Z.; Zeng, W.; Yang, Y.; Zhang, P.; Zhou, Z.; Li, Y.; Guo, Y.; Zhang, Y. Expression Profile Analysis of Circular RNAs in Leishmaniasis. *Trop. Med. Infect. Dis.* **2022**, *7*, 176. [CrossRef] [PubMed]
7. Solomon, M.; Fuchs, I.; Glazer, Y.; Schwartz, E. Gender and Cutaneous Leishmaniasis in Israel. *Trop. Med. Infect. Dis.* **2022**, *7*, 179. [CrossRef] [PubMed]
8. Van Herreweghe, M.; Breynaert, A.; De Bruyne, T.; Popescu, C.P.; Florescu, S.-A.; Lustig, Y.; Schwartz, E.; Gobbi, F.G.; Hermans, N.; Huits, R. Can Biomarkers of Oxidative Stress in Serum Predict Disease Severity in West Nile Virus Infection? A Pilot Study. *Trop. Med. Infect. Dis.* **2022**, *7*, 207. [CrossRef] [PubMed]
9. Zhong, Y.-M.; Zhang, X.-H.; Ma, Z.; Liu, W.-E. Prevalence of Escherichia coli ST1193 Causing Intracranial Infection in Changsha, China. *Trop. Med. Infect. Dis.* **2022**, *7*, 217. [CrossRef] [PubMed]
10. Zhang, X.S.; Xiong, H.; Chen, Z.; Liu, W. Importation, Local Transmission, and Model Selection in Estimating the Transmissibility of COVID-19: The Outbreak in Shaanxi Province of China as a Case Study. *Trop. Med. Infect. Dis.* **2022**, *7*, 227. [CrossRef] [PubMed]

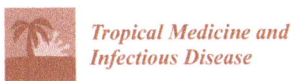 

*Article*

# Barriers and Facilitators to HIV Treatment Adherence in Indonesia: Perspectives of People Living with HIV and HIV Service Providers

Bona S. H. Hutahaean [1,2], Sarah E. Stutterheim [3] and Kai J. Jonas [1,*]

1. Department of Work and Social Psychology, Maastricht University, 6200 MD Maastricht, The Netherlands
2. Department of Clinical Psychology, Universitas Indonesia, Depok 16424, Indonesia
3. Department of Health Promotion & Care and Public Health Research Institute, Maastricht University, 6220 MD Maastricht, The Netherlands
* Correspondence: kai.jonas@maastrichtuniversity.nl

**Abstract:** HIV treatment adherence in Indonesia is a major challenge. Although previous studies have demonstrated several barriers and facilitators to adherence, studies providing a comprehensive analysis from both PLHIV and HIV service providers' perspectives are limited, especially in Indonesia. In this qualitative study with 30 people living with HIV on treatment (PLHIV-OT) and 20 HIV service providers (HSPs), we explored, via online interviews, the barriers and facilitators to antiretroviral therapy (ART) adherence using a socioecological approach. Both PLHIV-OT and HSPs reported stigma as a major barrier at each socioecological level, including public stigma at the societal level, stigma in healthcare settings, and self-stigma at the intrapersonal level. Stigma reduction must therefore be prioritized. PLHIV-OT and HSPs also reported support from significant others and HSPs as the foremost facilitators to ART adherence. The enablement of support networks is thus an important key to improved ART adherence. Overall, the societal level and health system barriers to ART adherence should be addressed in order to remove barriers and enhance the facilitators at the subordinate socioecological levels.

**Keywords:** HIV; antiretroviral (ARV); antiretroviral treatment (ART); adherence; socioecological approach; Indonesia

## 1. Introduction

Indonesia initiated the use of antiretroviral therapy (ART) for people living with HIV (PLHIV) in the late 1990s. HIV is now considered a manageable chronic illness as long as PLHIV adhere to treatment [1]. However, ART adherence among PLHIV in Indonesia is low [2]. In terms of the 95-95-95 targets, the UNAIDS data for 2021 indicated that, of the estimated 610.000 PLHIV in Indonesia, only 66% are aware of their HIV status, 26% on ART, and no 2021 data was available on viral suppression [3], but earlier data also showed very poor rates of viral suppression [4,5]. Clearly, Indonesia, as a whole, does not meet the 95-95-95 targets [6] despite efforts, such as the 2012 continuum of care government initiative (Layanan Komprehensif Berkesinambungan) [7] and regional activities, such as the governor of Jakarta having signed the Paris Declaration in 2015 [8]. A number of reasons have been brought forward, such as poor retention in care [2], but also stigma and discrimination in society, as well as criminalization of key populations (e.g., men who have sex with men {MSM}, trans women), which creates barriers for accessing HIV services [9–13].

Adherence to ART is challenging, mainly because PLHIV are required to have 95% or near-perfect adherence to achieve viral suppression [14]. In Indonesia, of the 21.347 individuals reported to be on treatment, only 55.7% had good adherence to ART [15,16]. Poor adherence can result in drug resistance, greater risk of onward HIV transmission, and health deterioration leading to AIDS-related diseases or death [16–18].

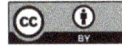

Good adherence can lead to viral suppression, and thus prevent onward transmission [1,18–21]. An undetectable viral load makes HIV untransmittable [19,22,23]. As such, good ART adherence benefits not only the health and well-being of PLHIV; it also supports HIV prevention. This is termed Treatment-as-Prevention (TasP) [19].

Consistent ART adherence has many advantages, but it is not easy. There are many individual and environmental factors that can impede ART adherence. To effectively support treatment adherence in countries like Indonesia, we need a comprehensive understanding of both that which hinders and that which enables ART adherence. For this reason, we set out to explore the multiplicity of barriers and facilitators to ART adherence among PLHIV in Indonesia using a socioecological approach as our framework.

The socioecological approach argues that behavior is impacted by societal, organizational, community, interpersonal, and intrapersonal factors [24–26]. Societal level influences include values and beliefs in the society, as well as legislation and policy. Organizational level influences, such as health systems, shape behavior indirectly through, for example, organizational policies, protocols, and bureaucratic processes. The interpersonal level entails the influence of direct interactions between individuals and others, such as friends, family, support groups, and individual HIV service providers. Lastly, the intrapersonal level reflects internal influences on an individual's nature in ways relating to their attitudes, beliefs, and knowledge [24].

Clearly, given the complexity of behavior and its influences, it is relevant to explore barriers and facilitators to ART adherence across socioecological levels. In addition, to gain a full understanding of the barriers and facilitators to ART adherence, it is also important to explore this from multiple perspectives. For this reason, we investigated barriers and facilitators to ART adherence in Indonesia from both the perspective of PLHIV on treatment (PLHIV-OT) and from the perspective of HIV service providers (HSPs), something that has not previously been done in the Indonesian context. In fact, to date, most studies investigating ART adherence in Indonesia focused only on one perspective, either the perspective of PLHIV or the perspective of HIV service providers [10,21,27–34]. We believe that understanding the barriers and facilitators from multiple perspectives is essential to effective interventions to improve ART adherence in Indonesia.

## 2. Materials and Methods

### 2.1. Study Design and Context

We conducted a qualitative study with semi-structured interviews among PLHIV-OT and HSPs to investigate barriers and facilitators of ART adherence. Data were collected in the greater Jakarta area, which covered five main areas of Jakarta as the capital (Central Jakarta, South Jakarta, West Jakarta, North Jakarta, East Jakarta) and the metro Jakarta area, namely Bogor, Depok, Tangerang, and Bekasi, abbreviated as Jabodetabek. Jakarta is characterized by a highly diverse population as well as a high proportion of growth every year due to migration from other provinces [35,36].

Ethical approval was provided by the Ethics Review Committee at Maastricht University's Faculty of Psychology and Neuroscience (reference number: 188_11_02_2018_S17) and by the Health Research Ethics Committee at the National Institute of Health Research and Development in Indonesia (Badan Penelitian dan Pengembangan Kesehatan; No: LB.02.01/2/KE.139/2020). Research permits were provided by Dinas Penanaman Modal dan Pelayanan Terpadu Satu Pintu, Pemerintah Provinsi Daerah Khusus Ibukota Jakarta (No: 60/AF.1/1/-1.862.9/e/2020) and Dinas Kesehatan Pemerintah Provinsi DKI Jakarta (No: 2271/-1.779.3).

### 2.2. Sampling and Recruitment

We recruited a convenience sample of 50 participants for semi-structured interviews. Thirty were PLHIV on ARV treatment (PLHIV-OT) and twenty were HIV service providers (HSPs) including physicians, nurse practitioners, psychologists, and treatment companions or counselors working voluntarily at NGOs. Inclusion criteria for PLHIV-OT were:

(1) having received an HIV diagnosis; (2) being on ART for at least one year; and (3) being willing and able to provide informed consent. Inclusion criteria for HSPs were: (1) working in HIV care for at least one year in a community health center, public hospital, or private clinic; (2) being willing and able to give informed consent.

Recruitment occurred initially purposively at community health centers (*Puskesmas*), public hospitals, and private HIV clinics, and then through snowball sampling from participants who had completed an interview. To recruit, we first sent documentation (i.e., research permits, ethical approval, and recruitment posters) to the targeted health centers, who put us in contact with eligible HIV service providers (e.g., physicians, nurse practitioners, treatment companions, and counselors) and PLHIV-OT. Once connected with potential participants, we explained the purpose and procedure for the study, the potential to withdraw at any time, and the fact that all data would be handled confidentially.

### 2.3. Participant Characteristics

The mean age of PLHIV-OT was 38.7 years with the average of 6.7 years for people on ARV treatment. Among them, more than half were cisgender men and self-identified as straight. The HIV service providers had a mean age of 34.7 years while more than half of them had between 7 to 14 years of professional experience in HIV care. In terms of formal educational attainment, 35% of the HSPs had vocational training and 25% had a bachelor's degree, with only one of them never received any HIV-related formal training. Additional details are depicted in Table 1.

**Table 1.** Participant characteristics.

| Characteristics | PLHIV-OT (n = 30) | | HIV Service Providers (n = 20) | |
|---|---|---|---|---|
| | N | % | N | % |
| *Age* | | | | |
| 25–35 | 12 | 40 | 11 | 55 |
| 36–45 | 11 | 37 | 8 | 40 |
| 46–59 | 7 | 23 | 1 | 5 |
| *Gender identity* | | | | |
| Cis male | 17 | 57 | 10 | 50 |
| Cis female | 10 | 33 | 10 | 50 |
| Trans woman | 3 | 10 | na | na |
| *Educational background* | | | | |
| Below High School | 2 | 7 | - | - |
| High School | 15 | 50 | 4 | 20 |
| Vocational School | 7 | 23 | 7 | 35 |
| Bachelor | 6 | 20 | 5 | 25 |
| Master | - | - | 4 | 20 |
| *Sexual orientation* | | | | |
| Straight | 19 | 63 | na | na |
| Gay | 6 | 33 | na | na |
| Bisexual | 5 | 17 | na | na |
| *Key population/most widely handled key population* | | | | |
| MSM (men who have sex with men) | 11 | 37 | 7 | 35 |
| PWID (people who inject drugs) | 7 | 23 | 6 | 30 |
| Female sex workers and their clients | 3 | 10 | 3 | 15 |
| Waria (trans women) | 2 | 7 | 2 | 10 |
| Others | 7 | 23 | 2 | 10 |

Table 1. *Cont.*

| Characteristics | PLHIV-OT (n = 30) | | HIV Service Providers (n = 20) | |
|---|---|---|---|---|
| | N | % | N | % |
| *HIV clinic location* | | | | |
| Central Jakarta | 11 | 37 | 6 | 30 |
| South Jakarta | 3 | 10 | 3 | 15 |
| East Jakarta | 6 | 20 | 7 | 35 |
| North Jakarta | 6 | 20 | 1 | 5 |
| Bekasi | 4 | 13 | - | - |
| Depok | - | - | 1 | 5 |
| Bogor | - | - | 1 | 5 |
| Tangerang | - | - | 1 | 5 |
| *Region of origin* | | | | |
| Java | 18 | 60 | 8 | 40 |
| Sumatera | 6 | 20 | 6 | 30 |
| Jakarta | 3 | 10 | 3 | 15 |
| Sulawesi | 2 | 7 | 2 | 10 |
| Nusa Tenggara | 1 | 3 | - | - |
| Bali | - | - | 1 | 5 |
| *Time since HIV diagnosis* | | | | |
| <10 years | 19 | 63 | na | na |
| >10 years | 11 | 37 | na | na |
| *ARV initiation (months after diagnosis)* | | | | |
| <1 month | 9 | 30 | na | na |
| <12 months | 12 | 40 | na | na |
| >12 months | 9 | 30 | na | na |
| *Time on ARV* | | | | |
| <10 years | 21 | 70 | na | na |
| >10 years | 9 | 30 | na | na |
| *ARV access/location of work* | | | | |
| Public hospital | 20 | 67 | 7 | 35 |
| Community health center (*Puskesmas*) | 9 | 30 | 10 | 50 |
| Private clinic | 1 | 3 | 3 | 15 |
| *Perceived health condition (past 4 weeks)* | | | | |
| Bad | 2 | 7 | na | na |
| Fair | 4 | 13 | na | na |
| Good | 7 | 23 | na | na |
| Very good | 7 | 23 | na | na |
| Extremely good | 3 | 10 | na | na |
| *Profession/role in HIV care* | | | | |
| GP (general practitioner) | na | na | 5 | 25 |
| Nurse | na | na | 5 | 25 |
| Treatment companion/buddy/counselor | na | na | 8 | 40 |
| Psychologist | na | na | 2 | 10 |
| *Professional experience in HIV care* | | | | |
| <7 years | na | na | 9 | 45 |
| >7 <14 years | na | na | 11 | 55 |
| *Received training/workshop regarding HIV/ARV* | | | | |
| Yes | na | na | 19 | 95 |
| No | na | na | 1 | 5 |

na = not assessed/not applicable.

*2.4. Data Collection*

Interview guides were first developed in English based on the socioecological approach [24,25]. For PLHIV-OT, the main topics were participants' experiences with an HIV diagnosis, and the barriers and facilitators to ART adherence at each socioecological level. For HSPs, the main topics were their views on their experiences caring for PLHIV, including challenges, and their views on barriers and facilitators to ART adherence.

The interview guides were then pre-tested with two English-speaking professionals working in HIV. After the pre-test, adjustments were made based on the feedback provided. Then, we translated the interview guides into Bahasa Indonesia and pre-tested them with two Indonesian colleagues, both of whom were HIV counselors, one of whom was also a researcher.

Single, face-to-face, semi-structured online interviews of approximately one hour were conducted between March and June of 2020 by the first author with assistance from four female postgraduate students who had extensive experience conducting qualitative research. Interviews were conducted in Bahasa Indonesia at a location chosen by the participants, usually the participant's house or bedroom for PLHIV-OT or at the HIV clinic for the HSPs. No other people were present at the time of the interview. Interviews were preceded by informed consent, guided by the semi-structured interview guide with follow-up probes, and followed by a short survey measuring demographic and HIV-related or occupational characteristics for PLHIV-OT and HSPs, respectively.

Data collection coincided with the beginning of the worldwide COVID-19 outbreak. As a result, Jakarta and the metro Jakarta area imposed a large-scale social restriction policy (*Pembatasan Sosial Berskala Besar* [PSBB]) in March of 2020. The new measures limited social contact, and the interviews thus needed to take place online or by telephone. We utilized online mobile applications such as WhatsApp audio or video call, or online chat and video telephony software platforms such as Zoom to avoid direct contact with participants and ensure their safety from any COVID-19 risks. The participants who were willing to be involved in this study could choose the online platform that was most suitable for them. All participants agreed to their interviews to be recorded with a digital voice recorder. Video was not recorded.

*2.5. Data Analyses*

All of the interview recordings were transcribed verbatim in Bahasa Indonesia. Subsequently, all of the HSP transcripts and two of the PLHIV-OT transcripts were translated into English by a professional translator. The first author and the translator also reviewed the translated transcripts to ensure that the translations adequately reflected the original text. All authors were involved in the coding of the English transcripts and the first author coded the rest of the transcripts. We coded all of the transcripts using Atlas Ti V.8.4.5.

Thematic analyses was employed to identify, analyze, and report the recurring pattern of themes within the data [37]. We followed all six stages of thematic analyses [37]. First, we familiarized ourselves with the data by transcribing, reading, and making notes of the initial codes. Second, after the initial codes emerged, we collated the relevant data with each code. Third, we organized the codes into potential themes and merged the relevant data to each potential theme. Fourth, we reviewed the themes, resulting in an analysis thematic 'map'. Fifth, we defined and gave names to each theme. Sixth, we generated the report of the analysis for this article. Selected quotes were translated to English and reviewed for the originality of meaning by the first author and the translator, who is fully bilingual in English and Bahasa Indonesia. An example of our theme development is provided in Table 2.

Table 2. Example of theme development.

| Quotes | | Category | Theme |
|---|---|---|---|
| PLHIV-OT | HSP | | |
| "We don't want to think of it (ARV) as a drug, but consider it a vitamin. If we take vitamins, we want to be healthy, right?" | "I've always told PLHIV that this drug is a 'vitamin'. Drug or medicine has such a bad stigma in their mind." | Lightening the "load" with euphemistic terminology | |
| "I told my friends in the peer support group, that ARV is ... beauty pills (laughing), because we can be beautiful and productive again with the pills." | "They (PLHIV-OT) need to think of it as doing daily activities such as brushing their teeth every night, having dinner, or taking daily vitamin." | | Intrapersonal level facilitators of treatment adherence at an advanced HIV age |
| "My kids, my mom. My kids mostly. I want to be able to watch them grow up, finish college. That's everyone hope I guess." | "Like I've said before, the things that can help them (PLHIV-OT) to comply is their desire to live, their desire to be productive, and their desire to live with their family." | Meaning-making through goals and spirituality | |
| "All I know that I'm committed to always pick up the ARV whenever it's available for me as I still want to be alive." | "When someone has a spirit of life, he must has a purpose in life. For example, he wants to have a family one day, or he wants to stay alive until the children get old. That's a motivation." | | |

## 3. Results

Various barriers and facilitators to ART adherence emerged, some cross-cutting and some particular to one or more socioecological levels. Stigma was the main barrier appearing at every level. It manifested as public stigma at the societal level, stigma in healthcare settings at the health system level, stigma toward PLHIV-OT from significant others at the interpersonal level, and self-stigma at the intrapersonal level. Below, we outline the barriers and facilitators from the perspectives of both PLHIV-OT and HSPs at each socioecological level and describe how barriers and facilitators were interrelated.

### 3.1. Societal Barriers and Facilitators

Public stigma and discrimination in society colored adherence to ART. PLHIV-OT stated that stigma and discrimination were the major barriers that they had to face. They reported that society has an insufficient and incorrect understanding about HIV and PLHIV, which results in substantial stigma and discriminatory attitudes against PLHIV.

> "The challenge is from the society. There are still many people who look down on PLHIV, many people who stay away when they hear (HIV), many people still discriminate ... We (PLHIV-OT) feel that we are just the same like everybody else, but they (society) still judge us." (PLHIV-OT, 31, public hospital)

> "Well, the things that prevent them (PLHIV-OT) from complying is their own fears about what they're going to deal with, including stigma and discrimination from the society in general." (Psychologist, 26, community health center)

Stigma and discrimination in society created fear of being ostracized among PLHIV-OT, resulting in the non-disclosure of HIV status or being secretive about ART. However, the collectivistic culture in Indonesia makes it difficult as people in one's neighborhood are likely to question why someone is secretive. This situation makes PLHIV-OT uncomfortable about doing anything related to HIV treatment (e.g., taking ARV medication, going to the clinic) around the neighborhood. They thus prefer to go to a clinic much further away, which leads to downstream hurdles that can potentially decrease their adherence. Moreover, PLHIV-OT who had already made an effort to adhere to ARV to reach viral suppression felt that their effort was unavailing when they were still being stigmatized and discriminated against.

> "... One of the challenges in undergoing the (ARV) treatment is the society. They still look us (PLHIV) one-sided or avoid us while we try to interact with them. Why is that a challenge? We (PLHIV-OT) take the meds, we cannot transmit the virus to others, but they (society) are afraid to shake our hands, let alone to have a conversation with us ... " (PLHIV-OT, 31, public hospital)

> "These patients' adherence can be influenced from the stigma in the society. All of this time, the neighborhood might not notice if this patient doesn't show any symptoms. But if he always goes to the hospital with his family for a routine check, there must be a question from the neighborhood: "Why does he always go to the hospital?" (GP, 52, public hospital)

> "Stigma from the society since they are lacking of understanding about HIV population. This stigma can weaken PLHIV (adherence), lower their motivation, and make them slide back to where they were before." (Counselor, 38, public hospital)

The substantial stigma and discrimination in society also creates fear of being condemned, which affected PLHIV-OT's willingness to continue ART, disclose their HIV status, or just be comfortable living with HIV. As a hope voiced by many PLHIV-OT and HSPs, less stigma and discrimination in society could contribute to better adherence. Moreover, less stigma and discrimination could contribute to support almost all of the facilitators at the subordinate levels, and certainly could help to overcome most of the barriers.

*3.2. Health System Barriers and Facilitators*

The health system barriers to adherence were stigma in healthcare settings, insufficient healthcare system coverage, complicated bureaucracy, and problems with ART access. Both PLHIV-OT and HSPs indicated that NGOs and HSPs have important roles in the provision of better healthcare coverage and easy access to ARV as the facilitator to adherence.

3.2.1. Stigma in Healthcare Settings

PLHIV-OT and HSPs reported that there were many stigma-free and discrimination-free HIV clinics. However, stigma and discrimination at certain HIV clinics was still reported.

> " ... I think some of them (HSP) still have stigma against PLHIV that it can make patients feel uncomfortable coming to the care center." (PLHIV-OT, 38, private clinic)

> "All I can think about is the healthcare providers who still have stigma against PLHIV. We have to be able to create a comfortable environment for PLHIV so that they'd feel welcome. If we fail to do that, then they will move somewhere else or find another center or hospital to get treatment, or worse, they completely stop the medication out of fear of being treated in the same manner as at the previous clinic they went to." (Nurse, 38, public hospital)

Even though many HSPs are knowledgeable about HIV and know standard procedures for interacting with PLHIV in the clinic, stigmatizing and discriminating attitudes and procedures in the health system were reported. These directly and indirectly affect adherence, particularly for men who have sex with men (MSM) and trans women. For example, trans women reported being called on by HSPs with their birth name listed on their identity card rather than their acquired name (i.e., deadnaming), and MSM who experienced stigmatization in clinics opted not to return and thus could not access ARV.

> "The transgender patients felt that they already put such effort to dress up like a lady so that people should address them as such. It's a discomfort for them, but we have rigid system. If system allowed some changes to the rule, then they could add 'alias'

*next to birth name on ID card so that there's option how or what to address a person."* (Psychologist, 31, community health center)

*"For example, there was an experience of my colleague who took my shift, I didn't really understand what happened, maybe she mistakenly said something that was considered as stigma for those MSM patients. They (MSM patients) didn't want to come (to the clinic) again."* (GP, 31, community health center)

3.2.2. Healthcare System Coverage

The HIV healthcare system in Indonesia has improved over the years, but our participants still hoped that the government would provide more solutions to overcome the insufficient universal coverage in HIV care. ARV medication is provided for free by the government, but PLHIV who do not have a social security card (BPJS Kesehatan) still need to pay an administration fee of around IDR 15.000 (+/− USD 1) when they come to the HIV clinic in the community health center or public hospital. This amount is considered high, and thus is certainly a barrier, especially for PLHIV-OT who live in remote areas and have financial difficulties, considering Indonesia's national income per capita in 2019 was around IDR 161.917 (+/− USD 11) per day, while the average national expenditure per capita was around IDR 40.195 (+/− USD 3) per day [38]. As a consequence, PLHIV-OT preferred to spend their money on groceries or basic needs rather than spending it on administration fees or transportation costs to get to their HIV clinic.

*"They (HIV patients) only pay retribution when they come into the clinic to register. It's quite cheap—only IDR 15.000. However, for some people in Indonesia, IDR 15.000 is a lot of money to spend, in addition to transport cost of going back and forth from clinic to home."* (Counselor, 38, community health center)

*" . . . It is really burdening for us (PLHIV-OT) when we have to pay for the CD4 and VL tests. Not everyone has enough money or BPJS . . . "* (PLHIV-OT, 37, public hospital)

In addition, those without social security have to pay for CD4 and viral load (VL) tests, which is often beyond their means. Even though there were some externally funded programs by the Indonesian AIDS Commission and other NGOs that provide free post-ARV tests, only a few PLHIV-OT could benefit from these programs. Moreover, the information available about these programs was not shared widely or came too late for them to make use of free tests.

*" . . . Indeed, the VL test is important, but I had an experience when they informed me about the free VL test two days before the event! It was definitely hard for the patients to get a permission from their daily job. If they want to make such an event, it will be better if they announce it weeks before the event . . . "* (PLHIV-OT, 26, community health center)

3.2.3. Bureaucracy

PLHIV-OT with more income reported more choices for accessing ART, including private clinics which charged more in terms of administration fees and other laboratory tests, but the bureaucracy was less complicated compared to HIV clinics in public hospitals or community health centers. Meanwhile, PLHIV-OT who accessed ART in public hospitals or community health centers had to deal with more complicated bureaucracy as a tradeoff for a more affordable service.

*"First, most hospitals still require PLHIV patients to pay for registration fee. We need to waive the registration fee as most PLHIV are poverty-stricken. Second, we need to cut down bureaucracy and find a simple way to let patients get medication in any community health center or hospitals they want. We need to integrate the reporting and filing system so that patients can just show their registration serial number to get access to medication everywhere . . . "* (Counselor, 38, public hospital)

Unsurprisingly, HSPs reported that having less bureaucracy by cutting certain procedures could certainly facilitate adherence. One example would be allowing trans women or anyone without an ID card to access ART without their ID card. Even though the regulations state that patients always need to show their ID card, in order to access ARV, some community health centers have chosen to not comply with this regulation so that trans women in particular can access ARV without having to show their ID card. Participants also reported that some HIV clinics, particularly private clinics, already tackled bureaucratic barriers and provided faster access to ART and less queueing. This would also help to overcome the stigma in healthcare settings that we mentioned earlier.

" . . . we (HIV service providers) also try to simplify the procedure. We have administration team who handle the (patient's) data in our clinic. I usually give the administration staff number to the patients, so that they don't have to queue every time they come to the clinic. These patients just have to make an agreement with my friend (the administration staff), and then he will register the patients. So, they don't need to queue . . . " (GP, 31, community health center)

"There are many community health centers running different procedures with ours. We have a more flexible procedure because we think of what's best for patients' health. We bend a couple of regulation here and there such as we allow patients to come for VCT and ARV at our clinic without ID card because we know a lot of transgender community don't have it." (Counselor, 38, community health center)

3.2.4. ART Access

Faster access to ART as a result of less bureaucracy would be more complete with easy access to ART, which could be implemented in three ways. First, based on the data, it is advisable to implement a one-stop service where PLHIV-OT could come to the clinic, register, consult with the doctor, do tests if necessary, and acquire ARV at the same time and in the same place. This way, PLHIV-OT could access the medication with minimal effort by picking up their ARV medication easily in the clinic instead of the pharmacy. This is not only advantageous because it is more efficient; PLHIV-OT also reported feeling more comfortable going to just one place, which reduces the chances of running into people they know. Evidently, internalized and anticipated stigma as barriers to ART can be minimized by enabling one-stop access to ARV medication in the clinic.

" . . . I've heard there is this Puskesmas which has a very simple system. It's really good. Starting from the registration, then the weight and blood pressure measurement, then directly to the consultation with the doctor, and the doctor gives the medication directly to the patient. All at one place. So, they don't have to pick up the medication at the pharmacy. That's really comfortable." (PLHIV-OT, 50, community health center)

" . . . At the time being, what is helpful is giving the medication at VCT clinic directly, not at the pharmacy counter . . . Most transgender patients, if not all, like to be called by their female's name, not with their old male's name on ID card. When they pick up medication at pharmacy, the counter will always use patient's real name from ID card, and transgenders population don't like that very much. So, they are very happy to pick up medication at our clinic because no one there is exposing their real male's name." (Nurse, 27, community health center)

" . . . One-door service! The medical devices should be provided more to be able to give 'one-door service'. The patients just have to come to 'one door' when they want to do an X-ray, VL, CD4 test, or get a TB and STDs treatment. They can feel more comfortable and don't have to run back and forth just to take those tests . . . Thank God we already have it all here in Puskesmas X." (GP, 38, community health center)

The second way in which access to ART can be facilitated at the health system level is by providing ARV supplies to PLHIV-OT for two or three months at once, instead of for only one month, so that the patients do not have to come to the clinic every month. This was really helpful for PLHIV-OT with financial constraints that limit their ability to travel back and forth to the clinic.

> " ... Nowadays, when the healthcare providers see good progress from a patient, they give meds for 2-month supply. It helps patient's adherence to the medication and avoid them coming every month ... ."
> (PLHIV-OT, 34, private clinic)

Third, easy access to ART can be implemented by allowing the patients with good adherence to have their ARV medication delivered using an online taxi bike application (ojek online). This ARV medication delivery service is an informal collaboration between HIV clinics and treatment companions from the NGOs (Pendamping Minum Obat; PMO). However, PLHIV still need to come and consult with an HIV physician one month after ARV medication delivery for a routine check. PLHIV-OT who have a good relationship with their health care provider can ask for their help for ARV medication delivery or ask the treatment companion to deliver it. Therefore, having a good client–provider relationship at the interpersonal level, which we will explain later, can support easier access to ART for better adherence.

> " ... We make things easier too nowadays. NGO also steps up and helps deliver the medication to them. So, there's no excuses to not taking it." (Counselor, 25, community health center)

> "We do have a lot of requests for delivery during this corona pandemic, but only with one condition: compliance to taking the medication regularly ... For example, if we see that the patient has a good viral load, then we will hire a delivery service to send the medication for him. But if we see that his last VL result is bad, and he is always a week or 2 weeks late to pick up medication, then we ask the patient to come to the clinic for re-consultation." (Nurse, 27, community health center)

Despite increased opportunities for easy access to ART, PLHIV-OT who experienced the ARV stock crisis in 2015 or 2017, and when the COVID-19 outbreak happened in early 2020, voiced concerns. Insufficient ARV stock made it difficult for them to access ART for a one-month supply as usual. Instead, physicians prescribed them for only one or two weeks with different types or amounts of ARV, which led to patients having to adjust to a new regimen, including side effects.

> " ... That's right, I got more than one pills (when there was ARV stock crisis). I was even a bit worried whether there would be another side effects or not ... " (PLHIV-OT, 28, public hospital)

It was very inefficient and time-consuming, especially for PLHIV-OT who had inflexible schedules but had to come to the clinic almost every week, which brought about extra transportation costs. PLHIV-OT with financial constraints often waited until the ARV stock was back to normal again before reinitiating ART. This created an adherence gap. Although the ARV stock crisis is not currently an ongoing barrier, it still can create lingering anxieties for PLHIV-OT.

> " ... I'm grateful for the free ARV, but I think the government needs to rethink its management plan on ARV national stock supply as these meds need to be taken for a lifetime. In addition, there's been rare stock supply in region of Aceh, Padang, Ambon, Bali, and Manado. Most PLHIV there only get 14-day supply and not a full 1-month supply." (PLHIV-OT, 30, private clinic)

In conclusion, health system level barriers to ART adherence include stigma, insufficient universal coverage in HIV care, and complicated bureaucracy. Informal collaboration between HSPs and NGOs that enables ARV medication delivery, as well as reduced bureaucracy and easy one-stop access to ART, can serve to overcome some of the barriers to ART.

### 3.3. Interpersonal Barriers and Facilitators

Interpersonal level barriers were stigma from the PLHIV-OT's significant others or their own HSP, which led to, among other things, poorer client–provider relationships and, consequently, lowered the adherence. PLHIV-OT reported support from significant others as a major facilitator and, surprisingly, HSPs mentioned that the use of fear appeals facilitates adherence.

### 3.3.1. Significant Others

Significant others, such as friends, family members, and (ex)partners, played important roles both as barriers and as facilitators to ART adherence. As a barrier, significant others who stigmatized and discriminated against PLHIV by rejecting or excluding them (i.e., enacted stigma) directly and indirectly affected adherence. For example, PLHIV-OT who were ostracized by their family or friends or rejected by a partner or potential partners after disclosing their HIV status were at risk of discontinuing ART because they would potentially feel depressed and thus did not come to the clinic to pick up their ARV medication.

> "I once dated a guy and just being straight forward by telling him my (HIV) status. He said: "Maybe I'm not your match. I hope you're healthy." And then he ran away (laugh). I thought I might just tell him than regret it, right?" (PLHIV-OT, 48, public hospital)

> " ... We have several patients who were shunned by their family. They got so depressed and never picked up medication again. That's how we lost contact with the patients. We don't know where they are until today." (Counselor, 38, community health center)

Significant others who accepted the HIV status of their partners functioned as a facilitator to ART adherence. They could provide sufficient emotional and instrumental support, but this was reported to not be immediate. PLHIV-OT who disclosed their HIV status to friends and family often reported initial difficulties gaining acceptance from others, but then receiving support later, and this helped facilitate their adherence to ART. Specifically, they described emotional support, such as acceptance and listening to treatment challenges, and instrumental support, such as accompaniment to the HIV clinic or pharmacy. According to HSPs, PLHIV-OT receiving support, particularly from their family, had a better adherence than those who did not.

> " ... The form of support is not only about reminding us to take the medicine on time, but also about accepting our condition, that we are different, we have a 'special' situation ... " (PLHIV-OT, 31, public hospital)

> "Family maybe is more important (than friends). Most patients are brought to the clinic by their family member, the closest family member ... I think they can help reminding patient to take medication." (Nurse, 27, community health center)

### 3.3.2. Client–Provider Relationships

Not surprisingly, given its presence at the societal and health system levels, stigma was also apparent in interactions between HSPs and PLHIV. A poor client–provider relationship, caused by patients who were not very communicative or stigmatizing HSPs, often led PLHIV-OT to discontinue consultation. Examples included HSPs who disrespectfully told a trans PLHIV that trans PLHIV almost always fail to adhere to ART and HSPs who expressed judgment about sex between men.

> "The doctor saw my ID card (listed as a male) and asked me why do I look like this (female appearance). He said that my chance (as a trans woman) of not complying to the treatment would be much greater throughout this lifetime treatment. He didn't respect me at all. And I think he did this not only to the trans patients, but also to the MSM community." (PLHIV-OT, 26, community health center)

> [Telling stories before moving to the current HIV clinic] "I realize that we (patients) have to be honest to our providers during consultation. So, I told my doctor that I am gay. He instantly said: "Why are you gay? Aren't you afraid of sins, being punished, this and that? You must repent from your sins!" I came to him not to listen to his religious lecture.

*If you are a healthcare provider, just do your job as a healthcare provider."* (PLHIV-OT, 31, public hospital)

To overcome poor client–provider relationships, HSPs encouraged their patients to be more proactive in asking questions and discussing matters regarding their treatment. They observed that the PLHIV-OT who speak up, ask questions, or complain more tended to have better adherence.

*" ... I noticed that the more they (PLHIV-OT) complain, the more adhere they are to the treatment. Because when they start to complain, they will text us through WhatsApp, asking lots of questions etc., and it's easier for us to do a little bit of counseling through the text and always remind them to adhere."* (GP, 38, community health center)

In other words, PLHIV-OT who felt comfortable being assertive showed that their providers facilitated a safe atmosphere for them to ask questions during clinic visits, by dedicating more time to patients, providing more information, and acting in a friendly manner. This safe atmosphere created a good client–provider relationship that motivated PLHIV-OT to interact more with their providers, come to the clinic, and adhere to treatment. This healthy relationship could also be a form of adherence support, which was a prominent facilitator mentioned by both PLHIV-OT and HSPs.

*"The truth is, when we're building a good relationship with patients, they'll be comfortable enough to talk about anything with us. We need to have that kind of relationship in order to keep this medication going. It's a way to reach out to them and support them."* (Counselor, 35, community health center)

Lastly, in addition to HSPs in the clinic, PLHIV-OT also needed to maintain a good relationship with other HSPs such as the NGOs that explicitly provided a "helping hand" to support adherence.

### 3.3.3. The Role of NGOs and Use of Fear Appeals

To be able to receive additional support from outside the clinic, PLHIV have to disclose their HIV status to people they can trust. Unfortunately, not all PLHIV-OT were willing to disclose their HIV status to family or friends, mostly because they, justifiably, feared being stigmatized and discriminated against. In order to overcome this, PLHIV-OT could join peer support groups (Kelompok Dukungan Sebaya) which commonly exist under the umbrella of certain NGOs. These groups usually comprise PLHIV who do not know each other before joining the group but that become friends who share treatment experiences and support one another. Having this opportunity to experience affinity with other PLHIV can make patients feel more comfortable sharing their stories and may help them feel supported. Within the context of these support groups (but also beyond), other PLHIV's success stories regarding ARV served as positive examples and were perceived to have an advantageous influence on adherence.

*" ... these support group and HIV organization can also be a support system. Some patients don't have any support at all; the family totally rejected them. In this case, the friends from NGO can be their support system - not in picking up their medication or anything, but in a sense of what support system really does."* (GP, 36, community health center)

*"I believe I'm most comfortable with the testimonial from the people living with HIV. They shared not only on their life story, but also the side effects of the ARV treatment. The doctor can only give me the explanation about it, but not actually feeling what I'm going through as none of them are HIV positive."* (PLHIV-OT, 35, private clinic)

*" ... I think they (peer support group) are great. When someone with HIV feels the world is rejecting them, it gives them a place to go when they want information or simply just to have a sanctuary, or to be comfortable knowing that they are not the only one."* (Psychologist, 26, community health center)

Nonetheless, HSPs reported that apprehensive stories or pictures, such as reminding a patient not to stop ARV by sending pictures of untreated PLHIV taken from the internet, could serve as "good" role models for the PLHIV-OT as it would keep them from discontinuing ART. HSPs felt that PLHIV-OT would be more likely to adhere if they were exposed to messages of how other PLHIV suffered after discontinuing treatment. These are termed, in psychology, fear appeals, and are known to be usually ineffective in the absence of self-efficacy and skills.

" ... I haven't found out how to manage boredom. I am now back to taking the medicine not because I am obedient, but because I am afraid ... Thankfully, my adherence is getting better these past two months because of fear, fear of death, fear of creating problems to other people ... " (PLHIV-OT, 45, public hospital)

" ... If we have a patient died, we share it on the group chat to encourage them not to forget to take medicine routinely ... If they (HIV patients) don't want to take it (ARV), we show them a picture of someone without taking medication. That usually does the trick. Thankfully, we have some that started taking it again yesterday." (Nurse, 28, community health center) (Nurse, 28, community health center)

3.3.4. Influence of (Social) Media

The content of some social media accounts was also reported to be a barrier to ART adherence. Unreliable social media accounts (e.g., the anti-ARV Facebook group called Mahastar) provided incorrect information regarding HIV and ART. They suggested PLHIV stop ARV and use alternative medication as the way to cure HIV so that PLHIV would not be dependent on it and provided testimonies from PLHIV who apparently discontinued ART but were still healthy.

" ... There are so many anti-ARV movements in Facebook. That kind of wrong information will make them unstable in making decisions to start or even to undergo the (ARV) treatment." (GP, 38, community health center)

"Nowadays, we can easily 'ask' Google about anything, even about the medicine to cure HIV, or herbal medicine. There were lots of unfortunate cases from our friends (PLHIV) who stopped taking ARV and decided to take the herbal medicine because they thought that it could cure them. In the end, they caught typhoid, got AIDS, and then regretted and realized that ARV was the only medicine that they needed, not the herbal medicine." (PLHIV-OT, 36, community health center)

"It's never proven successful clinically. I advise the patients to fight this notion on herbal medicine ... So, we do have a lot of challenges, and one of them is the anti-ARV." (Counselor, 35, community health center)

Despite the incorrect information about HIV and ART on social media, there were still credible HIV-related social media accounts on Instagram, Twitter, or other platforms that could facilitate PLHIV-OT to gain more reliable information and potentially help them adhere to ART. For example, participants described PLHIV disclosing their HIV status on Instagram or YouTube, sharing their stories of accepting HIV, talking about being on ART, and showing that they could live healthy lives with HIV by taking ART. By viewing these inspiring stories, PLHIV-OT felt they had more knowledge about HIV and ART, and looked up to the living-proof examples of ART adherence, which increased their own adherence. As an additional form of support, HSPs shared examples of credible social media accounts with PLHIV.

"I can ask them (social media accounts) about some things. For example, before I moved to Jakarta, I asked (certain social media) "Is there any HIV clinic in Jakarta that provides access to the medicine on weekends?" They gave me choices 'here, here, here' and so, I kept looking on the internet too, and it turns out that they (HIV clinics) have social media." (PLHIV-OT, 28, public hospital)

"... Most PLHIV know these accounts and the accuracy of the information there, therefore it can help PLHIV to comply with ARV medication. These accounts give a clear idea of the risk if they don't take the medication." (Nurse, 30, community health center)

Distributing correct information about HIV and ART through social media not only had a direct influence on the PLHIV-OTs' adherence; it also indirectly increased awareness in society, offering increased opportunities for the provision of better support to PLHIV and hopefully decreasing stigma and discrimination.

"... When the public has good education, they tend to be able to process new information logically. They will use critical thinking and they'll want to recheck the information given from those platforms further. It's absolutely beneficial having these platforms spreading news about it." (Psychologist, 31, community health center)

In sum, the interpersonal level barriers to ART adherence included poor client–provider relationships and incorrect information regarding HIV and ARV from unreliable social media accounts. Facilitators to ART adherence were often the opposite or the absence of the barriers and frequently took the form of support. Being proactive with HSPs was also a strong facilitator for improved client–provider relationships, and disclosure of HIV status, when safe, was claimed to be helpful in helping PLHIV gain more support outside the clinic. Internet or social media content also played an important role both as barriers and as facilitators, depending on the aim and content provided.

*3.4. Intrapersonal Barriers and Facilitators*

Intrapersonal level barriers and facilitators to ART adherence were the most mentioned by both groups of participants, starting from self-stigma, with barriers and facilitators starting from the moment they initiate treatment, but also occurring after years of treatment.

3.4.1. Self-Stigma

PLHIV-OT reported that HIV is often thought of as a "cursed disease" and, not unsurprisingly or unjustifiably, they were scared that people would ostracize them. This internalized and anticipated stigma made them approach treatment in a complicated way that required efforts to hide their HIV status so that others would not know they had HIV. For instance, PLHIV-OT reported choosing clinics much further from their home and disposing of empty ARV boxes in public waste bins away from their home so that others would not find out they have HIV. Clearly, PLHIV-OT spend subsantial time and effort concealing their HIV treatment.

"Every time I want to disclose or share my stories to others, I have an automatic answer in my head: "They will alienate me." That's why I choose to be secretive ... I don't want to be ostracized. If I disclose my (HIV) status, is it possible that people would accept me? I think it's impossible." (PLHIV-OT, 46, public hospital)

"... But not all patients want to get the treatment in their hometown, with many reasons, mostly because they feel ashamed.." (GP, 31, community health center)

"Every month, I never throw the ARV box in the household waste because I am afraid that my family would find the box and search the info about the medicine." (PLHIV-OT, 33, public hospital)

Self-stigma in PLHIV was driven by perceived stigma in society, having observed stigma in healthcare settings, and previous experiences with enacted stigma. By internalizing negative beliefs about HIV and PLHIV, PLHIV-OT often alienated themselves from their surroundings and did not see that there might be people who would not reject them and were even willing to support them. Self-stigma thus precluded them from seeing possibilities to gain acceptance and support from others.

### 3.4.2. Side Effects and Knowledge Gaps

Both PLHIV-OT and HSPs reported that challenges related to ART initiation were one of the major barriers to later ART adherence. Side effects (e.g., fever, nausea, vomiting, or feeling sluggish and tired), experienced by most PLHIV-OT, impacted their attitude towards ART adherence later.

> "A lot of patients complain about the horrible side effects they've been experiencing. There are some that cut the meds off completely, thus, lost to follow up due to the problematic side effects that they couldn't endure ... " (PLHIV-OT, 39, community health center)

> " ... Secondly, the side effects can stop their adherence. The patients who just start the treatment barely can stand the side effects; hence, it will make them stop to take the medication." (GP, 38, community health center)

HSPs believed that PLHIV-OT who had a better understanding of HIV and ART would also be more willing to continue ART despite initial side effects. PLHIV-OT commonly thought, upon receiving their HIV diagnosis, that they would have a short life and inevitably die. That changed after HSPs explained how ART could suppress their viral load and increase their life expectancy. Some PLHIV-OT then sought out more information on the internet or social media, and/or had more discussions with their HSP leading to better knowledge about HIV and ART.

> " ... the person's knowledge on HIV really affects his adherence to meds. Once he knows how to treat his illness, it's easier for him to adhere to the meds given." (PLHIV-OT, 34, private clinic)

> " ... By getting more information about HIV from social media, it empowers them more to stay healthy and therefore, adhering to the medication ... " (Counselor, 35, community health center)

### 3.4.3. Reduced Motivation

Problems with adherence can also arise later in life, long after HIV diagnosis. PLHIV-OT who had been on ART for five years or more said the major barriers were a lack of motivation to continue treatment or simply feeling lazy, bored, or forgetful. In general, taking ART on a daily basis for the entire duration of one's life was considered tedious.

> "I think it's really human when we (PLHIV-OT) are bored of taking these meds every day. It's the same feeling when we have with eating rice with the same side dish every day ... " (PLHIV-OT, 50, community health center)

> "I'm adhering to the meds, but still, I sometimes forget whether I have taken one in a day, so yes, I kind of skip a couple of times because I forget." (PLHIV-OT, 39, community health center)

According to HSPs, a lack of motivation, laziness, boredom, and forgetfulness might reflect mental health issues. HSPs claimed that many PLHIV develop depressive symptoms after HIV diagnosis and, correspondingly, ART initiation, but also much later in their care trajectories. It is possible that PLHIV-OT are also in denial about their HIV status, which leads to dissonance with ART adherence. Additional, ongoing substance use dependence can further impede ART adherence.

> " ... I think they (PLHIV-OT) are prone to experience a psychological disorder and when it's not properly treated, that will certainly affect how they're going to conduct their daily routines. That's why they need a well-balanced and stable mental health on day to day basis ... When there's hindrance psychologically to initiate or maintain medication, that can cause thought blocking. A negative behavior will create itself ... " (Psychologist, 30, community health center)

> "They (IDU) don't think the way normal people do. They only think about how to get to the next drug or syringe. They only come (to the clinic) when they're already in a bad

condition. Even then, they will discontinue the ARV medication once they don't feel the need of taking it again." (Counselor, 35, community health center)

3.4.4. Lightening the Load with Euphemistic Terminology

Some PLHIV-OT reported unique ways to make ART adherence more bearable and less tedious. For example, some used euphemistic terminology by addressing ARV as "vitamins", "supplements", or "beauty pills" because ARV medication, like vitamins or supplements, is taken every day, and because ARV medication can make PLHIV-OT healthier and physically more aligned with beauty ideals. Clearly, the use of euphemistic terminology was employed to 'lighten' the load of daily ART adherence.

" . . . We don't want to think of it as a drug, but consider it a vitamin. If we take vitamins, we want to be healthy, right?" (PLHIV-OT, 33, public hospital)

"I've always told PLHIV that this drug is a 'vitamin'. Drug or medication has such a bad stigma in their mind. By switching the term to 'vitamin', they don't really think of it as an obligation, rather, as daily activity that they need to do every day . . . ." (Nurse, 35, community health center)

3.4.5. Meaning-Making through Goals and Spirituality

Having clear goals or intentions, such as wanting to get married and have children, seeking a promotion at work, or pursuing higher education, was also reported to facilitate ART adherence. Having goals demonstrated hope for the future, feeling motivated, and having reasons to live through ART adherence.

[Talking about the things that can help to adhere to ART] " . . . My kids, my mom. My kids mostly. I want to be able to watch them grow up, finish college. That's everyone's hope, I guess. I'll use the rest of my time given by the highest power above to continue this therapy if that is what it takes to be with my kids." (PLHIV-OT, 39, community health center)

"Like I've said before, the things that can help them (PHIV-OT) to comply is their desire to live, their desire to be productive, and their desire to live with their family. For example, a sex worker patient has a desire to get married, to have a new life. That's really helpful for her to comply to ARV. Another example is from a housewife who has a child: She thinks that she has to stay healthy in order to work and raise her child. That's also really helpful for her to stay on ARV . . . " (GP, 38, community health center)

Having hope and a reason to live as the result of having goals was supported by other facilitators, namely religion and spirituality. Some PLHIV-OT believed that their HIV diagnosis provided them with a "second chance" in life, particularly for those who realized that their engagement with risky behaviors had led to their HIV diagnosis. These PLHIV-OT tended to view ART adherence as a necessary way to demonstrate their gratitude to God for their new 'chance' at a "second life". PLHIV-OT set goals after realizing that they could live long and healthy lives with HIV, and they reported trying to live life to the fullest.

" . . . In fact, I am increasingly convinced that this (ART) is proof of God's love for me. God's love is universal. I was given a second chance to continue living. So, I have to do my best (by adhering to the treatment)." (PLHIV-OT, 33, public hospital)

"I believe in God, and I believe God always ask us to cooperate. At least that's what they always remind us about during the worship session. We cannot just ask, ask, ask for a healthy life from God, but we don't try to live a healthy life." (PLHIV-OT, 37, public hospital)

3.4.6. Fatalism

Although having goals and spirituality brought about more hope and motivation to adhere to ART for some PLHIV-OT, for others, a belief that all things in life, including having HIV, is predetermined and therefore inevitable, served as a barrier to ART adherence.

HSPs reported that some PLHIV hold the fatalistic belief that their health destiny is in the hands of God and, because of that, there is no reason to take ARV medication.

> "... I heard couple of patients hopelessly said: "What will be, will be." Some undisciplined patients also tend to use the same tone of language and adding: "We all eventually will die anyway. I know there's a widely spread notion out there that there's no hope for them. That's why a lifetime commitment doesn't register well in their brain, especially for the depressed patients. They tend to say: "Why am I still not cured? I've been taking this medication for ages." (Psychologist, 28, community health center)

Similarly, PLHIV-OT experiencing depression and the impacts of stigmatization felt that lifetime treatment was useless and made them feel even more hopeless, which impeded adherence.

> "... Once, I had a difficult patient who liked to throw cynical remarks at us by saying: "Death is on God's hands ... so relax ... " Sometimes, that kind of remark hurts our feelings because it defies our continuous effort to keep them safe and alive ... Compliance is the ultimate challenge." (Nurse, 27, community health center)

In conclusion, intrapersonal level barriers to adherence included self-stigma, side effects, knowledge gaps, reduced motivation, mental health difficulties, and fatalistic beliefs. These barriers could be overcome by improving knowledge about HIV and ARV, referring to ART euphemistically, setting goals or intentions, and making meaning through religion and spirituality which provides a sense of hope for PLHIV-OT.

## 4. Discussion

This study presents, from the perspectives of both PLHIV-OT and HSPs, facilitators and barriers to ART adherence in Indonesia across socioecological levels. The findings clearly show that stigma and discrimination are the main barriers to ART adherence at each socioecological level, and that reduced stigma and discrimination in the future can facilitate ART adherence. Furthermore, the role of treatment companions or buddies from NGOs can help to reduce barriers at the health system level, and peer support groups can facilitate PLHIV-OTs' adherence at the interpersonal level. Additionally, intrapersonal level barriers such as side effects, knowledge gaps, reduced motivation, mental health difficulties, and fatalistic beliefs can be tackled by improving knowledge or lightening the 'load' of ART adherence by creating a sense of purpose through goal setting and spirituality.

Across the findings, participants reported perceiving substantial public stigma in society, institutional stigma in the health system, discrimination in contact with HSPs, enacted stigma from significant others, and anticipated and internalized stigma in PLHIV themselves. That HIV stigma is a major impediment to ART adherence is well established in the literature [9,13,39], as is the fact that HIV stigma in health care is highly prevalent and highly detrimental for PLHIV [40–43]. As such, our findings dovetail with previous studies reporting that stigma in any form hinders treatment adherence [3,11,27,30–32,42,44–59]. PLHIV also often experience intersectional stigma or stigmatization due to multiple identities within marginalized groups (e.g., gender or sexual orientation) [60,61].

Indeed, our study has shown that the many forms of stigma—perceived, enacted, anticipated, and internalized—serve as barriers to ART adherence and interact with one another [9,13,62]. Therefore, if we are to improve adherence, we must reduce HIV stigma and discrimination in Indonesia [48,60,63,64]. There are several ways to successfully reduce stigma [65]. Some include activating self-acceptance through empowerment and education to reduce self-stigma at the intrapersonal level, improving HIV and ART knowledge through peer support and training for HSPs at the interpersonal and health system level, and collaborating with community leaders (e.g., religious leaders) to implement a more humanistic approach towards PLHIV at the societal level [65,66]. The utilization of technology, such as the internet, social and mass media, in ways that provide more positive information, as well as articles reflecting a human perspective on HIV can bring about greater empathy in society and can actively help to alleviate public HIV stigma [41,67].

Additional efforts that seek to change beliefs, such as beliefs that HIV is highly contagious and a condemned disease, and breaking cultural taboos on HIV and sexuality, should also be embedded in stigma reduction interventions [43,65,68].

In addition, ascertaining that stigma is the foremost barrier to ART adherence, our findings have illuminated additional, sometimes temporary, barriers, such as the ARV stock crisis. During the initial outbreak of COVID-19 in Indonesia, significant delays in the ARV shipments from India to Indonesia occurred [69]. The pandemic had a substantial negative impact on PLHIV-OT who were prescribed different and often less ideal drug regimens. As a result, thousands of PLHIV-OT discontinued treatment [70]. Even though the pandemic is now well handled, our participants strongly voiced the need for better policies to ensure that ARV stock remains stable even when unforeseeable circumstances arise.

In terms of facilitators to ART adherence, our findings showed that support is a prominent facilitator to ART adherence at the interpersonal level. Previous studies have also reported that receiving sufficient support can, and does, facilitate adherence and can act as a buffer against psychological distress and other mental health issues (e.g., depression, anxiety) in PLHIV [11,12,21,71,72]. However, in order to receive support, disclosure of HIV status is often necessary [56]. This can be difficult, and potentially unsafe, for PLHIV-OT who anticipate stigma and discrimination from others. Several studies reported that PLHIV-OT who want to disclose their HIV status should receive counseling where they can weigh the risks and benefit of disclosure, and mentally prepare for a wide range of reactions to their status disclosure [73]. Furthermore, counseling can improve their ability to provide accurate information about HIV and ARV to others after disclosing their HIV status [12]. It is important to state that HSPs should not immediately think that a disclosure of HIV status is the best (and only) choice for PLHIV-OT [74,75].

Our interpersonal level findings on facilitators to ART adherence indicated that the HSPs in this study felt that PLHIV-OT could experience support and increased motivation through the provision of fear appeals. The WHO HIV treatment guidelines state that this is unethical [76], and a previous review has clearly demonstrated that it is generally ineffective in the absence of self-efficacy and skills [77]. We strongly advise against the use of fear appeals.

Overall, this study provides a comprehensive overview and interpretation of barriers and facilitators to ART adherence in Indonesia. We believe this study adds important theoretical and practical knowledge to previous studies on ART adherence, particularly in resource-limited settings such as Indonesia. We also hope that our findings can provide input and impetus to adjust policies on ART supply, stock, and treatment procedures, as well as non-discrimination of PLHIV. We further suggest that both PLHIV-OT and HSPs work on enhancing the facilitators described in our study and reducing the barriers. For example, HSPs can offer suggestions to PLHIV-OT, even practical and seemingly minor coping strategies such as speaking about ARV medication euphemistically. They can further help PLHIV-OT to set clear goals to increase hope and motivation to adhere to ART. PLHIV-OT can proactively seek out HIV and ARV knowledge through reliable sources to have a good understanding on why ART adherence is important. In addition, both PLHIV-OT and HSPs should work on establishing and maintaining a good relationship with one another.

Our findings also have additional implications for clinical practice. First, we strongly recommend that HCPs provide a reliable and easy to access, one-stop treatment service for PLHIV-OT with consistent long-term follow-up. This requires significant effort to address barriers to ART adherence that can be overcome (e.g., lack of discipline or forgetting to take the ARV, lack of knowledge and awareness). Additionally, it is advisable to create optimal conditions for the establishment and maintenance of a solid support system for PLHIV-OT either from their significant others or a peer support group. Furthermore, it is important that HSPs continuously improve their awareness and knowledge of HIV care and counseling, potentially through training sessions and workshops, so that they can provide the most optimal service.

Our study has several strengths. One is our comprehensive approach where we investigated barriers and facilitators to ART adherence from both the perspectives of PLHIV-OT and the perspectives of HSPs. This allowed us to effectively identify the overarching and unifying theme of stigma as the major barrier to ART adherence. We believe that our triangulation of data across PLHIV-OT and HSPs is a major strength. Both perspectives are extremely crucial for successful ART adherence. Another strength is our sample size. We successfully recruited and included a robust number of participants (n = 50), which provided the basis for comprehensive results, and offered insights into unexpected barriers and facilitators such as social media (both positive and negative) and spirituality (again with both facilitating and inhibiting effects).

In spite of these strengths, our study also has limitations. First, sampling occurred mostly in Jabodetabek, which is located in the metro Jakarta area, or inside and around the capital of Indonesia. We did not sample in other provinces. However, based on our noting of places of origin, our participants did represent the diversity of people in the Indonesian population relatively well. However, it would be advisable to conduct similar work in other provinces, particularly those with high HIV prevalence and/or low levels of adherence. A second limitation is the fact that our participants are a convenience sample. We recruited purposively based on inclusion and exclusion criteria and followed this up with snowball sampling. The risk of this approach is that new participants were referred by participants with similar opinions. However, it is important to note that generalizability is not the goal of qualitative research [78] and that our 50 participants were a diverse group in terms of age, gender, educational attainment, and professional and HIV-related characteristics. Another possible limitation was that PLHIV-OT, by virtue of them being on treatment, have experience with treatment and may have more favorable views on ART. It is therefore important to also explore barriers and facilitators to ART initiation.

## 5. Conclusions

Stigma is the foremost barrier to ART adherence across every socioecological level, and it converges with a number of other barriers starting from treatment initiation until after years of treatment. These barriers can be overcome by complementary facilitating factors that ameliorate the barriers at each socioecological level, and, for this to be effective, collaboration between PLHIV-OT, their significant others, HSPs, and NGOs is necessary. Overall, it is crucial to intervene by starting from the most abstract societal level, so that facilitators can be bolstered and barriers can be overcome at the subordinate levels.

**Author Contributions:** Conceptualization, B.S.H.H., S.E.S. and K.J.J.; methodology, B.S.H.H. and S.E.S.; formal analysis, B.S.H.H., S.E.S. and K.J.J.; data curation, B.S.H.H. and S.E.S.; writing—original draft preparation, B.S.H.H., S.E.S. and K.J.J.; writing—review and editing, B.S.H.H., S.E.S. and K.J.J.; funding acquisition, B.S.H.H. and K.J.J. All authors have read and agreed to the published version of the manuscript.

**Funding:** This research was funded by Indonesia Endowment Fund for Education or LPDP (Lembaga Pengelola Dana Pendidikan).

**Institutional Review Board Statement:** The study was conducted in accordance with the Declaration of Helsinki, and approved by the Health Research Ethics Committee, National Institute of Health Research and Development, or Badan Penelitian dan Pengembangan Kesehatan (protocol number LB.02.01/2/KE.139/2020 approved on 05-03-2020) and Ethics Review Committee of Faculty of Psychology and Neuroscience Maastricht University (reference number 188_11_02_2018_S17 approved on 04-02-2020) for studies involving humans.

**Informed Consent Statement:** Informed consent was obtained from all subjects involved in the study.

**Data Availability Statement:** Not applicable.

**Acknowledgments:** The authors wish to acknowledge the research team, interviewers, and translator in Indonesia: Ashma Nur Afifah, Dian Nur Halimah, Divani Aery Lovian, Josephine Indah Setyawati, Sustriana Saragih, and Melanesia Tamara Achta.

**Conflicts of Interest:** The authors declare no conflict of interest.

## References

1. UNAIDS. 90-90-90: An Ambitious Treatment Target to Help End the AIDS Epidemic. Available online: https://www.unaids.org/sites/default/files/media_asset/90-90-90_en.pdf (accessed on 14 December 2022).
2. Januraga, P.P.; Reekie, J.; Mulyani, T.; Lestari, B.W.; Iskandar, S.; Wisaksana, R.; Kusmayanti, N.A.; Subronto, Y.W.; Widyanthini, D.N.; Wirawan, D.N.; et al. The cascade of HIV care among key populations in Indonesia: A prospective cohort study. *Lancet HIV* **2018**, *5*, e560–e568. [CrossRef] [PubMed]
3. Ssekalembe, G.; Atoillah, M.; Isfandiari, M.A.; Suprianto, H. Current status towards 90-90-90 UNAIDS target and factors associated with HIV viral load suppression in Kediri City, Indonesia. *HIV/AIDS Res Palliat Care.* **2020**, *12*, 47–57. [CrossRef] [PubMed]
4. AIDS Data Hub. Cumulative Cross-Sectional Cascade for HIV Treatment and Care, Indonesia, 2021. Available online: https://www.aidsdatahub.org/country-profiles/indonesia (accessed on 14 December 2022).
5. Progress Report on HIV in the WHO South-East Asia Region 2016. 2016. Available online: https://apps.who.int/iris/handle/10665/251727 (accessed on 14 December 2022).
6. United Nations Programme on HIV/AIDS. UNAIDS. *UNAIDS Data 2021*, 2021, 4–38.
7. Innovations Map Indonesia. Available online: https://www.innovationsmap.asia/hivst_indonesia (accessed on 14 December 2022).
8. Paris Declaration Jakarta 2015. Available online: https://www.fast-trackcities.org/sites/default/files/Paris_Declaration_-_Jakarta_%282015%29.pdf (accessed on 19 December 2022).
9. Sweeney, S.M.; Vanable, P.A. The Association of HIV-Related Stigma to HIV Medication Adherence: A Systematic Review and Synthesis of the Literature. *AIDS Behav.* **2016**, *20*, 29–50. [CrossRef]
10. Baral, S.; Beyrer, C.; Muessig, K.; Poteat, T.; Wirtz, A.L.; Decker, M.R.; Sherman, S.G.; Kerrigan, D. Burden of HIV among female sex workers in low-income and middle-income countries: A systematic review and meta-analysis. *Lancet HIV* **2012**, *12*, 538–587. [CrossRef]
11. Mitchell, E.; Lazuardi, E.; Rowe, E.; Anintya, I.; Wirawan, D.N.; Wisaksana, R.; Subronto, Y.W.; Prameswari, H.D.; Kaldor, J.; Bell, S. Barriers and Enablers to HIV Care Among *Waria* (Transgender Women) in Indonesia: A Qualitative Study. *AIDS Educ. Prev.* **2019**, *31*, 538–552. [CrossRef]
12. Lazuardi, E.; Newman, C.E.; Anintya, I.; Rowe, E.; Wirawan, D.N.; Wisaksana, R.; Subronto, Y.W.; Kusmayanti, N.A.; Iskandar, S.; Kaldor, J.; et al. Increasing HIV treatment access, uptake and use among men who have sex with men in urban Indonesia: Evidence from a qualitative study in three cities. *Health Policy Plan.* **2019**, *35*, 16–25. [CrossRef]
13. Katz, I.T.; Ryu, A.E.; Onuegbu, A.G.; Psaros, C.; Weiser, S.D.; Bangsberg, D.R.; Tsai, A.C. Impact of HIV-related stigma on treatment adherence: Systematic review and meta-synthesis. *J. Int. AIDS Soc.* **2013**, *16*, 18640. [CrossRef]
14. Nelwan, E.J. Adherence to Highly Active Antiretroviral Therapy (HAART) in HIV/AIDS Patient. Available online: http://www.aidsinfo.nih.gov/contentfiles/ (accessed on 16 December 2022).
15. Kementerian Kesehatan Republik Indonesia. Estimasi Jumlah Populasi Kunci Terdampak HIV Tahun 2012. 2014.
16. Kementerian Kesehatan, RI. Infodatin HIV/AIDS. 2020, 1–8. Available online: https://pusdatin.kemkes.go.id/resources/download/pusdatin/infodatin/infodatin-2020-HIV.pdf (accessed on 16 December 2022).
17. Utami, S.; Sawitri, A.A.S.; Wulandari, L.P.L.; Putra, I.W.G.A.E.; Astuti, P.A.S.; Wirawan, D.N.; Causer, L.; Mathers, B. Mortality among people living with HIV on antiretroviral treatment in Bali, Indonesia: Incidence and predictors. *Int. J. STD AIDS* **2017**, *28*, 1199–1207. [CrossRef]
18. WHO. Guidelines for Managing Advanced HIV/AIDS. 2017. Available online: https://www.who.int/publications/i/item/9789241550062 (accessed on 14 December 2022).
19. Bor, J.; Fischer, C.; Modi, M.; Richman, B.; Kinker, C.; King, R.; Calabrese, S.K.; Mokhele, I.; Sineke, T.; Zuma, T.; et al. Changing Knowledge and Attitudes Towards HIV Treatment-as-Prevention and "Undetectable = Untransmittable": A Systematic Review. *AIDS Behav.* **2021**, *25*, 4209–4224. [CrossRef]
20. Hodgson, I. HIV Care: Learning from the Past, and the Right to Health. 2018. Available online: www.unaids.org/sites/default/files/ (accessed on 16 December 2022).
21. Suryana, K.; Suharsono, H.; Antara, I.G.P.J. Factors Associated with Adherence to Anti-Retroviral Therapy Among People Living With HIV/AIDS at Wangaya Hospital in Denpasar, Bali, Indonesia: A Cross-Sectional Study. *HIV/AIDS Res. Palliat. Care* **2019**, *11*, 307–312. [CrossRef]
22. Eisinger, R.W.; Dieffenbach, C.W.; Fauci, A.S. HIV viral load and transmissibility of HIV infection undetectable equals untransmittable. *J. Am. Med. Association. Am. Med. Assoc.* **2019**, *321*, 451–452. [CrossRef]
23. Myers, J.; Kobrak, P.; Daskalakis, D. U = U Guidance for Implementation in Clinical Settings. 2020.
24. Bronfenbrenner, U. The Ecology of Human Development. 1975.

25. Rosa, E.M.; Tudge, J. Urie Bronfenbrenner's Theory of Human Development: Its Evolution from Ecology to Bioecology. *J. Fam. Theory Rev.* **2013**, *5*, 243–258. [CrossRef]
26. Vélez-Agosto, N.M.; Soto-Crespo, J.G.; Vizcarrondo-Oppenheimer, M.; Vega-Molina, S.; Coll, C.G. Bronfenbrenner's Bioecological Theory Revision: Moving Culture from the Macro Into the Micro. *Perspect. Psychol. Sci.* **2017**, *12*, 900–910. [CrossRef]
27. Culbert, G.J.; Bazazi, A.R.; Waluyo, A.; Murni, A.; Muchransyah, A.P.; Iriyanti, M.; Finnahari; Polonsky, M.; Levy, J.; Altice, F.L. The Influence of Medication Attitudes on Utilization of Antiretroviral Therapy (ART) in Indonesian Prisons. *AIDS Behav.* **2016**, *20*, 1026–1038. [CrossRef]
28. Weaver, E.R.N.; Pane, M.; Wandra, T.; Windiyaningsih, C.; Herlina; Samaan, G. Factors that Influence Adherence to Antiretroviral Treatment in an Urban Population, Jakarta, Indonesia. *PLoS ONE* **2014**, *9*, e107543. [CrossRef]
29. Fauk, N.K.; Merry, M.S.; Siri, T.A.; Tazir, F.T.; Sigilipoe, M.A.; Tarigan, K.O.; Mwanri, L. Facilitators to Accessibility of HIV/AIDS-Related Health Services among Transgender Women Living with HIV in Yogyakarta, Indonesia. *AIDS Res. Treat.* **2019**, *2019*, 6045726. [CrossRef]
30. Ibrahim, K.; Lindayani, L.; Emaliyawati, E.; Rahayu, U.; Nuraeni, A. Factors Associated with Adherence to Antiretroviral Therapy among People Living with HIV Infection in West Java Province, Indonesia. *Malays. J. Med. Health Sci.* **2020**, *16*, 209–214.
31. Lumbantoruan, C.; Kermode, M.; Giyai, A.; Ang, A.; Kelaher, M. Understanding women's uptake and adherence in option b+ for prevention of mother-to-child hiv transmission in papua, Indonesia: A qualitative study. *PLoS ONE* **2018**, *13*, e0198329. [CrossRef]
32. Mitchell, E.; Lazuardi, E.; Anintya, I.; Rowe, E.; Whitford, K.; Wirawan, D.N.; Wisaksana, R.; Subronto, Y.W.; Prameswari, H.D.; Kaldor, J.; et al. A Qualitative Exploration of Family, Work, Community, and Health Service Influences on HIV Treatment Uptake and Adherence Among Female Sex Workers in Three Cities in Indonesia. *AIDS Educ. Prev.* **2020**, *32*, 243–259. [CrossRef]
33. Safira, N.; Lubis, R.; Fahdhy, M. Factors Affecting Adherence to Antiretroviral Therapy. *KnE Life Sci.* **2018**, *4*, 60. [CrossRef]
34. Suryana, K. The Impact of Universal Test and Treat Program on Highly Active Anti Retroviral Therapy Outcomes (Coverage, Adherence and Lost to Follow Up) at Wangaya Hospital in Denpasar, Bali-Indonesia: A Retrospective Cohort Study. *Open AIDS J.* **2021**, *15*, 28–34. [CrossRef]
35. Temple, G. Migration to Jakarta. *Bull. Indones. Econ. Stud.* **1975**, *11*, 76–81. [CrossRef]
36. McCarthy, P. The Case of Jakarta, Indonesia. 2020.
37. Braun, V.; Clarke, V. Using thematic analysis in psychology. *Qual. Res. Psychol.* **2006**, *3*, 77–101. [CrossRef]
38. Samudro, A.B.P. Pengeluaran Untuk Konsumsi Penduduk Indonesia per Provinsi. *Badan Pus. Stat. RI* **2022**, *4*, 88–100.
39. Been, S.K.; van de Vijver, D.A.M.C.; Nieuwkerk, P.T.; Brito, I.; Stutterheim, S.E.; Bos, A.E.R.; Wolfers, M.E.G.; Pogány, K.; Verbon, A. Risk Factors for Non-Adherence to cART in Immigrants with HIV Living in the Netherlands: Results from the Rotterdam Adherence (ROAD) Project. *PLoS ONE* **2016**, *11*, e0162800. [CrossRef]
40. Nyblade, L.; Stangl, A.; Weiss, E.; Ashburn, K. Combating HIV stigma in health care settings: What works? *J. Int. AIDS Soc.* **2009**, *12*, 1–7. [CrossRef]
41. Nyblade, L.; Stockton, M.A.; Giger, K.; Bond, V.; Ekstrand, M.L.; Mc Lean, R.; Mitchell, E.M.H.; Nelson, L.R.E.; Sapag, J.C.; Siraprapasiri, T.; et al. Stigma in health facilities: Why it matters and how we can change it. *BMC Med.* **2019**, *17*, 25. [CrossRef]
42. Stutterheim, S.E.; Sicking, L.; Brands, R.; Baas, I.; Roberts, H.; Van Brakel, W.H.; Lechner, L.; Kok, G.; Bos, A. Patient and Provider Perspectives on HIV and HIV-Related Stigma in Dutch Health Care Settings. *AIDS Patient Care STDs* **2014**, *28*, 652–665. [CrossRef]
43. Stutterheim, S.E.; Kuijpers, K.J.R.; Waldén, M.I.; Finkenflügel, R.N.N.; Brokx, P.A.R.; Bos, A.E.R. Trends in HIV Stigma Experienced by People Living with HIV in the Netherlands: A Comparison of Cross-Sectional Surveys Over Time. *AIDS Educ. Prev.* **2022**, *34*, 33–52. [CrossRef]
44. Sianturi, E.I.; Latifah, E.; Probandari, A.; Effendy, C.; Taxis, K. Daily struggle to take antiretrovirals: A qualitative study in Papuans living with HIV and their healthcare providers. *BMJ Open* **2020**, *10*, e036832. [CrossRef]
45. Shubber, Z.; Mills, E.J.; Nachega, J.B.; Vreeman, R.; Freitas, M.; Bock, P.; Nsanzimana, S.; Penazzato, M.; Appolo, T.; Doherty, M.; et al. Patient-Reported Barriers to Adherence to Antiretroviral Therapy: A Systematic Review and Meta-Analysis. *PLoS Med.* **2016**, *13*, e1002183. [CrossRef]
46. Mitchell, E.; Hakim, A.; Nosi, S.; Kupul, M.; Boli-Neo, R.; Aeno, H.; Redman-Maclaren, M.; Ase, S.; Amos, A.; Hou, P.; et al. A socio-ecological analysis of factors influencing HIV treatment initiation and adherence among key populations in Papua New Guinea. *BMC Public Health* **2021**, *21*, 2003. [CrossRef]
47. Gourlay, A.; Birdthistle, I.; Mburu, G.; Iorpenda, K.; Wringe, A. Barriers and facilitating factors to the uptake of antiretroviral drugs for prevention of mother-to-child transmission of HIV in sub-Saharan Africa: A systematic review. *J. Int. AIDS Soc.* **2013**, *16*, 18588. [CrossRef]
48. Wirawan, D.N. Stigma and discrimination: Barrier for ending AIDS by 2030 and achieving the 90–90-90 targets by 2020. *Public Health Prev. Med. Arch.* **2019**, *7*, 1–2. [CrossRef]
49. Nafisah, L.; Riono, P.; Muhaimin, T. Do stigma and disclosure of HIV status are associated with adherence to antiretroviral therapy among men who have sex with men? *HIV AIDS Rev.* **2021**, *19*, 244–251. [CrossRef]
50. Fauk, N.K.; Merry, M.S.; Ambarwati, A.; Sigilipoe, M.A.; Ernawati; Mwanri, L. A qualitative inquiry of adherence to antiretroviral therapy and its associated factors: A study with transgender women living with HIV in Indonesia. *Indian J. Public Health* **2020**, *64*, 116–123.
51. Wasti, S.P.; van Teijlingen, E.; Simkhada, P.; Randall, J.; Baxter, S.; Kirkpatrick, P.; Gc, V.S. Factors influencing adherence to antiretroviral treatment in Asian developing countries: A systematic review. *Trop. Med. Int. Health* **2012**, *17*, 71–81. [CrossRef]

52. Ameli, V.; Taj, L.; Barlow, J.; Sabin, L.; Meinck, F.; Haberer, J.; Mohraz, M. 'You just prefer to die early!': How socioecological context impedes treatment for people living with HIV in Iran. *BMJ Glob. Health* **2021**, *6*, e006088. [CrossRef]
53. Nuraidah, D.W.; Hayati, H.; Rachmawati, I.N.; Waluyo, A. "I can live a normal life": Exploring adherence to antiretroviral therapy in Indonesian adolescents living with HIV. *Belitung Nurs. J.* **2022**, *8*, 108–114. [CrossRef]
54. Sianturi, E.I.; Perwitasari, D.A.; Islam, A.; Taxis, K. The association between ethnicity, stigma, beliefs about medicines and adherence in people living with HIV in a rural area in Indonesia. *BMC Public Health* **2019**, *19*, 55. [CrossRef]
55. Msc, J.W.N.; Gichane, M.W.; Browne, F.A.; Bonner, C.P.; Zule, W.A.; Cox, E.N.; Smith, K.M.; Carney, T.; Wechsberg, W.M.; ScD, F.A.B.; et al. 'We have goals but [it is difficult]'. Barriers to antiretroviral therapy adherence among women using alcohol and other drugs living with HIV in South Africa. *Health Expect.* **2022**, *25*, 754–763. [CrossRef]
56. Lyimo, R.A.; Stutterheim, S.E.; Hospers, H.J.; de Glee, T.; van der Ven, A.; de Bruin, M. Stigma, Disclosure, Coping, and Medication Adherence among People Living with HIV/AIDS in Northern Tanzania. *AIDS Patient Care STDS* **2014**, *28*, 98–105. [CrossRef] [PubMed]
57. Sianturi, E.I.; Latifah, E.; Gunawan, E.; Sihombing, R.B.; Parut, A.A.; Perwitasari, D.A. Adaptive Stigma Coping Among Papuans Living with HIV: A Qualitative Study in One of the Indigenous People, Indonesia. *J. Racial Ethn. Health Disparities* **2022**, 1–8. [CrossRef] [PubMed]
58. Fauk, N.; Hawke, K.; Mwanri, L.; Ward, P. Stigma and Discrimination towards People Living with HIV in the Context of Families, Communities, and Healthcare Settings: A Qualitative Study in Indonesia. *Int. J. Environ. Res. Public Health* **2021**, *18*, 5424. [CrossRef]
59. Chijioke-Nwauche, I.N.; Akani, Y. Influencing Factors of Adherence to Antiretroviral Drugs among People Living with HIV in South-South Nigeria. *Saudi J. Med. Pharm. Sci.* **2021**, *7*, 145–152.
60. Andersson, G.Z.; Reinius, M.; Eriksson, L.E.; Svedhem, V.; Esfahani, F.M.; Deuba, K.; Rao, D.; Lyatuu, G.W.; Giovenco, D.; Ekström, A.M. Stigma reduction interventions in people living with HIV to improve health-related quality of life. *Lancet HIV* **2020**, *7*, e129–e140. [CrossRef]
61. Stutterheim, S.E.; van Dijk, M.; Wang, H.; Jonas, K.J. The worldwide burden of HIV in transgender individuals: An updated systematic review and meta-analysis. *PLoS ONE* **2021**, *16*, e0260063. [CrossRef]
62. van der Kooij, Y.L.; Kupková, A.; Daas, C.D.; Berk, G.E.V.D.; Kleene, M.J.T.; Jansen, H.S.; Elsenburg, L.J.; Schenk, L.G.; Verboon, P.; Brinkman, K.; et al. Role of Self-Stigma in Pathways from HIV-Related Stigma to Quality of Life Among People Living with HIV. *AIDS Patient Care STDs* **2021**, *35*, 231–238. [CrossRef]
63. Grossman, C.I.; Stangl, A.L. Editorial: Global action to reduce HIV stigma and discrimination. *J. Int. AIDS Soc.* **2013**, *16* (Suppl. 2), 1–6. [CrossRef]
64. Brown, L.; Macintyre, K.; Trujillo, L. Interventions to reduce HIV/AIDS stigma: What have we learned? *AIDS Educ. Prev.* **2003**, *15*, 49–69. [CrossRef]
65. Stutterheim, S.E.; Van Der Kooij, Y.L.; Crutzen, R.; Ruiter, R.A.C.; Bos, A.E.R.; Kok, G. A Systematic Approach to Stigma Reduction Intervention Mapping as a Guide to Developing, Implementing, and Evaluating Stigma Reduction Interventions. *Preprint* **2022**. [CrossRef]
66. Dunbar, W.; Labat, A.; Raccurt, C.; Sohler, N.; Pape, J.W.; Maulet, N.; Coppieters, Y. A realist systematic review of stigma reduction interventions for HIV prevention and care continuum outcomes among men who have sex with men. *Int. J. STD AIDS* **2020**, *31*, 712–723. [CrossRef]
67. He, A.; Liu, H.; Tian, Y. Reducing HIV public stigma through news information engagement on social media: A multi-method study of the role of state empathy. *Cyberpsychol. J. Psychosoc. Res. Cyberspace* **2022**, *16*. [CrossRef]
68. Stutterheim, S.E.; Bos, A.E.R.; van Kesteren, N.M.C.; Shiripinda, I.; Pryor, J.B.; de Bruin, M.; Schaalma, H.P. Beliefs Contributing to HIV-related Stigma in African and Afro-Caribbean Communities in the Netherlands. *J. Community Appl. Soc. Psychol.* **2012**, *22*, 470–484. [CrossRef]
69. Pangestika, D. Activists Urge Govt to Resolve HIV Drugs Shortage Amid COVID-19 Pandemic. 2020. Available online: https://www.thejakartapost.com/news/2020/03/20/activists-urge-govt-to-resolve-hiv-drugs-shortage-amid-covid-19-pandemic.html (accessed on 16 December 2022).
70. Cao, B.; Wang, Y.; Wen, D.; Liu, W.; Wang, J.; Fan, G.; Ruan, L.; Song, B.; Cai, Y.; Wei, M.; et al. A Trial of Lopinavir–Ritonavir in Adults Hospitalized with Severe COVID-19. *N. Engl. J. Med.* **2020**, *382*, 1787–1799. [CrossRef]
71. Stutterheim, S.E.; Bos, A.E.R.; Pryor, J.B.; Brands, R.; Liebregts, M.; Schaalma, H.P. Psychological and Social Correlates of HIV Status Disclosure: The Significance of Stigma Visibility. *AIDS Educ. Prev.* **2011**, *23*, 382–392. [CrossRef]
72. Been, S.K.; Van De Vijver, D.A.; Smit, J.; Bassant, N.; Pogány, K.; Stutterheim, S.E.; Verbon, A. Feasibility of Four Interventions to Improve Treatment Adherence in Migrants Living with HIV in The Netherlands. *Diagnostics* **2020**, *10*, 980. [CrossRef]
73. Rathore, M.A.; Rashid, Z.; Khushk, I.A.; Mashhadi, F.; Rathore, M.A.; Barnes, S. Exploring health seeking behaviour among incidentally diagnosed HIV cases in Rawalpindi, Pakistan: A qualitative perspective. *J. Pak. Med. Assoc.* **2022**, *72*, 2453–2458. [CrossRef]
74. Stutterheim, S.E.; Shiripinda, I.; Bos, A.E.; Pryor, J.B.; De Bruin, M.; Nellen, J.F.; Kok, G.; Prins, J.M.; Schaalma, H.P. HIV status disclosure among HIV-positive African and Afro-Caribbean people in the Netherlands. *AIDS Care* **2011**, *23*, 195–205. [CrossRef]
75. Dima, A.L.; Stutterheim, S.E.; Lyimo, R.; de Bruin, M. Advancing methodology in the study of HIV status disclosure: The importance of considering disclosure target and intent. *Soc. Sci. Med.* **2014**, *108*, 166–174. [CrossRef] [PubMed]

76. World Health Organization. Consolidated Guidelines on HIV Prevention, Diagnosis, Treatment and Care for Key Populations. WHO Guidel. 2014, 184. Available online: http://apps.who.int/iris/bitstream/10665/128048/1/9789241507431_eng.pdf?ua=1 (accessed on 16 December 2022).
77. Ruiter, R.A.; Abraham, C.; Kok, G. Scary warnings and rational precautions: A review of the psychology of fear appeals. *Psychol. Health* **2001**, *16*, 613–630. [CrossRef]
78. Stutterheim, S.E.; Ratcliffe, S.E. Understanding and addressing stigma through qualitative research: Four reasons why we need qualitative studies. *Stigma Health* **2021**, *6*, 8–19. [CrossRef]

**Disclaimer/Publisher's Note:** The statements, opinions and data contained in all publications are solely those of the individual author(s) and contributor(s) and not of MDPI and/or the editor(s). MDPI and/or the editor(s) disclaim responsibility for any injury to people or property resulting from any ideas, methods, instructions or products referred to in the content.

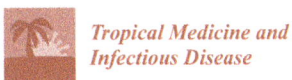

*Tropical Medicine and Infectious Disease*

Article

# Estimating Dengue Transmission Intensity in China Using Catalytic Models Based on Serological Data

Ning Li [1,2], Haidong Li [1,3], Zhengji Chen [1,4], Huan Xiong [1], Zhibo Li [1], Tao Wei [5], Wei Liu [1] and Xu-Sheng Zhang [6,*]

1. School of Public Health, Kunming Medical University, Kunming 650500, China
2. Centers for Disease Control and Prevention of Yunnan Province, Kunming 650118, China
3. The Affiliated Hospital of Stomatology, Chongqing Medical University, Chongqing 401147, China
4. Kunming Centers for Disease Control and Prevention, Kunming 650228, China
5. Library, Kunming Medical University, Kunming 650500, China
6. Statistics, Modelling and Economics Department, Data, Analytics & Surveillance, UK Health Security Agency, London NW9 5EQ, UK
* Correspondence: xu-sheng.zhang@ukhsa.gov.uk

**Abstract:** In recent decades, the global incidence of dengue has risen sharply, with more than 75% of infected people showing mild or no symptoms. Since the year 2000, dengue in China has spread quickly. At this stage, there is an urgent need to fully understand its transmission intensity and spread in China. Serological data provide reliable evidence for symptomatic and recessive infections. Through a literature search, we included 23 studies that collected age-specific serological dengue data released from 1980 to 2021 in China. Fitting four catalytic models to these data, we distinguished the transmission mechanisms by deviation information criterion and estimated force of infection and basic reproduction number ($R_0$), important parameters for quantifying transmission intensity. We found that transmission intensity varies over age in most of the study populations, and attenuation of antibody protection is identified in some study populations; the $R_0$ of dengue in China is between 1.04–2.33. Due to the scarceness of the data, the temporal trend cannot be identified, but data shows that transmission intensity weakened from coastal to inland areas and from southern to northern areas in China if assuming it remained temporally steady during the study period. The results should be useful for the effective control of dengue in China.

**Keywords:** Bayesian inference; catalytic model; dengue; mathematical modelling; serological data; transmission intensity

## 1. Introduction

### 1.1. Current Status of Dengue

Dengue is a mosquito-borne virus infectious disease mainly transmitted through the bites of female *Aedes aegypti* and *Aedes albopictus*. Dengue virus (DENV) has four different serotypes (DENV-1, 2, 3 and 4), and both infants and adults are susceptible. The incubation period is generally 4–10 days, and the infection period is 2–7 days [1]. Dengue is one of the 17 neglected tropical diseases in the Neglected Tropical Diseases (NTD) roadmap [2]. In recent decades, the incidence of dengue has risen dramatically. The World Health Organization (WHO) estimates 100 to 400 million cases of infection each year worldwide, and nearly half of the world's population is at risk of the infection [3]. Moreover, since most cases of dengue manifest as asymptomatic infections (recessive infections), the actual number may exceed the reported number. According to Bhatt et al. [4], about 390 (95% CI: 284, 528) million dengue infections occur each year, of which only about 96 (95% CI: 67, 136) million express clinical symptoms. Dengue has caused a huge burden of disease globally. The year 2019 saw the highest number of dengue cases reported globally in recent memory. Many countries and regions have been affected, with the first recorded transmission of dengue in Afghanistan. The United States alone has reported 3.1 million cases, with more than 25,000 severe cases, while large numbers of cases have also been reported in Bangladesh (101,000), Malaysia (131,000), the Philippines (420,000) and Vietnam (320,000) in Asia [3].

China is in eastern Asia and is adjacent to some Southeast Asia countries that have high dengue incidence. Its southeast coast is a high-incidence area of dengue, especially in Guangdong province [5]. Dengue cases were reported almost every year, and a large outbreak of 45,217 cases occurred in 2014 in China [6]. In addition, in the northern and inland regions, from 2018 to 2020, there were successive outbreaks of dengue in Hebei province [7], Yunnan province [8], Hunan province [9], Hubei province [10], with a total of more than 300 reported cases. China is not the original area of dengue, and most dengue outbreaks in China were caused by imported cases from abroad. Because recessive dengue infections are not detected by symptom screening, it is very likely that a large number of those infections [4] become a source of infection and lead to a significant increase in the positivity rate [11–14]. The social and economic burdens caused by dengue are getting heavier. In the specific measures to achieve the three major goals of dengue control, the WHO clearly proposed to conduct research on the transmission kinetics of dengue and develop models to quantify the joint method of vaccine and vector control in transmission [15]. In this paper, we used catalytic models based on serological data to estimate dengue transmission intensity and review the changes in dengue transmission in China over the past years.

*1.2. Dengue Data and Modelling*

In the modeling study of infectious diseases, the important parameters used to characterize transmission intensity are the force of infection (FOI, defined as the instantaneous per capita infection rate at which susceptible individuals acquire infection [16]), and basic reproductive number ($R_0$, defined as the average number of secondary cases caused by an infectious individual entering a susceptible population [17]). The role of FOI has greater significance than the widely used incidence rate because it can distinguish potential age-related changes in infection rates [16]. When an infectious disease first occurs, a patient must infect at least one individual; that is what keeps the epidemic going. However, not every susceptible person who comes into contact with an infected person will be infected, and the probability is determined by FOI. When the susceptible population within a region has got infected and then acquired immunity or died, the proportion of the susceptible population will decline; but due to the supplement of newborn babies and migrant susceptible people from external populations, the proportion of susceptible people may increase again. To characterize the spread potential of an infectious disease under the constantly changing susceptibility, the effective reproduction number, which is defined as a product of basic reproduction number and susceptibility (i.e., $R_0$ × susceptibility), is an appropriate measure. When a population reaches a steady-state for an infectious disease, its effective reproduction is equal to 1, implying the total number of infections is neither increasing nor decreasing. Therefore, $R_0$ determines not only the growth rate of the infectious disease but also the proportion ($1/R_0$) of the steady-state population infected by the disease [18].

In China, we learned through a literature search that there were few studies using serological data for dengue modeling. Due to the lag in the infectious disease surveillance and reporting system and the differences in regional regulatory systems, there is a problem with using case notification data in that the number of reports does not match the reality. The spread of dengue shows a high degree of geographic heterogeneity [19] and even needs to be measured in a very fine spatial range [20]. Moreover, in many situations, dengue cases show mild or asymptomatic [4] or are only diagnosed as another viral infection in the clinic, which may cause dengue to be misclassified or difficult to diagnose, even the highly sensitive disease surveillance systems may also underestimate the incidence of dengue [21,22]. Therefore, the use of dengue case notification data for research may underestimate dengue transmission intensity.

Using serological data to estimate dengue transmission intensity has great advantages because it can detect past symptomatic and asymptomatic infection cases [19] and more accurately reflect transmission intensity. A literature review of dengue studies in China showed that most studies used IgM and IgG ELISA (Enzyme-Linked Immunosorbent Assay) data. Although PRNT (Plaque Reduction Neutralization Test) and PCR (Polymerase Chain Reaction) can identify different serotypes of dengue virus, their difficulty and cost are relatively high, while ELISA has the advantages of low cost and high efficiency. Imai [19] used IgG and IgM ELISA, IE (Inhibition ELISA) and PRNT data to estimate dengue transmission intensity, and they showed that the FOI estimated by the ELISA data was equal to the sum of the FOI estimated from the specific serological data. In this study, we used non-serotype-specific data to estimate FOI and $R_0$.

## 2. Materials and Methods
### 2.1. Literature Search and Data

We searched multiple literature databases for potentially available studies related to dengue serology in China. Since we mainly studied the spread of dengue in China in recent years, articles published before 1980 and articles whose study areas are not in China were excluded. Since a wider age group may not accurately reflect the difference in the seropositivity rate of the age group [19], the studies that had at least five age groups were included. Based on these selection criteria (Figure 1), 23 studies [23–45] were finally included (Supplementary File S1).

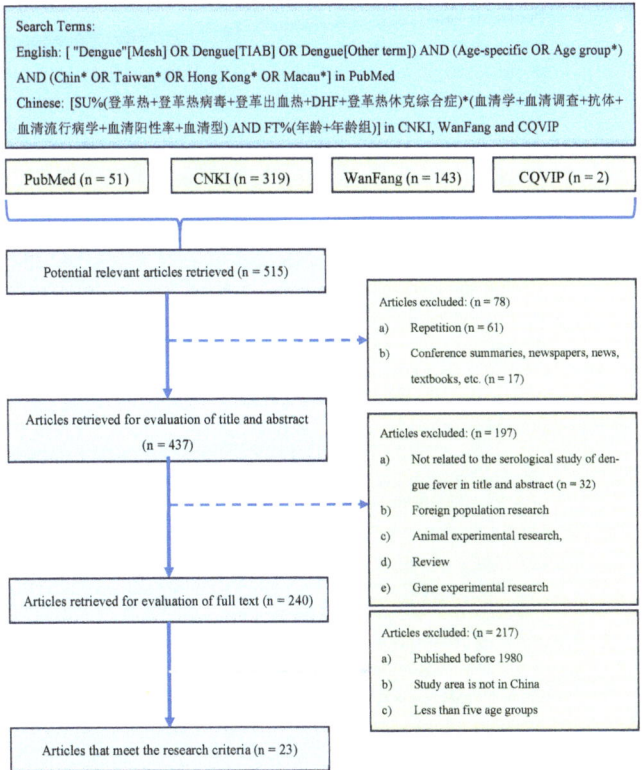

**Figure 1.** Literature search and screening process. Notice: (1) In the search query [ "Dengue"[Mesh] OR Dengue[TIAB] OR Dengue[Other term]) AND (Age-specific OR Age group*) AND (Chin* OR Taiwan* OR Hong Kong* OR Macau*], *, an asterisk, is the truncation symbol in PubMed, which

was used at the end of a word to search for all terms that begin with that basic word root. (2) The search query [SU%( 登革热+ 登革热病毒+ 登革出血热+DHF+ 登革热休克综合症)*( 血清学+ 血清调查+ 抗体+ 血清流行病学+ 血清阳性率+ 血清型) AND FT%( 年龄+ 年龄组)] in CNKI database can be translated into [SU%(Dengue + Dengue virus + Dengue hemorrhagic fever +DHF+ Dengue shock syndrome)*(Serology + serum survey + antibody + seroepidemiology + Seropositive rate + Serotype) AND FT%(age + age group)], where SU stands for subject, or TITLE, ABSTRACT, and/or KEYWORD; % stands for INCLUDE; + stands for the boolean operator OR; * stands for the boolean operator AND; FT stands for FULL TEXT. (3) The search queries for other two Chinese literature databases are similar to the one used in CNKI database.

The 23 studies involved eight provinces and one region in China, namely Guangdong, Guangxi, Zhejiang, Hunan, Guizhou, Hainan, Yunnan, Taiwan and Hong Kong, with a total of 18 study regions and 31 data sets (Table 1). They are all located south of the Yangtze River in China. Among them, Guangdong, Guangxi, Zhejiang, Hainan, Taiwan and Hong Kong are all coastal provinces, while Hunan, Guizhou and Yunnan are inland provinces. In addition, Yunnan Province and Guangxi Province are adjacent to Southeast Asian countries. Most of the eight provinces or regions are located between 20° and 30° north latitude, with tropical or subtropical seasonal characteristics, high temperature and humid climate.

Those studies reported the survey data on the age-stratified non-serotype-specific prevalence of dengue from 1980 to 2019. In the last column of Table 1, we use "Herd" to indicate that its sample is from the healthy general population; Use "Hospital/CDC" to indicate that the data was collected at the hospital and/or Centers for Disease Control and Prevention (CDC); "Blood donation center" means that the sample population is healthy blood donors in the blood donation center. "Health Checkup Center" means the sample population is the health checkup population at the port health checkup center. In addition, single-year cross-sectional data from 2011 to 2013 can be extracted from the study [27] and from 2013 to 2015 from the study [45]. The study [43] was based on the phased data collected at different stages of a dengue outbreak in the study area. For the three studies, we fitted our models to the data of each year.

2.2. Dengue Models

Due to the presence of dengue immune antibodies, the seroprevalence rate of the population increases with age. This rate of change with age can be interpreted as a measure of the "strength" of the spread of dengue in the past. The significant change in the seroprevalence rate of each age group may be further due to a unique change in the risk of infection in a certain age window or caused by a change in unique risk factors that are not related to age, or a combination of the two [46]. Therefore, the seroprevalence rate provides information about the overall cumulative risk of infection experienced by the entire age group [47]. In addition, the individual's dengue immune antibody level may also decrease with age (antibody protection decay effect). Here, we consider the impact of different infection mechanisms (Model A–D) on the dengue transmission intensity. For Model A, we assume that the FOI does not change with age; that is, the FOI is a constant. For Model B, since the seroprevalence rate of some data sets seems to decrease with age, we assume that antibody protection decays at a constant rate. For Models C and D, we consider that the seropositivity rate changed significantly at a certain age due to changes in the exposure levels or other reasons and introduced the concept of threshold age ($A_{crit}$). In view of that changes in population structure can greatly complicate mathematical models and require a large amount of longitudinal population data, we ignore demographic changes such as population mobility and natural birth/death rates. In the following, we give the details of the four models.

Table 1. 23 studies for estimation of dengue transmission intensity in China.

| Survey Region | Reference | Survey Year | Age Range | No. of Samples | No. of Positives | Testing Method | * Circulating Serotype | Source of Sample Population |
|---|---|---|---|---|---|---|---|---|
| **Guangdong Province** | | | | | | | | |
| Guangzhou | Huang Y et al. [23] | 1981 | 5–50+ | 174 | 86 | HI | DENV-1,2,3,4 | Herd |
| Zhuhai | Li Z et al. [24] | 1998 | 10–60+ | 374 | 4 | ELISA | NA | Herd |
| Zhuhai | Yang Z et al. [25] | 2001 | 10–50+ | 558 | 51 | ELISA | NA | Herd |
| # GZ Huangpu | Zheng X et al. [26] | 2008 | 0–71+ | 324 | 55 | ELISA/RT-PCR | NA | Herd |
| Guangzhou | Cao Y et al. [27] | 2011 | 0–60+ | 2075 | 200 | ELISA | NA | Hospital/CDC |
|  |  | 2012 | 0–60+ | 1201 | 192 | ELISA | NA | Hospital/CDC |
|  |  | 2013 | 0–60+ | 1235 | 124 | ELISA | NA | Hospital/CDC |
| Guangzhou | Li S et al. [28] | 2014 | 18–60 | 4000 | 131 | ELISA/PCR | DENV-1,2 | Blood Donation Center |
| Guangzhou | Jing Q et al. [29] | 2015 | 0–60+ | 850 | 56 | ELISA/IFA test | DENV-1,2,3,4 | Herd |
| **Guangxi Province** | | | | | | | | |
| Beihai | Tian X et al. [30] | 1980 | 0–40 | 435 | 116 | HI | DENV-2 | Sentinel Hospital |
| $ QZ/FCG/HP | Zhou K et al. [31] | 2010–2012 | 0–79 | 1800 | 37 | ELISA | NA | Herd |
| **Zhejiang Province** | | | | | | | | |
| Yiwu | Sun J et al. [32] | 2009 | 0–80+ | 365 | 102 | ELISA | DENV-3 | Herd |
| Cixi | Cen D et al. [33] | 2004 | 0–80+ | 520 | 35 | IFA | NA | Herd |
| **Hunan Province** | | | | | | | | |
| Chenzhou | Gao L et al. [34] | 2005 | 0–80+ | 488 | 7 | ELISA | NA | Herd |
| **Guizhou Province** | | | | | | | | |
| Guiyang | Gao R et al. [35] | 2004–2005 | 0–50+ | 2281 | 197 | ELISA | NA | Herd |
| Guiyang | Tian H et al. [36] | 2005 | 0–60+ | 755 | 55 | ELISA | NA | Herd |
| & GY/CJ/LD | Jiang W et al. [37] | 2011 | 5–60+ | 530 | 11 | ELISA | NA | Herd |
| **Hainan Province** | | | | | | | | |
| Danzhou | Jin Y et al. [38] | 2006 | 0–60+ | 431 | 7 | ELISA | NA | Herd |
| **Yunnan Province** | | | | | | | | |
| Mengla | Lu Y et al. [39] | 2014 | 0–60 | 182 | 3 | ELISA | NA | Health Checkup Center |
| Hekou | Pu L et al. [40] | 2016 | 0–60 | 203 | 9 | ELISA/RT-PCR | NA | Health Checkup Center |
| Xishuangbanna | Li L et al. [41] | 2019 | 18–60 | 2254 | 484 | ELISA | NA | Blood Donation Center |

Table 1. Cont.

| Survey Region | Reference | Survey Year | Age Range | No. of Samples | No. of Positives | Testing Method | *Circulating Serotype | Source of Sample Population |
|---|---|---|---|---|---|---|---|---|
| Taiwan Province % TP/TY/TN | Lee YH et al. [42] | 2010 | 0–70+ | 1308 | 44 | ELISA | NA | Herd |
| Kaohsiung | Tsai JJ et al. [43] | 2015.8–11 | 0–89 | 417 | 48 | ELISA | DENV-1,2 | Herd |
| | | 2016.2–5 | 0–89 | 294 | 36 | ELISA | DENV-1,2 | Herd |
| | | 2016.9–2017.1 | 0–59 | 226 | 23 | ELISA | DENV-1,2 | Herd |
| | | 2017.8–9 | 20–89 | 153 | 28 | ELISA | DENV-1,2 | Herd |
| Kaohsiung and Tainan | Pan YH et al. [44] | | | | | | | |
| Kaohsiung | | 2016 | 40–80+ | 1498 | 595 | ELISA | DENV-1,2,3, | Herd |
| Tainan | | 2016 | 40–80+ | 2603 | 291 | ELISA | DENV-1,2,3,4 | Herd |
| Hong Kong | Lee P et al. [45] | 2013 | 1–66+ | 700 | 24 | ELISA | NA | Hospital |
| | | 2014 | 1–66+ | 700 | 32 | ELISA | NA | Hospital |
| | | 2015 | 1–66+ | 700 | 31 | ELISA | NA | Hospital |

* Circulating serotype is the dengue serotype detected in the study or the main serotype currently circulating, and NA indicates the serotype that was not detected or mentioned in the study. # GZ Huangpu represents Huangpu District in Guangzhou city; $ QZ/FCG/HP stands for Qinzhou City, Fangchenggang City and Hepu County in Guangxi; & GY/CJ/LD represents Yunyan District of Guiyang City, Congjiang County of Southeast Guizhou Province and Luodian County of Guizhou Province; % TP/TY/TN indicates Taipei, Taoyuan and Tainan of Taiwan Province.

### 2.2.1. Model A: Constant Force of Infection

According to Muench's catalytic model [48], people in age group $i$ changes from a seronegative group to a seropositive group after infection at a rate $\lambda$, as shown in Figure 2. Here $\lambda$ is used to denote FOI, and the proportions of seronegative and seropositive in the age group $i$ are $x(a_i)$ and $z(a_i)$, respectively.

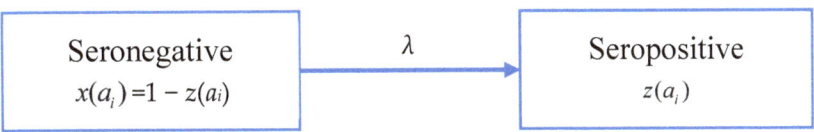

**Figure 2.** Model A: the catalytic model that assumes constant FOI without antibody decay.

Since the data is not serotype-specific, we assume that the total FOI of the four serotypes is constant and that individuals receive lifelong immunity after infection. Assuming that $\lambda$ is a constant, the proportion of the seropositive population in age group $i$, $z(a_i)$ is given by:

$$z(a_i) = 1 - \exp(-\lambda a_i) \quad (1)$$

Here $a_i$ is the median age of the age group $i$.

### 2.2.2. Model B: Antibody Protection Decay

There are four serotypes of the dengue virus. A person who is infected with one serotype will have acquired immunity. Although there is serotype cross-immunity, the duration of cross-immunity is very different from person to person [49–51]. Studies have shown that in the first six months after primary infection with dengue, the neutralizing antibody (NAb) titers against all serotypes are the highest [52], but after that, NAb titers gradually weaken, which mainly depends on the intensity of dengue and the degree of exposure [53–56]. According to the data we have obtained, the seroprevalence rate of some data sets decreases with age, which means that there may be a phenomenon that antibody levels decrease with age. Following [19], it is assumed that the immunity level of a seropositive group decays at a rate of $\alpha$, causing individuals to return to the seronegative group (Figure 3).

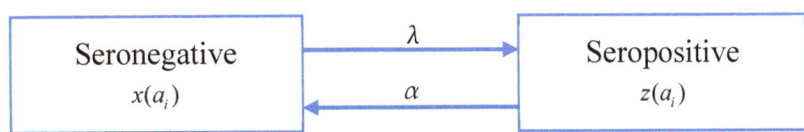

**Figure 3.** Model B: The catalytic model that assumes constant FOI and antibody decay.

As shown in Figure 3, the population is divided into the seropositive population ($z(a_i)$) and seronegative population ($x(a_i) = 1 - z(a_i)$); the antibody level of the seropositive population decays at a constant rate $\alpha$, while seronegative population may be infected to become seropositive people. By extending Model A, the change in the proportion of the seropositive population in age group $i$, $z(a_i)$ is given by:

$$\frac{dz(a_i)}{da} = \lambda[1 - z(a_i)] - \alpha z(a_i) = \lambda - (\lambda + \alpha)z(a_i) \quad (2)$$

Assuming that both $\lambda$ and $\alpha$ are constant, integrating the above formula gives,

$$z(a_i) = \{1 - \exp[-a_i(\lambda + \alpha)]\}\left(\frac{\lambda}{\lambda + \alpha}\right) \quad (3)$$

### 2.2.3. Models That Include Threshold Age

For people of different ages (such as the young and old), their risk of getting dengue may be different due to differences in the immune system, lifestyle, and other factors, even if they are exposed to the same environmental conditions. Assuming that the population is homogeneously mixed, for example, young people may reach a wider range of people, while the range of activities of the elderly is limited due to reasons such as study and work. Their potential exposure patterns are also different. In view of these potential factors, we assume that the seropositivity rate may change significantly in a certain age window due to changes in the exposure level or other reasons. We assume that there is a critical age ($A_{crit}$) by which the population is divided into two different age groups. Within each age group, the FOI is still assumed to be constant but varies between age groups. Based on this, Model A and Model B are extended to Model C and Model D as follows.

Model C: constant FOI is broken by a critical age

$$z(a_i) = 1 - \exp(-\lambda_1 a_i), \text{ when } a \leq A_{crit} \quad z(a_i) = 1 - \exp(-\lambda_2 a_i), \text{ when } a > A_{crit} \quad (4)$$

Model D: antibody protection decay with constant FOI broken by a critical age

$$\begin{aligned} z(a_i) &= \{1 - \exp[-a_i(\lambda_1 + \alpha)]\} \left(\frac{\lambda_1}{\lambda_1 + \alpha}\right), \text{ when } a \leq A_{crit} \\ z(a_i) &= \{1 - \exp[-a_i(\lambda_2 + \alpha)]\} \left(\frac{\lambda_2}{\lambda_2 + \alpha}\right), \text{ when } a > A_{crit} \end{aligned} \quad (5)$$

Here, $\lambda_1$ and $\lambda_2$ are the respective FOI when age $a$ is less than or equal to $A_{crit}$ or greater than $A_{crit}$, and the decay rate of antibody protection ($\alpha$) remains constant throughout all the age groups.

### 2.3. Inference Method

To estimate FOI and $R_0$, we fit the predicted seroprevalence rates of each age group to observed data, wherein the observed proportions of seropositivity in each age group are calculated based on the age-stratified seroprevalence survey data. In this study, we use Bayesian inference to estimate the model parameters [57]. The prior information on parameters is obtained through literature review and experience, and serological data are extracted from the literature as described in Section 2.1 (Supplementary File S1). Combining these with the likelihood function (see Section 2.4), the Markov Chain Monte Carlo (MCMC) method via normal random walk Metropolis-Hastings sampling method is used to generate the posterior distribution of model parameters [57], from which the median and its 95% credible interval (CrI) are obtained. The R statistical software (version 4.2.2 [58]) is used for calculations.

### 2.4. Negative Log-Likelihood (-LnL)

In Bayesian statistics, the likelihood function is calculated through the sample information (observation data). We assume that the probability of seropositive individuals in the age group $i$ obeys the Beta Binomial Distribution:

$$X_i \sim BetaBinomial(N_i, p_i, \gamma)$$

Here, $N_i$ is the total number of individuals in age group $i$, $p_i$ is the proportion of seropositive individuals observed in age group $i$, and $\gamma$ represents the overdispersion parameter of the beta-binomial distribution.

Following Imai et al. [19], the total negative log-likelihood function for all age groups, $-LnL(p)$, is given by:

$$-LnL(p) = -\left\{ \begin{array}{l} \sum_i \log\left\{ B\left[X_i + m_i(\frac{1}{\gamma} - 1), N_i - X_i + (1 - m_i)(\frac{1}{\gamma} - 1)\right] \right\} \\ -\log\left\{ B\left[m_i(\frac{1}{\gamma} - 1), (1 - m_i)(\frac{1}{\gamma} - 1)\right] \right\} \end{array} \right\} \quad (6)$$

where $B[a,b]$ is the beta function with standard parameters $a$ (predicted seropositive number) and $b$ (predicted seronegative number), $X_i$ is the number of seropositive individuals in age group $i$, $m_i$ is the predicted proportion of seropositive patients in the age group $i$.

2.5. Estimation of Basic Reproduction Number ($R_0$)

Assuming that FOI is constant for a certain amount of time, $R_0$ can be estimated from the formula [46]:

$$R_0 = \frac{1}{1 - \int_0^\infty f(a)z(a)da} \approx \frac{1}{1 - \sum_{i=1}^{na} f(a_i)z(a_i)} \quad (7)$$

Here $f(a)$ is the probability density function of the population age distribution, and $z(a)$ is the predicted seroprevalence from the proposed models. We collected the age distribution data of the population in each study area from the National Bureau of Statistics [59] of China and the website [60] of the Red and Black Population Database to calculate $f(a)$. In actual calculations, the age was divided into $n_a$ groups, and Formula (7) sums over these age groups. For the age group $i$, $a_i$ is its median age, and $f(a_i)$ is approximated by $f(a_i) = n_i/Total\_N$, with $n_i$ being the size in age group $i$ and $Total\_N$ being the total number of the population.

2.6. Deviation Information Criterion (DIC) and Model Selection

It should be borne in mind that the infectious disease system can be modeled because epidemics involve relatively simple processes that occur within a large number of individuals [18]. In the modeling studies of infectious diseases, models are used to simplify the complex real world, and the performance of model fitting varies among models. To compare model performance, we use the deviation information criterion (DIC) proposed by Spiegelhalter et al. [61], which combines the fit and complexity of the model and can compare models of any structure. The model that has the smallest DIC is the best and will be chosen [57].

Burnham and Anderson [62] suggested models receiving the Akaike Information Criterion (AIC) within 1–2 of the "best" deserve consideration, and 3–7 have considerably less support. According to Spiegelhalter et al. [61], these rules of thumb appear to work reasonably well for DIC. Therefore, in this study, we chose the critical value 3 as the criterion for DIC to select the best model. In other words, when comparing models, we believe that when the DIC difference between different models exceeds 3, there will be a performance difference. Considering that a simple model is more beneficial for result interpretation, for the data set whose DIC difference between the two models is less than 3, the model with a relatively simple structure is selected as the best model.

3. Results

Through the literature review, we selected 23 studies from 515 articles, and the study areas included 8 provinces, 14 cities or regions in China. Those studies reported the survey data of dengue age-stratified serological prevalence from 1980 to 2019. For each data set, we estimated its FOI and $R_0$ using the four models (the details are given in Tables S1–S4 in Supplementary File S2). The model fitting curves of the four models to 31 data sets are illustrated in Figures S1–S4 in Supplementary File S2. Figure 4 and Table S5 show the comparison results of DIC among the four models, and the final estimates (Table 2) are based on the best models that have the smallest values of DIC.

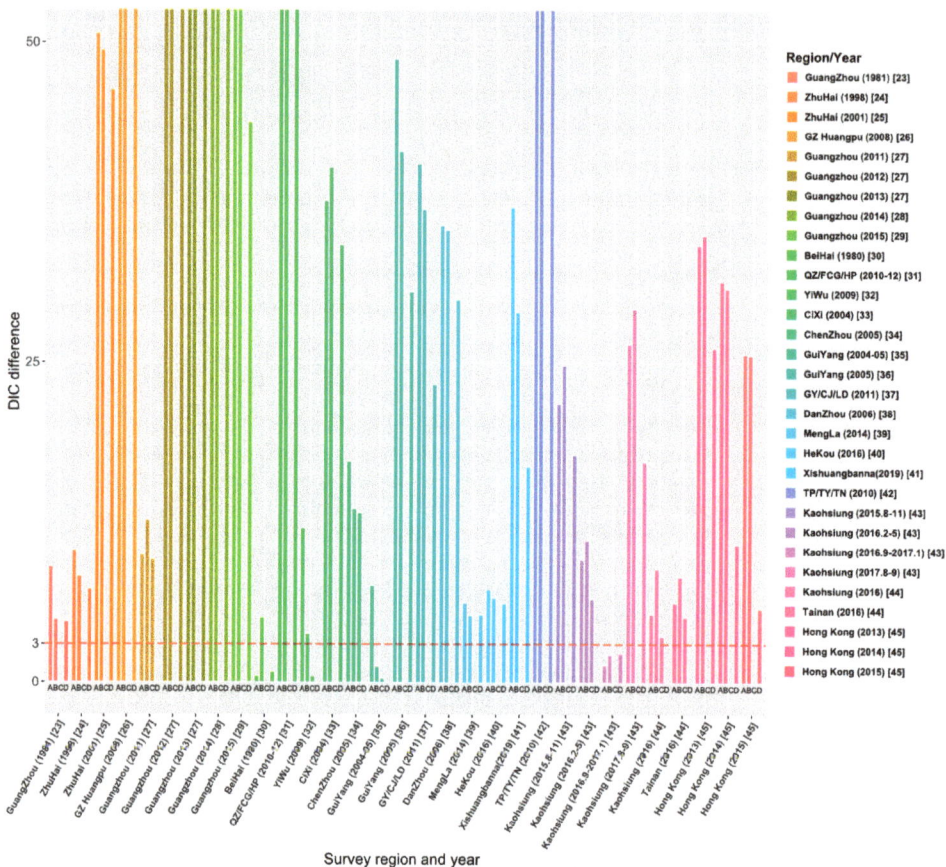

**Figure 4.** Comparison of DIC values over four models for 31 data sets. The ordinate 'DIC difference' is the difference between the DIC and the minimum DIC obtained by fitting the four models to data sets.

### 3.1. Model Comparison and Selection

Figure 4 demonstrates the relative DIC values to the best model for the 31 data sets. The results show that the best model for data sets [23–26,28,29,32,33,36–42,44,45] is Model C. In addition, Model C is also applicable to the data sets of 2012 and 2013 in the Guangzhou study [27] and the data sets from August to November 2015 and from August to September 2017 in the Kaohsiung study [43]. The best model for 25 data sets among the 31 data sets is Model C: constant FOI is broken by a critical age. This indicates the age effect on the intensity of dengue transmission among these study areas. Model D (Constant FOI broken by a threshold age with antibody protection decay) was applied to the data sets of 2011–2013 in the study of Guangzhou [27], Chenzhou in 2005 [34], and Kaohsiung in 2016 from February to May [43]. Model A (constant FOI without antibody protection decay) applies to data sets from September 2016 to January 2017 in the study in Kaohsiung [43] and the 1980 study in Beihai City, Guangxi [30]. Only the study [35] in Guiyang in 2004–05 is applied to Model B, which assumes constant FOI and antibody protection decay of dengue infection. Overall, model fittings illustrate that age has a universal effect on the transmission of dengue fever, but the protective attenuation effect of antibodies was not absent in the transmission of dengue fever.

**Table 2.** Summary of estimation results from the best model fitting to 31 data sets.

| Survey Region | Reference | Survey Year | $A_{crit}$ (95% CrI) | $\lambda_1$ | $\lambda$ (95% CrI) Year$^{-1}$ $\lambda_2$ | $R_0$ (95% CrI) | $\alpha$ (95% CrI) Year$^{-1}$ | Applicable Model |
|---|---|---|---|---|---|---|---|---|
| **Guangdong Province** | | | | | | | | |
| Guangzhou | Huang Y et al. [23] | 1981 | 20.7 (9.9, 82.1) | 0.0538 (0.0184, 0.1440) | 0.0269 (0.0094, 0.1348) | 2.33 (1.64, 3.50) | — | Model C |
| Zhuhai | Li Z et al. [24] | 1998 | 72.9 (11.6, 83.8) | 0.0009 (0.0003, 0.0236) | 0.0595 (0.0004, 0.1447) | 1.05 (1.02, 1.23) | — | Model C |
| Zhuhai | Yang Z et al. [25] | 2001 | 65.6 (10.3, 83.3) | 0.0034 (0.0021, 0.1238) | 0.0585 (0.0022, 0.1448) | 1.15 (1.09, 1.33) | — | Model C |
| #GZ Huangpu | Zheng X et al. [26] | 2008 | 78.1 (9.9, 84.1) | 0.0041 (0.0019, 0.0533) | 0.0428 (0.0028, 0.1446) | 1.15 (1.09, 1.25) | — | Model C |
| Guangzhou | Cao Y et al. [27] | 2011–2013 | 68.0 (15.5, 83.3)(15.5, 83.3) | 0.0085 (0.0040, 0.0237) | 0.0356 (0.0039, 0.1442) | 1.17 (1.12, 1.31) | 0.04 (0.00, 0.10) | Model D |
| | | 2012 | 39.7 (9.9, 83.1) | 0.0078 (0.0041, 0.0598) | 0.0071 (0.0034, 0.1400) | 1.22 (1.15, 1.40) | — | Model C |
| | | 2013 | 71.5 (12.2, 83.9) | 0.0037 (0.0024, 0.0175) | 0.0532 (0.0022, 0.1447) | 1.15 (1.09, 1.26) | — | Model C |
| Guangzhou | Li S et al. [28] | 2014 | 64.2 (10.4, 83.7) | 0.0014 (0.0007, 0.1331) | 0.0476 (0.0007, 0.1450) | 1.09 (1.04, 1.32) | — | Model C |
| Guangzhou | Jing Q et al. [29] | 2015 | 72.7 (11.7, 84.0) | 0.0027 (0.0014, 0.0308) | 0.0517 (0.0014, 0.1444) | 1.11 (1.06, 1.39) | — | Model C |
| **Guangxi Province** | | | | | | | | |
| Beihai | Tian X et al. [30] | 1980 | — | 0.0181 (0.0130, 0.0277) | | 1.73 (1.50, 2.19) | — | Model A |
| $QZ/FCG/HP | Zhou K et al. [31] | 2010–2012 | 78.7 (13.1, 84.2) | 0.0006 (0.0003, 0.0064) | 0.0606 (0.0003, 0.1450) | 1.04 (1.02, 2.10) | — | Model C |
| **Zhejiang Province** | | | | | | | | |
| Yiwu | Sun J et al. [32] | 2009 | 29.7 (16.1, 42.0) | 0.0252 (0.0122, 0.0559) | 0.0061 (0.0043, 0.0093) | 1.41 (1.25, 1.70) | — | Model C |
| Cixi | Cen D et al. [33] | 2004 | 14.0 (9.7, 81.9) | 0.0238 (0.0016, 0.1317) | 0.0029 (0.0015, 0.0205) | 1.13 (1.07, 1.32) | — | Model C |
| **Hunan Province** | | | | | | | | |
| Chenzhou | Gao L et al. [34] | 2005 | 51.7 (10.3, 83.7) | 0.0047 (0.0011, 0.0537) | 0.0061 (0.0006, 0.1033) | 1.04 (1.02, 1.25) | 0.08 (0.02, 0.10) | Model D |
| **Guizhou Province** | | | | | | | | |
| Guiyang | Gao R et al. [35] | 2004–2005 | — | 0.0092 (0.0038, 0.0358) | | 1.10 (1.06, 1.45) | 0.08 (0.02, 0.10) | Model B |
| Guiyang | Tian H et al. [36] | 2005 | 65.3 (11.4, 83.6) | 0.0047 (0.0014, 0.0669) | 0.0094 (0.0006, 0.1426) | 1.14 (1.06, 1.59) | — | Model C |
| & GY/CJ/LD | Jiang W et al. [37] | 2011 | 16.4 (9.9, 80.8) | 0.0469 (0.0020, 0.1449) | 0.0025 (0.0004, 0.1269) | 1.16 (1.03, 1.67) | — | Model C |
| **Hainan Province** | | | | | | | | |
| Danzhou | Jin Y et al. [38] | 2006 | 72.7 (11.3, 84.0) | 0.0017 (0.0004, 0.0706) | 0.0462 (0.0006, 0.1447) | 1.08 (1.02, 1.65) | — | Model C |
| **Yunnan Province** | | | | | | | | |
| Mengla | Lu Y et al. [39] | 2014 | 66.3 (11.1, 83.4) | 0.0024 (0.0007, 0.0554) | 0.0538 (0.0010, 0.1448) | 1.11 (1.03, 1.50) | — | Model C |
| Hekou | Pu L et al. [40] | 2016 | 66.5 (11.0, 83.7) | 0.0028 (0.0011, 0.0409) | 0.0551 (0.0012, 0.1441) | 1.12 (1.05, 1.42) | — | Model C |
| Xishuangbanna | Li L et al. [41] | 2019 | 60.5 (10.9, 83.3) | 0.0086 (0.0040, 0.1340) | 0.0199 (0.0031, 0.1439) | 1.34 (1.18, 1.71) | — | Model C |

Table 2. Cont.

| Survey Region | Reference | Survey Year | $A_{crit}$ (95% CrI) | λ (95% CrI) Year$^{-1}$ | $R_0$ (95% CrI) | α (95% CrI) Year$^{-1}$ | Applicable Model |
|---|---|---|---|---|---|---|---|
| Taiwan Province % TP/TY/TN | Lee YH et al. [42] | 2010 | 76.0 (10.2, 84.0) | 0.0021 (0.0008, 0.0545) | 0.0551 (0.0012, 0.1441) | 1.10 (1.04, 1.30) | — | Model C |
| Kaohsiung | Tsai JJ et al. [43] | 2015–2017 | | | | | | |
| | | 2015.8–11 | 68.1 (11.4, 83.1) | 0.0034 (0.0014, 0.0782) | 0.0099 (0.0031, 0.0419) | 1.19 (1.10, 1.57) | — | Model C |
| | | 2016.2–5 | 66.1 (11.0, 83.0) | 0.0155 (0.0046, 0.1169) | 0.0397 (0.0056, 0.1368) | 1.21 (1.12, 1.55) | 0.07 (0.01, 0.10) | Model D |
| | | 2016.9–2017.1 | — | 0.0052 (0.0021, 0.0203) | | 1.24 (1.09, 2.16) | — | Model A |
| | | 2017.8–9 | 31.6 (10.3, 81.5) | 0.0097 (0.0026, 0.1428) | 0.0089 (0.0039, 0.0370) | 1.33 (1.18, 1.82) | — | Model C |
| Kaohsiung and Tainan | Pan YH et al. [44] | 2016 | | | | | | |
| Kaohsiung | | | 30.9 (10.5, 74.3) | 0.0553 (0.0026, 0.1447) | 0.0073 (0.0043, 0.0133) | 1.50 (1.20, 2.56) | — | Model C |
| Tainan | | | 30.6 (10.2, 79.7) | 0.0617 (0.0015, 0.1461) | 0.0042 (0.0019, 0.0133) | 1.36 (1.10, 2.32) | — | Model C |
| Hong Kong | Lee P et al. [45] | 2013–2015 | | | | | | |
| | | 2013 | 71.9 (44.8, 83.8) | 0.0017 (0.0008, 0.0128) | 0.0299 (0.0013, 0.1450) | 1.12 (1.06, 1.23) | — | Model C |
| | | 2014 | 65.9 (30.2, 81.5) | 0.0010 (0.0005, 0.0037) | 0.0063 (0.0019, 0.1252) | 1.09 (1.06, 1.19) | — | Model C |
| | | 2015 | 65.7 (17.6, 81.8) | 0.0009 (0.0005, 0.0057) | 0.0070 (0.0019, 0.1263) | 1.10 (1.06, 1.18) | — | Model C |

Note: # GZ Huangpu represents Huangpu District in Guangzhou city; $ QZ/FCG/HP stands for Qinzhou City, Fangchenggang City and Hepu County in Guangxi; & GY/CJ/LD represents Yunyan District of Guiyang City, Congjiang County of Southeast Guizhou Province and Luodian County of Guizhou Province; % TP/TY/TN indicates Taipei, Taoyuan and Tainan of Taiwan Province.

## 3.2. Estimates of FOI and $R_0$

The estimates of the critical age ($A_{crit}$), FOI and $R_0$ from the best models selected for each data set are shown in Table 2 and Figure 5. Among the 28 data sets that have model C or D as their best models, they can be divided into two groups: For the 19 data sets that have estimated critical ages older than 60 years, the FOI for ages younger than the critical age ($\lambda_1$) is weaker than the FOI for ages older than the critical age ($\lambda_2$); while for the 9 data sets that have $A_{crit}$ < 60 years, $\lambda_1$ is greater than $\lambda_2$. Assuming that the spread of dengue in the study area is in a local potential endemic state, the estimates of $R_0$ would be greater than 1 (Figure 5). The estimate of $R_0$ obtained by the best model fittings of 31 data sets was between 1.04 and 2.33 (Table 2). The study [23] conducted in Guangzhou in 1981 had the largest estimate of $R_0$ = 2.33 (95% CrI: 1.64, 3.50), and the study conducted by Zhou et al. [31] and Gao et al. [34] had the smallest estimate of $R_0$ = 1.04 (95% CrI: 1.02, 1.10) and $R_0$ = 1.04 (95% CrI: 1.02, 1.25), respectively. The graph of estimates of $R_0$ versus the study year from 1980 to 2019 (see Supplementary File S2: Figure S5) showed that $R_0$ was over 1.5 in 1980 and 1981; since then, it dropped and fluctuated below 1.5.

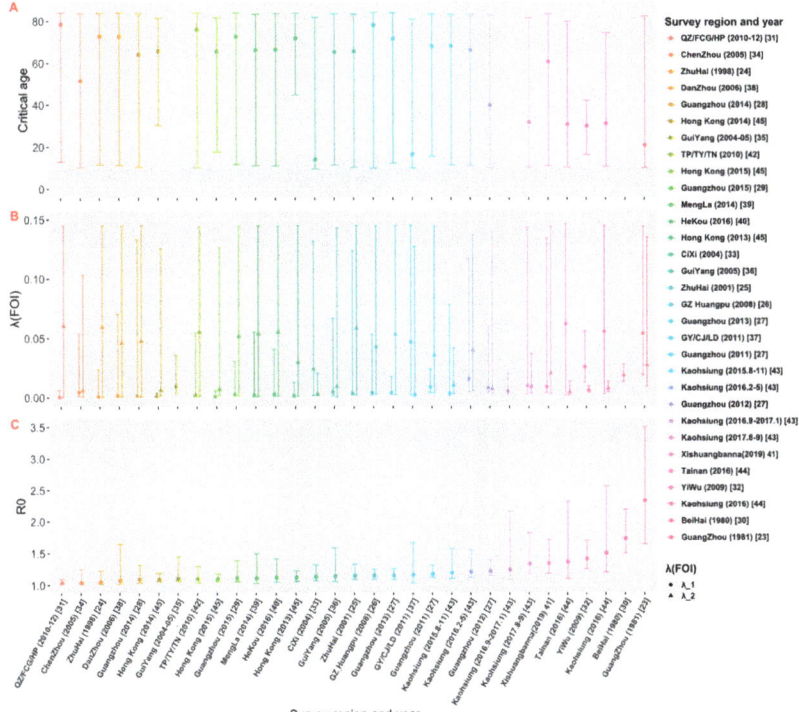

**Figure 5.** Estimates of (**A**) critical age ($A_{crit}$), (**B**) force of infection (FOI), and (**C**) basic reproduction number ($R_0$) based on the best model fittings to data sets. The estimates from 31 data sets are arranged in the ascending order of $R_0$.

## 3.3. Time-Space Comparison

Among 23 studies selected for this analysis, only three studies provided multiple years of data. We estimated FOI and $R_0$, respectively, by using their best models in different years (Figure 6). In the study conducted in Guangzhou [27] from 2011 to 2013, the estimate of $R_0$ in 2012 was the largest (1.22, 95% CrI: 1.15, 1.40). In the study [43] conducted in Kaohsiung from 2015 to 2017, the estimate of $R_0$ showed an upward trend, with $R_0$ = 1.33

(95% CrI: 1.18, 1.82) for the data set collected in August-September 2017. In the study [45] conducted in Hong Kong between 2013 and 2015, $R_0$ was estimated to be the largest in 2013 (1.12, 95% CrI: 1.06, 1.23). Figure 6 shows that there appears to be no significant time change trend in dengue transmission intensity in the three study areas.

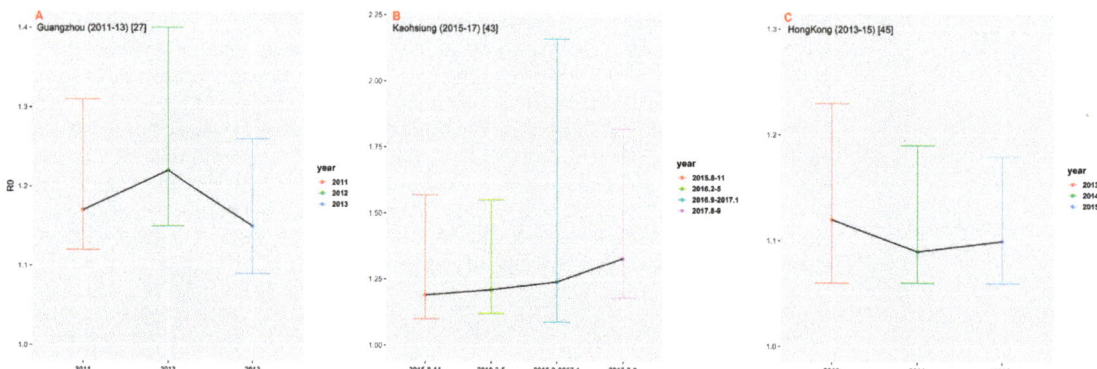

**Figure 6.** Comparison of $R_0$ in different time periods in the three regions: (**A**) Guangzhou; (**B**) Kaohsiung; and (**C**) Hong Kong.

The study areas included 8 provinces and 1 region in China with 31 data sets. These nine regions are geographically illustrated with their respective mean estimate of $R_0$ in Figure 7. The results suggested there may be an underlying spatial pattern of dengue spread in China: the intensity of dengue infection in coastal areas is generally higher than in inland areas, and the more it extends to the north, the lower the infection intensity.

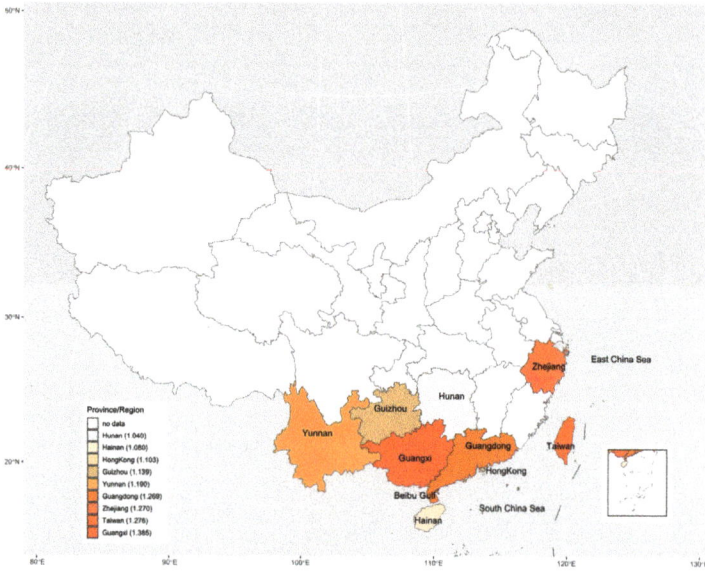

**Figure 7.** The geographic distribution of the basic reproduction number across the nine study areas. The legend indicates that from top to bottom, the darker the color is, the greater the basic reproduction number is. The numbers in legend brackets are the average of the basic reproduction numbers for each province/region.

## 4. Discussion

Based on dengue serological age stratification data extracted from 23 studies in China, we used four catalytic models to distinguish the potential transmission mechanisms of dengue and estimated dengue transmission intensity in study areas. We found that dengue transmission intensity varies among different age groups in most of the study populations, and attenuation of antibody protection is identified in some study populations. Furthermore, we found that $R_0$ of dengue in China was between 1.04–2.33, which agrees with that Imai's estimate for China (1.15–2.88) [63] and is comparable with that in Singapore (1.24–1.48) and Vietnam (1.76–1.85), but lower than that in Thailand (1.96–3.96) and Brazil (2.07–2.60) [19]. Our estimate of $R_0$ should provide useful information for the herd immunity threshold level and the effectiveness of vaccination or vector control measures required to control the spread of dengue in China [64].

Our study showed that there was a strong relationship between age and dengue transmission in the population. The model fitting indicated that the dengue transmission intensity changed at a critical age $A_{crit}$. Age could be used as a scale to quantify the exposure history in the past time, so we simply introduced $A_{crit}$ to model the potential change in transmission intensity with age. The performance of Model C and Model D, which include a critical age in transmission intensity, was better in 28 of the 31 data sets from the 23 studies. This suggests that populations in those study areas have generally experienced changes in the risk of dengue transmission over a period of time. The critical age might be the time when the risk of dengue transmission changed in the study population. In addition, the existence and identification of the critical age provide a basis for the optimal formulation of dengue prevention and control measures. For example, for the study [41] conducted in 2019 in Xishuangbanna, Yunnan Province, $A_{crit}$ was estimated to be 60.5 years (95% CrI: 10.9, 83.3), and the FOI was 0.0086 (95% CrI: 0.0040, 0.1340) and 0.0199 (95% CrI: 0.0031, 0.1439) for ages younger and older than the critical age, respectively; this indicates that the risk of dengue transmission was greater in the population aged older than 60.5 years, and the prevention and control of dengue fever should be focused on the elderly population. On the contrary, for the study [33] conducted in Cixi City, Zhejiang Province, in 2004, $A_{crit}$ was estimated to be 14 years (95% CrI: 9.7, 81.9), and the FOI was 0.0238 (95% CrI: 0.0016, 0.1317) and 0.0029 (95% CrI: 0.0015, 0.0205) for ages younger and older than 14 years, respectively, suggesting that children and adolescents were at greater risk of dengue transmission, and should be the focus of dengue prevention and control.

Primary infection with one serotype is often able to provide life-long immunity against the reinfection of the same serotype. However, cases of homotypic reinfection confirmed by reverse transcriptase-polymerase chain reaction (RT-PCR) have recently been observed in Nicaragua [65]. Severe DENV-2 transmission has also appeared in the DENV-2 antibody population in Iquitos, Peru [66,67]. The increase in infection in the older age group may be due to a significant change in the risk of dengue infection in the study group 51 years ago, as well as a decrease in antibody levels in the older age group. This indicates that isotype immunity may not be able to obtain complete protection, especially when the specific virulence of the virus strain is high, the infectivity is high, or the quality of host immunity is poor [68]. In addition, because there are four types of DENV, specific immune antibodies acquired through infection with one serotype might provide only partial protection against the other three serotypes, and it is still possible to infect a different serotype virus for a second time in the future. Due to the lack of specific serological data on dengue, it is difficult to estimate the transmission intensity of each serotype in this study. However, the potential relationship between the attenuation of antibody protection and the transmission of dengue fever in the population could be identified through mathematical modeling. Our comparison of model performance based on the DIC value illustrates this: The study [34] in Chenzhou, Zhejiang Province in 2005, provided evidence of this phenomenon. The applicable model for the data set from this study is Model D, with the estimated critical age being 51.7 years (95% CrI: 10.3, 83.7) and the FOI being 0.0047 (95% CrI: 0.0011, 0.0537) and 0.0061 (95% CrI: 0.0006, 0.1033) for ages younger and older than the critical age, respectively; its antibody protection is estimated to decay at a rate of 0.08 (95% CrI: 0.02, 0.10) per year.

Although we only estimated the total FOI of all serotypes in the study areas based on non-serotype-specific data, these data were still sufficient to assess the heterogeneity of overall dengue transmission intensity between different regions and populations. Related studies have demonstrated that FOI estimated from non-serotype-specific data is consistent with the sum of FOI estimated from PRNT data [27]. Although the data sets collected cover the period from 1981 to 2019, these data sets were obtained from different geographical locations across China. Among 23 studies collected, only three studies [27,43,45] provided the serological surveys over multiple years in the same locations; within the short time gaps only over 3 years, the data sets from the three studies cannot show any clear temporal changes in transmission intensity (Figure 6). If seroprevalence survey data over a long period, say more than 5 years were available, the potential periodicity or another temporal trend in dengue transmission intensity could be inferred (e.g., [19]). In view of temporally steady transmission intensity [19], the average transmission intensity over different locations within the same province and different study years (if there were more than one study in one province) showed the geographical patterns: It weakened from coastal areas to inland areas, and from southern areas to northern areas (Figure 7). This might reflect that the large and dense populations, including many foreigners in the southeast coastal areas of China, provided certain beneficial conditions for the spread of dengue. Compared to other inland provinces, Yunnan province had a relatively high transmission intensity. This might reflect its specialty: located in the southwest of China and bordered by Myanmar, Laos and Vietnam, which had a high incidence of dengue [19,20] and frequent population movements, trade, and cultural exchanges. The highest mean estimate of basic reproduction number comes from Guangxi Zhuang Autonomous Region; this could be the consequence of the following factors of the region: bordering with Vietnam and being parts of the coastline so that the pressure for imported cases to spread locally is enormous, and the hot and humid climate that is good for mosquitos to live and grow and therefore is more conducive to the spread of dengue fever.

It was reported that the force of infection has declined while the average age of dengue hemorrhagic fever (DHF) cases in Thailand has increased from 8.1 to 24.3 years over the last four decays. This is mainly driven by the decreased birth and death rate [69,70]. The limited data we collected in this study cannot show any clear temporal change in transmission intensity in China, as shown in Figure 6 and Figure S5. Further, our data are age-stratified serological data and cannot directly be used for analyzing the age of dengue hemorrhagic fever (DHF) cases. With the similar demographic transition due to decreased birth and death rates, it is interesting to investigate whether a similar change pattern in the age of dengue cases also occurred in China. This information is important for the control and prevention of dengue in China and is surely a future topic of investigation.

The advantage of using serological data for inferring the burden and transmission intensity of dengue is that it is not affected by infectious disease surveillance systems and case reporting systems. With more than 75% of people infected with dengue having no clinical symptoms [4], serological data can more accurately estimate the actual number of cases. However, there are still some problems. The main problem lies in the differences in the methods used in the studies included. In the 23 studies, seroprevalence surveys sampled different populations and used serum samples collected for different purposes, which might not be representative of the total population in the study area. For example, the sample populations of the studies [24,25] were entry and exit personnel at Zhuhai Port; the sample populations of studies [28,41] were the blood donors in the blood donation center; the sample populations of studies [39,40] were entry-exit personnel at port health examination centers; the sample population of the study [45] was patients sent to the Prince of Wales Hospital in Hong Kong for diagnosis. The use of convenient serum samples could increase the amount of serological data, but the potential bias introduced by such sampling must be considered when analyzing such data.

There are some other limitations in our research. First, when using the models to estimate $R_0$ through FOI, we assumed that dengue was in endemic balance, which means that the estimates of $R_0$ for all data sets were greater than 1. However, this was obviously not applicable to areas where dengue was not endemic or the cases were mainly imported from outside. Secondly, the literature review for dengue showed that there were still few studies in China using serological data as a tool to monitor dengue transmission. Most model studies used case notification data, and its reliability largely depended on the quality of the infectious diseases surveillance system and reporting system [71]. A better understanding of changes in transmission intensity can not only improve estimates of the burden of disease caused by dengue but also help policymakers develop effective prevention and control plans. Therefore, we advocate the more extensive and routine use of serological surveys as a monitoring tool to provide valuable data for the study of infectious disease as dengue.

**Supplementary Materials:** The following supporting information can be downloaded at: https://www.mdpi.com/article/10.3390/tropicalmed8020116/s1, Figure S1: The fitting curves of Model A to 31 datasets; Figure S2: The fitting curves of Model B to 31 datasets; Figure S3: The fitting curves of Model C to 31 datasets; Figure S4: The fitting curves of Model D to 31 datasets; Figure S5: Distribution of R0 in different study years; Table S1: Summary of model parameter estimates for Model A; Table S2: Summary of model parameter estimates for Model B; Table S3: Summary of model parameter estimates for Model C; Table S4: Summary of model parameter estimates for Model D; Table S5: Comparison of DIC among four models.

**Author Contributions:** Conceptualization, N.L. and X.-S.Z.; data Curation, N.L. and T.W.; formal Analysis, N.L., H.L., Z.C. and X.-S.Z.; funding acquisition, W.L.; investigation, N.L., H.X. and Z.L.; methodology: N.L., H.L. and X.-S.Z.; project administration: W.L.; visualization: N.L.; writing—original draft preparation, N.L.; writing—review & editing, N.L. and X.-S.Z. All authors have read and agreed to the published version of the manuscript.

**Funding:** The work was jointly supported by the National Nature Science Foundation of China (No. 81860607) and the Innovative Research Team of Yunnan Province (No. 2019(6)), China. The funders had no role in study design, data collection and analysis, the decision to publish, or the preparation of the manuscript.

**Institutional Review Board Statement:** Ethical review and approval were waived for this study since this is a theoretical study with personal identifications being removed from the survey data.

**Informed Consent Statement:** Patient consent was waived due to patients' identification being removed from the survey data.

**Data Availability Statement:** Data from previously published studies are all listed in the references and provided in Supplementary File S1.

**Conflicts of Interest:** The authors declare no conflict of interest. The funders had no role in the design of the study; in the collection, analyses, or interpretation of data; in the writing of the manuscript; or in the decision to publish the results.

# References

1. World Health Organization (WHO). *Dengue: Guidelines for Diagnosis, Treatment, Prevention and Control: New Edition*; World Health Organization: Geneva, Switzerland, 2009.
2. World Health Organization (WHO). *Accelerating Work to Overcome the Global Impact of Neglected Tropical Diseases*; World Health Organization: Geneva, Switzerland, 2007; Volume 7, p. 596.
3. World Health Organization. Dengue and Severe Dengue, 10 January 2022. Available online: https://www.who.int/news-room/fact-sheets/detail/dengue-and-severe-dengue (accessed on 22 October 2022).
4. Bhatt, S.; Gething, P.W.; Brady, O.J.; Messina, J.P.; Farlow, A.W.; Moyes, C.L.; Drake, J.M.; Brownstein, J.S.; Hoen, A.G.; Sankoh, O.; et al. The global distribution and burden of dengue. *Nature* **2013**, *496*, 504–507. [CrossRef] [PubMed]
5. Yang, F.; Huang, Y.; Zhang, X.; Xiong, L.; Li, Y.; Zhang, R. Epidemiology and genotyping of dengue fever in Shenzhen City in 2018. *Chin. J. Infect. Dis.* **2020**, *38*, 342–347. [CrossRef]
6. Wu, T.; Qin, N.; Zhang, J.; Wang, W.; Li, J. Dengue fever epidemic risk in Tianjin from 2009 to 2015. *Mod. Prev. Med.* **2016**, *43*, 1925–1927+1943.

7. Cai, Y.; Liu, S.; Wei, Y.; Han, X.; Han, Z.; Zhang, Y.; Xu, Y.; Qi, S.; Li, Q. Epidemic characteristics and prevention and control Strategies of imported Dengue fever in Hebei province from 2011 to 2018. *Pract. Prev. Med.* **2022**, *27*, 798–801.
8. Li, H.; Jiang, J.; Do, L.; Chen, Z.; Chen, S.; Li, J.; Liu, H. Emergency monitoring and analysis of the epidemiological characteristics and vectors of a dengue fever outbreak in Mengla County in 2018. *J. Parasit. Biol.* **2020**, *15*, 83–85+90. [CrossRef]
9. Feng, S.; Guan, J.; Chen, J.; Rao, Q.; Sun, Q. Clinical and laboratory characteristics of 96 cases of dengue fever in Qiyang County, Hunan Province, China in 2018. *Chin. J. Biol.* **2020**, *33*, 423–428+433.
10. Dai, B.; Wang, F.; Pan, J.; Han, C.; Huang, K. Epidemic characteristics and treatment effect of the first dengue fever outbreak in Hubei Province. *J. Public Health Prev. Med.* **2020**, *31*, 62–65. [CrossRef]
11. Ning, D.; Sun, J.; Peng, Z.; Wu, D. The epidemiological situation and epidemiological characteristics of dengue fever in Guangdong Province. *South China Prev. Med.* **2017**, *43*, 368–372.
12. Cai, W.; Jing, Q.; Liu, W.; Chen, C. Analysis of epidemiological characteristics of local dengue fever cases in Guangzhou from 2015 to 2019. *South China Prev. Med.* **2020**, *46*, 138–140.
13. Yang, J.; Chen, M.; Wang, H.; Zhang., S. Analysis of epidemiological characteristics of dengue fever outbreak in Fuzhou in 2016. *Chin. Trop. Med.* **2017**, *17*, 795–797+805.
14. Mai, G.; He, Y.; Chen, Z. Analysis of the epidemiological characteristics of dengue antibody positive in Gaoming District, Foshan City from 2015 to 2019. *Public Health Prev. Med.* **2020**, *31*, 122–124.
15. World Health Organization (WHO). *Global Strategy for Dengue Prevention and Control, 2012–2020*; World Health Organization: Geneva, Switzerland, 2012.
16. Grenfell, B.T.; Anderson, R.M. The estimation of age-related rates of infection from case notifications and serological data. *J. Hyg.* **1985**, *95*, 419–436. [CrossRef] [PubMed]
17. Anderson, R.M.; May, R.M. *Infectious Diseases of Humans: Dynamics and Control (Oxford Science Publications)*; OUP Oxford: Oxford, UK, 1992.
18. Ferguson, N.M. Mathematical prediction in infection. *Medicine* **2009**, *37*, 507–509. [CrossRef]
19. Imai, N.; Dorigatti, I.; Cauchemez, S.; Ferguson, N.M. Estimating dengue transmission intensity from sero-prevalence surveys in multiple countries. *PLoS Negl. Trop. Dis.* **2015**, *9*, e0003719. [CrossRef]
20. Thai, K.T.; Nagelkerke, N.; Phuong, H.L.; Nga, T.T.; Giao, P.T.; Hung, L.Q.; Binh, T.Q.; Nam, N.V.; De Vries, P.J. Geographical heterogeneity of dengue transmission in two villages in southern Vietnam. *Epidemiol. Infect.* **2010**, *138*, 585–591. [CrossRef] [PubMed]
21. Gordon, A.; Kuan, G.; Mercado, J.C.; Gresh, L.; Avilés, W.; Balmaseda, A.; Harris, E. The Nicaraguan pediatric dengue cohort study: Incidence of inapparent and symptomatic dengue virus infections, 2004–2010. *PLoS Negl. Trop. Dis.* **2013**, *7*, e2462. [CrossRef]
22. Endy, T.P.; Chunsuttiwat, S.; Nisalak, A.; Libraty, D.H.; Green, S.; Rothman, A.L.; Vaughn, D.W.; Ennis, F.A. Epidemiology of inapparent and symptomatic acute dengue virus infection: A prospective study of primary school children in Kamphaeng Phet, Thailand. *Am. J. Epidemiol.* **2002**, *156*, 40–51. [CrossRef] [PubMed]
23. Huang, Y.; Liang, J.; Lin, Z. Survey of dengue anti-antibody level in population after dengue fever epidemic in Guangzhou. *Guangzhou Med. J.* **1983**, *20–25*.
24. Li, Z.; Zhang, J.; Ma, H. Surveillance of Dengue Fever Antibody Levels in People in Zhuhai Port Area. *Chin. J. Front. Health Quar.* **1999**, *22*, 141–143. [CrossRef]
25. Yang, Z.; Zhu, H.; Lin, G.; Zeng, W.; Tu, C.; Ye, L.; Zhao, J.; Yao, R. Analysis of dengue antibody levels and related factors in different populations. *Mod. Prev. Med.* **2002**, *29*, 694–695. [CrossRef]
26. Zheng, X.; Wu, Y.; Zhang, M.; He, A.; Li, Z.; Qu, Z.; Zhan, X. Sero-epidemiological Investigation of Dengue Fever in Guangzhou. *J. Trop. Med.* **2009**, *9*, 1397–1399+1404.
27. Cao, Y.; Jiang, L.; Xu, Y.; Jing, Q.; Cao, Q.; Di, B.; Yang, Z. Monitoring and analysis of dengue fever serum antibody levels in Guangzhou from 2011 to 2013. *South China J. Prev. Med.* **2015**, *41*, 364–366. [CrossRef]
28. Li, J.; Liao, Q.; Liang, Y.; Chen, J.; You, R.; Xiong, H.; Huang, K.; Rong, X. Study on the risk of dengue virus transmission by blood transfusion in Guangzhou area. *Guangdong Med. J.* **2017**, *38*, 1064–1067. [CrossRef]
29. Jing, Q.; Li, Y.; Liu, J.; Jiang, L.; Chen, Z.; Su, W.; Birkhead, G.S.; Lu, J.; Yang, Z. Dengue Underestimation in Guangzhou, China: Evidence of Seroprevalence in Communities with No Reported Cases Before a Large Outbreak in 2014. *Open Forum Infect. Dis.* **2019**, *6*, ofz256. [CrossRef] [PubMed]
30. Tian, X.; Ai, C.; Li, C.; Wen, Y.; Liu, Y.; Xia, H. Epidemiological surveillance of dengue fever in Beihai City, Guangxi. *J. Mil. Med. Sci.* **1985**, *38*, 387–392.
31. Zhou, K.; Chen, M.; Tan, Y.; Mo, Y.; Bi, Y. Serological surveillance of healthy population in Guangxi dengue surveillance sites. *J. Appl. Prev. Med.* **2013**, *19*, 236–237. [CrossRef]
32. Sun, J.; Luo, S.; Lin, J.; Chen, J.; Hou, J.; Fu, T.; Lv, H.; Chen, Z.; Cong, L.; Ling, F.; et al. Inapparent infection during an outbreak of dengue fever in Southeastern China. *Viral Immunol.* **2012**, *25*, 456–460. [CrossRef] [PubMed]
33. Cen, D.; Wu, J.; Xu, Y. Application of Serum Bank in the Investigation and Analysis of Dengue Fever Antibody Level. *Chin. Prev. Med.* **2007**, *8*, 734–735. [CrossRef]
34. Gao, L.; Xiao, J.; Zhang, H.; Duan, L.; Liu, F.; Dai, D.; Li, J.; Deng, Z. Sero-epidemiology investigation of dengue fever in Chenzhou. *South China J. Prev. Med.* **2007**, *33*, 34–35. [CrossRef]

35. Gao, R.; Zhou, X.; Zhou, C.; Han, Y.; Luo, J.; Qin, J. Serological Epidemiological Research on Dengue Virus Antibodies among Personnel at Guiyang Port. *Chin. J. Front. Health Quar.* **2006**, *29* (Suppl. S1), 57–59. [CrossRef]
36. Tian, H.; Han, Y.; Dai, A.; Fu, D.; Zhou, Y.; Zhou, N.; Gao, R. The Investigation of the Population Infected with Dengue Virus at Guiyang Port and other Close Areas. *J. Travel Med. Sci.* **2007**, *13*, 28–29. [CrossRef]
37. Jiang, W.; Zhou, J.; Tang, G.; Zhuang, Y.; Yun, C.; Fu, L. Investigation on Dengue Fever Infection among Healthy Population in Some Counties and Cities in Guizhou Province. *Guizhou Med. J.* **2013**, *37*, 164–165. [CrossRef]
38. Jin, Y.; Sun, L.; Zeng, X.; Wu, W.; Ma, Y.; Su, X.; Lao, S.; Chen, Y.; Li, Z. Sero-epidemiological survey and analysis on dengue fever in Hainan Province. *China Trop. Med.* **2007**, *7*, 2007–2008. [CrossRef]
39. Lu, Y.; Liu, Y.; Ji, R.; Luo, Z.; Zhang, Q.; Zhou, L.; Yang, X. Serological surveillance on arboviral diseases among exit-entry population at Sino-Laos port. *Chin. J. Front. Health Quar.* **2016**, *39*, 180–182. [CrossRef]
40. Pu, L.; Chen, J.; Zhang, Q.; Zhang, C.; Li, Z.; Liu, W.; Wu, Z. Aedes surveillance and dengue fever serological survey at Sino-Vietnam Hekou-Laocai ports. *Chin. J. Front. Health Quar.* **2018**, *41*, 255–257+268. [CrossRef]
41. Li, L.; Li, Y.; Lu, S.; Dong, J.; Xu, H.; Zhang, Q.; Weng, R.; Yin, Y.; He, R.; Fang, P.; et al. Epidemiological survey and screening strategy for dengue virus in blood donors from Yunnan Province. *BMC Infect. Dis.* **2021**, *21*, 104. [CrossRef]
42. Lee, Y.H.; Hsieh, Y.C.; Chen, C.J.; Lin, T.Y.; Huang, Y.C. Retrospective Seroepidemiology study of dengue virus infection in Taiwan. *BMC Infect. Dis.* **2021**, *21*, 96. [CrossRef]
43. Tsai, J.J.; Liu, C.K.; Tsai, W.Y.; Liu, L.T.; Tyson, J.; Tsai, C.Y.; Lin, P.C.; Wang, W.K. Seroprevalence of dengue virus in two districts of Kaohsiung City after the largest dengue outbreak in Taiwan since World War II. *PLoS Negl. Trop. Dis.* **2018**, *12*, e0006879. [CrossRef]
44. Pan, Y.H.; Liao, M.Y.; Chien, Y.W.; Ho, T.S.; Ko, H.Y.; Yang, C.R.; Chang, S.F.; Yu, C.Y.; Lin, S.Y.; Shih, P.W.; et al. Use of seroprevalence to guide dengue vaccination plans for older adults in a dengue non-endemic country. *PLoS Negl. Trop. Dis.* **2021**, *15*, e0009312. [CrossRef]
45. Lee, P.; Yeung, A.C.M.; Chen, Z.; Chan, M.C.W.; Sze, K.H.; Chan, P.K.S. Age-specific seroprevalence of dengue infection in Hong Kong. *J. Med. Virol.* **2018**, *90*, 1427–1430. [CrossRef]
46. Ferguson, N.M.; Donnelly, C.A.; Anderson, R.M. Transmission dynamics and epidemiology of dengue: Insights from age-stratified sero-prevalence surveys. *Philos Trans. R. Soc. Lond. B Biol. Sci.* **1999**, *354*, 757–768. [CrossRef] [PubMed]
47. Becker, N.G. Martingale methods for the analysis of epidemic data. *Stat. Methods Med. Res.* **1993**, *2*, 93–112. [CrossRef] [PubMed]
48. Muench, H. *Catalytic Models in Epidemiology*; Harvard University Press: Cambridge, MA, USA; London, UK, 1959. [CrossRef]
49. Salje, H.; Lessler, J.; Endy, T.P.; Curriero, F.C.; Gibbons, R.V.; Nisalak, A.; Nimmannitya, S.; Kalayanarooj, S.; Jarman, R.G.; Thomas, S.J.; et al. Revealing the microscale spatial signature of dengue transmission and immunity in an urban population. *Proc. Natl. Acad. Sci. USA* **2012**, *109*, 9535–9538. [CrossRef]
50. Reich, N.G.; Shrestha, S.; King, A.A.; Rohani, P.; Lessler, J.; Kalayanarooj, S.; Yoon, I.K.; Gibbons, R.V.; Burke, D.S.; Cummings, D.A. Interactions between serotypes of dengue highlight epidemiological impact of cross-immunity. *J. R. Soc. Interface* **2013**, *10*, 20130414. [CrossRef] [PubMed]
51. OhAinle, M.; Balmaseda, A.; Macalalad, A.R.; Tellez, Y.; Zody, M.C.; Saborío, S.; Nuñez, A.; Lennon, N.J.; Birren, B.W.; Gordon, A.; et al. Dynamics of dengue disease severity determined by the interplay between viral genetics and serotype-specific immunity. *Sci. Transl. Med.* **2011**, *3*, 114ra128. [CrossRef]
52. Gibbons, R.V.; Kalanarooj, S.; Jarman, R.G.; Nisalak, A.; Vaughn, D.W.; Endy, T.P.; Mammen, M.P., Jr.; Srikiatkhachorn, A. Analysis of repeat hospital admissions for dengue to estimate the frequency of third or fourth dengue infections resulting in admissions and dengue hemorrhagic fever, and serotype sequences. *Am. J. Trop. Med. Hyg.* **2007**, *77*, 910–913. [CrossRef]
53. Puschnik, A.; Lau, L.; Cromwell, E.A.; Balmaseda, A.; Zompi, S.; Harris, E. Correlation between dengue-specific neutralizing antibodies and serum avidity in primary and secondary dengue virus 3 natural infections in humans. *PLoS Negl. Trop. Dis.* **2013**, *7*, e2274. [CrossRef]
54. Lai, C.Y.; Williams, K.L.; Wu, Y.C.; Knight, S.; Balmaseda, A.; Harris, E.; Wang, W.K. Analysis of cross-reactive antibodies recognizing the fusion loop of envelope protein and correlation with neutralizing antibody titers in Nicaraguan dengue cases. *PLoS Negl. Trop. Dis.* **2013**, *7*, e2451. [CrossRef]
55. Katzelnick, L.C.; Montoya, M.; Gresh, L.; Balmaseda, A.; Harris, E. Neutralizing antibody titers against dengue virus correlate with protection from symptomatic infection in a longitudinal cohort. *Proc. Natl. Acad. Sci. USA* **2016**, *113*, 728–733. [CrossRef]
56. Guzman, M.G.; Alvarez, M.; Rodriguez-Roche, R.; Bernardo, L.; Montes, T.; Vazquez, S.; Morier, L.; Alvarez, A.; Gould, E.A.; Kouri, G.; et al. Neutralizing antibodies after infection with dengue 1 virus. *Emerg. Infect. Dis.* **2007**, *13*, 282–286. [CrossRef]
57. Zhang, X.S.; Xiong, H.; Chen, Z.; Liu, W. Importation, Local Transmission, and Model Selection in Estimating the Transmissibility of COVID-19: The Outbreak in Shaanxi Province of China as a Case Study. *Trop. Med. Infect. Dis.* **2022**, *7*, 227. [CrossRef]
58. R Core Team. *R: A language and Environment for Statistical Computing*; R Foundation for Statistical Computing: Vienna, Austria, 2022; Available online: https://www.R-project.org/ (accessed on 25 December 2022).
59. National Bureau of Statistics of China. Census Data. Available online: http://www.stats.gov.cn/tjsj/pcsj/ (accessed on 25 December 2022).
60. The Red and Black Population Database. Ranking of Each Province by Region. Available online: https://www.hongheiku.com/ (accessed on 25 December 2022).

61. Spiegelhalter, D.J.; Best, N.G.; Carlin, B.; Linde, A. Bayesian measures of model complexity and fit. *J. R. Stat. Soc. Ser. B Stat. Methodol.* **2001**, *64*. [CrossRef]
62. Burnham, K.P.; Anderson, D.R. *Model Selection and Inference*; Springer: New York, NY, USA, 1998.
63. Imai, N.; Dorigatti, I.; Cauchemez, S.; Ferguson, N.M. Estimating Dengue Transmission Intensity from Case-Notification Data from Multiple Countries. *PLoS Negl. Trop. Dis.* **2016**, *10*, e0004833. [CrossRef] [PubMed]
64. Fine, P.; Eames, K.; Heymann, D.L. "Herd immunity": A rough guide. *Clin. Infect. Dis.* **2011**, *52*, 911–916. [CrossRef] [PubMed]
65. Waggoner, J.J.; Balmaseda, A.; Gresh, L.; Sahoo, M.K.; Montoya, M.; Wang, C.; Abeynayake, J.; Kuan, G.; Pinsky, B.A.; Harris, E. Homotypic Dengue Virus Reinfections in Nicaraguan Children. *J. Infect. Dis.* **2016**, *214*, 986–993. [CrossRef]
66. Williams, M.; Mayer, S.V.; Johnson, W.L.; Chen, R.; Volkova, E.; Vilcarromero, S.; Widen, S.G.; Wood, T.G.; Suarez-Ognio, L.; Long, K.C.; et al. Lineage II of Southeast Asian/American DENV-2 is associated with a severe dengue outbreak in the Peruvian Amazon. *Am. J. Trop. Med. Hyg.* **2014**, *91*, 611–620. [CrossRef]
67. Forshey, B.M.; Reiner, R.C.; Olkowski, S.; Morrison, A.C.; Espinoza, A.; Long, K.C.; Vilcarromero, S.; Casanova, W.; Wearing, H.J.; Halsey, E.S.; et al. Incomplete Protection against Dengue Virus Type 2 Re-infection in Peru. *PLoS Negl. Trop. Dis.* **2016**, *10*, e0004398. [CrossRef] [PubMed]
68. Rico-Hesse, R. Dengue virus virulence and transmission determinants. *Curr. Top. Microbiol. Immunol.* **2010**, *338*, 45–55. [CrossRef]
69. Cummings, D.A.T.; Iamsirithaworn, S.; Lessler, J.T.; McDermott, A.; Prasanthong, R.; Nisalak, A.; Jarman, R.G.; Burke, D.S.; Gibbons, R.V. The Impact of the Demographic Transition on Dengue in Thailand: Insights from a Statistical Analysis and Mathematical Modeling. *PLoS Med.* **2009**, *6*, e1000139. [CrossRef] [PubMed]
70. Huang, A.T.; Takahashi, S.; Salje, H.; Garcia-Carreras, B.; Anderson, K.; Endy, T.; Thomas, S.; Rothman, A.L.; Klungthong, C.; Jones, A.R.; et al. Assessing the role of multiple mechanisms increasing the age of dengue cases in Thailand. *Proc. Natl. Acad. Sci. USA* **2022**, *119*, e2115790119. [CrossRef]
71. Doherty, J.A. Final report and recommendations from the National Notifiable Diseases Working Group. *Can. Commun. Dis. Rep.* **2006**, *32*, 211–225; Erratum in *Can. Commun. Dis. Rep.* **2008**, *34*, 24–25. (In English and French) [PubMed]

**Disclaimer/Publisher's Note:** The statements, opinions and data contained in all publications are solely those of the individual author(s) and contributor(s) and not of MDPI and/or the editor(s). MDPI and/or the editor(s) disclaim responsibility for any injury to people or property resulting from any ideas, methods, instructions or products referred to in the content.

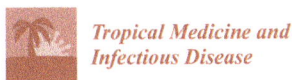

Tropical Medicine and
Infectious Disease

Article

# Rationality of Prescriptions by Rational Use of Medicine Consensus Approach in Common Respiratory and Gastrointestinal Infections: An Outpatient Department Based Cross-Sectional Study from India

Debjit Chakraborty [1], Falguni Debnath [1,*], Suman Kanungo [1], Sandip Mukhopadhyay [1], Nabanita Chakraborty [1], Rivu Basu [2], Palash Das [3], Kalpana Datta [4], Suman Ganguly [5], Prithwijit Banerjee [3], Nilima Kshirsagar [6] and Shanta Dutta [1]

[1] ICMR—National Institute of Cholera and Enteric Disease, Kolkata 700010, India
[2] R. G Kar Medical College & Hospital, Kolkata 700004, India
[3] College of Medicine and Sagar Dutta Hospital, Kolkata 700058, India
[4] Medical College & Hospital, Kolkata 700073, India
[5] West Bengal State AIDS Prevention & Control Society, Kolkata 700091, India
[6] Indian Council of Medical Research, New Delhi 110029, India
* Correspondence: falgunidebnath@yahoo.in

**Abstract:** Background: Drug utilisation studies are relevant for the analysis of prescription rationality and are pertinent in today's context of the increasing burden of antimicrobial resistance. Prescriptions for patients with diarrhoea or Acute Respiratory Infection (ARI) have been analysed in this study to understand the prescription pattern among various categories of prescribers in two tertiary care centers. Methods: This cross-sectional study was conducted from August 2019 to December 2020 in the medicine and pediatrics outpatient departments of two government teaching hospitals in West Bengal, India. A total of 630 prescriptions were evaluated against WHO standards. Prescriptions were assessed by a 'Rational Use of Medicine Consensus committee' approach. Results: The Fixed Dose Combination (FDC) was used in half of the patients (51%). Both the generic prescription (23.3%) and adherence to hospital formulary rates (36.5%) were low. The antibiotics prescription rate was high (57%), and it was higher for diarrhoea than ARI. Deviations from the standard treatment guidelines were found in 98.9% of prescriptions. Deviations were commonly found with prescriptions written by the junior doctors (99.6%). Conclusion: Irrational prescribing patterns prevail in tertiary care centers and indicate the necessity of awareness generation and capacity building among prescribers regarding AMR and its unseen consequences.

**Keywords:** prescription pattern; diarrhoea; acute respiratory infection; antibiotics prescription rate; rational use of medicine; antimicrobial resistance

## 1. Introduction

Rational use of medicine (RUM) is an extremely desirable requirement in the healthcare delivery system. The World Health Organization (WHO) has defined RUM as "patients receive medications appropriate to their clinical needs, in doses that meet their own individual requirements, for an adequate period of time, and at the lowest cost to them and their community" [1]. RUM not only reduces the chance of adverse drug reactions, undesirable drug interactions, mortality, morbidity, and the cost of treatment, but also helps in better utilization of resources, prevents 'financial toxicity', antimicrobial overuse, and hence, may prevent antimicrobial resistance (AMR) [1,2]. However, it was noted that, globally, even up to 50% of prescriptions suffer from irrationality [3]. Several factors were noted behind the irrational use of drugs, ranging from poor knowledge to pharmaceutical promotions [4,5].

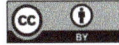

RUM is strongly promoted by the WHO, and a set of 'recommended optimums' were set by the WHO as indicators of rational prescriptions [1].

Evaluation of prescription patterns comprises studies mentioning drug utilization, with the main emphasis on rational use of medicine. The problem of irrational use of drugs, especially antibiotics, is prevalent worldwide [6,7]. The problem is further complicated in developing countries [8]. In developing countries, respiratory illnesses and diarrhoeal diseases remain the main causes of morbidity and mortality, particularly in children, accounting for one in five deaths and resulting in 1.5 million annual fatalities [9]. The majority of diarrhoea cases in children, especially under the age of five, are caused by viruses, whereas both bacterial and viral diarrhoeas are found in adults. Although it has been estimated that antibiotics are required in 5% of diarrhoea cases, the use of antibiotics in practise is rampant [10]. According to the WHO, in developing countries, half of all viral respiratory tract infections and viral diarrhoea were treated with antibiotics. Furthermore, antibiotics were not found to be prescribed in 70% of pneumonia cases where their use was an absolute necessity [11]. However, overuse or underuse of medicines, prescribing wrong or ineffective medicines, polypharmacy practices, use of expensive fixed-dose combination products, and misuse of antibiotics are the common forms of irrational prescription [12,13]. Since both diarrhoea and acute respiratory infections are major public health problems, particularly in children, specific management guidelines were developed by the WHO. Countries such as India came up with their own guidelines to be used in different State Government Health Departments as well [9,14,15]. However, such guidelines are actually tailormade for public health practitioners practicing in low-resource peripheral health settings. In a country such as India, where both the government and private healthcare systems look at the health issues of its 1.3 billion population, achieving RUM remains a daunting task. The primary objectives of this study were to assess prescribing patterns using the WHO criteria for prescription evaluation and to determine the appropriateness of the prescription and the acceptability of the deviations from standard guidelines through a consensus committee approach.

## 2. Materials and Methods

### 2.1. Study Design, Setting

This multicentre cross-sectional study was conducted at two Government teaching hospitals in West Bengal, India from August 2019 to December 2020. The prescriptions were collected from the OPDs of Medicine, Pediatrics, and the Urban Health Training Centre (UHTC) clinic.

### 2.2. Sample Size Calculation

For prescription evaluation studies, according to the WHO, a minimum of 600 prescriptions [16] are required to be studied. Consecutive sampling was conducted to collect the required number of prescriptions.

### 2.3. Study Enrolment

#### 2.3.1. Inclusion & Exclusion Criteria

We included the prescriptions of patients (adults or children) presenting with symptoms of acute diarrhoea or ARI in the OPD of the study sites and provided written consent to capture and copy the prescription for review. The prescriptions included in the study had details such as the signs and symptoms and/or provisional or final diagnosis of acute diarrhoea/ARI. Prescriptions from critically ill patients or those who did not give consent were excluded.

#### 2.3.2. Data Collection

Prescriptions of the patients attending the study sites were screened for eligibility and enrolled for the study after application of inclusion criteria by capturing a photograph of it. The photographed prescription, demographic details, relevant clinical information, diagnosis, and medication details were abstracted in the case record forms.

2.3.3. Data Management and Analysis Plan

The data management system is comprised of data entry, cleaning, back-up, and the generation of regular reports. Built-in quality control mechanisms were developed to ensure data quality and confidentiality. Prescriptions were analysed using the mentioned WHO indicators. Information was collected about the prescriber also in terms of their hierarchical designation, e.g., general resident doctors, post-graduate residents, and senior doctors (Medical officer/Demonstrator/Clinical Tutor, Assistant Professor, Associate Professor and Professor).

A house staff is a junior resident who has completed undergraduate medical degree (MBBS) and internship but yet to join for a post graduate course. Faculty in clinical disciplines include Residential Medical Officer (RMO) cum Clinical Tutor, Assistant Professor, Associate Professor, and Professor. All have qualified with post-graduate medical degrees (MD).

All the above proportions were compared across age groups (pediatric and adult) and different categories of prescribers. The prescriptions were assessed using a "Consensus Committee approach".

2.3.4. Assessment of Prescription through Consensus Committee Approach

A Rational Use of Medicine Consensus Committee was formed, including clinicians and clinical pharmacologists, with the objective of developing the assessment framework for diarrhoea and ARI prescriptions. Both clinicians and pharmacologists evaluated the prescriptions independently for appropriateness and the identification of deviation from the standard treatment guidelines (WHO, Ministry of Health & Family Welfare, Government of India, ICMR, 2019 and Standard Treatment Guideline, Institute of Health & Family Welfare, Govt. of West Bengal, 2011) [9,14,15,17].

Since all the guidelines are mostly targeted at general practitioners in public health settings, they do not cover many additional drugs, such as probiotics, antihistamines, leukotriene receptor antagonists, bronchodialators, mucolytics, etc., which are commonly prescribed in medical college settings. In such cases, both pharmacologist and clinician performed the assessment based on the scientific rationale and their clinical expertise.

Furthermore, the pharmacologist judged the prescriptions as appropriate or inappropriate on the basis of the signs and symptoms prescribed, the adverse effects of drugs, the route of administration, the dose (appropriate as per age and body weight, individualization, and the maximum dose per day mentioned for acute drugs), duration being correct as per documented indication, the possibility of drug interaction, and the prescription of generic names. The clinician judged the prescriptions independently as appropriate or inappropriate according to the above criteria as well as their clinical judgement, particularly optimising symptom remission and tolerating adverse effects. Acceptability of Deviation was determined using the Table 1:

**Table 1.** Assessment framework for deviation of prescription through Rational Use of Medicine Consensus Approach.

|  |  | Clinician | |
|---|---|---|---|
|  |  | Appropriate | Inappropriate |
| Pharmacologist | Appropriate | Acceptable/No deviation | Ref to Consensus committee |
|  | Inappropriate | Ref to Consensus committee | Unacceptable |

In case of a disagreement between pharmacologist and clinician, acceptability of the prescription was discussed in the RUMC committee and a case-to-case decision was taken based on the understanding of significant harm over benefit.

Statistical Analysis: descriptive statistics were used to analyse and present the data in terms of proportion (percentage), and mean with standard deviation (SD). The percentage of prescriptions adhering to each indicator was calculated overall and in the subgroups of patient age (below and above 18 years) and different types of prescribers. Agreement between clinicians and pharmacologists for the appropriateness of prescriptions was determined by Cohen's Kappa statistics.

## 3. Results

Out of total collected 630 prescriptions, 37.3%, 47.5%, and 15.2% were from medicine OPDs, Paediatric OPDs, and UHTC OPD. The prescriber pattern obtained showed a majority of prescriptions (42.9%) written by senior doctors, followed by 39.7% written by general resident doctors, and 17.5% written by post-graduate residents.

ARI was more common among the collected prescriptions, with 511 (81.1%) prescriptions, and 119 (18.9%) prescriptions were for diarrhoea. It was found that the majority of the patients (63.2%—ARI and 64.7%—diarrhoea) were below the 18-year age group. Around 56% and 49.6% of patients suffering from ARI and diarrhoea, respectively, were female. The majority of ARI prescriptions were written by faculties (43.8%), while maximum diarrhoea prescriptions were written by interns and housestaff (42.9%).

Assessments of prescribing patterns were completed utilizing the WHO criteria. Deviation from WHO criteria were notable in one or more criteria in majority prescriptions (Table 2). Some of the major contributors to deviations were "no mention of signs and symptoms" (90%), "antibiotic prescription rate" (57%), "no mention of body weight" (56%) and Use of FDC (51%).

Table 2. Completeness of prescriptions as per different criteria according to disease and comparison with WHO core indicators.

| Broad Group | Criteria Mentioned in Prescription | Total ($n$ = 630) | WHO Core Indicators |
|---|---|---|---|
| | | $n$ (%) | (%) |
| Patient and Disease Related Information | Body weight | 354 (56.2) | |
| | Signs and symptoms | 569 (90.3) | |
| | Provisional diagnosis | 31 (4.9) | |
| | Follow up | 302 (48.0) | |
| Drug related information | Mean (SD) no.of drugs prescribed per prescription | 4.2 ± 1.9 | ≤2 |
| | Prescription having all Drugs with generic name | 147 (23.3) | 100 |
| | Prescription of all Drugs from Hospital schedule list | 230 (36.5) | 100 |
| | Prescription of all drugs having Fixed Dose Combiation | 321 (51.0) | |
| | Drug formulation not mentioned | 4 (0.6) | |
| | Drug frequency not mentioned | 45 (7.2) | |
| | Drug duration not mentioned | 96 (15.3) | |
| Injectables and antibiotics related information | Prescriptions with injectables | 0 (0.0) | 13.4–21.1 |
| | Antibiotic Prescription Rate | 359 (57.0) | <30 |

The antibiotic prescription rate (APR) was observed to be higher for diarrhoea (65.5%) than ARI (55.2%). The multiple antibiotic prescription rate (MPR) was also high in cases of diarrhoea (30%) as compared to ARI (3.9%). Among the diarrhoea cases, antibiotics were prescribed in 64.4% of acute watery diarrhoea and 66.7% in dysentery. Antibiotics of nitroimidazole class followed by quinolones, cephalosporins were mostly prescribed. Fixed Dose Combination of ciprofloxacin, tinidazole/ofloxacin, ornidazole and ofloxacin, metronidazole was also used. The antibiotics most commonly used in ARI were a combination of Amoxycillin and Clavulinic acid (Beta lactamase inhibitor), followed by Azithromycin, Cephalexin, Cefixime, Co-trimoxazole and Amoxycillin alone.

*3.1. Appropriateness of the Prescription and Acceptability of the Deviations through a Consensus Committee Approach*

Deviation from the standard guideline as evaluated by the RUMC consensus committee was present in 623 (98.9%) prescriptions (Figure 1). Among them, only 60 (9.5%) were found acceptable. Out of 563 unacceptable deviations, 357 (63.4%) suffered the possibility of Adverse Drug Reactions (ADR), whereas 421 (74.8%) prescriptions had inconsistent or irrational indications. The majority of the unacceptable deviations were due to antibiotics, followed by bronchodilators, antihistaminics, Proton Pump Inhibitor/H 2 receptor blocker/Antacids, Probiotics (Table 3).

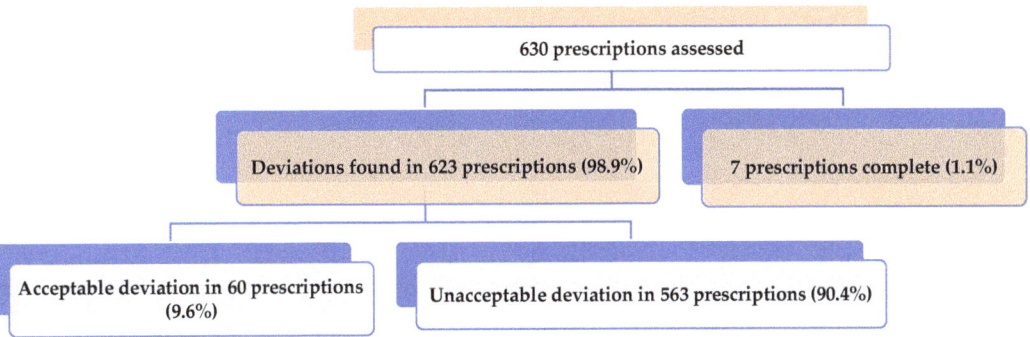

**Figure 1.** Acceptability of the deviations in assessed prescriptions through a consensus committee approach.

The appropriateness of prescriptions as per clinician and pharmacologist revealed an "agreement between them" in 90.4% of prescriptions (Kappa—0.14) (Table 4). However, only 1.1% of total prescriptions were appropriate according to both clinicians and pharmacologists. There were 9.6% prescriptions that were inappropriate as per a pharmacologist's recommendation but appropriate as per a clinician's recommendation. Some common points of disagreement were:

(a) The prescription of antihistaminics in ARI in children has been identified as inappropriate by pharmacologists; however, a 2nd generation antihistaminic (cetirizine) may be considered an acceptable deviation, but a 1st generation (Chlorpheniramine) is unacceptable due to excessive sedation.
(b) The prescription of Azithromycin in URTI was identified as inappropriate by the pharmacologist, as Azithromycin is not a first-line antibiotic, but it was considered an acceptable deviation by the clinician as standard practice.
(c) Drugs prescribed by brand names are considered inappropriate by the pharmacologist, but it was considered an acceptable deviation.
(d) Prescription of albendazole in children or Vitamin D in infants less than 6 months of age, though considered inappropriate by pharmacologists when there is no indication, is considered as acceptable deviation by consensus and adheres to the national program guideline.
(e) ORS prescribed without specific indication is also an acceptable deviation as it causes no apparent harm.

**Table 3.** Distribution of Drug responsible for unacceptable prescription. (*n* = 563 prescriptions, proportions are not mutually exclusive).

| Drug Group | Specific Agents Prescribed | No | % |
|---|---|---|---|
| Antibiotics | Amoxycillin, Cefuroxime, Azithromycin, Ofloxacin, Co-trimoxazole. | 246 | 43.7 |
| Bronchodilators | Salbutamol, Terbutaline, Theophylline | 240 | 42.6 |
| H1-Antihistaminics | Chlorpheniramine, Cetrizine, Fexofenadine | 128 | 22.7 |
| Probiotics | Lactobacillus, Bifidobacterium | 87 | 15.4 |
| Proton pump inhibitors | Omeprazone, Pantoprazole, Esomeprazole | 70 | 12.4 |
| Vitamins and mineral supplements | Water soluble vitamins, Iron, Calcium, Zinc. | 56 | 9.9 |
| Leukotrine receptor antagonists | Montelukast | 49 | 8.7 |
| Rehydrating agent | Oral rehydrating salt | 44 | 7.8 |
| H2 receptor blockers | Ranitidine, Famotidine | 31 | 5.5 |
| Non-steroidal anti-inflammatory drugs | Paracetamol, Nimesulide, Diclofenac | 28 | 4.9 |
| Antacids | Magaldrate, Aluminium hydroxide | 15 | 2.6 |
| Anti spasmodic agents | Dicylomine, Drotavarine | 15 | 2.6 |
| Anti-emetic agents | Ondansetron, Domperidone | 12 | 2.1 |
| Corticosteroids | Prednisolone, Deflazacort | 7 | 1.2 |
| Digestive enzymes | Amylase, Lipase | 6 | 1 |
| Nasal decongestants | Oxymetazoline, Xylometazoline | 4 | 0.7 |
| Mucolytic agents | Ambroxol, Guiaphenesin | 2 | 0.3 |
| Non-specific anti-diarrhoeal agent | Racecodotril | 1 | 0.2 |

**Table 4.** Appropriateness of prescriptions according to clinician and pharmacologist.

| Pharmacologist | Clinician | | Total | Kappa |
|---|---|---|---|---|
| | Appropriate | Inappropriate | | |
| Appropriate | 7 (1.1) | 0 (0.0) | 7 (1.1) | 0.14 |
| Inappropriate | 60 (9.5) | 563 (89.4) | 623 (98.9) | |
| Total | 67 (10.6) | 563 (89.4) | 630 (100.0) | |

*3.2. Completeness of Prescriptions—'Age-Wise'*

Body weight was mentioned in 88.5% of prescriptions of patients below 18 years age group. None of the adult prescriptions had body weight mentioned in them. Higher proportion of prescriptions with generic name (27% vs. 17%), and from hospital schedule list (41% vs. 29%) and lower FDC (44% vs. 63%) were observed in prescriptions of <18 years as compared to adults. APR was also lower for children than adults (48% vs. 71%).

Prescriptions with deviations were slightly lower in children (98.5% vs. 99.5%). However, proportion of acceptable deviations were more in <18 years age group (12% vs. 6%).

*3.3. Completeness of Prescriptions across Types of Prescribers*

Body weight, signs and symptoms, follow up visit was mentioned most commonly by residents while provisional diagnosis was commonly mentioned by faculties. Prescriptions of all drugs with generic names and from the hospital schedule list were mostly prescribed by residents, while fixed-dose combinations and antibiotics were mostly prescribed by faculties. Deviations were most commonly observed in the prescriptions of junior residents (99.6%), whereas acceptable deviations were more common among the PG residents (15%) (Table 5).

**Table 5.** Completeness of prescriptions as per different criteria across types of prescriber.

| Criteria Mentioned in Prescription | Intern & Housestaff (n = 250) | Residents (n = 110) | Faculty (n = 270) |
|---|---|---|---|
| | n (%) | n (%) | n (%) |
| Body weight | 106 (42.4) | 89 (80.9) | 159 (58.9) |
| Signs and symptoms | 247 (98.8) | 109 (99.0) | 213 (78.8) |
| Provisional diagnosis | 5 (2.0) | 1 (0.9) | 25 (9.2) |
| Follow up | 146 (58.4) | 92 (83.6) | 64 (23.7) |
| Prescription having all Drugs with generic name | 41 (16.4) | 59 (53.6) | 47 (17.4) |
| Prescription of all Drugs from Hospital schedule list | 81 (32.4) | 61 (55.5) | 88 (32.6) |
| Prescription of all drugs having FDC | 132 (52.8) | 29 (26.4) | 160 (59.2) |
| Prescription with antibiotics | 133 (45.2) | 29 (26.4) | 197 (73.0) |
| Drug formulation not mentioned | 1 (0.4) | 1 (0.9) | 2 (0.7) |
| Drug frequency not mentioned | 20 (8.0) | 3 (2.7) | 22 (8.2) |
| Drug duration not mentioned | 45 (18.0) | 14 (12.8) | 37 (13.7) |
| Prescription With ORS * | n = 51 | n = 22 | n = 46 |
| | 43 (84.3) | 19 (86.3) | 35 (76.0) |
| Prescriptions with deviations | 249 (99.6) | 106 (96.3) | 268 (99.2) |
| Prescriptions with acceptable deviations ** | n = 249 | n = 106 | n = 268 |
| | 11 (4.4) | 16 (15.0) | 33 (12.3) |
| Prescriptions with chance of ADR *** | n = 238 | n = 90 | n = 235 |
| | 156 (65.5) | 66 (73.3) | 131 (55.7) |
| Prescriptions with inconsistent/irrational indication *** | n = 238 | n = 90 | n = 235 |
| | 163 (68.4) | 45 (50.0) | 213 (90.6) |

* Proportion of prescriptions with ORS has been computed for diarrhoea cases only. ** Proportion of acceptable deviations have been computed out of total deviations in each category. *** Proportion of prescriptions with chances of ADR and inconsistent/irrational indication have been computed out of Unacceptable deviations in each category.

## 4. Discussion

In this study, polypharmacy emerged as a major concern as the average number of drugs prescribed per patient was 4.2 ± 1.9 which is much higher than the WHO standard of ≤2 [18]. However, a few studies have also mentioned a higher average number of drug prescriptions [10,19] per patient, whereas much lower estimates (1.5) were also observed [20]. Several other studies also reported an average range of 2.8–3.2 drugs per patient [21–25]. The higher number of drugs may enhance the chance of adverse drug reactions, antimicrobial resistance, healthcare expenditure and also interfere with prescription adherence.

Only 23.3% drugs were prescribed by generic names in this study. This is much lower than the standard cut-off of 100% [18]. Higher proportions of generic names were found in studies by Viswanath et al. [26] (62.3%) and Shankar PR et al. [19] (58.1%). Furthermore, in various other studies the proportion of generic names in the prescriptions ranged from 46.2–100% [21,22,27]. The use of generic names is recommended by the government to reduce healthcare costs. It was observed that 53.6% of residents prescribed generic names, compared with only 18% for interns and faculties. However, drugs with Fixed Dose

Combinations (FDC) were prescribed in little more than half of the prescriptions and similar findings had been reported by others also [27].

Injectable drugs were not prescribed in any of the prescriptions in this study, as the patients were first-time OPD attendees. The standard value of the proportion of prescriptions where injectables can be prescribed lies between 13.4% and 24.1% [18]. The WHO also recommends lesser use of injectable medications as it increases the cost as well as morbidity and mortality from infections viz. HIV, Hepatitis B and C, air embolism etc. [28].

Overall, 57.0% of prescriptions have at least one antibiotic prescribed. Considering the higher magnitude of infectious diseases in developing countries, WHO has limited the use of antibiotics to <30% of prescriptions for all infectious diseases [18,29]. Consequently, we observed a very high APR and significantly higher in case of diarrhoea and adult patients compared to their counterparts in the study ($p < 0.05$). In India, irrational antibiotic prescription is a serious concern, as reflected by the rates (20% to 72.8%) reported by different studies [21–24,27]. Antibiotic prescriptions without a provisional diagnosis in a first-time patient support the notion that physicians should cover for immediate medical catastrophes rather than consider backing up antibiotics for future implications in the era of rapidly emerging antimicrobial resistance. We reported a MPR of 10%, which is much lower than studies by Ashraf et al. [30] and Panchal et al. [10]; however, much lower usage of antibiotics of 1 per prescription was reported by Bordoloi et al. [31]. In most of the prescriptions, antibiotics have been prescribed as an empirical therapy without mentioning any provisional diagnosis. A study by Hekster et al. also reported similar findings, where diagnosis was not the deciding factor for prescribing antibiotics in half of the prescriptions [32]. Most episodes of watery diarrhoea in children and sometimes in adults are supposed to be of viral aetiology, where the use of antibiotics is inappropriate; even Acute Respiratory Infection may also be of a viral origin with no indication for antibiotic prescription. This will ultimately contribute to antimicrobial resistance [33–36]. Also according to ICMR guidelines, antibiotics should not be used for viral respiratory infections and watery diarrhoea and their use should be limited to Streptococcal pharyngitis, bacterial sinusitis and diarrhoea caused due to cholera, amoebiosis, Giarrdiasis, Shigellosis and those caused by Campylobacter or Aeromonas [17]. The Guidelines issued by the State of West Bengal in 2011 also inhibit the inadvertent empirical use of antibiotics [15]. However, our observations are not in accordance with those guidelines.

The most commonly used antibiotic for respiratory infections was a combination of Amoxycillin and Clavulinic Acid, which was corroborated by other studies [37,38]. The most commonly used antibiotics for diarrhoea were Metronidazole alone or with Ciprofloxacin. The easy availability of metronidazole and ciprofloxacin combined with prescriber's inclination towards a broad spectrum to eliminate the possibility of mixed infection may drive such type of prescriptions.

Deviations from the available treatment guidelines were found in 98.9% of prescriptions, with 90.3% being unacceptable deviations. The unacceptable deviations were in the form of preventable ADR, documentation errors, or drugs prescribed for which rationality could not be explained. A study completed at outpatient clinics in Saudi Arabia reported omissions of various components of the treatment regimen, with some reaching up to 91% incompleteness [39]. Higher adherence to guidelines will actually lead to treatment regimen completion, possibly because of the institutional culture of emphasising the treatment regimen prescription writing [40].

In conclusion, the pattern of prescriptions for diarrhoea and ARI revealed inappropriate practises and non-adherence to the available guidelines (ICMR, state, and WHO). Some common forms of inappropriateness were the use of multiple drugs, the use of brand names, prescribing fixed dose combinations, and the overuse of antibiotics without any rationale.

At the same time, it came to our attention that the available guidelines are more suitable for 'primary care settings' where simpler cases are expected to be managed, and probably not the best for managing the 'complicated' or 'referred cases' in the 'higher tiers of healthcare'. Hence, healthcare tier specific, evidence-based treatment guidelines may be formulated to minimise the subjective variations in the management approach.

However, the outcome of irrational prescriptions, such as cure rate, drug-drug interaction, or adverse events, was beyond the scope of the present study. Moreover, diarrhoea and ARI cases are mostly self-limiting and viral in nature. Irrational antimicrobial prescription and consumption not only affect human health adversely but also contribute to environmental contamination with antibiotic residues, Antibiotic Resistant Bacteria (ARBs) and Antibiotic Resistant Genes (ARGs). Judicious use of antibiotics is a prerogative in not only the human health sector but also in animal sectors such as animal husbandry, fisheries, poultry, etc. Unless the problem of Antimicrobial Resistance is tackled through multisectoral involvement, the problem of One Health cannot be fully addressed. In this study, we identified a need for training and education among junior doctors, particularly interns and house staff, regarding rational antibiotic practices, and the findings can be applied to similar practises in other sectors as well. Holistically, in order to establish a One Health approach for the problem of AMR, it requires standardised guidelines, regular capacity strengthening, behaviour change communication, and periodic evaluation at all levels. Our study is a small attempt towards achieving this larger goal.

**Author Contributions:** Conceptualization, S.K., N.K. and S.D.; Methodology, D.C., F.D., R.B., P.D., K.D., N.K. and S.D.; Formal analysis, D.C., F.D., S.M., N.C., K.D., S.G. and P.B.; Investigation, N.C., R.B., S.G. and P.B.; Resources, S.K.; Data curation, D.C., F.D., S.M., N.C. and P.D.; Writing—original draft, D.C.; Writing—review & editing, F.D., S.M., R.B., S.G., P.B., N.K. and S.D.; Supervision, N.C., R.B, P.D and N.K.; Project administration, S.K. and N.K.; Funding acquisition, S.K. and S.D. All authors have read and agreed to the published version of the manuscript.

**Funding:** The study was funded by Indian Council of Medical Research, New Delhi (Grant Letter No. 65/11/2018/BMS/RUD/NICED dated 2 July 2019).

**Institutional Review Board Statement:** Approval was obtained from ethics committee of ICMR-NICED and the participating hospitals. Written consent or verbal consent.

**Informed Consent Statement:** Informed written consent was obtained from all subjects involved in the study.

**Data Availability Statement:** The data presented in this study are available on request from the corresponding author.

**Acknowledgments:** The authors sincerely acknowledge Indian Council of Medical Research task force members for providing valuable inputs in designing the protocol and providing guidance towards enriching the manuscript. We acknowledged the Medical colleges admiistrations for their support to conduct the study.

**Conflicts of Interest:** The authors declare no conflict of interest.

# References

1. Promoting Rational Use of Medicines. Available online: https://www.who.int/activities/promoting-rational-use-of-medicines (accessed on 11 July 2022).
2. Ofori-Asenso, R.; Agyeman, A.A. Irrational Use of Medicines—A Summary of Key Concepts. *Pharmacy* **2016**, *4*, 35. [CrossRef] [PubMed]
3. Bigdeli, M.; Peters, D.H.; Wagner, A.K. *Medicines in Health Systems: Advancing Access, Affordability and Appropriate Use*; World Health Organization: Geneva, Switzerland, 2014; Available online: https://apps.who.int/iris/handle/10665/179197 (accessed on 8 December 2022).
4. Holloway, K.A. Combating inappropriate use of medicines. *Expert Rev. Clin. Pharmacol.* **2011**, *4*, 335–348. [CrossRef] [PubMed]
5. Sema, F.D.; Asres, E.D.; Wubeshet, B.D. Evaluation of Rational Use of Medicine Using WHO/INRUD Core Drug Use Indicators at Teda and Azezo Health Centers, Gondar Town, Northwest Ethiopia. *Integr. Pharm. Res. Pract.* **2021**, *10*, 51–63. [CrossRef] [PubMed]
6. Ahmad, A.; Parimalakrishnan, S.; Mohanta, G.P.; Patel, I.; Manna, P.K. A study on utilization pattern of higher generation antibiotics among patients visiting community pharmacies in Chidambaram, Tamil Nadu at South India. *Int. J. Pharm.* **2012**, *2*, 466–471.

7. Sharma, S.; Sethi, G.R.; Gupta, U. *Standard Treatment Guidelines—A Manual for Medical Therapeutics*, 3rd ed.; Delhi Society for Promotion of Rational Use of Drugs, B I Publishing House Pvt. Ltd.: New Delhi, India, 2009; pp. 116–124. Available online: https://scholar.google.com/scholar_lookup?title=Standard+Treatment+Guidelines+%E2%80%93+A+Manual+for+Medical+Therapeutics&author=S+Sharma&author=GR+Sethi&author=U+Gupta&publication_year=2009& (accessed on 11 July 2022).
8. Ghimire, S.; Nepal, S.; Bhandari, S.; Nepal, P.; Palaian, S. A prospective surveillance of drug prescribing and dispensing in a teaching hospital in Western Nepal. *J. Pak. Med. Assoc.* **2009**, *59*, 726–731.
9. *The Treatment of Diarrhoea: A Manual for Physicians and Other Senior Health Workers*, 4th ed.; Department of Child and Adolescent Health and Development, World Health Organization: Geneva, Switzerland, 2005; Available online: http://www.whqlibdoc.who.int/publications/2005/9241593180.pdf (accessed on 2 December 2022).
10. Panchal, J.R.; Desai, C.K.; Iyer, G.S.; Patel, P.P.; Dikshit, R.K. Prescribing pattern and appropriateness of drug treatment of diarrhoea in hospitalised children at a tertiary care hospital in India. *Int. J. Med. Public Health* **2013**, *3*, 335–341. [CrossRef]
11. *The World Medicines Situation 2011—Access to Controlled Medicines*, 3rd ed.; World Health Organization: Geneva, Switzerland, 2011; Available online: https://www.who.int/publications/i/item/WHO-EMP-MIE-2011-2.4 (accessed on 6 December 2022).
12. Ahmad, A.; Parimalakrishnan, S.; Patel, I.; Praveen Kumar, N.V.; Balkrishnan, R.; Mohanta, G.P. Evaluation of self-medication antibiotics use pattern among patients attending community pharmacies in rural India, Uttar Pradesh. *J. Pharm. Res.* **2012**, *5*, 765–768.
13. Blum, N.L. *Drug Information Development. A Case Study Nepal. Rational Pharmaceutical Management Project*; Online; United States Pharmacopoeia: Rockville, MD, USA, 2000; Available online: http://www.usp.org/pdf/EN/dqi/nepalCaseStudy (accessed on 20 July 2020).
14. *Standard Treatment Guidelines—Management of Common Respiratory Infections in Children in India*; Ministry of Health and Family Welfare, Government of India: New Delhi, India, 2016. Available online: http://clinicalestablishments.gov.in/WriteReadData/4671.pdf (accessed on 23 July 2020).
15. *Standard Treatment Guidelines—Manual for Physician*; Goverment of West Bengal: Kolkata, India, 2011; Available online: www.ihfwkolkata.org/stg/index.html (accessed on 7 October 2020).
16. WHO. Study design and sample size. In *How to Investigate Drug Use in Health Facilities: Selected Drug Use Indicators*, 1st ed.; World Health Organization: Geneva, Swtzerland, 1993; 92p.
17. *Treatment Guidelines for Antimicrobial Use in Common Syndromes*; ICMR: New Delhi, India, 2019; Available online: https://main.icmr.nic.in/sites/default/files/guidelines/Treatment_Guidelines_2019_Final.pdf (accessed on 5 October 2020).
18. Isah, A.O.; Ross-Degnan, D.; Quick, J.; Laing, R.; Mabadeje, A.F. *The Development of Standard Values for the WHO Drug Use Prescribing Indicators*; ICUM/EDM/WHO: Geneva, Switzerland, 2001; Available online: http://www.archives.who.int/prduc2004/rducd/ICIUM_Posters/1a2_txt.htm. (accessed on 20 July 2020).
19. Shankar, P.R.; Upadhyay, D.K.; Subish, P.; Dubey, A.; Mishra, P. Prescription patterns among paediatric inpatients in a teaching hospital in Western Nepal. *Singapore Med. J.* **2006**, *47*, 261–264.
20. Alam, M.B.; Ahmed, F.U.; Rahman, M.E. Misuse of drugs in acute diarrhoea in under five children. *Bangladesh Med. Res. Counc. Bull.* **1998**, *24*, 27–31.
21. Karande, S.; Sankhe, P.; Kulkarni, M. Patterns of prescription and drug dispensing. *Indian J. Pediatr.* **2005**, *72*, 117–121. [CrossRef]
22. Hazra, A.; Tripathi, S.K.; Alam, M.S. Prescribing and dispensing activities at the health facilities of a non-governmental organization. *Natl. Med. J. India* **2000**, *13*, 177–182.
23. Krishna, J.; Goel, S.; Singh, A.; Roy, A.; Divya, D.C.; Shamsi, M.S. Evaluation of prescription pattern and drug dispensing from a pediatric outpatient department of a tertiary care hospital. *Indian J. Sci. Res.* **2015**, *6*, 113–117.
24. Tekur, U.; Kalra, B.S. Monitoring an interventional programme of drug utilization in a health facility of Delhi. *Indian J. Med. Res.* **2012**, *135*, 675–677.
25. Kumar, A.; Jain, P.; Upadhyaya, P.; Jain, S. A study monitoring prescription pattern of antibiotics in a tertiary care hospital in North India. *Int. J. Basic Clin. Pharmacol.* **2014**, *3*, 1006–1011. [CrossRef]
26. Vishwanath, M.; Reddy, S.N.; Devadas, S. Assessment of drug utilization in hospitalized children at a tertiary care teaching hospital. *J. Chem. Pharm. Res.* **2014**, *6*, 592–598.
27. Lalan, B.K.; Hiray, R.S.; Ghongane, B.B. Drug prescription pattern of outpatients in a tertiary care teaching hospital in Maharashtra. *Int. J. Pharm. Biol. Sci.* **2012**, *3*, 225–229.
28. Hussain, S.; Yadav, S.S.; Sawlani, K.K.; Khatri, S. Assessment of drug prescribing pattern using world health organization indicators in a tertiary care teaching hospital. *Indian J. Public Health* **2018**, *62*, 156–158. [CrossRef]
29. Sumaila, A.N.; Tabong, P.T.N. Rational prescribing of antibiotics in children under 5 years with upper respiratory tract infections in Kintampo Municipal Hospital in Brong Ahafo Region of Ghana. *BMC Res. Notes* **2018**, *11*, 443. [CrossRef]
30. Ashraf, H.; Handa, S.; Khan, N.A. Prescribing pattern of drugs in out-patient department of Child Care Centre in Moradabad city. *Int. J. Pharm. Sci. Rev. Res.* **2010**, *3*, 1–5.
31. Bordoloi, P. Drug utilization study in the management of acute diarrhoea in the Paediatrics department at a tertiary health care institution. *Br. J. Med. Health Res.* **2016**, *3*, 46–55.

32. Hekster, Y.A.; Vree, T.B.; Goris, R.J.; Boerema, J.B. The defined daily dose per 100 bed-days as a unit of comparison and a parameter for studying antimicrobial drug use in a university hospital. A retrospective study of the effects of guidelines and audit on antimicrobial drug use. *J. Clin. Hosp. Pharm.* **1982**, *7*, 251–260. [CrossRef] [PubMed]
33. Schindler, C.; Krappweis, J.; Morgenstern, I.; Kirch, W. Prescriptions of systemic antibiotics for children in Germany aged between 0 and 6 years. *Pharmacoepidemiol. Drug Saf.* **2003**, *12*, 113–120. [CrossRef] [PubMed]
34. World Health Organization. *Pocket Book of Hospital Care for Children Guidelines for the Management of Common Illnesses with Limited Resources*; World Health Organization: Geneva, Switzerland, 2007; pp. 72–81.
35. Sahoo, K.C.; Tamhankar, A.J.; Johansson, E.; Lundborg, C.S. Antibiotic use, resistance development and environmental factors: A qualitative study among healthcare professionals in Orissa, India. *BMC Public Health* **2010**, *10*, 629. [CrossRef]
36. Chukwuani, C.M.; Onifade, M.; Sumonu, K. Survey of drug use practices and antibiotic prescribing pattern at a general hospital in Nigeria. *Pharm. World Sci.* **2002**, *24*, 188–195. [CrossRef]
37. Das, B.; Sarkar, C.; Majumder, A.G. Medication use for pediatric upper respiratory tract infections. *Fundam. Clin. Pharmacol.* **2006**, *20*, 385–390. [CrossRef]
38. Beg, M.A.; Dutta, S.B.; Bawa, S.; Kaur, A.; Vishal, S.; Kumar, U. Prescribing trends in respiratory tract infections in a tertiary care teaching hospital. *Int. J. Res. Med. Sci.* **2017**, *5*, 2588–2591. [CrossRef]
39. Irshaid, Y.M.; Al Homrany, M.; Hamdi, A.A.; Adjepon-Yamoah, K.K.; Mahfouz, A.A. Compliance with good practice in prescription writing at outpatient clinics in Saudi Arabia. *East. Mediterr. Health J.* **2005**, *11*, 922–928.
40. Nkera-Gutabara, J.G.; Ragaven, L.B. Adherence to prescription-writing guidelines for outpatients in Southern Gauteng district hospitals. *Afr. J. Prim. Health Care. Fam. Med.* **2020**, *12*, e1–e11. [CrossRef]

**Disclaimer/Publisher's Note:** The statements, opinions and data contained in all publications are solely those of the individual author(s) and contributor(s) and not of MDPI and/or the editor(s). MDPI and/or the editor(s) disclaim responsibility for any injury to people or property resulting from any ideas, methods, instructions or products referred to in the content.

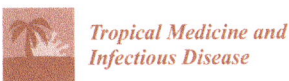 Tropical Medicine and Infectious Disease

*Article*

# Human and Livestock Surveillance Revealed the Circulation of Rift Valley Fever Virus in Agnam, Northern Senegal, 2021

Moufid Mhamadi [1,2,†], Aminata Badji [3,†], Mamadou Aliou Barry [4,†], El Hadji Ndiaye [3], Alioune Gaye [3], Mignane Ndiaye [1], Moundhir Mhamadi [5], Cheikh Talibouya Touré [1], Oumar Ndiaye [1,5], Babacar Faye [2,*], Boly Diop [6], Mamadou Ndiaye [6], Mathioro Fall [7], Andy Mahine Diouf [1], Samba Niang Sagne [4], Cheikh Loucoubar [4], Hugues Fausther-Bovendo [8], Ara XIII [9], Amadou Alpha Sall [1], Gary Kobinger [9], Ousmane Faye [1], Mawlouth Diallo [3] and Oumar Faye [1,*]

1. Virology Department, Institut Pasteur de Dakar, Dakar 12900, Senegal
2. Parasitology Department, Université Cheikh Anta Diop de Dakar, Dakar 10700, Senegal
3. Medical Zoology Department, Institut Pasteur de Dakar, Dakar 12900, Senegal
4. Epidemiology, Clinical Research and Data Science Department, Institut Pasteur de Dakar, Dakar 12900, Senegal
5. Institut Pasteur de Dakar, DIATROPIX, Dakar 12900, Senegal
6. Ministry of Health and Social Action, Dakar 12900, Senegal
7. Ministry of Livestock and Animal Production, Dakar 12900, Senegal
8. Global Urgent and Advanced Research and Development, Batiscan, QC G0X 1A0, Canada
9. University of Texas Medical Branch, Galveston, TX 77555-0132, USA
* Correspondence: babacar2.faye@ucad.edu.sn (B.F.); oumar.faye@pasteur.sn (O.F.)
† These authors contributed equally to this work.

**Abstract:** The mosquito-borne disease caused by the Rift Valley Fever Virus (RVFV) is a viral hemorrhagic fever that affects humans and animals. In 1987, RVFV emerged in Mauritania, which caused the first RVFV outbreak in West Africa. This outbreak was shortly followed by reported cases in humans and livestock in Senegal. Animal trade practices with neighboring Mauritania suggest northern regions of Senegal are at high risk for RVF. In this study, we aim to conduct a molecular and serological survey of RVFV in humans and livestock in Agnam (northeastern Senegal) by RT-PCR (reverse transcription real-time polymerase chain reaction) and ELISA (Enzyme-Linked Immunosorbent Assay), respectively. Of the two hundred fifty-five human sera, one (0.39%) tested RVFV IgM positive, while fifty-three (20.78%) tested positive for RVFV IgG. For animal monitoring, out of 30 sheep recorded and sampled over the study period, 20 (66.67%) showed seroconversion to RVFV IgG antibodies, notably during the rainy season. The presence of antibodies increased significantly with age in both groups ($p < 0.05$), as the force of RVF infection (FOI), increased by 16.05% per year for humans and by 80.4% per month for livestock sheep. This study supports the usefulness of setting up a One Health survey for RVF management.

**Keywords:** Rift Valley Fever Virus; survey; humans; livestock; northeastern Senegal

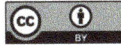

## 1. Introduction

Rift Valley Fever Virus (RVFV) is an arthropod-borne virus belonging to the *Phlebovirus* order in the *Phenuiviridae* family which infects humans and animals, including animal livestock. The virus is transmitted mainly by infected mosquito bites during a blood meal, yet humans can also acquire RVFV infection through contact with an infected animal or handling of contaminated animal products, as well as in the healthcare setting during the care of infected patients [1].

RVF was first documented in 1930 in the Rift Valley region of Kenya in East Africa [2]; the disease has since been reported throughout Africa and the Arabic peninsula, and the diffusion is likely attributed to livestock trade. In 1987, RVFV emerged in Mauritania and caused the first RVFV outbreak in West Africa [3]. Due to the high risk of RVF introduction by livestock trade with neighboring Mauritania, Senegal's northern regions are the most exposed. In Senegal, serological and molecular evidence of RVFV circulation has been reported in humans, livestock, and mosquitoes [4–11]. *Aedes vexans*, *Culex quinquefasciatus*, and *Culex poicilipes* can transmit the disease [12].

In humans, after infection and a few days of incubation, clinical signs and symptoms such as fever, headache, backache, vertigo, anorexia, and photophobia appear. In a few cases, additional severe clinical manifestations can appear, including hepatitis, jaundice, further neurological disease, and hemorrhagic disease [13]. RVFV infects a wide range of animals with signs including fever, bloody diarrhea, and abortion, as well as behaviors indicative of listlessness, loss of appetite, disinclination to move, and abdominal pain [13]. A differential influence of age on mortality was reported, with juveniles more susceptible to severe outcomes than adults [13]. RVFV remains detectable by reverse transcription real-time polymerase chain reaction (RT-PCR) 10 days after symptom onset. Antibody levels start to increase at day four (4) after symptom onset for immunoglobulin M (IgM) and on day seven (7) after symptom onset for immunoglobulin G (IgG). These antibodies remain detectable by serological assay for at least forty-two (42) days for IgM and several years for IgG [14].

The RVFV genome is a ribonucleic (RNA) genome that is composed of three segments: small (S), medium (M), and large (L). The S segment encodes the nucleocapsid (N) protein and non-structural proteins (NS), which are translated from overlapping open reading frames (ORF). The M segment encodes for the glycoproteins (Gn and Gc) and a non-structural protein (NSm). Lastly, the L segment encodes the RNA-dependent RNA polymerase (RDRP) [15].

Several commercialized vaccines are available to protect against RVFV infection, including the live attenuated MP-12 and the inactivated vaccine TSI-GSD-200 for human immunization [16], as well as the ancestral live attenuated vaccine Smithburn strain and the newly developed live attenuated vaccine Clone 13 for livestock animal vaccination [17]. Even so, thus far, no specific pharmaceutical treatment for RVF exists, which prompts an urgency to assess the circulation of the disease. Here we used a One Health site to assess the circulation of RVFV in Agnam, an area near Mauritania at risk of infection in animals and humans related to the importation of infected livestock.

## 2. Materials and Methods

### 2.1. Study Sites

This survey was established in the Matam region (15°06′18″ N and 13°38′30″ W), more particularly in Agnam, in the villages located around Agnam Civol (16°00′18″ N, 13°41′35″ W) and Idite (15°55′09.5″ N 13°43′05.1″ W) (Figure 1). These Sudano-Sahelian areas are located in the northeast of the country on the border of Mauritania with an estimated population of 654,951 inhabitants. Within Agnam, Agnam Civol constitutes the urban environment, which includes markets and hospitals. In contrast, Idite contains pastoral activities such as grazing and livestock breeding.

In Agnam, the rainy season starts in June and ends in October, with a low amount of 369 mm of rainfall per year.

### 2.2. Blood Sampling in Humans and Animals

During this study, to assess the potential circulation of RVFV in Agnam, human and animal samples were collected.

Every febrile patient who signed their consent was blood sampled in the Agnam Civol healthcare sentinel site between June 2021 and December 2021 as already described [18]. Blood samples were transiently conserved at +4 °C then transferred to the arbovirus and viral hemorrhagic fever virus unit at the Institut Pasteur de Dakar as part of the ongoing Syndromic Sentinel Surveillance network in Senegal (4S network) [19]. In the laboratory, arboviral and viral hemorrhagic fever infections were tested by RT-PCR (reverse transcription real-time polymerase chain reaction) and ELISA (Enzyme-Linked Immunosorbent Assay) for the research of the antibodies immunoglobulin M (IgM) and immunoglobulin G (IgG).

**Figure 1.** Study sites (Idite for animal survey represented by the black dot and Agnam Civol for human survey represented by the red dot) located in Matam (colored in green) in Northern Senegal. Download from (https://d-maps.com/carte.php?num_car=25271&lang=fr, accessed on 7 January 2023) and edit.

For the animal survey, 30 sheep located in Idite (15°55′09.5″ N 13°43′05.1″ W) were blood sampled by jugular routes and tested for RVFV infection by RT-PCR and anti-RVFV IgG by ELISA in February 2021 to include individuals without any contact with the virus. Only the sheep that tested negative for RVFV infection were included in this subsequent study. These sheep were blood sampled every 2 weeks up to day 56 and then monthly from February to December 2021 to monitor RVFV infection. The sheep were also monitored for typical signs of RVFV infection, symptoms such as abortion and an increased mortality rate in young animals.

### 2.3. Serological Assay for RVFV

The presence of anti-RVFV immunoglobulin M (IgM) was tested in human sera with an in-house immunocapture Enzyme-Linked Immunosorbent Assay (ELISA) [18]. Goat anti-human IgM (Sera care, Milford, MA, USA) was diluted at 1/1000 in carbonate–bicarbonate buffer (0.015 M sodium carbonate, 0.035 M sodium bicarbonate, pH 9.6) as coating buffer. Coated plates (Immulon II 96-well microtiter plates; Dynatech Industries, Inc., Rockdale, Australia) were incubated overnight at 4 °C. After the incubation step, the plates were washed thrice using phosphate-buffered saline (PBS, Gibco, Ph 7.4) 1X at 0.05% Tween 20. Sera and homologous positive and negative antibody controls were added to the wells at a dilution of 1:100. The diluent used was phosphate-buffered saline with 0.05% Tween 20 and 1% non-fat dry milk. After one-hour incubation at 37 °C and 3 washing steps, viral and normal antigens of infected suckling mouse liver obtained from the WHOCC collection were added at dilutions of 1:100. After one-hour incubation at 37 °C and 3 washing steps, polyclonal Mouse Ascitic Fluids specific to RVF Ag were prepared at 1:1000 in diluent solution. Plates were incubated for a further 1 h at 37 °C and washed 3 times. Peroxidase-conjugated anti-mouse IgG horseradish was subsequently added at a dilution of 1/30,000 in the diluent buffer.

After one-hour incubation at 37 °C and 3 washing steps, 3, 3′, 5, 5′-tetramethylbenzidine (TMB SIGMA Aldrich, USA) was used as a substrate and the reaction was stopped 5 min later with 1 N sulfuric acid. Reactions were measured using a MultiSkan microplate reader (Thermofisher Scientific, Waltham, MA, USA) at an absorbance of 450 nm with 620 nm as a passive reference.

The difference ($\Delta DO$) was measured between the optical density yielded by the sample viral antigen OD and the sample negative antigen OD; any $\Delta DO > 0.2$ was considered positive and any lower value was considered negative.

For anti-RVFV IgG detection in human and animal sera, we used an indirect in-house Enzyme-Linked Immunosorbent Assay (ELISA) test [18]. Plate wells were sensitized by adding 100 µL per well of 50 ng of RVF glycoprotein (Abcam) diluted in phosphate-buffered saline (phosphate-buffered saline (PBS, Gibco, Ph 7.4)) 1X and incubated overnight at 4 °C. Plate wells were then washed 3 times with a washing buffer composed of PBS 1X and 0.005% Tween 20. After this washing step, the antigen residues were blocked by adding 200 µL per well of a blocking buffer composed of PBS 1x, 0.05% Tween 20, and 5% non-fat skimmed milk. After 1 h of incubation at 37 °C, the plate wells were washed thrice with the washing buffer, and 1/100 diluted sera and antibody controls (negative and positive) were added to the plate wells. Then, the plates were incubated at 37 °C for 1 h. After a washing step, 100 µL of a species-specific antibody conjugated with horseradish peroxidase (rabbit anti-sheep IgG (Biorad) or a goat anti-human IgG (KPL)) was added to each well, then the plates were incubated for 1 h at 37 °C. The Tetramethylbenzidine (TMB) substrate was added after three final washing steps, and then the reaction was stopped with 1 N sulfuric acid. The plate well was read using the absorbance 450/620 filters using a Multiskan microplate reader, and the generated data were processed in Microsoft Excel. RVFV glycoprotein ELISA cut-off was determined with a finite mixture model.

### 2.4. Reverse Transcription Real-Time Polymerase Chain Reaction for RVFV

Ribonucleic acid (RNA) was extracted from human and sheep sera sampling using the QIAamp RNA Viral Kit (Qiagen GmbH, Heiden, Germany). Briefly, RNA was extracted from 140 µL of sera using AVL lysing buffer and eluted in 60 µL using AVE buffer according to the manufacturer's instructions. Then, extracted RNA was immediately stored at −80 °C until further use. The presence of the RVFV virus non-structural (NSs) gene of the small segment was tested by RT-PCR using the AgPath-ID One-step RT-PCR kit (Thermofisher) mixed with primers (forward primer TGCCACGAGTYAGAGCCA and reverse primer GTGGGTCCGAGAGTYTGC) and probe (probe TCCTTCTCCCAGTCAGCCCCAC), as previously described [20]. The reaction mixture consisted of 5 µL RNA, 12.5 µL of buffer, 4 µL of RNase-free water, 1 µL of each primer at 10 µm, 0.5 µL of the probe at 10 µm, and 1 µL of enzymes for a total volume of 25 µL. The RVFV NSs gene detection was performed on QuantStudio 5 (Applied Biosystems, Foster City, CA, USA) thermocycler platform using the following cycling conditions: reverse transcription step at 50.0 °C for 10 min, denaturation at 95.0 °C for 15 min, 40 cycles' hybridization for 15 s at 95.0 °C, and elongation for 1 min at 60 °C.

### 2.5. Statistical Analysis

Data were processed in Microsoft Excel. Data analysis was carried out in R software version 4.1.1 (2009–2022 RStudio, PBC). The risk of RVFV exposure was evaluated by logistic regression with statistical significance set up as $p < 0.05$. The rate at which susceptible individuals become infected, which is called the force of infection (FOI), was evaluated as previously described [21]. The FOI is an important public health parameter for measuring the weight or the burden of disease and the effect of outbreak management programs. The analysis of the human survey (one serosurvey) replicated the methodology of the Colombo survey as previously described [21]. Alternatively, the animal survey (multiple serosurveys) replicated the methodology of the Medellin survey as previously described [21].

We use the finite mixture model to determine the cut-off of RVFV glycoprotein ELISA assay. Finite mixture models are classes of statistical models for addressing the heterogeneity of data and characterizing the unobserved class of each observation. It is well-studied in the field of statistics and has a wide range of applications in the fields of biostatistics, bioinformatics, medical care, and computer science. Particularly, the finite mixture model can be used to model bimodal data and derive a cut-off value that separates the two peaks. In this case, the main task of data analysis is clustering, i.e., using numerical vectors (IgG concentration, Optic Density (OD) ELISA) to identify positive and negative samples. We can model such a bimodal distribution by a finite mixture model that uses continuous distributions from the exponential family [22]. In the absence of clear expectations on the shape of these distributions, we can consider the normal, the gamma, and the Weibull distributions. In this paper we use the normal distribution. The normal distribution is defined on all real numbers and is characterized by 2 parameters: a location parameter μ and a scale parameter σ. The first parameter accounts for the location of most of the data and corresponds to the mean of the normal distribution. The second parameter accounts for the spread of the data around the location parameter and corresponds to the standard deviation. We refer to μ1 and σ1 for the location and scale parameters of the peak of the lower optic density (OD ELISA) and μ2 and σ2 for the location and scale parameters of the peak of the higher optic density (OD ELISA). The density of the bimodal distribution of optic density ELISA thus reads as follows.

$$f(x|\lambda, \mu1, \sigma1, \mu2, \sigma2) = \lambda \times D1(x|\mu1, \sigma1) + (1-\lambda) \times D2(x|\mu2, \sigma2)$$

The parameters of the finite mixture model are estimated by the expectation maximization algorithm [23] as coded by the function. These parameters include two parameters for each of the two probability distributions and a mixture parameter.

We use the fitted finite mixture model to identify a cut-off value that discriminates the two modes of the dataset. For that, we compute the probability for a datum to belong to distribution D1 as

$$p1 = \frac{\lambda \times D1(x|\mu1, \sigma1)}{\lambda \times D1(x|\mu1, \sigma1) + (1-\lambda) \times D2(x|\mu2, \sigma2)}$$

and the probability for a datum to belong to distribution D1 as

$$p2 = \frac{(1-\lambda) \times D2(x|\mu2, \sigma2)}{\lambda \times D1(x|\mu1, \sigma1) + (1-\lambda) \times D2(x|\mu2, \sigma2)}$$

We equate this probability to the type I error we aim at to find the cut-off value.

## 3. Results

### 3.1. Human Survey

During the survey, 255 human sera were collected from febrile patients between June 2021 and December 2021. The median temperature was 38.5 °C with a sex ratio of 0.84 (46.27% for men and 53.73% for women). The patient's median age was 19 years, with a minimum age of 2 months and a maximum age of 98 years. Analysis of the signs and symptoms shows that headache (91.78%) was the most documented sign/symptom followed by myalgia (65.72%), arthralgia (30.87%), asthenia (7.36%), and rashes (5.66%). The most sampled age group was 0–20 years, and the most febrile patients sampled were in October (81/255 or 31.76%).

One febrile patient tested positive for a recent RVFV infection by testing positive for the anti-RVFV IgM test. We noticed that 53 were positive for anti-RVFV IgG, and none of the collected human sera were positive by RVFV NSs RT-PCR test. The anti-RVFV IgM-positive patient was a 60-year-old woman from Bagonde village located in Idite, and she had contact with livestock animals. She had a consultation 2 days after the symptoms' onset. Her clinical signs and symptoms were headache and arthralgia with a temperature of 38.6 °C, and her malaria histidine rich protein (HRP) rapid diagnostic test (RDT) was negative. The anti-RFVV IgG detection test performed 20 days later was positive, and the patient regained good health without any complications. We also noticed that 30 years old was the median age of the positive tested (IgM and IgG) patients, with comparable rates between women and men (sex ratio = 0.89). The overall seroprevalence (IgM + IgG) was 21.17% in this study.

We estimated the force of infection to be 16.05% per year with a credible interval of 11.22 to 22.11%, with sensitivity and specificity both varying (Figure 2).

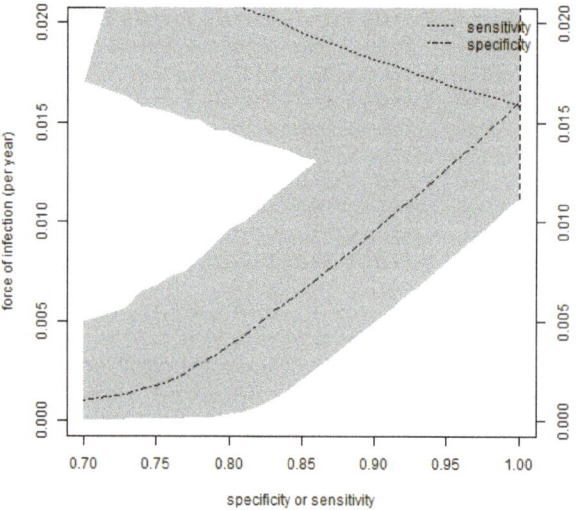

**Figure 2.** The force of infection among Agnam's tested human population is calculated for each value of sensitivity or specificity, which is considered to be fixed. Figure 2 shows that the 95% credible intervals are represented in the grey zones. When specificity reaches 100% sensitivity is less than 100%, with the converse also being true. On the right side of the plot of Figure 2, as accuracy approaches 100%, the credible interval approaches the statistical significance of 5% from the standard binomial (vertical dashed line).

The seropositivity rates between men and women did not show a statistical difference. Still, the RVFV exposure or infection risk becomes significatively higher with increasing age ($p$-value = 0.027), and anti-RVFV immunoglobulins (IgM + IgG) rates were significatively higher in Bele village (Table 1), which is a pastoral area like Idite.

*3.2. Animal Survey*

From February to December 2021, 314 sera were sampled from a study group of 30 sheep located in Idite. This population principally consisted of females (94.11%), and the ages ranged from a minimum of four (4) months to a maximum of eighteen (18) months, with a median age of eight (8) months. The analysis shows that 20 of the 30 (66.67%) animals seroconverted to RVFV during the eleven (11) monthly surveys (Figure 3).

Table 1. Risk factors of RVF infection among the human study group. N IgG (%) = number of people with anti-RVFV IgG antibodies (percentage of people with anti-RVFV IgG).

|  | N IgG (%) | OR (CI, 95%) | $p$-Value |
|---|---|---|---|
| **Sex** | | | |
| Male | 25 (47.17%) | 1.04 (0.56, 1.91) | 0.883 |
| Female | 28 (52.83%) | | |
| **Age** | | | |
| | NA | 1.02 (1.00, 1.04) | 0.027 |
| **Season** | | | |
| Rainy | 36 (67.92%) | 1.36 (0.72, 2.63) | 0.348 |
| Dry | 17 (32.08%) | | |
| **Months** | | | |
| June | 4 (7.54%) | 1.27 (0.28, 5.22) | 0.736 |
| July | 2 (3.77%) | 1.91 (0.22, 13.74) | 0.515 |
| August | 8 (15.09%) | 0.65 (0.22, 2.00) | 0.445 |
| September | 7 (13.20%) | 0.69 (0.21, 2.20) | 0.534 |
| October | 17 (32.07%) | 0.76 (0.29, 2.08) | 0.548 |
| November | 9 (16.98%) | 0.60 (0.20, 1.80) | 0.356 |
| December | 6 (11.32%) | 0.55 (0.16, 1.81) | 0.335 |
| **Location** | | | |
| Agnam Civol | 22 (41.50%) | 1.75 (0.63, 5.69) | 0.308 |
| Agnam Godo, Agnam Sinthou Cire, Badiya, Idite, Ngouloum, Thilogne, Yero Yabe | 1 (1.88%) | 8.50 (0.04 6.32) | 0.888 |
| Agnam Ouro Ciré | 13 (24.52%) | 2.94 (0.98, 1.00) | 0.063 |
| Bagonde | 5 (9.43%) | 2.61 (0.63, 1.09) | 0.176 |
| Bele | 4 (7.54%) | 6.80 (1.26, 3.89) | 0.024 |
| Toulel Thiale | 2 (3.77%) | 1.51 (0.19, 8.40) | 0.652 |

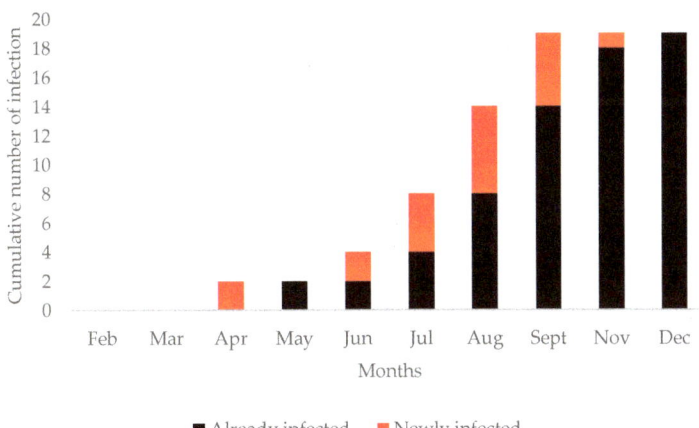

Figure 3. Temporal occurrence of anti-RVFV IgG among Sheep.

Furthermore, the typical clinical signs of RVFV infection, such as abortion storm among pregnant females, were not observed in the sentinel sheep. Additionally, mortality rates did not abnormally increase among lambs or young sheep during the livestock sheep survey. Reverse transcription real-time polymerase chain reaction (RT-PCR) for RVFV NSs detection shows that no sheep was positive for RVFV infection. We noticed that RVFV seroconversion occurred mostly in the rainy season ($p$ = 0.0152), particularly in August ($p$ = 0.002786) and

September ($p$ = 0.000191). The presence of anti-RVFV IgG was significatively higher in adult sheep ($p$ = 0.0000000387) (Table 2). During the survey, two deaths were recorded, but neither was positive for RVFV by RT-PCR and Enzyme-Linked Immunosorbent Assay (ELISA) tests (Table 2).

**Table 2.** Risk factors for RVF in livestock sheep. N IgG (%) = sheep with anti-RVFV IgG antibodies (percentage of sheep with anti-RVFV IgG).

|  | N IgG (%) | OR (CI, 95%) | $p$-Value |
|---|---|---|---|
| **Age** | | | |
| Juvenile | 2 (10%) | 1.21 (1.14, 1.31) | 0.0000000387 |
| Adult | 18 (90%) | | |
| **Season** | | | |
| Dry | 3 (15%) | 1.84 (1.12, 3.03) | 0.0152 |
| Rainy | 17 (85%) | | |
| **Months** | | | |
| February | 0 | 1.38 (7.96, 1.33) | 0.988 |
| March | 0 | 1.38 (2.19, 6.91) | 0.988 |
| April | 2 (10%) | 2.13 (3.86, 1.62) | 0.401 |
| May | 0 | 1.00 (1.14, 8.75) | 1 |
| June | 2 (10%) | 2.13 (3.86, 1.62) | 0.401 |
| July | 4 (20%) | 4.14 (9.12, 2.94) | 0.0915 |
| August | 6 (30%) | 1.12 (2.75, 7.62) | 0.002786 |
| September | 5 (25%) | 2.02 (5.03, 1.38) | 0.000191 |
| November | 1 (5%) | 2.02 (5.03, 1.38) | 0.000191 |
| December | 0 | 2.02 (5.03, 1.38) | 0.000191 |
| **Sex** | | | |
| Male | 0 (0%) | 6.39 (NA, 1.30) | 0.985 |
| Female | 20 (100%) | | |

Analysis shows that the force of infection (FOI) increased by 80.4% per month (CI: 53.6 to 100%) (Figure 4).

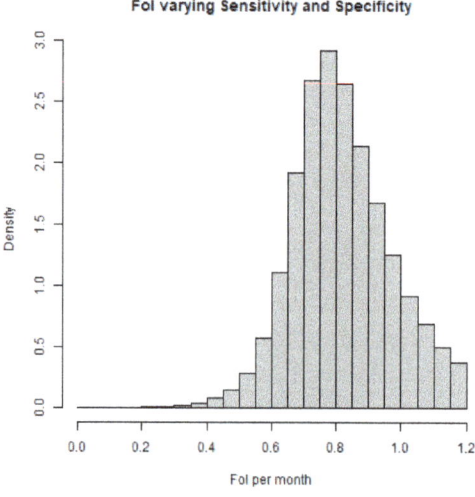

**Figure 4.** Force of infection (FOI) among livestock sheep. The density is determined by the proportion of individuals (sheep) contained in each age group.

## 4. Discussion

Rift Valley Fever Virus (RVFV) remains a major threat to human and livestock health. To survey RVFV emergence, a molecular and serological pilot survey study of RVF was undertaken in Agnam, a northern Senegal area with a high risk of RVFV emergence. Among the two hundred fifty-five human patients tested, one (1) was positive for anti-RVFV immunoglobulin M (IgM) (0.39%), and the anti-RVFV IgG test performed 20 days after the anti-RVFV IgM test became positive. To our knowledge, this patient represents the first ever reported case of acute human RVFV infection in the Agnam area and shows the usefulness of monitoring emerging disease surveillance through a human survey. The anti-RVFV IgM patient reported having contact with livestock animals such as cattle, goats, sheep, horses, and donkeys, which classed her at high risk of RVF infection or exposure. Ultimately, this woman recovered without complications. Importantly, our results show that 53 (20.78%) patients presented anti-RVFV IgG, which means they were already exposed to RVFV. This finding shows that RVFV actively circulates among the human population in this area. Human overall seroprevalence (IgM + IgG) is 21.17%, which is a comparable rate to the 21.30% found in Rosso (northern Senegal) [24], the 22.30% found in Yonofere (central Senegal) [25], and the 21% found in Moudjeria (Mauritania) [26]. However, the 20.78% rate is lower than the seroprevalence reported in Kenya [27], at a rate of 36.40%. This difference could be explained by the fact that during the Kenyan study, they sampled a high-risk population, unlike our study where only febrile patients were tested. Still, our seroprevalence is higher than those found in Nigeria (5.3% [28]) and in Senegal (6.5% in Linguere (central Senegal), Mbour (western Senegal), and Kedougou (southern Senegal) [29], 0.89% in Kedougou (southern) [30], and 5.2% in Diawara (southern Senegal) [31]). This difference could be due to the different epidemic factors or profiles between our study areas. Historically, northern Senegal including Agnam is known to be at high risk for RVFV emergence because of its proximity to endemic areas. Furthermore, Agnam is located in the Matam region, one of the main paths of human transport of livestock into Senegal, Mauritania, and Mali [32]. Interestingly, previous studies show that transboundary livestock trade between countries has been related to the Comoros island RVFV outbreak [33] and the reemergence of RVFV in Somalia [34]. Indeed, epizootics (amplification of the virus in an animal population such as livestock animals) acting as a vector have usually preceded human RVFV epidemics [22].

The animal survey showed that seroconversion to RVFV occurred in 20 of the 30 livestock sheep (66.67%), and anti-RVFV IgG persisted until the end of the study (December 2021). Furthermore, high mortality rates among the sheep, including abortion storms, were not observed during the livestock animal survey. These results could indicate that RVFV circulates sub-clinically in our livestock sheep. The high seroprevalence (66.67%) found in this study is comparable to the 75% reported in Senegal [29], 55% from Mauritania [35], and 45% from Uganda [34]. Our prevalence is higher than that reported in Senegal (14.3%) [8], Mauritania (3.8%) [36], the Central African Republic (12.9%) [37], and Uganda (4%) [38], which could be explained by the long exposure time (11 months) of the sentinel sheep in natural settings. The increasing seroprevalence in sheep (Figure 3) has preceded the only anti-RVFV IgM human case found in this study (Figure 2), which, in conjunction with her contact with livestock, suggests RVFV replication in sheep could have also led to the first human acute case of RVFV.

Our results show that seropositivity was significatively higher in the older population in both humans and sheep, which supports previously documented studies [16,22,38]. A study conducted in the lower Senegal river basin demonstrated that children born after the 1987 RVF outbreak have a small anti-RVFV IgG antibody rate (5%) compared to the elder population (25.3%) [22]. Our age-associated results are supported by the increased FOI with time (years or months in each group). The first recorded human acute case of RVF in Agnam is a 60-year-old woman in our study whose disease was detected in October 2021, which is in line with age and rainfall being major factors in RVF epidemiology. Likewise, nearly all seroconversion occurred in adult animals and during the rainy season (28 of 30 animals).

## 5. Conclusions

This study provided evidence of RVF circulation in humans and livestock. These results highlighted the importance of RVFV surveys in both humans and animals for averting potential RVF outbreaks. Our findings show that in Agnam, the highest RVFV seroconversion rates occur in the rainy season, and the elder population is the most at risk of RVFV exposure. Accordingly, an immunization campaign for RVFV vaccine implementation should be established in the dry season. Lastly, to improve RVFV epidemiological studies in Agnam, a survey of mosquitoes/vectors and other hosts needs to be conducted alongside human and animal surveys for the elucidation of the mechanisms underlying RVFV emergence in the northern Senegal area and beyond.

**Author Contributions:** Conceptualization, O.F. (Oumar Faye) and M.D.; methodology, O.F. (Oumar Faye), M.D., O.N., M.M. (Moufid Mhamadi), M.M. (Moundhir Mhamadi), M.N. (Mignane Ndiaye) and C.T.T.; software, M.M. (Moundhir Mhamadi); validation, O.F. (Oumar Faye), M.D. and O.F. (Ousmane Faye); formal analysis, M.M. (Moufid Mhamadi), A.B., M.N. (Mignane Ndiaye), M.M. (Moundhir Mhamadi) and C.T.T.; investigation, M.A.B., S.N.S., M.M. (Moufid Mhamadi), M.N. (Mamadou Ndiaye), B.D., M.F. and C.L.; resources, M.M. (Moundhir Mhamadi); data curation, M.M. (Moufid Mhamadi), H.F.-B., O.F. (Oumar Faye), M.D., A.G. and E.H.N.; writing—original draft preparation, M.M. (Moufid Mhamadi), A.B., O.F. (Oumar Faye), M.D., A.G., E.H.N. and B.F.; writing—review and editing, M.M. (Moufid Mhamadi), A.B., O.F. (Oumar Faye), M.D., A.G., A.M.D., A.XIII and E.H.N.; visualization, M.M. (Moufid Mhamadi), A.B., H.F.-B., O.F. (Oumar Faye) and M.D.; supervision, H.F.-B., O.F. (Oumar Faye) and M.D.; project administration, H.F.-B., O.F. (Oumar Faye), M.D., O.F. (Ousmane Faye), A.A.S. and G.K.; funding acquisition, H.F.-B. and G.K. All authors have read and agreed to the published version of the manuscript.

**Funding:** This research was funded by the International Development Research Center (grant 109075-001) and the Canadian Department of Global Affairs (grant BIO-2019-005).

**Institutional Review Board Statement:** The study was conducted according to the Declaration of Helsinki and approved by the National Ethical Committee for Health Research in Senegal (# 00000806 MSAS/DPRS/DR) for studies involving humans and animals.

**Informed Consent Statement:** Informed consent was obtained from all subjects involved in the study.

**Data Availability Statement:** Not applicable.

**Acknowledgments:** We acknowledge our colleagues of the IPD Virology Department and the Medical Zoology Department for their tremendous scientific and technical support.

**Conflicts of Interest:** The authors declare no conflict of interest. The funders had no role in the design of the study; in the collection, analysis, or interpretation of data; in the writing of the manuscript; or in the decision to publish the results.

## References

1. Wright, D.; Kortekaas, J.; Bowden, T.A.; Warimwe, G.M. Rift Valley Fever: Biology and epidemiology. *J. Gen. Virol.* **2019**, *100*, 1187–1199. [CrossRef] [PubMed]
2. Daubney, R.; Hudson, J.R. Enzootic hepatitis or Rift Valley Fever. An undescribed virus disease of sheep cattle and man from East Africa. *J. Pathol. Bacteriol.* **1931**, *34*, 545–579. [CrossRef]
3. Digoutte, J.P.; Peters, C.J. General aspects of the 1987 Rift Valley Fever epidemic in Mauritania. *Res. Virol.* **1989**, *140*, 27–30. [CrossRef]
4. Ba, Y.; Sall, A.A.; Diallo, D.; Mondo, M.; Girault, L.; Dia, I.; Diallo, M. Re-emergence of Rift Valley Fever virus in Barkedji (Senegal, West Africa) in 2002-2003: Identification of new vectors and epidemiological implications. *J. Am. Mosq. Control Assoc.* **2012**, *28*, 170–178. [CrossRef] [PubMed]
5. Bob, N.S.; Barry, M.A.; Diagne, M.M.; Faye, M.; Ndione, M.H.D.; Diallo, A.; Diop, M.; Diop, B.; Faye, O.; Loucoubar, C.; et al. Detection of Rift Valley Fever Virus Lineage H from South Africa through Syndromic Sentinel Surveillance Network in Senegal. *Open Forum Infect. Dis.* **2021**, *9*, ofab655. [CrossRef] [PubMed]

6. Bob, N.S.; Bâ, H.; Fall, G.; Ishagh, E.; Diallo, M.Y.; Sow, A.; Sembene, P.M.; Faye, O.; El Kouri, B.; Sidi, M.L.; et al. Detection of the Northeastern African Rift Valley Fever Virus Lineage During the 2015 Outbreak in Mauritania. *Open Forum Infect. Dis.* **2017**, *4*, ofx087. [CrossRef] [PubMed]
7. Diallo, D.; Talla, C.; Ba, Y.; Dia, I.; Sall, A.A.; Diallo, M. Temporal distribution and spatial pattern of abundance of the Rift Valley Fever and West Nile fever vectors in Barkedji, Senegal. *J. Vector Ecol. J. Soc. Vector Ecol.* **2011**, *36*, 426–436. [CrossRef]
8. Durand, B.; Lo Modou, M.; Tran, A.; Ba, A.; Sow, F.; Belkhiria, J.; Fall, A.G.; Biteye, B.; Grosbois, V.; Chevalier, V. Rift Valley Fever in northern Senegal: A modelling approach to analyse the processes underlying virus circulation recurrence. *PLoS Negl. Trop. Dis.* **2020**, *14*, e0008009. [CrossRef]
9. Monlun, E.; Zeller, H.; Le Guenno, B.; Traoré-Lamizana, M.; Hervy, J.P.; Adam, F.; Ferrara, L.; Fontenille, D.; Sylla, R.; Mondo, M. Surveillance of the circulation of arbovirus of medical interest in the region of eastern Senegal. *Bull. Soc. Pathol. Exot.* **1990**, *86*, 21–28.
10. Saluzzo, J.F.; Chartier, C.; Bada, R.; Martinez, D.; Digoutte, J.P. La Fièvre de la Vallée du Rift en Afrique de l'Ouest. *Rev. D'élevage Médecine Vétérinaire Pays Trop.* **1987**, *40*, 215–223.
11. Thiongane, Y.; Gonzalez, J.P.; Fati, A.; Akakpo, J.A. Changes in Rift Valley Fever neutralizing antibody prevalence among small domestic ruminants following the 1987 outbreak in the Senegal River basin. *Res. Virol.* **1991**, *142*, 67–70. [CrossRef] [PubMed]
12. Ndiaye, E.H.; Fall, G.; Gaye, A.; Bob, N.S.; Talla, C.; Diagne, C.T.; Diallo, D.; BA, Y.; Dia, I.; Kohl, A.; et al. Vector competence of Aedes vexans (Meigen), Culex poicilipes (Theobald) and Cx. quinquefasciatus Say from Senegal for West and East African lineages of Rift Valley Fever virus. *Parasites Vectors* **2016**, *9*, 94. [CrossRef]
13. Ikegami, T.; Makino, S. The pathogenesis of Rift Valley Fever. *Viruses* **2011**, *3*, 493–519. [CrossRef] [PubMed]
14. Paweska, J.T.; Burt, F.J.; Anthony, F.; Smith, S.J.; Grobbelaar, A.A.; Croft, J.E.; Ksiazek, T.G.; Swanepoel, R. IgG-sandwich and IgM-capture enzyme-linked immunosorbent assay for the detection of antibody to Rift Valley fever virus in domestic ruminants. *J. Virol. Methods* **2003**, *113*, 103–112. [CrossRef]
15. Ikegami, T. Molecular biology and genetic diversity of Rift Valley Fever virus. *Antiviral Res.* **2012**, *95*, 293–310. [CrossRef] [PubMed]
16. Dungu, B.; Lubisi, B.A.; Ikegami, T. Rift Valley Fever vaccines: Current and future needs. *Curr. Opin. Virol.* **2018**, *29*, 8–15. [CrossRef]
17. Von Teichman, B.; Engelbrecht, A.; Zulu, G.; Dungu, B.; Pardini, A.; Bouloy, M. Safety and efficacy of Rift Valley fever Smithburn and Clone 13 vaccines in calves. *Vaccine* **2011**, *29*, 5771–5777. [CrossRef]
18. Mhamadi, M.; Badji, A.; Dieng, I.; Gaye, A.; Ndiaye, E.H.; Mignane, N.; Mhamadi, M.; Touré, C.T.; Mbaye, M.R.; Barry, M.A.; et al. Crimean–Congo Hemorrhagic Fever Virus Survey in Humans, Ticks, and Livestock in Agnam (Northeastern Senegal) from February 2021 to March 2022. *Trop. Med. Infect. Dis.* **2022**, *7*, 324. [CrossRef]
19. Barry, M.A.; Arinal, F.; Talla, C.; Hedible, B.G.; Sarr, F.D.; Ba, I.O.; Diop, B.; Dia, N.; Vray, M. Performance of case definitions and clinical predictors for influenza surveillance among patients followed in a rural cohort in Senegal. *BMC Infect. Dis.* **2021**, *21*, 31. [CrossRef]
20. Weidmann, M.; Sanchez-Seco, M.P.; Sall, A.A.; Ly, P.O.; Thiongane, Y.; Lô, M.M.; Schley, H.; Hufert, F.T. Rapid detection of important human pathogenic Phleboviruses. *J. Clin. Virol.* **2008**, *41*, 138–142. [CrossRef]
21. Alexander, N.; Carabali, M.K.; Lim, J. Estimating force of infection from serologic surveys with imperfect tests. *PLoS ONE* **2021**, *16*, e0247255. [CrossRef] [PubMed]
22. Schlattmann, P. *Medical Applications of Finite Mixture Models, Statistics for Biology and Health*; Springer: Berlin/Heidelberg, Germany, 2009. [CrossRef]
23. Do, C.B.; Batzoglou, S. What is the expectation maximization algorithm? *Nat. Biotechnol.* **2008**, *26*, 897–899. [CrossRef] [PubMed]
24. Thonnon, J.; Picquet, M.; Thiongane, Y.; Lo, M.; Sylla, R.; Vercruysse, J. Rift Valley Fever surveillance in the lower Senegal river basin: Update 10 years after the epidemic. *Trop. Med. Int. Health* **1999**, *4*, 580–585. [CrossRef] [PubMed]
25. Wilson, M.L.; Chapman, L.E.; Hall, D.B.; Dykstra, E.A.; Ba, K.; Zeller, H.G.; Traore-Lamizana, M.; Hervy, J.P.; Linthicum, K.J.; Peters, C.J. Rift Valley Fever in rural northern Senegal: Human risk factors and potential vectors. *Am. J. Trop. Med. Hyg.* **1994**, *50*, 663–675. [CrossRef]
26. Sow, A.; Faye Ousmane Ba, Y.; Ba, H.; Diallo, D.; Faye Oumar Loucoubar, C.; Boushab, M.; Barry, Y.; Diallo, M.; Sall, A.A. Rift Valley Fever outbreak, southern Mauritania, 2012. *Emerg. Infect. Dis.* **2014**, *20*, 296–299. [CrossRef]
27. Tigoi, C.; Sang, R.; Chepkorir, E.; Orindi, B.; Arum, S.O.; Mulwa, F.; Mosomtai, G.; Limbaso, S.; Hassan, O.A.; Irura, Z.; et al. High risk for human exposure to Rift Valley Fever virus in communities living along livestock movement routes: A cross-sectional survey in Kenya. *PLoS Negl. Trop. Dis.* **2020**, *14*, e0007979. [CrossRef]
28. Opayele, A.V.; Odaibo, G.N.; Olaleye, O.D. Rift Valley Fever virus infection among livestock handlers in Ibadan, Nigeria. *J. Immunoass. Immunochem.* **2018**, *39*, 609–621. [CrossRef]
29. Sow, A.; Faye Ousmane Ba, Y.; Diallo, D.; Fall, G.; Faye Oumar Bob, N.S.; Loucoubar, C.; Richard, V.; Dia, A.T.; Diallo, M.; Malvy, D.; et al. Widespread Rift Valley Fever Emergence in Senegal in 2013–2014. *Open Forum Infect. Dis.* **2016**, *3*, ofw149. [CrossRef]
30. Sow, A.; Faye, O.; Faye, O.; Diallo, D.; Sadio, B.D.; Weaver, S.C.; Diallo, M.; Sall, A.A. Rift Valley Fever in Kedougou, southeastern Senegal, 2012. *Emerg. Infect. Dis.* **2014**, *20*, 504–506. [CrossRef]
31. Marrama, L.; Spiegel, A.; Ndiaye, K.; Sall, A.A.; Gomes, E.; Diallo, M.; Thiongane, Y.; Mathiot, C.; Gonzalez, J.P. Domestic transmission of Rift Valley Fever virus in Diawara (Senegal) in 1998. *Southeast Asian J. Trop. Med. Public Health* **2005**, *36*, 1487–1495.

32. ONUAA. La transhumance transfrontalière en Afrique de l'Ouest Proposition de plan d'action 5, 764. 2012. Available online: https://www.inter-reseaux.org/wp-content/uploads/Transhumance_Transfrontalier_en_AO_Rapport_FAO.pdf (accessed on 7 January 2023).
33. Roger, M.; Girard, S.; Faharoudine, A.; Halifa, M.; Bouloy, M.; Cetre-Sossah, C.; Cardinale, E. Rift Valley Fever in Ruminants, Republic of Comoros, 2009. *Emerg. Infect. Dis.* **2011**, *17*, 1319–1320. [CrossRef] [PubMed]
34. Birungi, D.; Aceng, F.L.; Bulage, L.; Nkonwa, I.H.; Mirembe, B.B.; Biribawa, C.; Okethwangu, D.; Opio, N.D.; Monje, F.; Muwanguzi, D.; et al. Sporadic Rift Valley Fever Outbreaks in Humans and Animals in Uganda, October 2017–January 2018. *J. Environ. Public Health* **2021**, *2021*, 8881191. [CrossRef] [PubMed]
35. Jäckel, S.; Eiden, M.; El Mamy, B.O.; Isselmou, K.; Vina-Rodriguez, A.; Doumbia, B.; Groschup, M.H. Molecular and serological studies on the Rift Valley Fever outbreak in Mauritania in 2010. *Transbound. Emerg. Dis.* **2013**, *60* (Suppl. 2), 31–39. [CrossRef] [PubMed]
36. Rissmann, M.; Eiden, M.; El Mamy, B.O.; Isselmou, K.; Doumbia, B.; Ziegler, U.; Homeier-Bachmann, T.; Yahya, B.; Groschup, M.H. Serological and genomic evidence of Rift Valley Fever virus during inter-epidemic periods in Mauritania. *Epidemiol. Infect.* **2017**, *145*, 1058–1068. [CrossRef] [PubMed]
37. Nakouné, E.; Kamgang, B.; Berthet, N.; Manirakiza, A.; Kazanji, M. Rift Valley Fever Virus Circulating among Ruminants, Mosquitoes and Humans in the Central African Republic. *PLoS Negl. Trop. Dis.* **2016**, *10*, e0005082. [CrossRef] [PubMed]
38. Nyakarahuka, L.; de St Maurice, A.; Purpura, L.; Ervin, E.; Balinandi, S.; Tumusiime, A.; Kyondo, J.; Mulei, S.; Tusiime, P.; Lutwama, J.; et al. Prevalence and risk factors of Rift Valley Fever in humans and animals from Kabale district in Southwestern Uganda, 2016. *PLoS Negl. Trop. Dis.* **2018**, *12*, e0006412. [CrossRef] [PubMed]

**Disclaimer/Publisher's Note:** The statements, opinions and data contained in all publications are solely those of the individual author(s) and contributor(s) and not of MDPI and/or the editor(s). MDPI and/or the editor(s) disclaim responsibility for any injury to people or property resulting from any ideas, methods, instructions or products referred to in the content.

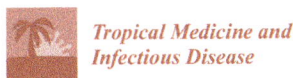 *Tropical Medicine and Infectious Disease*

*Article*

# The COVID-19 Infodemic on Twitter: A Space and Time Topic Analysis of the Brazilian Immunization Program and Public Trust

Victor Diogho Heuer de Carvalho [1,*], Thyago Celso Cavalcante Nepomuceno [2], Thiago Poleto [3] and Ana Paula Cabral Seixas Costa [4]

1. Eixo das Tecnologias, Campus do Sertão, Universidade Federal de Alagoas, Delmiro Gouveia 57480-000, Brazil
2. Núcleo de Tecnologia, Centro Acadêmico do Agreste, Universidade Federal de Pernambuco, Caruaru 55014-900, Brazil
3. Departamento de Administração, Instituto de Ciências Sociais Aplicadas, Universidade Federal do Pará, Belém 66075-110, Brazil
4. Departamento de Engenharia de Produção, Centro de Tecnologia e Geociências, Universidade Federal de Pernambuco, Recife 50740-550, Brazil
* Correspondence: victor.carvalho@delmiro.ufal.br

**Citation:** de Carvalho, V.D.H.; Nepomuceno, T.C.C.; Poleto, T.; Costa, A.P.C.S. The COVID-19 Infodemic on Twitter: A Space and Time Topic Analysis of the Brazilian Immunization Program and Public Trust. *Trop. Med. Infect. Dis.* **2022**, *7*, 425. https://doi.org/10.3390/tropicalmed7120425

Academic Editor: Yannick Simonin

Received: 31 October 2022
Accepted: 3 December 2022
Published: 9 December 2022

**Publisher's Note:** MDPI stays neutral with regard to jurisdictional claims in published maps and institutional affiliations.

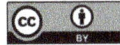

**Copyright:** © 2022 by the authors. Licensee MDPI, Basel, Switzerland. This article is an open access article distributed under the terms and conditions of the Creative Commons Attribution (CC BY) license (https:// creativecommons.org/licenses/by/ 4.0/).

**Abstract:** The context of the COVID-19 pandemic has brought to light the infodemic phenomenon and the problem of misinformation. Agencies involved in managing COVID-19 immunization programs are also looking for ways to combat this problem, demanding analytical tools specialized in identifying patterns of misinformation and understanding how they have evolved in time and space to demonstrate their effects on public trust. The aim of this article is to present the results of a study applying topic analysis in space and time with respect to public opinion on the Brazilian COVID-19 immunization program. The analytical process involves applying topic discovery to tweets with geoinformation extracted from the COVID-19 vaccination theme. After extracting the topics, they were submitted to manual annotation, whereby the polarity labels pro, anti, and neutral were applied based on the support and trust in the COVID-19 vaccination. A space and time analysis was carried out using the topic and polarity distributions, making it possible to understand moments during which the most significant quantities of posts occurred and the cities that generated the most tweets. The analytical process describes a framework capable of meeting the needs of agencies for tools, providing indications of how misinformation has evolved and where its dissemination focuses, in addition to defining the granularity of this information according to what managers define as adequate. The following research outcomes can be highlighted. (1) We identified a specific date containing a peak that stands out among the other dates, indicating an event that mobilized public opinion about COVID-19 vaccination. (2) We extracted 23 topics, enabling the manual polarity annotation of each topic and an understanding of which polarities were associated with tweets. (3) Based on the association between polarities, topics, and tweets, it was possible to identify the Brazilian cities that produced the majority of tweets for each polarity and the amount distribution of tweets relative to cities populations.

**Keywords:** COVID-19; infodemic; misinformation; Twitter; topic analysis; immunization program; public trust; Brazil

## 1. Introduction

The pandemic has significantly impacted people's daily lives worldwide, affecting work, education, and social interactions and leading to the enforcement of distancing measures worldwide [1–3]. Physical distancing made people interact predominantly through virtual and online platforms such as social networks, video-conference software, and instant messenger applications [4]. In addition to adopting home-based work [5], these interactions generated large volumes of data that can be retrieved for various types of analysis [6,7], supporting strategies to mitigate the COVID-19 outbreak, from early detections to monitoring infodemic phenomena based on people's opinions and emotions, and the misinformation spread through the social web [8].

The opinions and sentiments expressed by people about aspects of the pandemic have triggered worldwide research seeking to analyze the associated patterns and generate informational inputs to support actions in favor of combating the social effects of COVID-19 [9]. Among the themes studied by researchers worldwide based on opinions and sentiment analysis, the construction of corpora about the pandemic can be considered a starting point for any related analysis (see, for instance, [10–14]).

In this context, Cotfas et al. [15] analyzed public opinion about COVID-19 vaccination in the United Kingdom. Topics were extracted using latent Dirichlet allocation (LDA) to support the analysis of the opinions. The authors suggested that their findings can be used to combat public hesitation with respect to vaccines, as information about the causes of such hesitation can be extracted through topics.

Abdulaziz et al. [10] also focused on sentiment analysis of COVID-19, using LDA to extract topics from Twitter texts and the Valence Aware Dictionary and Sentiment Reasoner (VADER) lexicon model to classify text sentiments. Using these techniques, they identified trending topics during the pandemic, including "drugs research", "news", "losses", 'economy", "lockdown", "updated cases", "school closures", and "rules", separating the topics according to positive, neutral, and negative labels.

Melton et al. [16] applied public sentiment analysis using information shared in Reddit communities about COVID-19 vaccines, using the LDA to model and extract topics, classifying them according to their sentiment polarity ("positive", "negative", or "neutral"). The study results showed that Reddit communities expressed more positive than negative opinions about vaccine-related content, maintaining this tendency over time.

Shi et al. [17] developed a study on emotional analysis based on public opinion among the Chinese population, using posts from the Weibo microblog platform. In their analytical process, they applied LDA for topic discovery and text emotion extraction using a pre-existing emotional ontology vocabulary and analyzed the evolution of emotional timelines for Chinese cities, in addition to identifying the most discussed topics during the first wave of the COVID-19 pandemic.

In a study with a medical infoveillance orientation, Mackey et al. [18] applied topic modeling using the Biterm Topic Model (BTM) to detect and characterize conversations among Twitter users that were COVID-19-related. The authors reported that tweets could be separated into five kinds: those related to reports of symptoms, those involving symptom reporting concurrent with lack of testing, those containing discussions about recovery, those containing discussions about test confirmations reporting a negative COVID-19 diagnosis, and those recalling symptoms and questioning whether they had already contracted the disease.

Daradkeh [19] presented an analytical framework for topic modeling COVID-19 misinformation on social media using LDA, sentiment analysis, and VADER. The topic model consisted of vaccination policy and strategy, society and community, organizations and institutions, family and friends, vaccination behavior, and vaccination experience. Sentiment analysis separated tweets into four classes: misinformation combined with positive sentiment, misinformation combined with negative sentiment, non-misinformation with positive sentiment, and non-misinformation with negative sentiment, enabling the generation of a sentiment trend timeline over six months.

Wang et al. [20] analyzed topic and feature distribution relative to the need for public information on COVID-19 using texts extracted from a Chinese online question-and-answer community. Their methodology applied LDA and the *k*-means clustering algorithm, obtaining as results keywords related to the public information about vaccination, a co-keywords network, and an "information needs framework" based on the results of both methods, elucidating, for instance, the information needs of various social groups.

Zhu et al. [21] developed a public opinion analysis framework based on LDA for topic modeling and Bidirectional Encoder Representations from Transformers (BERT) with Functional Data Analysis (FDA) for sentiment classification using data collected from Weibo platform in China. A remarkable result of their research was the distinction between positive and negative posts, revealing differences in the topics with vaccine-support and vaccine-hesitant orientations.

Xie et al. [22] reviewed the Chinese government's information about COVID-19 to identify scientific communication topics. They applied LDA, correlation analysis, and analysis of variance (ANOVA) on a collection of news briefings composing a science-related corpus. They found topics related to communication about (1) prevention, control, epidemiological investigation, and personal health according to the popularization of scientific knowledge models; (2) research on Chinese medicine, vaccines, and medical resources according to the public understanding of scientific knowledge; and (3) citizen, community, and enterprise participation in scientific knowledge co-production.

Another interesting study related to the pandemic was developed by Zhou et al. [23] in China to assess the spatio-temporal characteristics of public sentiments about COVID-19 in small cities, supporting public agencies to decide on anti-pandemic measures. They applied a dictionary-based sentiment analysis, local Moran's index, and kernel-density analysis to support analyzing non-linear evolution and clustering characteristics of public sentiment in space and in time.

The vaccination campaign against COVID-19 in Brazil was marked by the division of public opinion, with discussions and confrontations between pro- and anti-vaccination groups on social networks and the notable dissemination of misinformation about vaccines [24,25]. Political interference in support of both movements in Brazil took this discussion to a different level, leading to an investigation by the Brazilian Senate into potential crimes committed throughout the entire process of fighting COVID-19, from sanitary and isolation measures to the vaccines' purchasing [26] and even considering politicians' negationism about the pandemic [27].

The dissemination of misinformation about COVID-19 vaccination in Brazil and the world brought to light the need for immunization program management agencies to properly analyze the infodemic phenomenon [27]. It includes analytical tools able to demonstrate how misinformation evolves in time and space, ensuring the understanding of where and when it emerged, understanding the effects on the population, and making it possible to replace "wrong" with "right" information [24,28,29].

Some recent studies have indicated paths to be followed to address this need. We highlight those that are most associated with the research we carry out: applying methods to discover patterns in comments and opinions indicating the commenter's behavior [30]; systematizing the assessment of underlying exogenous variables related to people's belief in misinformation [31]; building datasets with significant amounts of texts to be used by analytical tools, providing reliable results, considering texts with geographic information, and obtaining them from multiple channels to extend the studies validity [10,25,32].

The present article reports a new study expanding the findings of de Carvalho et al. [33], who applied temporal opinion analysis to tweets about COVID-19 vaccination in Brazil. The main objective is to present the results of a spatio-temporal analysis of a set of geocoded tweets, demonstrating which topics were discussed between 2020 and 2021 through an interface that considers the distribution of posts over time and the Brazilian geographic space.

This study attempts to address the needs identified above by applying a methodological approach that public agencies managing the COVID-19 immunization program can use to combat the spread of misinformation, considering natural language processing tools, text mining, and machine learning to provide structured and helpful information.

Four research questions can be defined regarding our research problem:

(1) What topics were discussed during 2020 and 2021 on COVID-19 immunization in Brazil?

(2) What can be understood/interpreted about the extracted topics?
(3) How did topics evolve over time?
(4) How are they distributed in Brazilian territory, and which places have generated the most tweets?

Among the research findings, we highlight the most interesting: (1) the highest peak in the number of tweets for most of the topics and all polarities on 17 January 2021, the date of the first COVID-19 vaccine applied in Brazil; (2) twenty-three topics were extracted and, after manual annotation, fifteen of them received the pro-vaccination label, five the neutral label, and three the anti-vaccination label, indicating a predominance of topics supporting vaccination in Brazil within the period studied, according to the annotators' judgments; (3) through the association *polarity* → *topic* → *tweet*, it was possible to identify the Brazilian cities that produced the most tweets according to each polarity, and the distribution of the number of tweets according to the cities' population.

## 2. Methods

The methodological approach applied in our research was based on a social web mining framework [34] with the following main elements:

(1) Texts collection from Twitter
(2) Texts preprocessing
(3) Feature selection
(4) Topic modeling and discovery
(5) Spatio-temporal topic analysis

Figure 1 describes the workflow of this framework, divided into four parts, starting with the data acquisition and ending with the exploration of topic distribution in space and time.

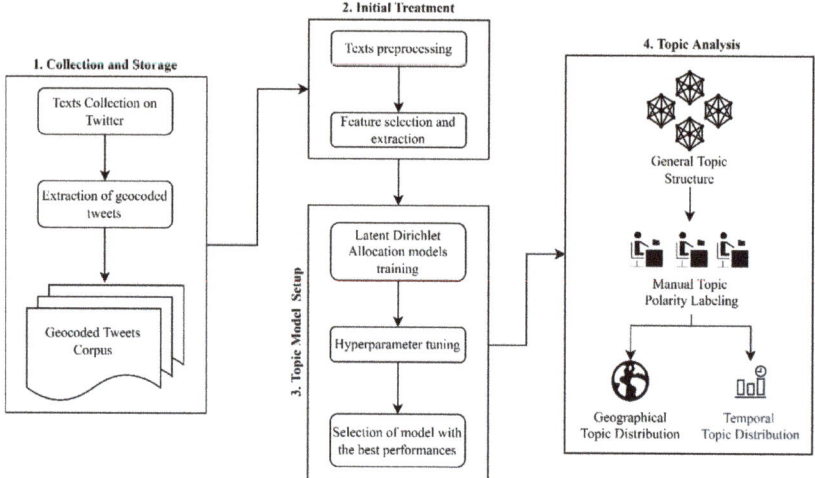

**Figure 1.** Workflow for the spatio-temporal topic analysis.

### 2.1. Texts Collection and Storage

The texts were collected using Twitter API 2.0 through a scraping script developed in Python, applying functions from the "requests" library. Larger corpora were constructed, as reported in de Carvalho et al. [33], but a subset containing only geocoded tweets was extracted, composing a georeferenced corpus. Table S1 in the Supplementary Materials presents the parameters used in the scraping script. The blocks of keywords applied for scraping are based on the studies by de Oliveira et al. [35] and de Carvalho et al. [33,36].

In the final steps of the scraping process, there is a preliminary treatment to exclude fields from tweets unrelated to this search. The final georeferenced corpus was stored in a comma-separated values (csv) file with the following fields:

(1) Tweet text (*text* field)
(2) Place name (*place_name* field)
(3) Country name (*country* field)
(4) Geographic coordinates (*point* field)
(5) Creation date (*created_at* field)

The geographic coordinates field consists of *latitude* and *longitude*, and it was later decomposed into specific vectors for each part of the coordinate. The dates were transformed into a readable format by the temporal analysis scripts.

## 2.2. Initial Treatment

A set of preprocessing functions was applied to minimize textual noise effects: case folding; duplicities exclusion; tasks for eliminating punctuation, emojis/emoticons, numbers, stop words, links/URLs; and tokenization. The preprocessing was developed through another Python script using mainly the Spacy library [37], which implements all the listed functions, and the Pandas library [38] for data frame manipulation and to convert data frames to the final storage file format (csv).

After preprocessing, the texts were vectorized using simple term counting (defining the frequency of the term) and the term frequency-inverse document frequency (TF-IDF). Both vectorization processes were applied using the respective functions available through the Scikit-Learn framework [39].

Each vectorization method received the lemmatized tokens extracted from the tweets. So, for the subsequent topic modeling and analysis phases, the words (treated as uni-grams) were the selected features.

## 2.3. Topic Model Setup

Topic modeling methods consist of converting numeric (document × term) vectors representing documents to (topic × term) and (document × topic) vectors [40]. The topic modeling applied in our study was based on the Latent Dirichlet Allocation (LDA), a hierarchical probabilistic model to decompose a collection of documents in topics based on probability distributions of vocabularies [41].

The model was proposed and described by Blei et al. [42] and can be represented by the generative process in Algorithm 1, where $N$ denotes a sequence of words $w = (w_1, w_2, \ldots, w_n)$, $\theta$ is a $k$-dimensional Dirichlet random variable that can assume values in the $(k-1)$-*simplex* vector. In our study, we used Scikit-Learn's LDA implementation considering the online variational Bayes method [43], using mini-batches of training data to update the number of components incrementally.

**Algorithm 1** Latent Dirichlet Allocation Generative Process

| | |
|---|---|
| 1. | For each document $w$ in a corpus $D$: |
| 1.1 | Choose $N \sim Poisson(\xi)$ |
| 1.2 | Choose $\theta \sim Dirichlet(\alpha)$ |
| 1.3 | For each of the $N$ words $w_n$: |
| 1.3.1 | Choose a topic $z_n \sim Multinomial(\theta)$ |
| 1.3.2 | Choose a word $w_n$ from $p(w_n|z_n, \beta)$, a multinomial probability related to the topic $z_n$ |

A hyperparameter tuning using Scikit-Learn's Grid Search function was performed, considering learning decays of 0.5, 0.7, and 0.9 for between 3 and 30 topics. The learning decays are parameters that control the learning rate when using the LDA online variational Bayes method and can vary from 0.3 to 1.0.

The Grid Search can deliver test scores such as the model perplexity and the log-likelihood ($\log p(w_d)$) for hyperparameter combinations. We can interpret the perplexity as a measure of the possibilities of the collection of unseen words of a text belonging to a topic, and the lower it is, the better the LDA model's performance [44]; the higher the log-likelihood, the better the model [42]. Scikit-Learn's perplexity function calculates the related score as $exp(-1 \times \log p(w_d))$.

*2.4. Topic Analysis*

The previous phase outputs enable the topic analysis. For the overall topic visualization, we used (1) intertopic distance mapping, (2) the most salient terms evidencing, and (3) topic segregation. For the intertopic distance mapping and the most salient terms, we used a Python library called pyLDAvis [45,46], automatically creating dashboards for topic visualization.

In the intertopic distance map, the extracted topics are represented by circles, and their area corresponds to each topic's term prevalence. The center of each topic is defined by calculating the distance between the topics, using a multidimensional scaling process to represent the distances on a two-dimensional plane [47]. The process to obtain the most salient terms consists of applying a saliency measure to filter and rank the terms, considering Equations (2) and (3) described by Chuang et al. [48]:

$$istinctiveness(w) = \sum_T P(T|w) \times \log \frac{P(T|w)}{P(T)} \qquad (2)$$

$$saliency(w) = P(w) \times distinctiveness(w) \qquad (3)$$

According to Chuang et al. [48], Equation (2) describes how informative the specific term $w$ is for determining the generating topic $T$, versus a randomly-selected term $w'$. Equation (3) describes how to calculate the salience measure, considering that given the number of words, the list of the most probable terms contains more generic words than the list of specific terms [48].

For topic segregation, we used the *t*-distributed stochastic neighbor embedding (*t*-SNE) implemented in Scikit-Learn and the Bokeh library [49] for plotting. The *t*-SNE was designed to alleviate the crowding problem in the traditional stochastic neighbor embedding (SNE) using a symmetric version of the SNE cost function [50]. Joint probabilities $p_{ij}$ described by Equations (4) and (5) are defined to measure similarities between objects $x_i$ and $x_j$, symmetrizing two conditional probabilities, where $\sigma_i$ represents the bandwidth of Gaussian kernels defined so that the perplexity of the conditional distribution $P_i$ is equal to a predefined perplexity $u$ [50,51].

$$p_{i|j} = \frac{\exp(-d(x_i, x_j)^2 / 2\sigma_i^2)}{\sum_{k \neq i} \exp\left(-d(x_i, x_k)^2 / 2\sigma_i^2\right)} \qquad (4)$$

$$p_{i|j} = \frac{p_{j|i} + p_{i|j}}{2N} \qquad (5)$$

The final part of the methodologic workflow is the space and time topic analysis. Using the results of the previous phase, we can perform the following tasks:

(1) Manual topic polarity labeling, dedicated to annotating the polarity trend associated with each topic into three types:

    (1) Supportive topic (pro), with positive relation, denoting trust about the COVID-19 vaccination.

    (2) Negationist or unsupportive topic (anti), with negative relation, denoting mistrust about vaccination.

    (3) Neutral topic (neutral), not associated with the types above.

(2) Geographical Topic Analysis is dedicated to visualizing and understanding the topics' distribution in a geographic area. There are two possible ways to perform this analy-

sis [52]: (1) discovering different topics of interest that are coherent across geographic regions and (2) comparing several topics across different geographical locations.

(3) Time Topic Analysis is dedicated to visualizing and understanding the topics' distribution over time. One example of this application can be seen in the study by Martin et al. [53].

In our research, the manual topic polarity annotation was performed by an initial group of three scholars, from different research areas, with different backgrounds: Informatics, Economics, and Life/Health Sciences. This manual labeling becomes necessary to ensure an alignment based on human knowledge and the consequent reliability of the topics concerning their positioning on the investigated theme. The use of three annotators is a way to ensure that, if there is a disagreement between the labels of two of them, the labeling of a third one can serve as a basis to define which polarity label will be defined [54]. If there is still a tie, even with the judgments of the three annotators, a fourth annotator will be invited to perform the tiebreakers only for the topics that caused indecision.

The Brazilian geographic space is considered for the analysis performed in this study, and the geographical topic analysis is aligned with the idea of discovering topics of interest across the Brazilian geographic regions. Using data collected from June 2020 to October 2021, we could perform the time topic analysis, demonstrating the evolution of the discussions. Graphs were developed using the Python Matplotlib library [55], and the geographical features were handled using the GeoPandas library [56].

## 3. Results and Discussion

The results will be presented following, divided into (1) the general findings, considering initial data about the corpus constructed for the spatio-temporal analysis; (2) the topic modeling results according to the Grid Search applied; and (3) topic analysis findings, considering the manual labeling, and the spatio-temporal analysis.

### 3.1. General Findings

Considering the geocoded tweets extracted from one of the corpora presented by de Carvalho et al. [33], the initial corpus composition for the present study contained 62,873 tweets. We applied a cleaning process to eliminate tweets that escaped location and language filters, resulting in 55,758 tweets. Table S2 in the Supplementary Materials contains an example of georeferenced corpus content, with its first five lines. Figure 2 presents the tweets' amounts over the seventeen months (from June 2020 to October 2021).

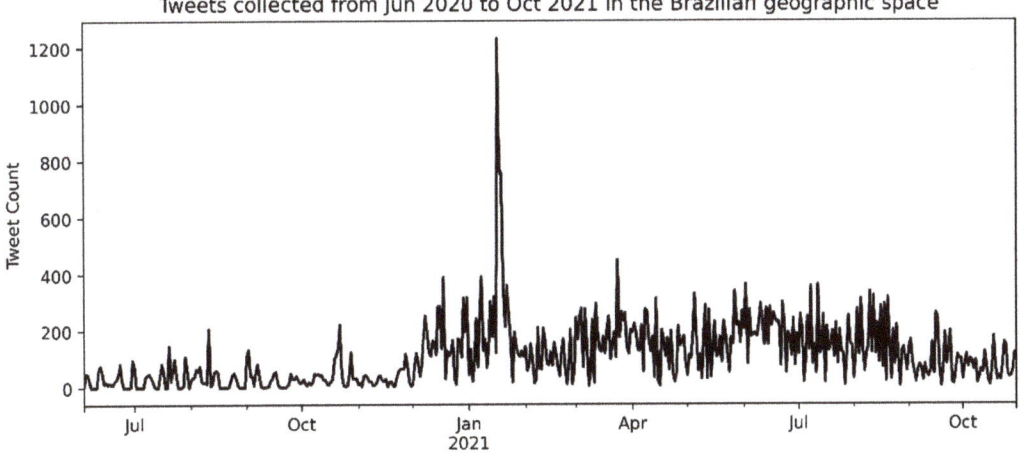

**Figure 2.** Overall tweets distribution over 17 months.

The number of tweets started to increase in mid-December 2020; in addition, there was a peak with 1224 tweets on 17 January 2021, identified by analyzing the collected data. Both situations were also noted in the study by de Carvalho et al. [33]. Figure 3 presents the general distribution of tweets according to the cities that generated them in the Brazilian municipal grid.

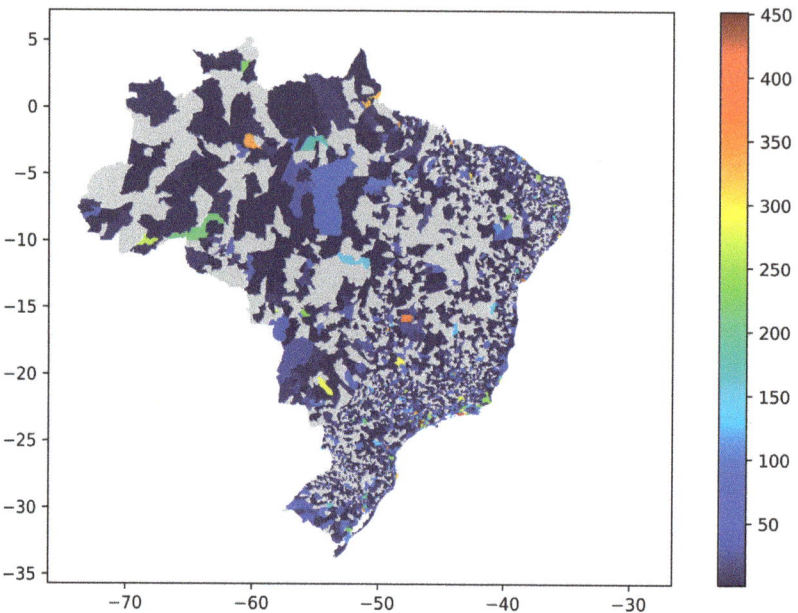

**Figure 3.** Overall tweets distribution in Brazilian territory.

There are twenty-five cities with at least 300 tweets registered in the corpus; among them, twenty cities are state capitals, including Brasília (the country capital), and the others are major urban centers in their respective states. Table S3 in the Supplementary Materials presents the list of these twenty-five cities with the associated number of tweets. In this map and all the others along the results, the cities are represented in the Brazilian municipal grid. In other words, for figures with maps, although we refer to the cities, the graphical representations are the municipalities.

*3.2. Topic Modeling Results*

The topic modeling process considered two word-vectors, one obtained using the count vectorizer and the other the TF-IDF vectorizer. The main results for the Grid Searches using these vectors were:

(1) For the words vector obtained with the count method: a topic model with only three components (topics), using a learning decay equals 0.7. This result is corroborated by the best log-likelihood of $-840{,}183.6751$ and perplexity of 1479.7684.
(2) For the words vector obtained with TF-IDF method, a topic model with only three components, and in this case, using a leaning decay equals 0.5. This result is corroborated by the log-likelihood of $-281{,}057.5610$ and perplexity of 4225.0856.

However, the results of this test require a sensitivity analysis that can be applied using the learning decay's performance graphs. This analysis can help define a more significant number of topics within the determined limits. Although the increase in the number of topics for each learning decay may cause a decrease in the log probability (whose values are negative) regardless of the applied vectorization, there will be a better margin of topics for analysis based on the diversification of the sub-themes involved. The graph grid in Figure 4 contains the overall performance curves for each of the three learning decays.

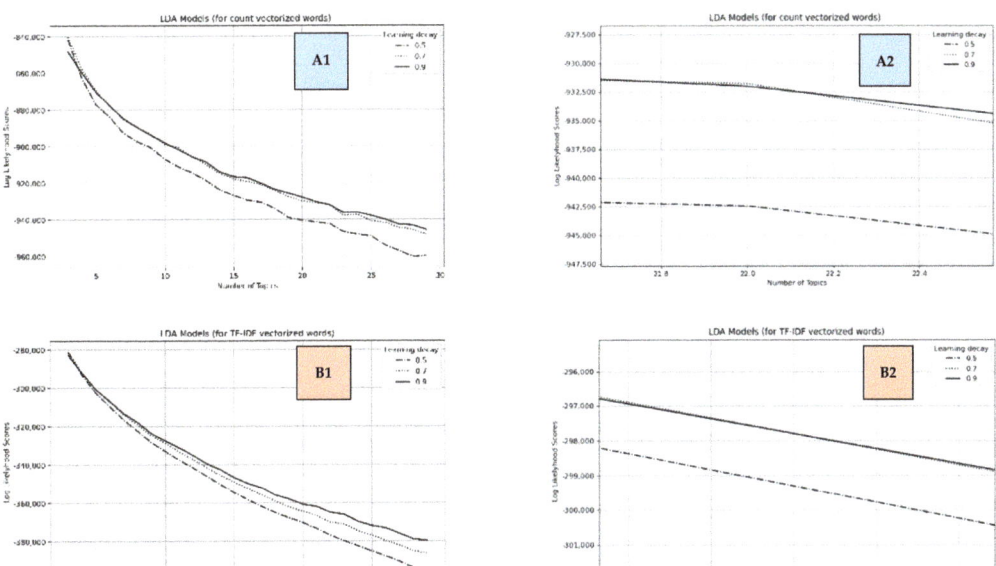

**Figure 4.** Learning decay curves for both words' vectors: graphs (**A1,B1**) contain the overall curves for the traditional count (frequency), and the TF-IDF vectorized words, successively; graphs (**A2,B2**) present the regions where the last overcome between the curves occurred, supporting defining the best topic model.

Graphs A1 and B1 in Figure 4 corroborate the best topic models with only three topics, but we can refine these results by looking for the graphs' regions where the initial best-performing learning decay curves are overcome.

Learning decay curves for the words vector obtained using the count vectorizer presented the definitive overcoming of the learning decay curve of 0.7 between 22 and 22.5 for the number of topics. The curve initially containing the best result was surpassed by the learning decay curve of 0.9, as presented in Graph A2 (Figure 4). So, for this case, we can define 23 as the number of topics, rounding this number after 22.5. The learning decay curve of 0.5 in this analysis always remained below the other two.

For the learning decay curves related to the words' vectors obtained using the TF-IDF vectorizer, there were several points where the curves of 0.5 and 0.7 crossed each other. For instance, the first time was between 3.10 and 3.15 topics, where the learning curve of 0.5 (containing the initial best model) was overcome by the curve of 0.7. However, as recorded in Graph B2 (Figure 4), the learning curve of 0.7 was overcome by 0.9 between 4.60 and 4.70 topics. After this, there was no other overcoming among the curves. It indicated a model with five topics, rounding this number of topics immediately after 4.7 and the learning decay of 0.9.

Based on this sensitivity analysis, we opted to use a model with 23 topics according to the words' vector obtained through the count method.

### 3.3. Topic Analysis Findings

The initial output of the topic modeling and extraction is the overall topic structure. There are several forms to present this structure. Table S4 in the Supplementary Materials presents the 15 most frequent terms for each topic, and Table S5 translates these terms into English. A graphical visualization for the topics is given in Figure 5.

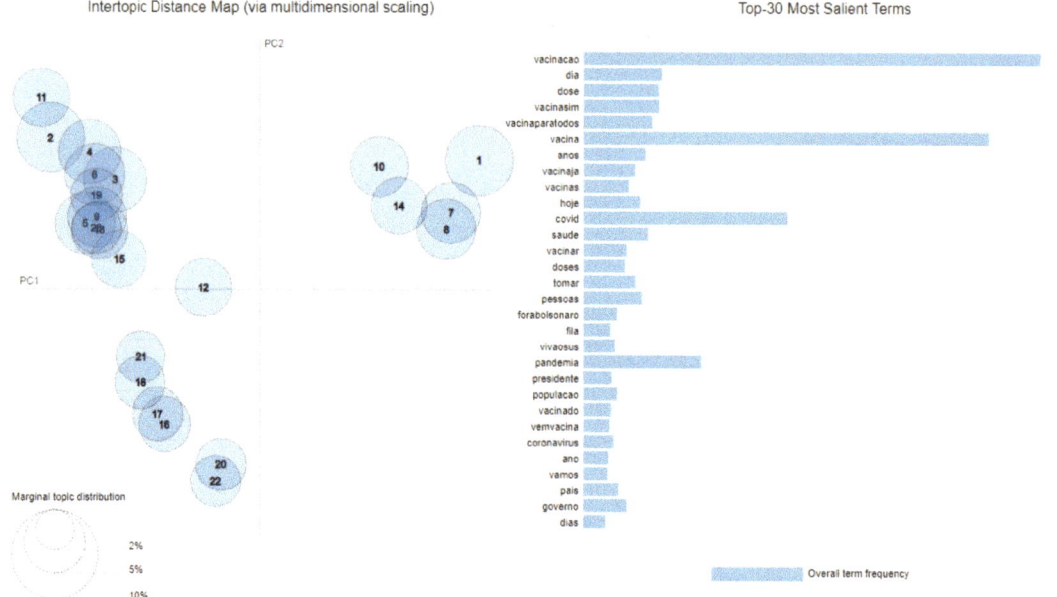

**Figure 5.** Intertopic distance map and the most salient terms found in the extraction process [45,48].

The graphs in Figure 5 support understanding the distribution and proximity of each topic in a two-dimensional projection and the most salient terms that can be interpreted as the most frequent words between all the topics. The thirty most salient terms, translated to English, are: vaccination, day, shot, vaccineyes, vaccineforeverybody, vaccine, years, vaccinenow, vaccines, today, covid, health, to vaccinate, shots, to take, people, outbolsonaro, queue, hailthesus, pandemic, president, population, vaccinated, comevaccine, coronavirus, year, [we] will, country, government, and days. Some of these terms, before preprocessing, contained hashtags (#):

- vaccineyes → vaccine yes
- vaccineforeverybody → vaccination for everybody
- vaccinenow → vaccine now
- outbolsonaro → out Bolsonaro (the family name of the Brazilian president at the time this study was carried out)
- hailthesus → hail the SUS (the last part is the acronym for *Sistema Unico de Saúde*, the Brazilian Public Health System)
- comevaccine → come vaccine

See Table S6 in the Supplementary Materials for the interpretations of what each topic can mean. The number of tweets on each topic is presented in Table S7 in the Supplementary Materials. Figure 6 presents the distribution of tweets among topics.

For each topic, we also could extract the weights of the terms presented in Table S4 in the Supplementary Materials. Figure 7 presents the plot of the 15 terms with the highest weights in each topic (see the translations to English in Table S5).

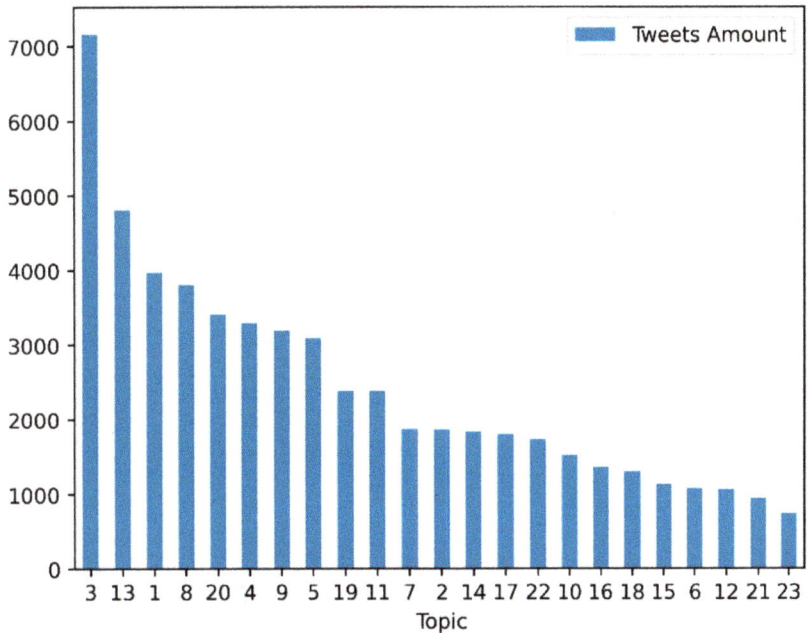

**Figure 6.** Tweets distributions among the 23 extracted topics.

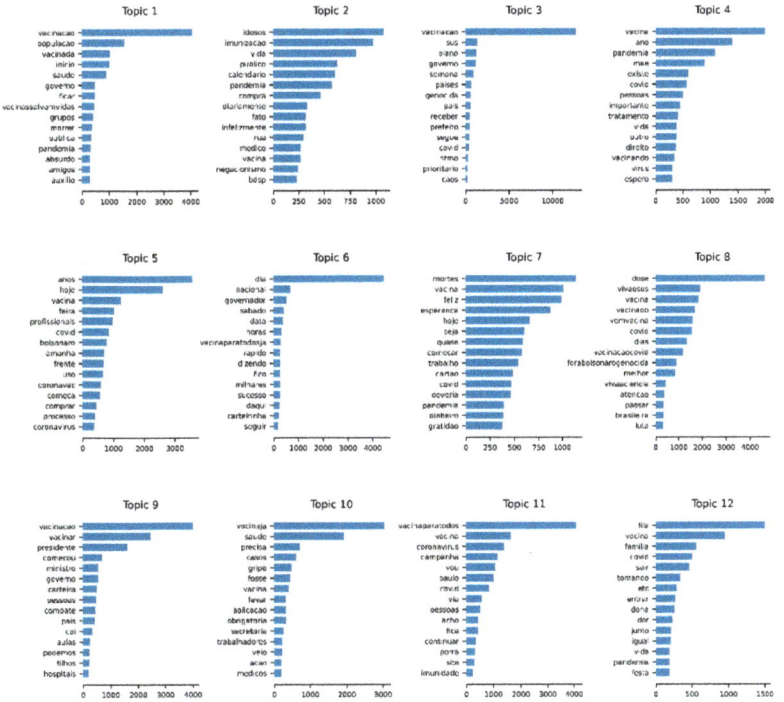

**Figure 7.** *Cont.*

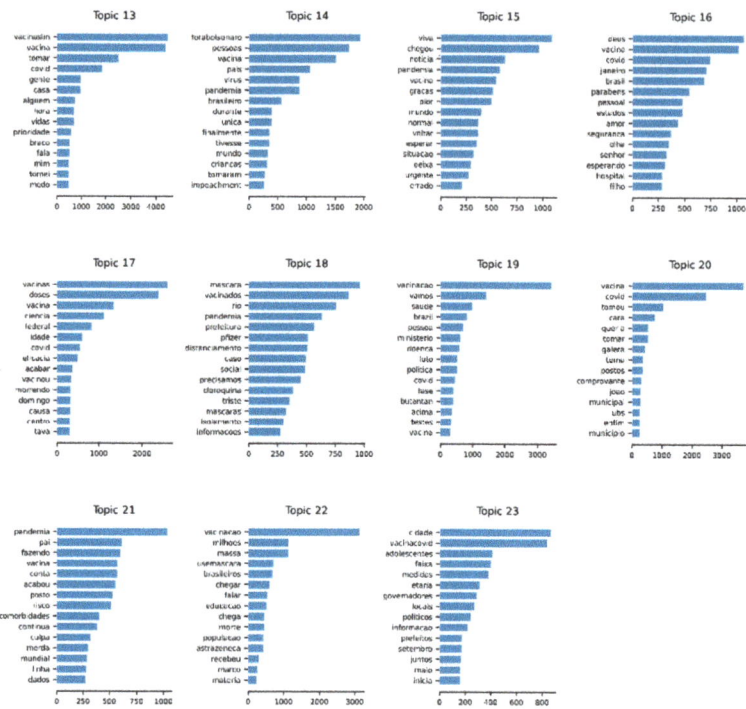

**Figure 7.** The fifteen terms with the highest weights in each topic.

The segregation of clusters of tweets according to related topics was generated from the results of the *t*-SNE method, allowing another kind of visualization of the topics' distributions in a two-dimensional projection. These clusters are shown in Figure 8.

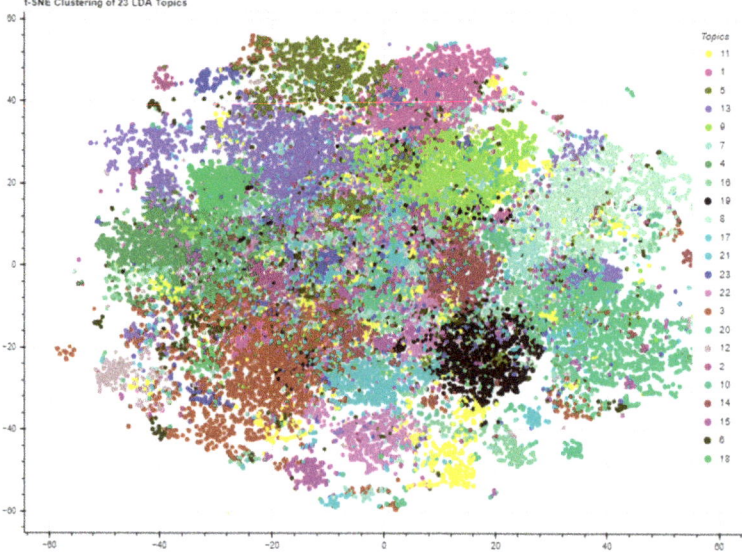

**Figure 8.** Tweets' clusters in a two-dimensional plane, according to the topics they are related.

3.3.1. Manual Annotation Results

The manual annotation of topics according to the three defined polarities did not generate ties for most topics. Only two topics (9 and 17) presented label ties as each of the three annotators applied a different label. A fourth annotator (an Engineering researcher) was invited to support resolving the indecision in the two topics. The results of the polarity label annotation are shown in Table 1.

Table 1. Results of the manual annotation process.

| Topic | Label   | Topic | Label   |
|-------|---------|-------|---------|
| 1     | Pro     | 13    | Pro     |
| 2     | Pro     | 14    | Pro     |
| 3     | Pro     | 15    | Neutral |
| 4     | Pro     | 16    | Neutral |
| 5     | Neutral | 17    | Anti    |
| 6     | Pro     | 18    | Anti    |
| 7     | Pro     | 19    | Pro     |
| 8     | Pro     | 20    | Pro     |
| 9     | Neutral | 21    | Neutral |
| 10    | Pro     | 22    | Pro     |
| 11    | Pro     | 23    | Pro     |
| 12    | Anti    | -     | -       |

After resolving the ties, the labels' distribution defined fifteen pro-vaccination topics, five neutral, and only three anti-vaccination. These labels enable the visualization of opinion distributions associated with the topics in space and time, helping to complete the analysis of the support and trust orientation regarding the COVID-19 immunization program in Brazil. After applying these labels to the corpus, the tweets' counts were: 41,868 pro-vaccination, 9725 neutral, and 4165 anti-vaccination.

3.3.2. Topics Timeline

The topic extraction process allowed the determination of the timelines for each of the 23 topics according to the number of tweets posted over the 17 months. As we obtained the topic → tweet association, it was possible to compute the totals of tweets collected according to each day for each topic.

The graph grid in Figure 9 presents the timelines, sharing the same axes (for the $x$-axis, the dates, and the $y$-axis, the tweets count). Each topic showed different peaks in the number of tweets on specific dates, with the highest peak in Topic 3 between January and February 2021, specifically on January 17, which is in line with the peak in the overall timeline of tweets (see Figure 2). Several smaller peaks in this same period can be observed in all other topics, whether they are the most significant peaks or not when we look inside each one.

The topic analysis over the seventeen months showed the trend of a significant peak in the count of tweets on several topics between January and February 2021. On 17 January 2021, the first vaccine application was carried out in Brazil, which had repercussions on social media and may be associated with this peak. Among the topics with peaks in this period, Topic 13 had the highest among all peaks, reaching 150 tweets.

All graphs show a trend toward fewer tweets between June and December 2020. As of December, the number of tweets on each topic started to grow. The month of December was marked by the launch of the National Vaccination Campaign against COVID-19, precisely on 16 December 2020. Therefore, from that date onwards, an intensification of online discussions on the subject was expected.

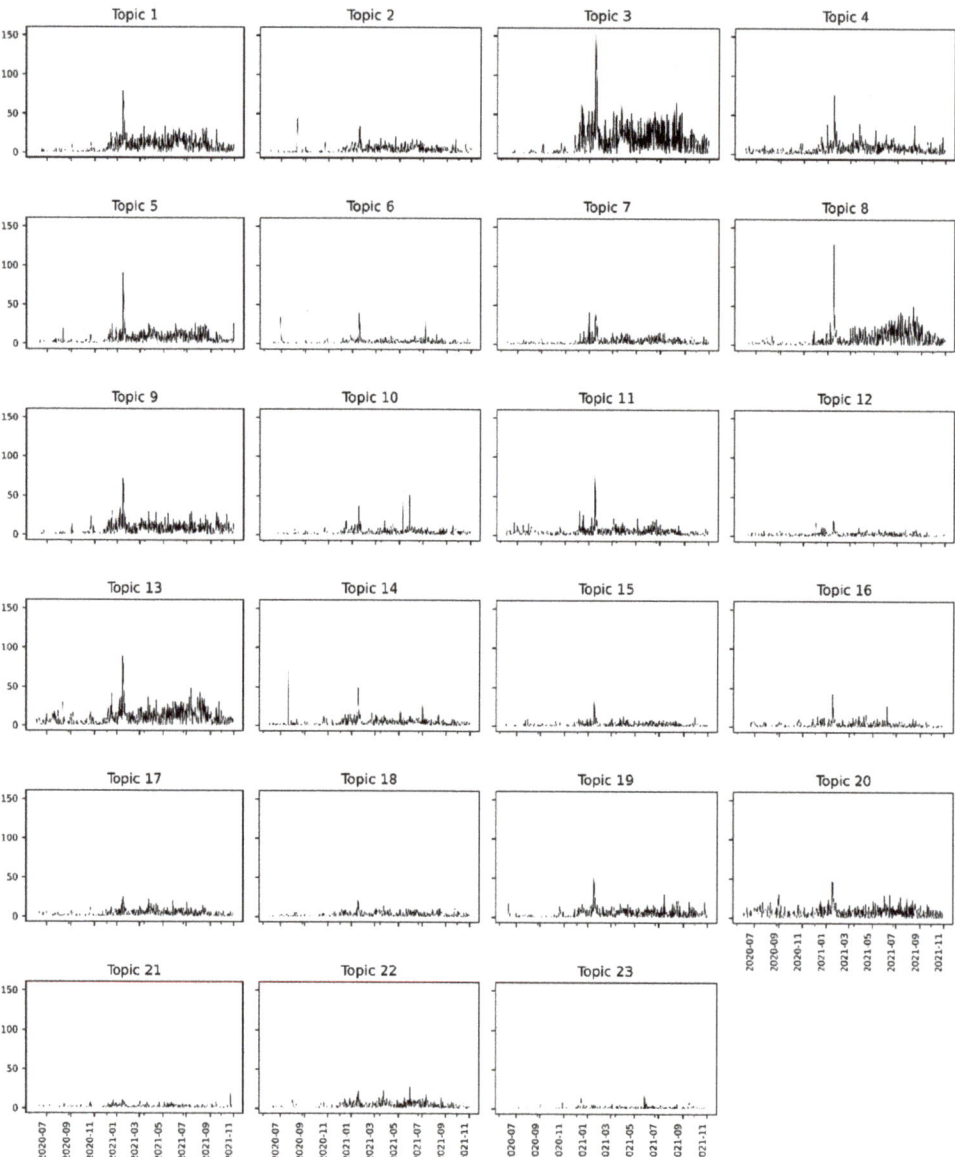

**Figure 9.** Timeline for each extracted topic, counting the number of tweets per day within the considered period.

It is interesting to note that in the period between June and December 2020, some topics had salient peaks in the number of tweets: Topic 2 between August and September 2020, Topic 6 between June and July 2020, and Topic 14 between July and August 2020. These peaks may indicate, for instance, periods of interest in more specific investigations, supporting the discovery of public discussion trends.

It was possible to create a timeline for each label based on the association between polarities and topics. The graph grid in Figure 10 presents these timelines.

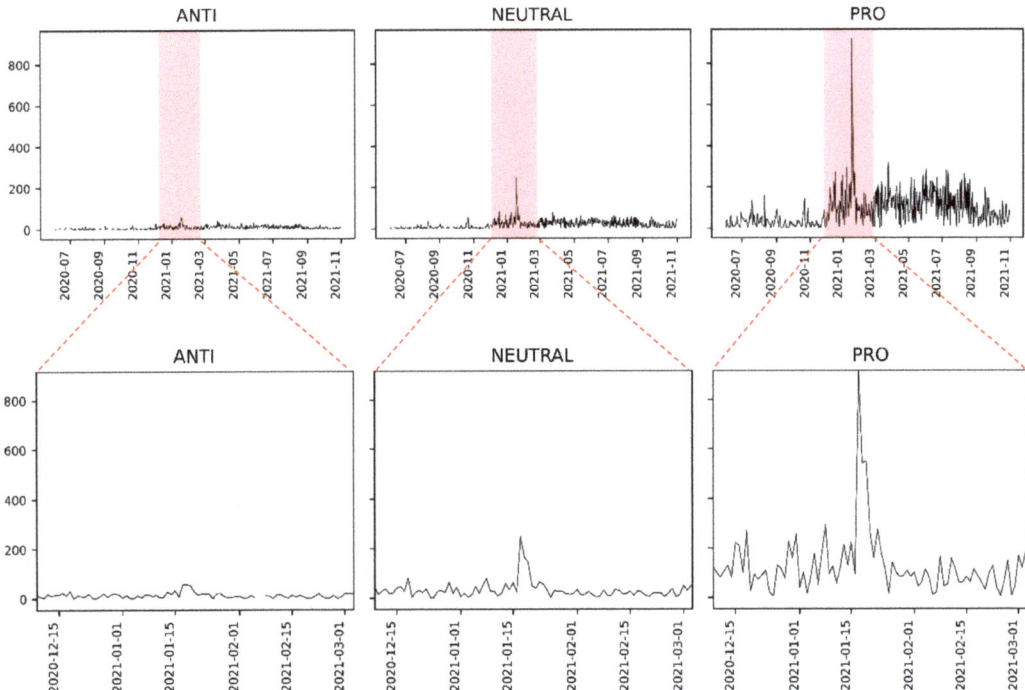

**Figure 10.** Timeline for each polarity, counting the number of tweets per day within the considered period.

The graphs show that most tweets are pro-vaccination according to the topic-polarity association. Each polarity presented a most significant peak in the tweets number which we zoomed to show more detail. Note that the peaks occurred on 17 January 2021.

3.3.3. Topics in Brazilian Geographic Space

The topic analysis in a geographic space has several levels of scope, ranging from the analysis of cities and neighborhoods to entire regions of a country. The granularity of the geographic information collected through the tweets allowed us to reach the municipal level, as seen in Figure 3.

Altogether, tweets from 3917 cities were retrieved, but not all of them had all the associated topics. It is also important to remember that only twenty-five cities had at least 300 tweets. As it is impossible to analyze the geographic distribution of all twenty-three topics in a shorter and more objective text such as this, we selected the two with the highest number of tweets to exemplify the analysis. Figures S1–S21 in the Supplementary Materials present the other topics' spatial distributions.

Topic 3, "Vaccination as a priority government action to combat COVID-19", with pro-vaccination polarity, has the most significant number of tweets (n = 7165). The map in Figure 11 presents the distribution of Topic 3 in Brazilian cities. In the areas with darker red, there are the highest amounts of tweets from Topic 3.

Topic 13, about "Vaccine saving lives concerning COVID-19" also with pro-vaccination polarity, has the second most significant number of tweets (n = 4815). Figure 12 contains the distribution of this topic in the Brazilian territory.

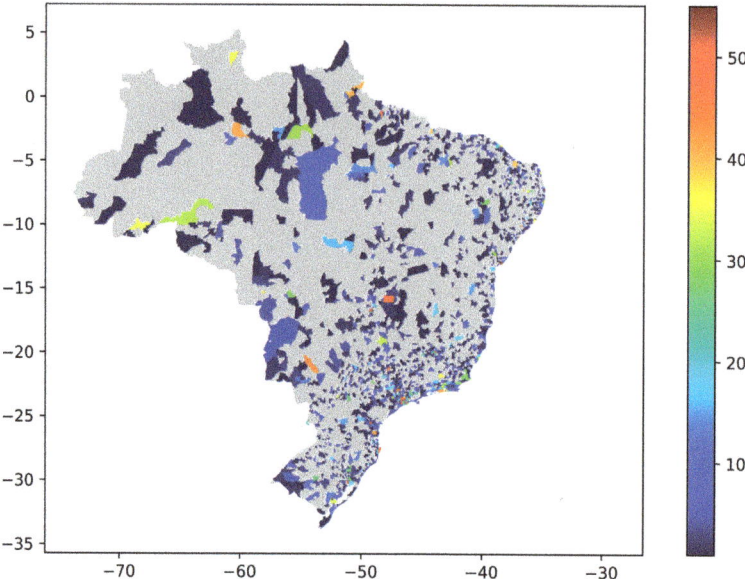

**Figure 11.** Topic 3 distribution on the Brazilian territory.

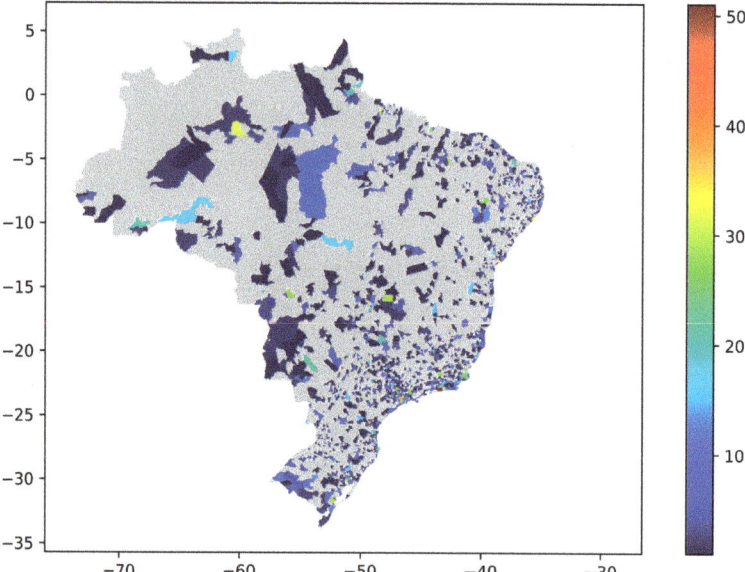

**Figure 12.** Topic 13 distribution on the Brazilian territory.

From the topic polarity annotation, in addition to analyzing the evolution of these polarities over 17 months, it is possible to visualize the geographic distribution of tweets according to the labels applied. The grid in Figure 13 contains maps according to polarity, making the distribution of tweets per city.

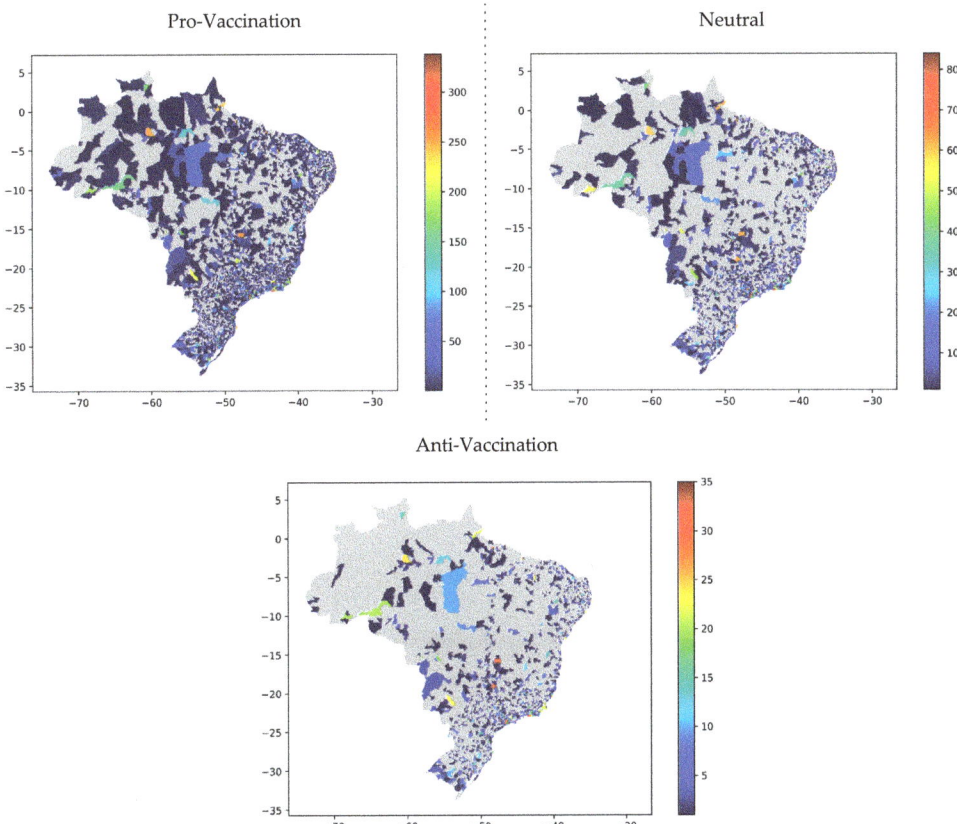

**Figure 13.** Distribution of tweets throughout the Brazilian territory according to polarities.

It was also possible to extract the ten cities with the highest number of tweets on each map according to polarities. Table 2 details these cities, separating them according to the polarity labels and presenting the tweets counting and percentual distributions. The populations presented for the cities came from the last population census of the Brazilian Institute of Geography and Statistics, which occurred in 2010.

The data in Table 2 highlights that São Paulo and Rio de Janeiro (both capitals of homonymous states and the two biggest cities in terms of population) had the highest number of pro-vaccination and neutral tweets. However, compared to other cities, which have smaller populations, they also have the smallest distribution of the amounts according to the population size, as seen through the percentual distribution column in the table. In the anti-vaccination polarity, Porto Alegre (capital of Rio Grande do Sul) had the highest number of tweets and the third highest percentual distribution score. São Paulo, followed by Rio de Janeiro, had the smallest distribution scores for the same polarity.

The percentual distribution scores represent interesting information to understand the opinions' penetration according to each city's population size. In cities with large populations, such as São Paulo and Rio de Janeiro, which also had some of the highest numbers of tweets, it is noted lower percentual distributions of tweets, a fact that may indicate that the extension of opinion effects is smaller than in cities with smaller populations and large amounts of tweets.

**Table 2.** Tweets' counts and percentual distributions for each of the ten cities with the highest number of tweets by polarity.

| Pro | | | | Neutral | | | |
|---|---|---|---|---|---|---|---|
| City | Population | Count | Distribution * (%) | City | Population | Count | Distribution * (%) |
| São Paulo | 11,253,503 | 338 | 0.00300 | São Paulo | 11,253,503 | 84 | 0.00075 |
| Rio de Janeiro | 6,320,446 | 321 | 0.00508 | Rio de Janeiro | 6,320,446 | 78 | 0.00123 |
| Curitiba | 1,751,907 | 279 | 0.01593 | Belém | 1,393,399 | 67 | 0.00481 |
| Salvador | 2,675,656 | 276 | 0.01032 | Campinas | 1,080,113 | 66 | 0.00611 |
| São Luís | 1,014,837 | 273 | 0.02690 | Fortaleza | 2,452,185 | 65 | 0.00265 |
| Belo Horizonte | 2,375,151 | 269 | 0.01133 | Florianópolis | 421,240 | 64 | 0.01519 |
| Porto Alegre | 1,409,351 | 267 | 0.01894 | Brasília | 2,570,160 | 63 | 0.00245 |
| Goiânia | 1,302,001 | 266 | 0.02043 | Uberlândia | 604,013 | 63 | 0.01043 |
| Brasília | 2,570,160 | 265 | 0.01031 | Macapá | 398,204 | 63 | 0.01582 |
| Recife | 1,537,704 | 265 | 0.01723 | Salvador | 2,675,656 | 62 | 0.00232 |

| Anti | | | |
|---|---|---|---|
| City | Population | Count | Distribution * (%) |
| Porto Alegre | 1,409,351 | 35 | 0.0025 |
| Brasília | 2,570,160 | 32 | 0.0012 |
| Uberlândia | 604,013 | 32 | 0.0053 |
| Rio de Janeiro | 6,320,446 | 31 | 0.0005 |
| Belo Horizonte | 2,375,151 | 30 | 0.0013 |
| Aracaju | 571,149 | 30 | 0.0053 |
| Vila Velha | 414,586 | 29 | 0.0070 |
| São Paulo | 11,253,503 | 29 | 0.0003 |
| Recife | 1,537,704 | 29 | 0.0019 |
| Belém | 1,393,399 | 28 | 0.0020 |

* Defined in the form of percentages according to the population of each city.

For example, looking at the pro-vaccination polarity, the city with the smallest population, São Luís (capital of the state of Maranhão), had a higher percentual distribution than São Paulo and Rio de Janeiro, indicating that the opinions may have had better penetration. Regarding opinions supporting vaccination, it is potentially desirable for the agencies managing the programs.

On the other hand, Porto Alegre, the city with the second highest population in the southern Brazilian region and the highest number of anti-vaccination tweets, had the third highest percentual distribution, demonstrating a greater tendency for penetration of negationist opinions. Still within the anti-vaccination polarity, the city of Vila Velha, despite having the smallest population among the ten cities listed, has the highest percentual distribution score, indicating that there may be a potential domain of negationist opinions shared by Twitter users.

Considering the ten cities with the highest number of tweets for each polarity, we can see that all cities are state capitals for the pro-vaccination polarity. In the neutral polarity, there is a predominance of capitals, except for two cities: Campinas and Uberlândia. Campinas has the third-largest population in the state of São Paulo, and Uberlândia has the second-largest population in the state of Minas Gerais. Finally, for the anti-vaccination polarity, there is also a predominance of the capital, except for two cities: Uberlândia and Vila Velha. Vila Velha is the second largest city in terms of population of the state of Espirito Santo, even ahead of the state capital, Vitória, which does not appear in Table 2.

*3.4. Theoretical and Practical Implications*

From a theoretical point of view, our study provides a methodological approach to analyze topics in space and time, using data obtained from Twitter about the Brazilian COVID-19 immunization program. However, the methodology was designed to be independent of research themes, contributing to the development of other research to understand how public opinion on the subject of interest evolves in space and time. There are other methods specifically for topic modeling and extraction; however, we rely on the literature when using LDA (see, for instance, [10,15,57–59]) since it corrects problems that occur in other similar methods, enabling us to achieve our study's objectives.

From a practical point of view, this work follows the same line as de Carvalho et al. [33]. It intends to present solutions for agencies and authorities related to immunization campaigns, to carry out analyzes to identify foci of misinformation, applying measures to mitigate the damage caused in the long-term public opinion. We presented a toolbox with a coherent and well-interconnected stepwise to generate reliable results in combating misinformation. This toolbox is a highlighted practical implication in infodemic-related research [60].

Authorities focused on combating this negative aspect of the large data volumes have the potential benefits of understanding the opinions distribution, the topics discussed, and analyzing the evolution of these discussions from the desired point in time, in addition to identifying which locations generate the most misinformation. Identifying which entities (people or organizations) are responsible for creating and spreading misinformation also becomes possible, delimiting the analysis to more particular levels. Based on these last comments, the infodemic opening space for cybercrimes or generating situations of civil danger is an issue to be explored by further studies [61,62].

In this context, while in our previous study we dealt only with the opinion classification based on a textual training dataset containing tweets with pro, anti-vaccination, or neutral orientation, manually searching for correlated events on social web and news search engines, in the current work we sought to deepen the investigation with new elements. We identified the main topics discussed so that researchers from different areas can apply manual annotation of polarity labels, no longer using machine classification, but now classification based on human judgment, for later automation of the hierarchical association *polarity* → *topic* → *tweet*.

From the previous work, we only used two sets of informational elements that we consider fundamental: (1) a part of one of the textual bases that contained geocoded tweets so that we could expand our developments with the distribution of topics in the Brazilian geographic space; and (2) the three-category classification scheme, with the pro, anti, and neutral labels.

The framework in the current study used different models than the previous one, although they were machine learning models in both cases. The present study applied topic modeling, using the Latent Dirichlet Allocation, and consequently clustering for visualization, with the *t*-SNE, enabling a more detailed view of the distribution of topics and polarities, according to the number of tweets, in time and Brazilian geographic space. In contrast, our previous work applied only classification models allowing the polarities evolution over time. The use of topic modeling was fundamental to increasing the specificity of the results obtained concerning the previous study.

One last implication to be mentioned is the development of new epidemiologic analyses of the COVID-19 outbreak [63]: infodemic and misinformation analysis can bring exciting findings about how people's opinions evolved in association with the evolution of the disease, using the numbers of infections and deaths over the time, for instance, as parameters to be associated with the collected opinion and related trust. It also should be noted that although we have dedicated the study to vaccination against COVID-19 in Brazil, the analytical framework can be used for other purposes in other domains, considering the guarantee of public health and security. We understand that even the private sector can use this process, for example, to understand how opinions about brands or products evolve over time and in a given geographic space.

*3.5. Difficulties, Challenges, and Limitations*

Although our methodological approach is based on techniques and tools implemented through secure and robust software, there is a need for subsequent refinements, especially in the text preprocessing and the definition and extraction of the features used in the process. There are several difficulties involved, listing some of them: we need to deal with texts outside the formal standard of the Portuguese language, which generates several noises such as abbreviations, the use of emojis/emoticons, and even the expansion of the stop words lists to include also associated abbreviations, and grammatical errors [64].

In this way, the construction of preprocessing scripts becomes challenging [65], even though there are already methods implemented in libraries and frameworks such as those applied in this study. There is a need to define a viable strategy for texts to be processed and transformed into a workable format by topic modeling methods. There are important decisions to be made about what should remain in the text and what should be removed, especially if we consider the indication made by Silva et al. [66] to keep the text as close as possible to the usage pattern from which it was extracted.

Another difficulty is related to the geocoding of tweets. We extracted geographic information as described in the methodological section, but we need to complete the information about the coordinates through points with latitude and longitude using Google's geographic API. The geographic information we could extract directly via the Twitter API brought us polygonal coordinates when our objective was the points referring to cities. As we also obtained the names of cities through Twitter API, we developed a process that retrieves the geographic points referring to these cities via Google API. Furthermore, the number of tweets obtained with geocoding was much lower than the number of tweets we parameterized to be searched and retrieved, as we reported in our previous work [33], implying that we obtained all the geocoded tweets according to the defined scraping parameters.

Thus, a critical limitation was the low number of geocoded tweets, with information from specific points to determine which cities generated the posts. It is crucial to retrieve more extensive amounts of geocoded tweets, to ensure statistical significance to the corpus to train topic extraction methods and consequently to ensure reliable analyses and results. Using tweets containing geographic information allows new studies to apply methods for analyzing correlations between variables identified through the texts with the variables traditionally used by management agencies, as in the case of vaccination programs. For example, the influence that pro- and anti-vaccination texts can exert on the flow of people receiving vaccinations can be studied using methods such as those applied by Huang et al. [67].

Even though the LDA fixes existing problems in methods prior to it [68], there are criticisms of its performance when applied to short texts, caused by the sparseness problem, which occurs with this kind of text [69]. Other models, more suitable for short texts, can be used as substitutes for the LDA in our framework: the Dual-sparse Topic Model (Dsparse TM) proposed by Lin et al. [70], the Biterm Topic Model (BTM) proposed by Cheng et al. [71], and the Pseudo-document-based Maximum entropy discrimination Latent Dirichlet Allocation model (PSLDA) proposed by Sun et al. [72] are three state-of-art examples.

Another issue that still needs further development concerns the psychological effects of COVID-19 and related issues on people and the way they manifest on the social web. In this study, although we are considering people's opinions, we have not developed any analysis of psychological effects in parallel with the study of opinions. Several studies have demonstrated the need to investigate the effects of the pandemic on people's mental health, evaluating, for example, effects such as anxiety and the causes of hesitation to receive the vaccine (see, for instance, [23,31,73,74]).

Although our study sought the judgments of researchers from different areas to act as polarity labels annotators, there are still many gaps about this type of annotation to be addressed, including the annotators' suggestions for refining the process we intend to follow for future research. Using only three labels on topic polarity also restricted the scope of related analyses. A more extensive list of labels referring to the emotions perceived by the annotators concerning the topics can improve the analyses.

## 4. Final Considerations

This article presented a study developed to identify topics discussed on Twitter between 2020 and 2021 about the COVID-19 immunization program in Brazil. The main contribution of the research was the definition of a framework containing a set of tools to deliver structured and helpful information, supporting agencies and authorities involved in the immunization program to understand the evolution of public opinion on vaccination and identifying cities with significant numbers of posts according to the extracted topics.

The methodology considered a manual annotation process on the topics, attributing polarity labels concerning support and trust in vaccination. Based on this labeling, it was possible to present both the evolution of polarities over time and their geographic distribution in Brazilian cities.

Interesting results were obtained regarding information surveillance (or infoveillance) about vaccination on social networks in the infodemic context, which can help guide efforts to combat potentially harmful information (or misinformation, as we have been calling it) to society and vaccination programs.

The temporal evolution analysis allowed the visualization of the moment when Brazilian posts started intensifying on the explored theme: from the launch of the national vaccination campaign in December 2020. It was also possible to detect when the highest peak of posts occurred: on 17 January 2021, when the first vaccine was applied in Brazil. There was a tendency for most of the topics to present peak on the same date.

Regarding the evolution of tweets for polarities, the peak on 17 December 2021, was more marked in the pro-vaccination orientation. However, they are also perceived in the anti-vaccination and neutral polarities on minor scales.

In the analysis of the distribution in the Brazilian geographic space, a greater concentration of tweets was identified in large cities, especially in the two largest cities in the country: São Paulo and Rio de Janeiro. However, based on the data collected, these two cities also had the lowest tweet percentual distributions according to their populations. The spatial analysis of the hierarchical association polarity → topic → tweet allowed the observation of the potential of some cities concerning the penetration of each opinion polarity in their populations.

It is worth mentioning that any other immunization program for other diseases can use the methodological approach presented. If we further expand this vision, the agencies involved in managing any crisis in any critical public sector are potential methodology users.

*Further Research*

As directions for further research, we highlight: (1) improvement of the technical data scraping process to extract more significant amounts of geocoded tweets about the desired topic; (2) development of an improved process for manual annotation on the opinion polarities, also considering labels referring to emotions such as happiness, anger, anguish, anxiety, fear, sadness, surprise, etc. Additionally, we highlight [75] for new space and time analyses; (3) testing and comparing the performance of other topic modeling algorithms specifically designed to work with short texts; (4) combining prospects of social distancing and mobility restrictions in different categories within the geographical locations [76]; and (5) analysis from the perspective of the psychological effects of public discussion on the social web on how the individual develops his opinion on the immunization programs.

**Supplementary Materials:** The following supporting information can be downloaded at: https://www.mdpi.com/article/10.3390/tropicalmed7120425/s1, Table S1: Parameters used in the scraping script; Table S2: Example of the georeferenced corpus, containing the first five rows; Table S3: Cities with at least 300 tweets retrieved; Table S4: The 23 topics extracted using LDA algorithm; Table S5: The 23 topics terms translations (or approximated translations) to English; Table S6: Possible interpretations for each topic; Table S7: Tweets amounts according to each topic; Figure S1: Topic 1 distribution on the Brazilian territory; Figure S2: Topic 2 distribution on the Brazilian territory; Figure S3: Topic 4 distribution on the Brazilian territory; Figure S4: Topic 5 distribution on the Brazilian territory; Figure S5: Topic 6 distribution on the Brazilian territory; Figure S6: Topic 7 distribution on the Brazilian territory; Figure S7: Topic 8 distribution on the Brazilian territory; Figure S9: Topic 10 distribution on the Brazilian territory; Figure S10: Topic 11 distribution on the Brazilian territory; Figure S11: Topic 12 distribution on the Brazilian territory; Figure S12: Topic 14 distribution on the Brazilian territory; Figure S13: Topic 15 distribution on the Brazilian territory; Figure S14: Topic 16 distribution on the Brazilian territory; Figure S15: Topic 17 distribution on the Brazilian territory; Figure S16: Topic 18 distribution on the Brazilian territory; Figure S17: Topic 19 distribution on the Brazilian territory; Figure S18: Topic 20 distribution on the Brazilian territory; Figure S19: Topic 21 distribution on the Brazilian territory; Figure S20: Topic 22 distribution on the Brazilian territory; Figure S21: Topic 23 distribution on the Brazilian territory.

**Author Contributions:** Conceptualization, V.D.H.d.C. and T.C.C.N.; methodology, V.D.H.d.C.; software, V.D.H.d.C.; validation, A.P.C.S.C., T.P. and V.D.H.d.C.; formal analysis, V.D.H.d.C. and T.C.C.N.; investigation, V.D.H.d.C. and T.P.; resources, A.P.C.S.C.; data curation, V.D.H.d.C.; writing—original draft preparation, V.D.H.d.C., T.C.C.N. and T.P.; writing—review and editing, V.D.H.d.C., T.C.C.N., T.P., and A.P.C.S.C.; visualization, V.D.H.d.C.; supervision A.P.C.S.C.; project administration, V.D.H.d.C. All authors have read and agreed to the published version of the manuscript.

**Funding:** This research received no external funding.

**Data Availability Statement:** The corpora files are not publicly available because of Twitter's Developer Agreement; however, we can make them available upon request, for academic research purposes.

**Acknowledgments:** We want to acknowledge the work of the anonymous annotators for their support in refining the topic analysis, with the labeling performed manually. We also want to acknowledge the support from the Coordenação de Aperfeiçoamento de Pessoal de Nível Superior (CAPES, Brazil), the Conselho Nacional de Desenvolvimento Científico e Tecnológico (CNPq, Brazil), and the Universidade Federal de Alagoas (UFAL, Brazil).

**Conflicts of Interest:** The authors declare no conflict of interest.

## References

1. Dwivedi, Y.K.; Hughes, D.L.; Coombs, C.; Constantiou, I.; Duan, Y.; Edwards, J.S.; Gupta, B.; Lal, B.; Misra, S.; Prashant, P.; et al. Impact of COVID-19 Pandemic on Information Management Research and Practice: Transforming Education, Work and Life. *Int. J. Inf. Manag.* **2020**, *55*, 102211. [CrossRef]
2. Venkatesh, V. Impacts of COVID-19: A Research Agenda to Support People in Their Fight. *Int. J. Inf. Manag.* **2020**, *55*, 102197. [CrossRef] [PubMed]
3. Boullosa, P.; Garea, A.; Area, I.; Nieto, J.J.; Mira, J. Leveraging Geographically Distributed Data for Influenza and SARS-CoV-2 Non-Parametric Forecasting. *Mathematics* **2022**, *10*, 2494. [CrossRef]
4. Islam, A.K.M.N.; Mäntymäki, M.; Laato, S.; Turel, O. Adverse Consequences of Emotional Support Seeking through Social Network Sites in Coping with Stress from a Global Pandemic. *Int. J. Inf. Manag.* **2022**, *62*, 102431. [CrossRef] [PubMed]
5. Chamakiotis, P.; Panteli, N.; Davison, R.M. Reimagining E-Leadership for Reconfigured Virtual Teams Due to COVID-19. *Int. J. Inf. Manag.* **2021**, *60*, 102381. [CrossRef]
6. González-Padilla, D.A.; Tortolero-Blanco, L. Social Media Influence in the COVID-19 Pandemic. *Int. Braz. J. Urol.* **2020**, *46*, 120–124. [CrossRef] [PubMed]
7. Gupta, P.; Kumar, S.; Suman, R.R.; Kumar, V. Sentiment Analysis of Lockdown in India during COVID-19: A Case Study on Twitter. *IEEE Trans. Comput. Soc. Syst.* **2021**, *8*, 939–949. [CrossRef]
8. Huang, X.; Wang, S.; Zhang, M.; Hu, T.; Hohl, A.; She, B.; Gong, X.; Li, J.; Liu, X.; Gruebner, O.; et al. Social Media Mining under the COVID-19 Context: Progress, Challenges, and Opportunities. *Int. J. Appl. Earth Obs. Geoinf.* **2022**, *113*, 102967. [CrossRef]
9. Imran, A.S.; Daudpota, S.M.; Kastrati, Z.; Batra, R. Cross-Cultural Polarity and Emotion Detection Using Sentiment Analysis and Deep Learning on COVID-19 Related Tweets. *IEEE Access* **2020**, *8*, 181074–181090. [CrossRef]
10. Abdulaziz, M.; Alotaibi, A.; Alsolamy, M.; Alabbas, A. Topic Based Sentiment Analysis for COVID-19 Tweets. *Int. J. Adv. Comput. Sci. Appl.* **2021**, *12*, 626–636. [CrossRef]
11. Alliheibi, F.M.; Omar, A.; Al-Horais, N. Opinion Mining of Saudi Responses to COVID-19 Vaccines on Twitter: A Computational Linguistic Approach. *Int. J. Adv. Comput. Sci. Appl.* **2021**, *12*, 72–78. [CrossRef]
12. Aparicio, J.T.; Salema de Sequeira, J.; Costa, C.J. Emotion Analysis of Portuguese Political Parties Communication over the COVID-19 Pandemic. In Proceedings of the 2021 16th Iberian Conference on Information Systems and Technologies (CISTI), Chaves, Portugal, 23–26 June 2021; pp. 1–6.
13. Cheng, I.K.; Heyl, J.; Lad, N.; Facini, G.; Grout, Z. Evaluation of Twitter Data for an Emerging Crisis: An Application to the First Wave of COVID-19 in the UK. *Sci. Rep.* **2021**, *11*, 19509. [CrossRef] [PubMed]
14. Naseem, U.; Razzak, I.; Khushi, M.; Eklund, P.W.; Kim, J. COVIDSenti: A Large-Scale Benchmark Twitter Data Set for COVID-19 Sentiment Analysis. *IEEE Trans. Comput. Soc. Syst.* **2021**, *8*, 976–988. [CrossRef] [PubMed]
15. Cotfas, L.-A.; Delcea, C.; Gherai, R. COVID-19 Vaccine Hesitancy in the Month Following the Start of the Vaccination Process. *Int. J. Environ. Res. Public Health* **2021**, *18*, 10438. [CrossRef]

16. Melton, C.A.; Olusanya, O.A.; Ammar, N.; Shaban-Nejad, A. Public Sentiment Analysis and Topic Modeling Regarding COVID-19 Vaccines on the Reddit Social Media Platform: A Call to Action for Strengthening Vaccine Confidence. *J. Infect. Public Health* **2021**, *14*, 1505–1512. [CrossRef]
17. Shi, W.-z.; Zeng, F.; Zhang, A.; Tong, C.; Shen, X.; Liu, Z.; Shi, Z. Online Public Opinion during the First Epidemic Wave of COVID-19 in China Based on Weibo Data. *Humanit. Soc. Sci. Commun.* **2022**, *9*, 159. [CrossRef]
18. Mackey, T.; Purushothaman, V.; Li, J.; Shah, N.; Nali, M.; Bardier, C.; Liang, B.; Cai, M.; Cuomo, R. Machine Learning to Detect Self-Reporting of Symptoms, Testing Access, and Recovery Associated With COVID-19 on Twitter: Retrospective Big Data Infoveillance Study. *JMIR Public Health Surveill.* **2020**, *6*, e19509. [CrossRef]
19. Daradkeh, M. Analyzing Sentiments and Diffusion Characteristics of COVID-19 Vaccine Misinformation Topics in Social Media: A Data Analytics Framework. *Int. J. Bus. Anal.* **2022**, *9*, 1–22. [CrossRef]
20. Wang, L.; Xian, Z.; Du, T. The Public Information Needs of COVID-19 Vaccine: A Study Based on Online Q&A Communities and Portals in China. *Front. Psychol.* **2022**, *13*, 961181. [CrossRef]
21. Zhu, J.; Weng, F.; Zhuang, M.; Lu, X.; Tan, X.; Lin, S.; Zhang, R. Revealing Public Opinion towards the COVID-19 Vaccine with Weibo Data in China: BertFDA-Based Model. *Int. J. Environ. Res. Public Health* **2022**, *19*, 13248. [CrossRef]
22. Xie, Q.; Xue, Y.; Zhao, Z. Understanding the Scientific Topics in the Chinese Government's Communication about COVID-19: An LDA Approach. *Sustainability* **2022**, *14*, 9614. [CrossRef]
23. Zhou, Y.; Xu, J.; Yin, M.; Zeng, J.; Ming, H.; Wang, Y. Spatial-Temporal Pattern Evolution of Public Sentiment Responses to the COVID-19 Pandemic in Small Cities of China: A Case Study Based on Social Media Data Analysis. *Int. J. Environ. Res. Public Health* **2022**, *19*, 11306. [CrossRef] [PubMed]
24. Leach, M.; MacGregor, H.; Akello, G.; Babawo, L.; Baluku, M.; Desclaux, A.; Grant, C.; Kamara, F.; Nyakoi, M.; Parker, M.; et al. Vaccine Anxieties, Vaccine Preparedness: Perspectives from Africa in a COVID-19 Era. *Soc. Sci. Med.* **2022**, *298*, 114826. [CrossRef] [PubMed]
25. Luo, C.; Chen, A.; Cui, B.; Liao, W. Exploring Public Perceptions of the COVID-19 Vaccine Online from a Cultural Perspective: Semantic Network Analysis of Two Social Media Platforms in the United States and China. *Telemat. Inform.* **2021**, *65*, 101712. [CrossRef] [PubMed]
26. da Fonseca, E.M.; Shadlen, K.C.; Bastos, F.I. The Politics of COVID-19 Vaccination in Middle-Income Countries: Lessons from Brazil. *Soc. Sci. Med.* **2021**, *281*, 114093. [CrossRef] [PubMed]
27. Biancovilli, P.; Makszin, L.; Jurberg, C. Misinformation on Social Networks during the Novel Coronavirus Pandemic: A Quali-Quantitative Case Study of Brazil. *BMC Public Health* **2021**, *21*, 1200. [CrossRef] [PubMed]
28. Caldarelli, G.; De Nicola, R.; Petrocchi, M.; Pratelli, M.; Saracco, F. Flow of Online Misinformation during the Peak of the COVID-19 Pandemic in Italy. *EPJ Data Sci.* **2021**, *10*, 34. [CrossRef] [PubMed]
29. Germani, F.; Biller-Andorno, N. The Anti-Vaccination Infodemic on Social Media: A Behavioral Analysis. *PLoS ONE* **2021**, *16*, e247642. [CrossRef]
30. Obadimu, A.; Khaund, T.; Mead, E.; Marcoux, T.; Agarwal, N. Developing a Socio-Computational Approach to Examine Toxicity Propagation and Regulation in COVID-19 Discourse on YouTube. *Inf. Process. Manag.* **2021**, *58*, 102660. [CrossRef]
31. Stoler, J.; Klofstad, C.A.; Enders, A.M.; Uscinski, J.E. Sociopolitical and Psychological Correlates of COVID-19 Vaccine Hesitancy in the United States during Summer 2021. *Soc. Sci. Med.* **2022**, *306*, 115112. [CrossRef]
32. Cotfas, L.-A.; Delcea, C.; Gherai, R.; Roxin, I. Unmasking People's Opinions behind Mask-Wearing during COVID-19 Pandemic—A Twitter Stance Analysis. *Symmetry* **2021**, *13*, 1995. [CrossRef]
33. de Carvalho, V.D.H.; Nepomuceno, T.C.C.; Poleto, T.; Turet, J.G.; Costa, A.P.C.S. Mining Public Opinions on COVID-19 Vaccination: A Temporal Analysis to Support Combating Misinformation. *Trop. Med. Infect. Dis.* **2022**, *7*, 256. [CrossRef] [PubMed]
34. de Carvalho, V.D.H.; Costa, A.P.C.S. Public Security Sentiment Analysis on Social Web: A Conceptual Framework for the Analytical Process and a Research Agenda. *Int. J. Decis. Support Syst. Technol.* **2020**, *13*, 1–20. [CrossRef]
35. Oliveira, W.C.C.d.; Reis, J.C.S.; Moro, F.B.M.M.; Almeida, V. Detecção de Posicionamento Em Tweets Sobre Política No Contexto Brasileiro. In *Anais do Brazilian Workshop on Social Network Analysis and Mining (BraSNAM)*; Sociedade Brasileira de Computação—SBC: Natal, Brazil, 2018.
36. de Carvalho, V.D.H.; Nepomuceno, T.C.C.; Poleto, T.; Turet, J.G. Ana Paula Cabral Seixas Costa Analyzing the Public Opinion Polarization about COVID-19 Vaccines in Brazil Through Tweets. In *Proceedings of the 2021 International Conference on Decision Support System Technology*; Choudhary, A., Jayawickrama, U., Spanaki, K., Delias, P., Eds.; EWG-DSS: Loughborough, UK, 2021.
37. Honnibal, M.; Montani, I.; Van Landeghem, S.; Boyd, A. SpaCy: Industrial-Strength Natural Language Processing (NLP) in Python 2020. Available online: https://spacy.io/ (accessed on 24 November 2022).
38. McKinney, W. Data Structures for Statistical Computing in Python. In Proceedings of the 9th Python in Science Conference (SciPy 2010), Austin, TX, USA, 28 June–3 July 2010; pp. 56–61.
39. Pedregosa, F.; Varoquaux, G.; Gramfort, A.; Michel, V.; Thirion, B.; Grisel, O.; Blondel, M.; Prettenhofer, P.; Weiss, R.; Dubourg, V.; et al. Scikit-Learn: Machine Learning in Python. *J. Mach. Learn. Res.* **2011**, *12*, 2825–2830.
40. Papadia, G.; Pacella, M.; Giliberti, V. Topic Modeling for Automatic Analysis of Natural Language: A Case Study in an Italian Customer Support Center. *Algorithms* **2022**, *15*, 204. [CrossRef]
41. Blei, D.; Carin, L.; Dunson, D. Probabilistic Topic Models. *IEEE Signal Process. Mag.* **2010**, *27*, 55–65. [CrossRef] [PubMed]
42. Blei, D.M.; Ng, A.Y.; Jordan, M.I. Latent Dirichlet Allocation. *J. Mach. Learn. Res.* **2003**, *3*, 993–1022.

43. Hoffman, M.D.; Blei, D.M.; Bach, F. Online Learning for Latent Dirichlet Allocation. In *Advances in Neural Information Processing Systems*; Lafferty, J., Williams, C., Shawe-Taylor, J., Zemel, R., Culotta, A., Eds.; Curran Associates, Inc.: Red Hook, NY, USA, 2010.
44. Srinivasan, B.; Mohan Kumar, K. Flock the Similar Users of Twitter by Using Latent Dirichlet Allocation. *Int. J. Sci. Technol. Res.* **2019**, *8*, 1421–1425.
45. Sievert, C.; Shirley, K. LDAvis: A Method for Visualizing and Interpreting Topics. In *Proceedings of the Workshop on Interactive Language Learning, Visualization, and Interfaces*; Association for Computational Linguistics: Stroudsburg, PA, USA, 2014; pp. 63–70.
46. Mabey, B.; English, P. PyLDAvis: Python Library for Interactive Topic Model Visualization 2015. Available online: https://pyldavis.readthedocs.io/en/latest/index.html (accessed on 24 November 2022).
47. Liu, Q.; Chen, Q.; Shen, J.; Wu, H.; Sun, Y.; Ming, W.-K. Data Analysis and Visualization of Newspaper Articles on Thirdhand Smoke: A Topic Modeling Approach. *JMIR Med. Inform.* **2019**, *7*, e12414. [CrossRef]
48. Chuang, J.; Manning, C.D.; Heer, J. Termite: Visualization Techniques for Assessing Textual Topic Models. In Proceedings of the International Working Conference on Advanced Visual Interfaces—AVI '12, Capri Island, Italy, 21–25 May 2012; ACM Press: New York, NY, USA, 2012; p. 74.
49. Bokeh Development Team Bokeh: Python Library for Interactive Visualization 2018. Available online: https://docs.bokeh.org/en/latest/ (accessed on 24 November 2022).
50. van der Maaten, L.; Hinton, G. Visualizing Data Using T-SNE. *J. Mach. Learn. Res.* **2008**, *9*, 2579–2605.
51. Maaten Van Der, L. Accelerating T-SNE Using Tree-Based Algorithms. *J. Mach. Learn. Res.* **2014**, *15*, 3221–3245.
52. Yin, Z.; Cao, L.; Han, J.; Zhai, C.; Huang, T. Geographical Topic Discovery and Comparison. In Proceedings of the 20th International Conference on World Wide Web, Hyderabad, India, 28 March–1 April 2011; pp. 247–256. [CrossRef]
53. Martin, S.; Kilich, E.; Dada, S.; Kummervold, P.E.; Denny, C.; Paterson, P.; Larson, H.J. "Vaccines for Pregnant Women . . . ?! Absurd"—Mapping Maternal Vaccination Discourse and Stance on Social Media over Six Months. *Vaccine* **2020**, *38*, 6627–6637. [CrossRef] [PubMed]
54. Vitório, D.; Souza, E.; Oliveira, A.L.I. Evaluating Active Learning Sampling Strategies for Opinion Mining in Brazilian Politics Corpora. In *Progress in Artificial Intelligence*; Moura Oliveira, P., Novais, P., Reis, L.P., Eds.; Lecture Notes in Computer Science; Springer International Publishing: Cham, Switzerland, 2019; Volume 11805, pp. 695–707.
55. Hunter, J.D. Matplotlib: A 2D Graphics Environment. *Comput. Sci. Eng.* **2007**, *9*, 90–95. [CrossRef]
56. Jordahl, K.; den Bossche, J.V.; Fleischmann, M.; Wasserman, J.; McBride, J.; Gerard, J.; Tratner, J.; Perry, M.; Badaracco, A.G.; Farmer, C.; et al. GeoPandas: V0.8.1 2020. Available online: https://geopandas.org/en/stable/ (accessed on 24 November 2022).
57. Jelodar, H.; Wang, Y.; Yuan, C.; Feng, X.; Jiang, X.; Li, Y.; Zhao, L. Latent Dirichlet Allocation (LDA) and Topic Modeling: Models, Applications, a Survey. *Multimed. Tools Appl.* **2019**, *78*, 15169–15211. [CrossRef]
58. Kalepalli, Y.; Tasneem, S.; Phani Teja, P.D.; Manne, S. Effective Comparison of LDA with LSA for Topic Modelling. In Proceedings of the 2020 4th International Conference on Intelligent Computing and Control Systems (ICICCS), Madurai, India, 13–15 May 2020; pp. 1245–1250.
59. Feng, Y.; Zhou, W. Work from Home during the COVID-19 Pandemic: An Observational Study Based on a Large Geo-Tagged COVID-19 Twitter Dataset (UsaGeoCov19). *Inf. Process. Manag.* **2022**, *59*, 102820. [CrossRef] [PubMed]
60. Varma, R.; Verma, Y.; Vijayvargiya, P.; Churi, P.P. A Systematic Survey on Deep Learning and Machine Learning Approaches of Fake News Detection in the Pre- and Post-COVID-19 Pandemic. *Int. J. Intell. Comput. Cybern.* **2021**, *14*, 617–646. [CrossRef]
61. Bahja, M.; Safdar, G.A. Unlink the Link between COVID-19 and 5G Networks: An NLP and SNA Based Approach. *IEEE Access* **2020**, *8*, 209127–209137. [CrossRef]
62. Smith, R.B.; Smith, N.N. A Tale of Two Pandemics: Fake News and COVID-19. *Kasetsart J. Soc. Sci.* **2022**, *43*, 677–682. [CrossRef]
63. Zhang, X.S.; Xiong, H.; Chen, Z.; Liu, W. Importation, Local Transmission, and Model Selection in Estimating the Transmissibility of COVID-19: The Outbreak in Shaanxi Province of China as a Case Study. *Trop. Med. Infect. Dis.* **2022**, *7*, 227. [CrossRef]
64. de Carvalho, V.D.H.; Costa, A.P.C.S. Towards Corpora Creation from Social Web in Brazilian Portuguese to Support Public Security Analyses and Decisions. *Libr. Hi Tech*, 2022; *in press*. [CrossRef]
65. Kumar, K.; Pande, B.P. Analysis of Public Perceptions Towards the COVID-19 Vaccination Drive: A Case Study of Tweets with Machine Learning Classifiers. In *Disease Control through Social Network Surveillance*; Bourlai, T., Karampelas, P., Alhajj, R., Eds.; Springer: Cham, Switzerland, 2022; pp. 1–30. ISBN 9783031078699.
66. Silva, R.M.; Santos, R.L.S.; Almeida, T.A.; Pardo, T.A.S. Towards Automatically Filtering Fake News in Portuguese. *Expert Syst. Appl.* **2020**, *146*, 113199. [CrossRef]
67. Huang, X.; Lu, J.; Gao, S.; Wang, S.; Liu, Z.; Wei, H. Staying at Home Is a Privilege: Evidence from Fine-Grained Mobile Phone Location Data in the United States during the COVID-19 Pandemic. *Ann. Am. Assoc. Geogr.* **2022**, *112*, 286–305. [CrossRef]
68. Noel, G.E.; Peterson, G.L. Applicability of Latent Dirichlet Allocation to Multi-Disk Search. *Digit. Investig.* **2014**, *11*, 43–56. [CrossRef]
69. Qiang, J.; Qian, Z.; Li, Y.; Yuan, Y.; Wu, X. Short Text Topic Modeling Techniques, Applications, and Performance: A Survey. *IEEE Trans. Knowl. Data Eng.* **2022**, *34*, 1427–1445. [CrossRef]
70. Lin, T.; Tian, W.; Mei, Q.; Cheng, H. The Dual-Sparse Topic Model. In Proceedings of the 23rd International Conference on World Wide Web—WWW '14, Seoul, Republic of Korea, 7–11 April 2014; ACM Press: New York, NY, USA, 2014; pp. 539–550.
71. Cheng, X.; Yan, X.; Lan, Y.; Guo, J. BTM: Topic Modeling over Short Texts. *IEEE Trans. Knowl. Data Eng.* **2014**, *26*, 2928–2941. [CrossRef]

72. Sun, M.; Zhao, X.; Lin, J.; Jing, J.; Wang, D.; Jia, G. PSLDA: A Novel Supervised Pseudo Document-Based Topic Model for Short Texts. *Front. Comput. Sci.* **2022**, *16*, 166350. [CrossRef]
73. Babicki, M.; Malchrzak, W.; Hans-Wytrychowska, A.; Mastalerz-Migas, A. Impact of Vaccination on the Sense of Security, the Anxiety of COVID-19 and Quality of Life among Polish. A Nationwide Online Survey in Poland. *Vaccines* **2021**, *9*, 1444. [CrossRef]
74. Murphy, J.; Vallières, F.; Bentall, R.P.; Shevlin, M.; McBride, O.; Hartman, T.K.; McKay, R.; Bennett, K.; Mason, L.; Gibson-Miller, J.; et al. Psychological Characteristics Associated with COVID-19 Vaccine Hesitancy and Resistance in Ireland and the United Kingdom. *Nat. Commun.* **2021**, *12*, 1–15. [CrossRef]
75. Batra, R.; Imran, A.S.; Kastrati, Z.; Ghafoor, A.; Daudpota, S.M.; Shaikh, S. Evaluating Polarity Trend amidst the Coronavirus Crisis in Peoples' Attitudes toward the Vaccination Drive. *Sustainability* **2021**, *13*, 5344. [CrossRef]
76. Nepomuceno, T.C.C.; Garcez, T.V.; e Silva, L.C.; Coutinho, A.P. Measuring the mobility impact on the COVID-19 pandemic. *Math. Biosci. Eng.* **2022**, *19*, 7032–7054. [CrossRef]

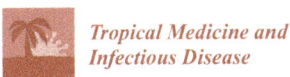

Article

# Identification of Bacterial Communities and Tick-Borne Pathogens in *Haemaphysalis* spp. Collected from Shanghai, China

Wenbo Zeng [1], Zhongqiu Li [1], Tiange Jiang [2], Donghui Cheng [1], Limin Yang [1], Tian Hang [2], Lei Duan [1], Dan Zhu [1], Yuan Fang [1,2] and Yi Zhang [1,2,*]

[1] National Institute of Parasitic Diseases, Chinese Center for Disease Control and Prevention (Chinese Center for Tropical Diseases Research), NHC Key Laboratory of Parasite and Vector Biology, WHO Collaborating Center for Tropical Diseases, National Center for International Research on Tropical Diseases, Shanghai 200025, China

[2] School of Global Health, Chinese Center for Tropical Diseases Research, Shanghai Jiao Tong University School of Medicine, Shanghai 200025, China

* Correspondence: zhangyi@nipd.chinacdc.cn

**Abstract:** Ticks can carry and transmit a large number of pathogens, including bacteria, viruses and protozoa, posing a huge threat to human health and animal husbandry. Previous investigations have shown that the dominant species of ticks in Shanghai are *Haemaphysalis flava* and *Haemaphysalis longicornis*. However, no relevant investigations and research have been carried out in recent decades. Therefore, we investigated the bacterial communities and tick-borne pathogens (TBPs) in *Haemaphysalis* spp. from Shanghai, China. Ixodid ticks were collected from 18 sites in Shanghai, China, and identified using morphological and molecular methods. The V3–V4 hypervariable regions of the bacterial 16S rRNA gene were amplified from the pooled tick DNA samples and subject to metagenomic analysis. The microbial diversity in the tick samples was estimated using the alpha diversity that includes the observed species index and Shannon index. The Unifrac distance matrix as determined using the QIIME software was used for unweighted Unifrac Principal coordinates analysis (PCoA). Individual tick DNA samples were screened with genus-specific or group-specific nested polymerase chain reaction (PCR) for these TBPs and combined with a sequencing assay to confirm the results of the V3–V4 hypervariable regions of the bacterial 16S rRNA gene. We found *H. flava* and *H. longicornis* to be the dominant species of ticks in Shanghai in this study. Proteobacteria, Firmicutes, Bacteroidetes and Actinobacteria are the main bacterial communities of *Haemaphysalis* spp. The total species abundances of Proteobacteria, Firmicutes and Bacteroidetes, are 48.8%, 20.8% and 18.1%, respectively. At the level of genus analysis, *H. longicornis* and *H. flava* carried at least 946 genera of bacteria. The bacteria with high abundance include *Lactobacillus*, *Coxiella*, *Rickettsia* and *Muribaculaceae*. Additionally, *Rickettsia rickettsii*, *Rickettsia japonica*, *Candidatus Rickettsia jingxinensis*, *Anaplasma bovis*, *Ehrlichia ewingii*, *Ehrlichia chaffeensis*, *Coxiella* spp. and *Coxiella*-like endosymbiont were detected in *Haemaphysalis* spp. from Shanghai, China. This study is the first report of bacterial communities and the prevalence of some main pathogens in *Haemaphysalis* spp. from Shanghai, China, and may provide insights and evidence for bacterial communities and the prevalence of the main pathogen in ticks. This study also indicates that people and other animals in Shanghai, China, are exposed to several TBPs.

**Keywords:** Ixodidae; bacteria; TBPs; metagenomics; PCR; China

Citation: Zeng, W.; Li, Z.; Jiang, T.; Cheng, D.; Yang, L.; Hang, T.; Duan, L.; Zhu, D.; Fang, Y.; Zhang, Y. Identification of Bacterial Communities and Tick-Borne Pathogens in *Haemaphysalis* spp. Collected from Shanghai, China. *Trop. Med. Infect. Dis.* **2022**, *7*, 413. https://doi.org/10.3390/tropicalmed7120413

Academic Editor: Yannick Simonin

Received: 31 October 2022
Accepted: 30 November 2022
Published: 1 December 2022

**Publisher's Note:** MDPI stays neutral with regard to jurisdictional claims in published maps and institutional affiliations.

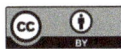

**Copyright:** © 2022 by the authors. Licensee MDPI, Basel, Switzerland. This article is an open access article distributed under the terms and conditions of the Creative Commons Attribution (CC BY) license (https://creativecommons.org/licenses/by/4.0/).

## 1. Introduction

Ticks are the second largest infectious agent in the world after mosquitoes, with a wide variety of species and a wide range of animal hosts [1]. They can carry and transmit a large number of pathogens, including bacteria, viruses and protozoa, posing a huge threat to human health and animal husbandry [2]. Ticks are known to harbor a number of veterinary and medically important bacterial species within the *Rickettsia*, *Anaplasma*, *Bartonella*, *Coxiella* and *Ehrlichia* genera [2,3]. As most ticks exhibit two-host or three-host life cycles, they are capable of supporting the transmission of pathogens between hosts, in which humans frequently serve as accidental hosts [4]. Multiple pathogenic agents may also be carried by an individual tick, which could transmit these pathogens to the human hosts bitten by ticks [3,4]. The main tick-borne diseases reported in China are forest encephalitis, Crimean Congo hemorrhagic fever, Lyme disease, rabbit fever, Q fever, North Asian tick-borne spotted fever, rickettsiosis, ehrlichiosis, anaplasmosis, babesiosis and Taylor disease [5–8]. Ticks of *Haemaphysalis* spp. have been implicated as potential disease vectors to humans and animals worldwide [3,9]. Various pathogenic bacteria have been previously detected in *Haemaphysalis* spp., including the disease agents for rickettsia spotted fever, tick typhus, anaplasmosis and ehrlichiosis [3,10–12].

Traditional detection methods (PCR, culture and serological methods), which have played a very important role in previous pathogen detection and identification, cannot detect all pathogens, especially when in low abundance and with unknown pathogens. Additionally, traditional detection methods are extremely dependent on known pathogens. However, metagenomic sequencing can identify a large number of micro pathogens, including unknown pathogens, in tick microflora captured in the field and does not depend on known nucleic acid sequences [13–15]. This method can be used not only to monitor microbial communities in infectious insect vectors but also as an ideal tool for monitoring emerging tick-borne diseases [13,15]. It can also provide a more thorough understanding of the ecological factors related to the prevalence and persistence of the vector-related microbial pedigree, which will help to predict and prevent the spread of diseases [13,15–17].

More and more tick-borne diseases and pathogens have been discovered. Recently, a new species of Yezo virus of the genus Nairobi virus was discovered in ticks in Hokkaido, Japan, and caused multiple infections [18]. Since the early 1980s, 34 pathogens of tick-borne diseases have been identified in mainland China, including eight species of spotted fever group *Rickettsia*, seven species of *Anaplasma*, six species of *Borrelia burgdorferi*, 11 species of *Babesia* and severe fever with thrombocytopenia syndrome new Bunyavirus (SFTSV) and Alongshan Virus (ALSV) [7,19]. Tick-borne diseases and tick bites frequently occur in provinces and cities around Shanghai, China, which seriously endangers the life and health of local residents. Human granulocytic anaplasmosis was first reported in Anhui Province in 2006. From 2010 to 2015, 286 cases of severe fever with thrombocytopenia syndrome (SFTS) were diagnosed in Jiangsu and Anhui provinces, with a fatality rate of 16.1% [20]. Li et al. (2021) predicted that most areas of Shanghai are highly suitable for ticks, and previous investigations have shown that the dominant ticks in Shanghai are *H. flava* and *H. longicornis* [21]. However, no relevant investigations and research have been undertaken in recent decades. Therefore, we expect that the metagenomic analysis of *Haemaphysalis* spp. in this region may provide an extensive list of pathogens carried by this important vector, thereby highlighting the potential risk of human infection caused by tick bites.

In our study, we first investigate the bacterial variability between populations of *H. flava* and *H. longicornis* from Shanghai, China. We sequenced the amplicons of the eubacterial 16S rRNA to (1) determine the baseline bacterial diversity from ticks collected from within a relatively small geographic area, (2) confirm the species identity of key taxa using taxon-specific PCR and Sanger sequencing and (3) estimate the relative abundance of the key bacterial taxa by PCR in the pooled DNA of ticks collected from Shanghai, China.

## 2. Materials and Methods

### 2.1. Study Area

These ticks were collected from 18 sampling sites in Shanghai. Shanghai, China, is located in the front of the alluvial plain of the Yangtze River Delta, with soft soil and low and flat topography, with an average elevation of 4 m from east to west. Except for a few hills nearly 100 m above sea level in the west, Shanghai is a large and low-level plain, and the whole plain river port is similar to a net. Shanghai, China, belongs to the northern subtropical humid monsoon climate zone, warm, humid and rainy, with four distinct seasons. A suitable natural environment provides favorable conditions for the survival of ticks. The sample points are selected from random sites in each functional area of the city (Figure 1). (Central cities (CC): 121°45′ E, 31°16′ N; 121°37′ E, 31°19′ N; 121°47′ E, 31°22′ N; 121°45′ E, 31°28′ N; 121°41′ E, 31°23′ N; 121°48′ E, 31°24′ N; Out suburban districts (OSD): 121°21′ E, 31°11′ N; 121°19′ E, 31°08′ N; 121°48′ E, 30°92′ N; 121°18′ E, 31°07′ N; Inner suburban districts (ISD): 121°33′ E, 31°14′ N; 121°21′ E, 31°37′ N; 121°52′ E, 31°41′ N; 121°38′ E, 31°15′ N and Chongming island (CMI): 121°49′ E, 31°71′ N; 121°51′ E, 31°72′ N; 121°47′ E, 31°69′ N; 121°52′ E, 31°73′ N).

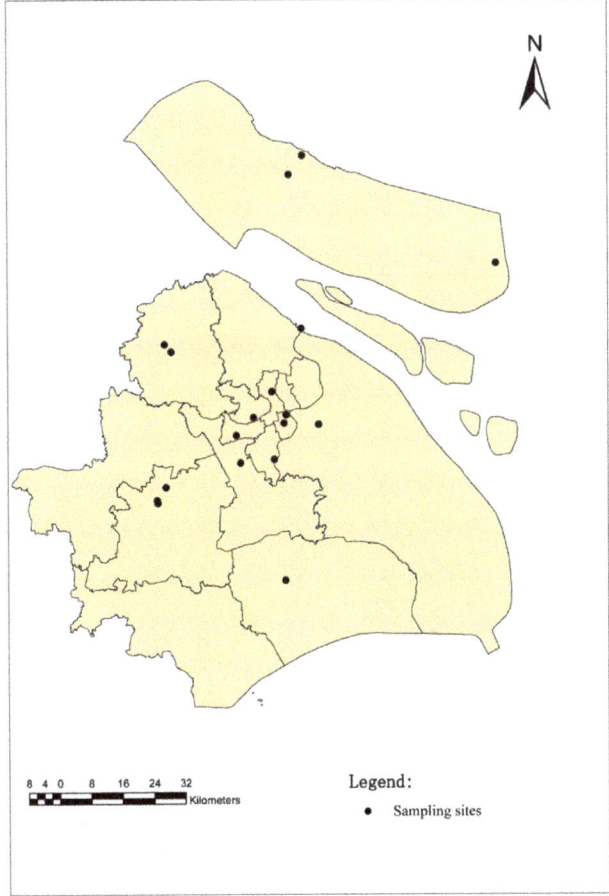

**Figure 1.** Map of the sampling sites in Shanghai, China. The black dots indicate the sampling regions in this study.

*2.2. Ticks Collection and Species Identification*

Wild ticks were collected by dragging flags on the vegetation layer during the day. Additionally, parasitic ticks (90 *H. flava* and 22 *H. longicornis*) were collected from animals (dogs, goats, sheep, cows, etc.). For the first step, different morphological characteristics were observed to identify the species and development stages of the collected ticks by an entomologist (Zhu Dan) [22], and then 12S rDNA [23] and Cytochrome C oxidase subunit I (CO I) gene [24] identification was used to further determine the species of ticks, as previously described. All ticks of the genus *Haemaphysalis* from each site were included in the study. Secondly, in the lab stage, the ticks were rinsed with 75% ethanol for 1 min to remove any environmental contaminants; then, they were rinsed with deionized water for 5 min to remove 75% ethanol and finally stored in a refrigerator (−80 °C).

## 2.3. DNA Extraction

After morphological identification, the ticks collected from the same site were pooled according to developmental stages. Overall, 2102 *H. flava* (80 adults, 295 nymphs and 1727 larvae) were divided into 211 pools, and 151 *H. longicornis* (65 adults, 8 nymphs and 78 larvae) were divided into 15 pools. The total genomic DNA was extracted using the DNeasy Blood & Tissue Kit (Qiagen, Hilden, Germany) following the manufacturer's instructions. The DNA concentration and integrity were measured using a NanoDrop 2000 spectrophotometer (Thermo Fisher Scientific, Waltham, MA, USA) and agarose gel electrophoresis, respectively.

## 2.4. Molecular Identification of Tick Vectors by PCR

To further confirm the results of the morphological classification of *Haemaphysalis* spp., multi-locus sequence typing depending on five tick's genomic DNA markers amplified fragments was carried out, which included: one nuclear gene CO I gene and a mitochondrial gene 12S rRNA. The PCR primers for the two genes are presented in Table 1.

**Table 1.** Primers used in this study.

| Target | Gene | Primer Name | Sequence (5′-3′) | Reference |
|---|---|---|---|---|
| Tick | 12S rDNA | T1B | AAACTAGGATTAGATACCCT | [23] |
|  |  | T2A | AATGAGAGCGACGGGCGATGT |  |
| Tick | CO I | HCO2198 | TAAACTTCAGGGTGACCAAAAAATCA | [24] |
|  |  | LCO1490 | GGTCAACAAATCATAAAGATATTGG |  |
| Microbiome | 16S rDNA | 343F | TACGGRAGGCAGCAG | [25] |
|  |  | 798R | AGGGTATCTAATCCT |  |
| *Coxiella* spp. | 16S rDNA | Cox16SF1 | CGTAGGAATCTACCTTRTAGWGG | [16] |
|  |  | Cox16SR1 | ACTYYCCAACAGCTAGTTCTCA |  |
|  |  | Cox16SF2 | TGAGAACTAGCTGTTGGRRAGT |  |
|  |  | Coc16SR2 | GCCTACCCGCTTCTGGTACAATT |  |
| *Rickettsia* spp. | ompA | Rr190.70p | ATGGCGAATATTTCTCCAAAA | [26] |
|  |  | Rr190.602n | AGTGCAGCATTCGCTCCCCCT |  |
| *Ehrlichia* spp. | 16S rRNA | Eh-out1 | TTGAGAGTTTGATCCTGGCTCAGAACG | [16,27] |
|  |  | Eh-out2 | CACCTCTACACTAGGAATTCCGCTATC |  |
|  |  | Eh-gs1 | GTAATACTGTATAATCCCTG |  |
|  |  | Eh-gs2 | GTACCGTCATTATCTTCCCTA |  |
| *Anaplasma* spp. | 16S rRNA | Eh-out1 | TTGAGAGTTTGATCCTGGCTCAGAACG | [27] |
|  |  | Eh-out2 | CACCTCTACACTAGGAATTCCGCTATC |  |
|  |  | HGA1 | GTCGAACGGATTATTCTTTATAGCTTG |  |
|  |  | HGA2 | TATAGGTACCGTCATTATCTTCCCTAC |  |

## 2.5. DNA Amplification

PCR amplification of the V3–V4 hypervariable regions of the bacterial 16S rRNA gene was carried out in a 25 µL reaction system using universal primer pairs (343F and 789R) (Table 1). The reverse primer contained a sample barcode, and both primers were connected with an Illumina sequencing adapter (Illumina Inc., San Diego, CA, USA).

## 2.6. Library Construction and Sequencing

The Amplicon quality was visualized using gel electrophoresis. The PCR products were purified with Agencourt AMPure XP beads (Beckman Coulter Co., Breya, CA, USA) and quantified using a Qubit dsDNA assay kit. The concentrations were then adjusted for sequencing. The sequencing was performed on an Illumina NovaSeq6000 with two paired-end read cycles of 250 bases each (Illumina Inc.; OE Biotech Company, Shanghai, China).

*2.7. Bioinformatics Analysis*

Raw sequencing data were in the FASTQ format. Paired-end reads were then pre-processed using cutadapt software to detect and cut off the adapter. After trimming, the paired-end reads were filtered for low-quality sequences, denoised, merged and detected and cut off the chimera reads using DADA2 [28] with the default parameters of QIIME2 [29] (November 2020); last, the software outputs, the representative reads and the ASV abundance table was generated. The representative read of each ASV was selected using the QIIME 2 package. All of the representative reads were annotated and blasted against Silva database Version 138 using q2-feature-classifier with the default parameters. The microbial diversity in the tick samples was estimated using the alpha diversity that includes the observed species index and Shannon index. The Unifrac distance matrix performed by QIIME software was used for unweighted Unifrac Principal coordinates analysis (PCoA).

*2.8. Specific PCR for Detection of Some Pathogens in Ticks*

Based on the results of 16S rRNA gene amplicon sequencing, genus-/group-specific PCR was performed to confirm the presence of TBPs in individual ticks. PCR was performed using a PCR System 9700 (Applied Biosystems, GeneAmp®, Carlsbad, CA, USA). For PCR, 2 µL of each DNA sample (150–330 ng) was used as the template for the first round, and 1 µL of the primary PCR product was used as the template for the second round. For the first round, a negative control (ddwater) and an extraction control mentioned above were included in each PCR experiment. Tube strips with individual caps were used in the amplification steps to prevent cross-contamination, and all PCR amplifications were carried out using PrimeSTAR® HS (Premix) (TaKaRa, Beijing, China). All of the operations were carried out in a biological safety cabinet. The amplified products were then electrophoresed on a 1.5% agarose gel, and the positive amplicons were sent to TSINGKE Biological Technology (Beijing, China) for sequencing. The PCR primers for *Rickettsia* spp., *Anaplasma* spp. and *Ehrlichia* spp. and *Coxiella* spp. are presented in Table 1.

*2.9. Phylogenetic Analysis*

The obtained nucleotide sequences were compared with those available in GenBank using the National Center for Biotechnology Information (NCBI; Bethesda, MD, USA) Basic Local Alignment Search Tool (BLAST) search engine (http://blast.ncbi.nlm.nih.gov/blast.cgi, accessed on 30 October 2022), and multiple sequence alignment was performed using the MEGA X (version 10.0) multiple alignment tool with the default parameters in MEGA X. The phylogenetic analysis was performed using MEGA X, and the tree was constructed using neighbor-joining (NJ) methods. The phylogenetic analysis of 12S rRNA and CO I gene for ticks, *ompA* for *Rickettsia* spp., 16S rRNA for *Anaplasma* spp., 16S rRNA for *Ehrlichia* spp., and 16S rRNA for *Coxiella* spp. was performed using the neighbor-joining method (NJ method) based on MEGA X. Bootstrap values were estimated for 1000 replicates.

## 3. Results

*3.1. Taxonomic Classification and Sequencing Data Statistics*

A total of 2253 hard ticks were identified as *H. flava* ($n$ = 2102) and *H. longicornis* ($n$ = 151) based on morphological identifications and confirmed by species-specific PCR and sequencing assays. There were 20 groups of *H. flava* (CCF1-5, OSDF1-5, ISDF1-5 and CMIF1-5) and 10 groups of *H. longicornis* (CCL1-5 and CMIL1-5) analyzed by amplicon sequencing on an Illumina NovaSeq6000 platform. The raw read data of the sequencing machine were distributed between 78,084 and 81,941, and the clean tag data after quality control were distributed between 4449 and 67,697. The valid tags (the final data used for analysis) data of clean tags were distributed between 4395 and 64,359, and the Amplicon Sequence Variant (ASV) numbers of each sample were distributed between 16 and 1191.

## 3.2. Alpha Diversity

Rarefaction curves were obtained for each tick group to determine if the sequencing depth was sufficient for each sample. Although the rarefaction curves for the observed ASVs approached saturation (Figure 2A), the Shannon diversity index curves reached a stable value (Figure 2B). The Good's coverage values for each group of samples ranged from 91.69% to 100%, indicating that the majority of the ASVs had been discovered. Altogether, these results suggest that the sequencing depth was sufficient to represent the majority of bacterial communities in these samples.

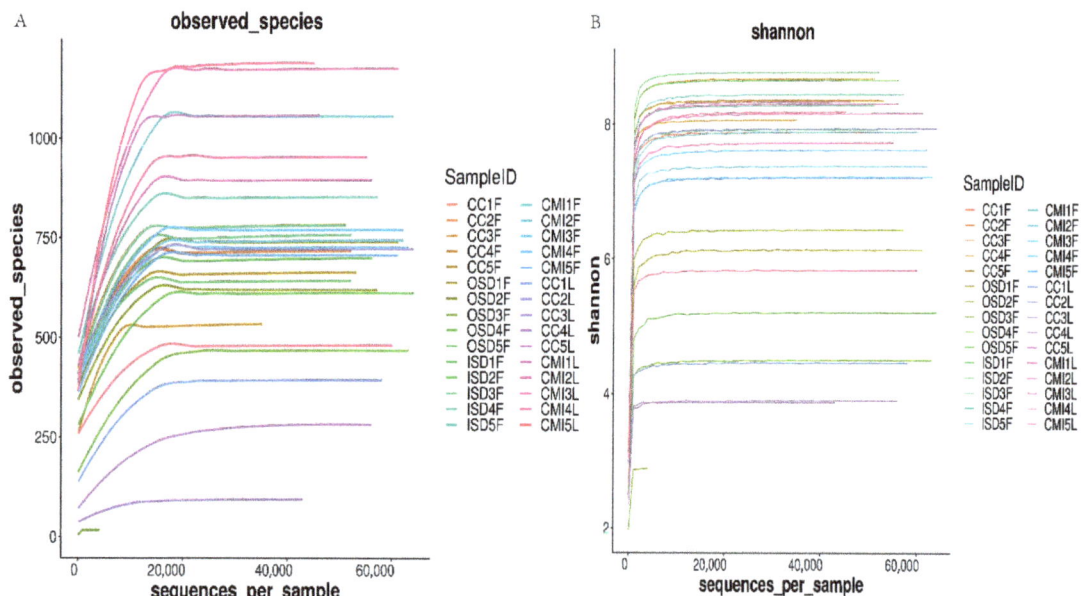

**Figure 2.** Rarefaction curves of observed species (**A**) and Shannon diversity index (**B**) for group tick samples.

## 3.3. Bacterial Microbiome Composition

All of the valid sequences were classified with 100% identity, and species information was obtained by comparison with the SILVA-138SSUrRNA database. A total of 15,903 ASVs were detected in this study, with a total of 1872 species belonging to 33 phyla, 91 classes, 235 orders, 403 families and 946 genera. A total of 10674ASVs were detected in *H. flava*, with a total of 1872 species belonging to 32 phyla, 84 classes, 209 orders, 358 families and 801 genera. A total of 6010ASVs were detected in *H. longicornis*, with a total of 1162 species belonging to 31 phyla, 81 classes, 201 orders, 333 families and 696 genera.

Proteobacteria, Firmicutes, Bacteroidetes and Actinobacteria are the main components of bacterial communities of *Haemaphysalis* spp. The total species abundances of Proteobacteria, Firmicutes and Bacteroidetes, are 48.80%, 20.80% and 18.10%, respectively.

The bacteria in *H. flava* with high abundance include Proteobacteria, 48.80%; Firmicutes, 21.60%; Bacteroidetes, 17.70% and Actinobacteria, 6.70%. The bacteria in *H. longicornis* with high abundance include Proteobacteria, 48.8%; Firmicutes, 19.20%; Bacteroidetes, 19.00% and Actinobacteria, 9.00% (Figure 3).

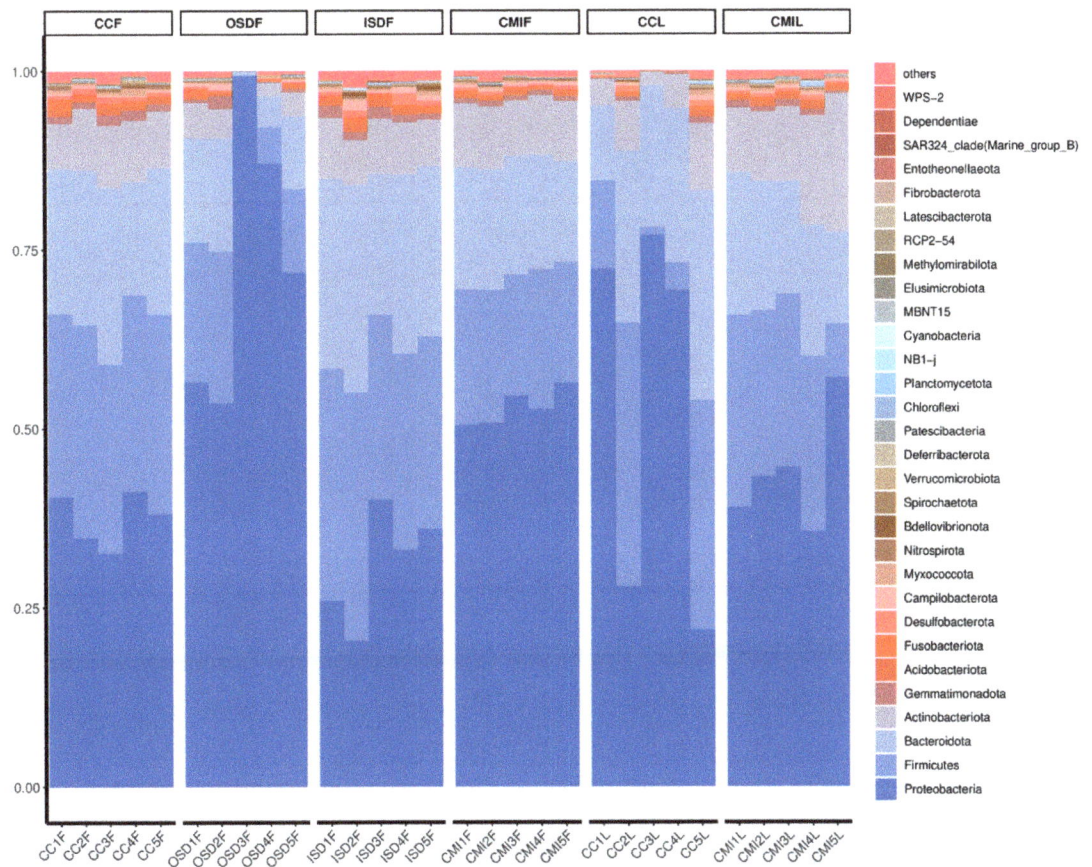

**Figure 3.** Relative abundances of potential top 30 pathogens at the phylum level in grouped *H. flava* and *H. longicornis* samples. The groups of *H. flava* are CCF, OSDF, ISDF and CMIF, and the groups of *H. longicornis* are CCL and CMIL.

At the level of genus analysis, *H. longicornis* and *H. flava* carried at least 946 genera of bacteria. The bacteria in *H. flava* with high abundance include *Lactobacillus*, *Rickettsia*, *Coxiella*, *Serratia* and *Muribaculaceae*. The bacteria in *H. longicornis* with high abundance include *Ochrobactrum*, *Coxiella*, *Lactobacillus* and *Sphingobacterium*. Additionally, some groups of OSDF, CCF and CCL include *Serratia* (Figure 4).

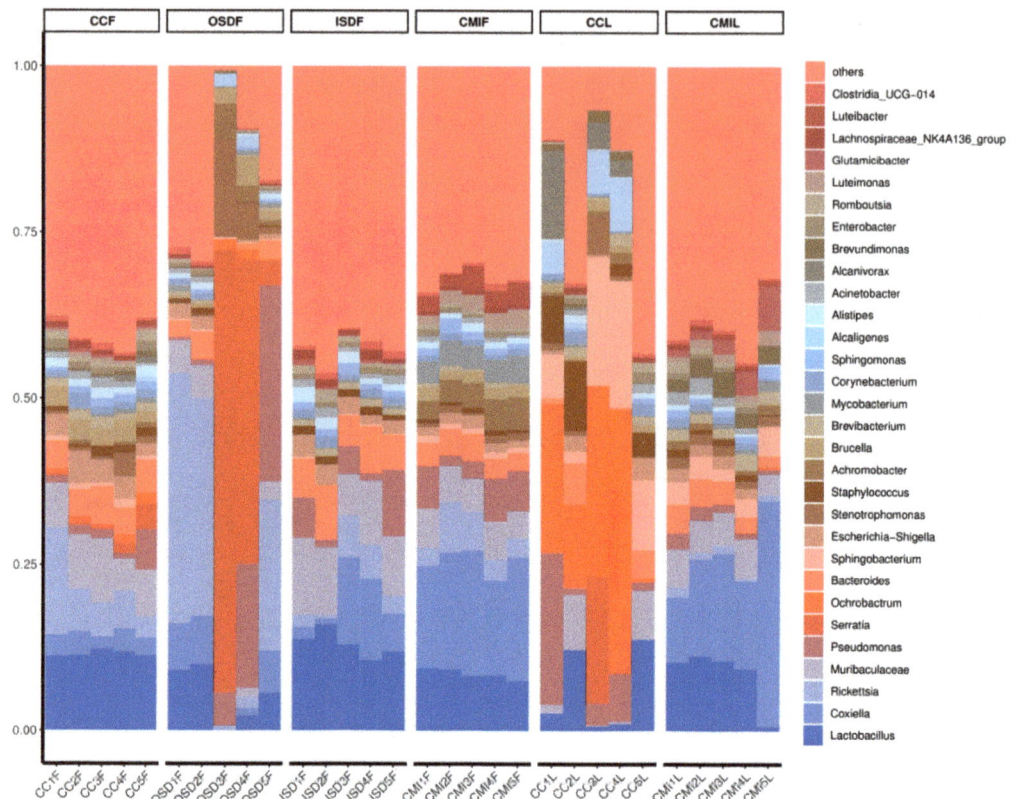

**Figure 4.** Relative abundances of potential top 30 pathogens at genus level in grouped *H. flava* and *H. longicornis* samples. The groups of *H. flava* are CCF, OSDF, ISDF and CMIF and the groups of *H. longicornis* are CCL and CMIL.

*3.4. Species and Location-Specific Differences in Microbial Diversity*

We examined the effects of location and tick species on the bacterial diversity of the grouped samples. Diversity indices CCF, ISDF, CMIF and CMIL clustered tightly, while OSDF and CCL were more diffused (Variable), and some of them were significant (Figure 5). In the principal coordinates analysis, decreased variability could be accounted for across two axes (6.05% × 4.42%) (Figure 6). We detected a significant difference in the bacterial community between locations and species.

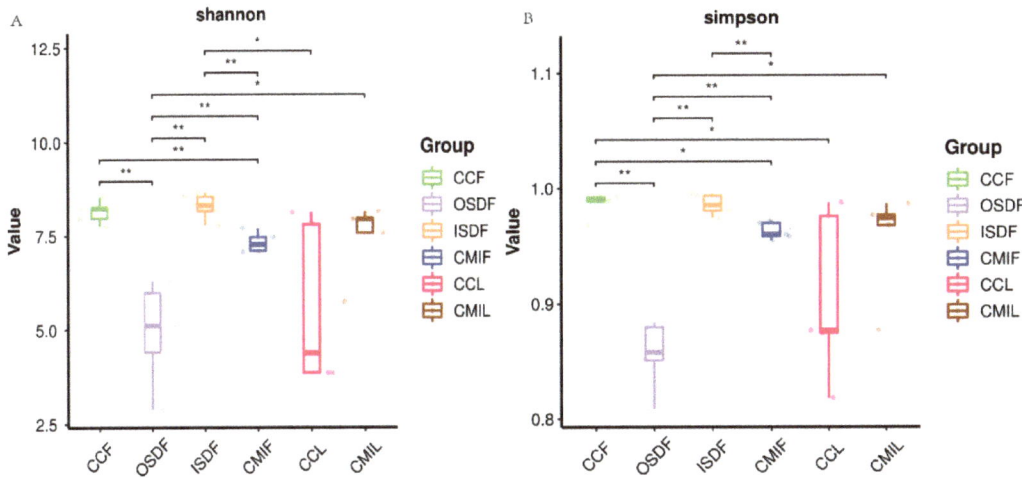

**Figure 5.** Plots of Alpha diversity indices of grouped *H. flava* and *H. longicornis* samples. Plot (**A**) the Shannon diversity index and plots (**B**) the Simpson diversity index (* $p < 0.05$, ** $p < 0.01$). The groups of *H. flava* are CCF, OSDF, ISDF and CMIF and the groups of *H. longicornis* are CCL and CMIL.

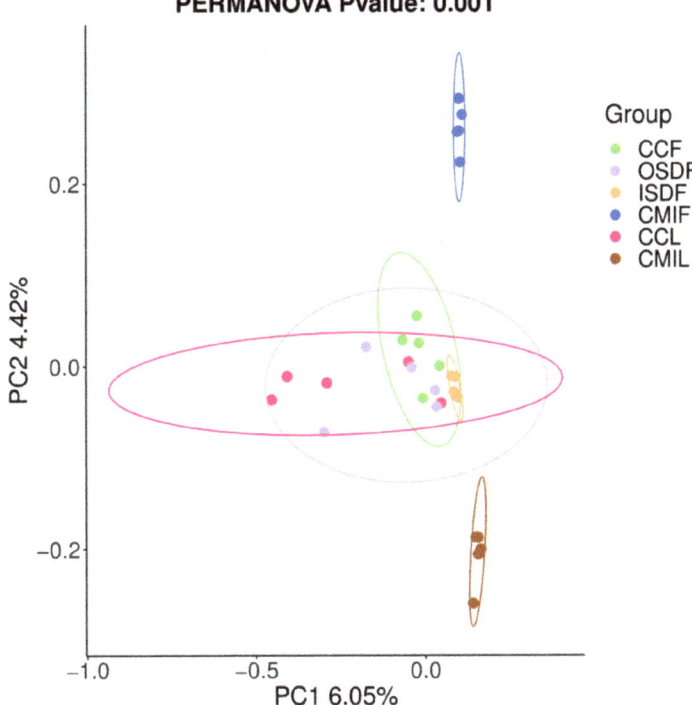

**Figure 6.** Principal coordinates analysis (PCoA) plot of 16SrRNA data from grouped samples of *H. flava* and *H. longicornis* samples of sample-based ecological distance. The groups of *H. flava* are CCF, OSDF, ISDF and CMIF and the groups of *H. longicornis* are CCL and CMIL.

## 3.5. Bacterial Relative Abundance Differences

Of special interest is the identification of members of the genera *Coxiella*, *Legionella*, *Anaplasma*, *Ehrlichia*, *Rickettsia* and *Sphingomonas*, some of which are pathogenic and can be transmitted by ticks. The relative abundances of *Lactobacillus*, *Coxiella*, *Sphingobacterium* and *Rickettsia* differed significantly between the two groups (Figure 7).

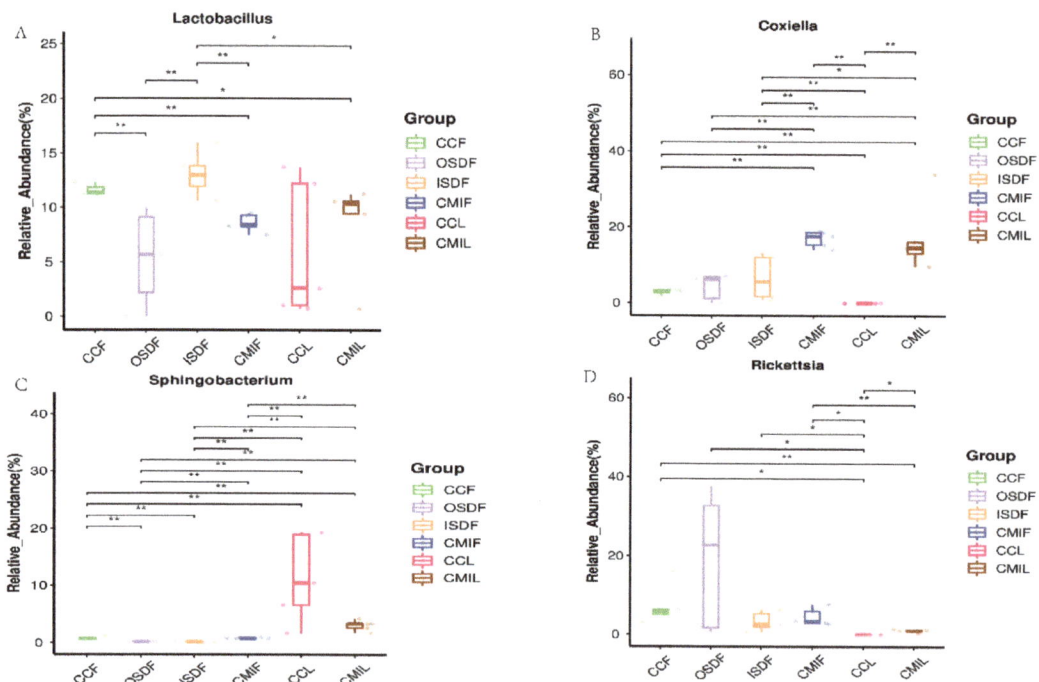

**Figure 7.** Relative titers of bacterial 16SrRNA gene from *Lactobacillus* (**A**), *Coxiella* (**B**), *Sphingobacterium* (**C**) and *Rickettsia* (**D**) between groups of *H. flava* and *H. longicornis* samples (* $p < 0.05$, ** $p < 0.01$). The groups of *H. flava* are CCF, OSDF, ISDF and CMIF and the groups of *H. longicornis* are CCL and CMIL.

## 3.6. Prevalence of Tick-Borne Pathogens in Individual Pools

The important pathogenic bacterial genera *Rickettsia* and *Coxiella* were found in the grouped tick samples. Each pool was detected by the genus-/species-specific PCR combined with sequencing in order to identify the TBPs carried by it. In addition, *Anaplasma* and *Ehrlichia* were often detected in ticks, so each pool was screened by *Anaplasma*/*Ehrlichia*-specific PCR.

As a result, *R. rickettsii* (2.37%, 5/211), *R. japonica* (3.32%, 7/211), *Candidatus R. jingxinensis* (16.59%, 35/211), *A. bovis* (1.42%, 3/211), *E. ewingii* (0.95%, 2/211), *E. chaffeensis* (1.90%, 4/211), *Coxiella* spp. (1.90%, 4/211), *C.*-like endosymbiont (2.37%, 5/211) were detected in *H. flava*. from Shanghai and *R. rickettsii* (20.00%, 3/15), *R. japonica* (20.00%, 3/15), *Candidatus R. jingxinensis* (20.00%, 3/15), *A. bovis* (26.67%, 4/15), *E. ewingii* (13.33%, 2/15), *E. chaffeensis* (6.67%, 1/15), *Coxiella* spp. (6.67%, 1/15), *C.*-like endosymbiont (20.00%, 3/15) were also detected in *H. longicornis* from Shanghai (Table 2).

Table 2. Prevalence of *Rickettsia*, *Anaplasma*, *Ehrlichia* and *Coxiella* in *H. flava* and *H. longicornis*.

|  | *H. flava* | *H. longicornis* |
|---|---|---|
| *R. rickettsii* | 2.37% (5/211) | 20.00% (3/15) |
| *R. japonica* | 3.32% (7/211) | 20.00% (3/15) |
| Candidatus *R. jingxinensis* | 16.59% (35/211) | 20.00% (3/15) |
| *A. bovis* | 1.42% (3/211) | 26.67% (4/15) |
| *E. ewingii* | 0.95% (2/211) | 13.33% (2/15) |
| *E. chaffeensis* | 1.90% (4/211) | 6.67% (1/15) |
| *Coxiella* spp. | 1.90% (4/211) | 6.67% (1/15) |
| *C.*-like endosymbiont | 2.37% (5/211) | 20.00% (3/15) |

*3.7. Symbiotic Interaction of Bacterial Communities*

The study also predicted the correlation among the top 30 genera in abundance. There is a positive correlation between *Acinetobacter*, *Clostridia_UGG-014*, *Romboutsia*, *Corynebacterium*, *Enterobacter*, *Escherichia-Shigella*, *Lactobacillus*, *Bacteroides*, *Muribaculaceae*, *Alistipes* and *Lachnospiraceae_NK4A136_group*. There is a negative correlation between one of *Alcaligenes*, *Orchrobactrum*, *Achromobacter*, *Serratia*, *Stenotrophomonas* and one of the above that has a positive correlation between them. There also is a positive correlation between *Achromobacter*, *Serratia*, *Stenotrophomonas* and *Brucella*, and there is a positive correlation between *Coxilla*, *Luteimonas*, *Luteibacter* and *Mycobacterium* (Figure 8).

*3.8. Phylogenetic Analysis*

The phylogenetical analyses of 12S rDNA and CO I of the two tick species sequences (*H. flava* and *H. longicornis*) agreed with their morphological identification. Constructing a phylogenetic tree based on 12S rDNA, *H. flava* and *H. longicornis* were placed in the same clades with *H. flava* (OK054521, ON954856, KJ747360, JQ625665, MT013252, OM368276) and *H. longicornis* (JQ346678, KF583588, OM368281), respectively (Figure 9), and *H. flava* and *H. longicornis* were also placed in a clade with *H. flava* (MN066331, JQ737097, MN784164, MN650208) and *H. longicornis* (JQ737092), respectively, in the COI tree (Figure 10). By phylogenetic analysis, *Coxiella* spp. and *C.*-like endosymbiont, identified in both *H. flava* and *H. longicornis*, were shown to be clustered with *Coxiella* spp. (KC776319, MG906671) and *C.*-like endosymbiont (JQ480822), respectively (Figure 11). *E. ewingii* and *E. chaffeensis*, identified in both tick species in the study, were also placed in a clade with *E. ewingii* (NR_044747, U96436) and *E. chaffeensis* (AF147752, NR_074500, MZ433238) (Figure 12). *A. bovis*, identified in *H. flava* and *H. longicornis*, were shown to be clustered with *A. bovis* (GU556626) (Figure 13). *R. japonica*, *R. rickettsii* and Candidatus *R. jingxinensis*, identified in both tick species in the study, were also placed in a clade with *R. japonica* (U83440), *R. rickettsii* (AY319290) and Candidatus *R. jingxinensis* (MN550905) (Figure 14).

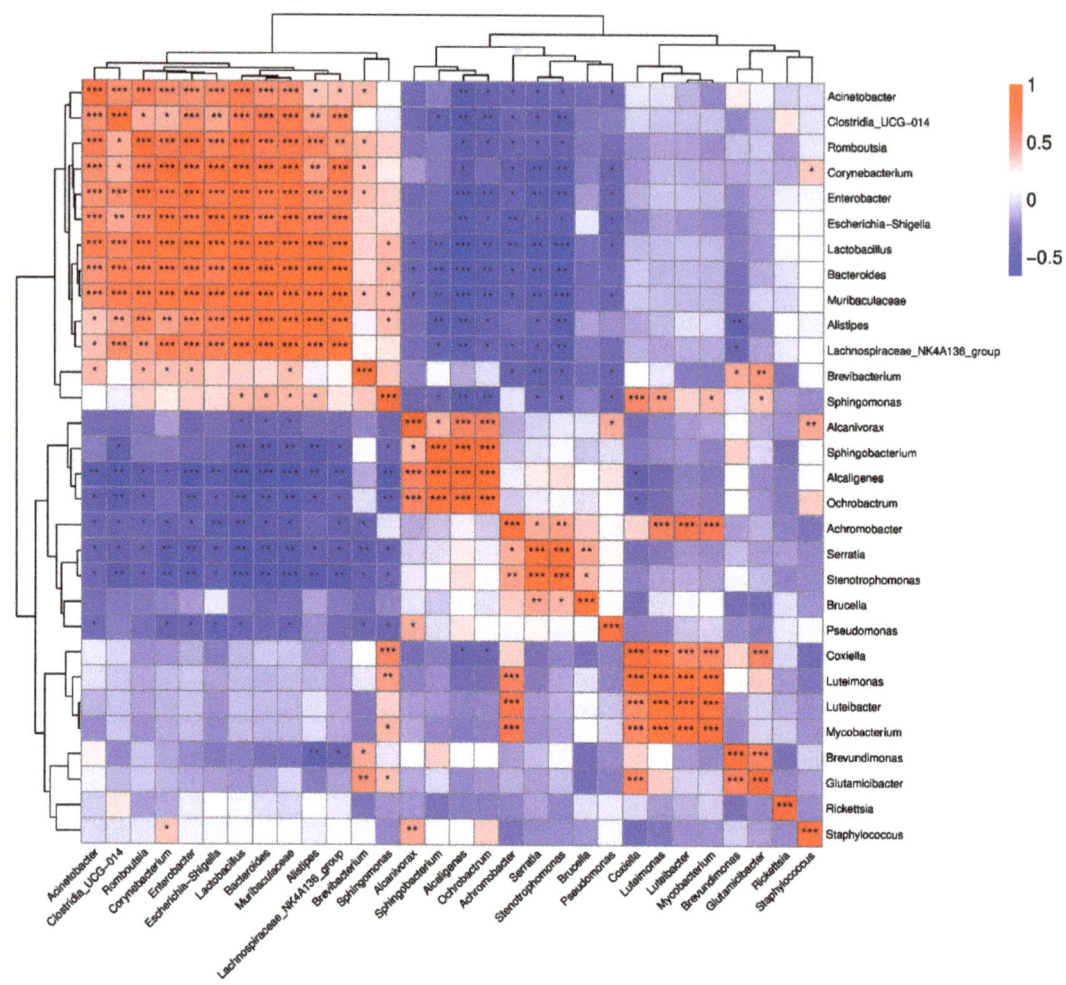

**Figure 8.** Correlation heatmap of Spearman coefficient of the top 30 genera of the groups of *H. flava* and *H. longicornis* samples (* $p < 0.05$, ** $p < 0.01$, *** $p < 0.001$). The groups of *H. flava* are CCF, OSDF, ISDF and CMIF and the groups of *H. longicornis* are CCL and CMIL.

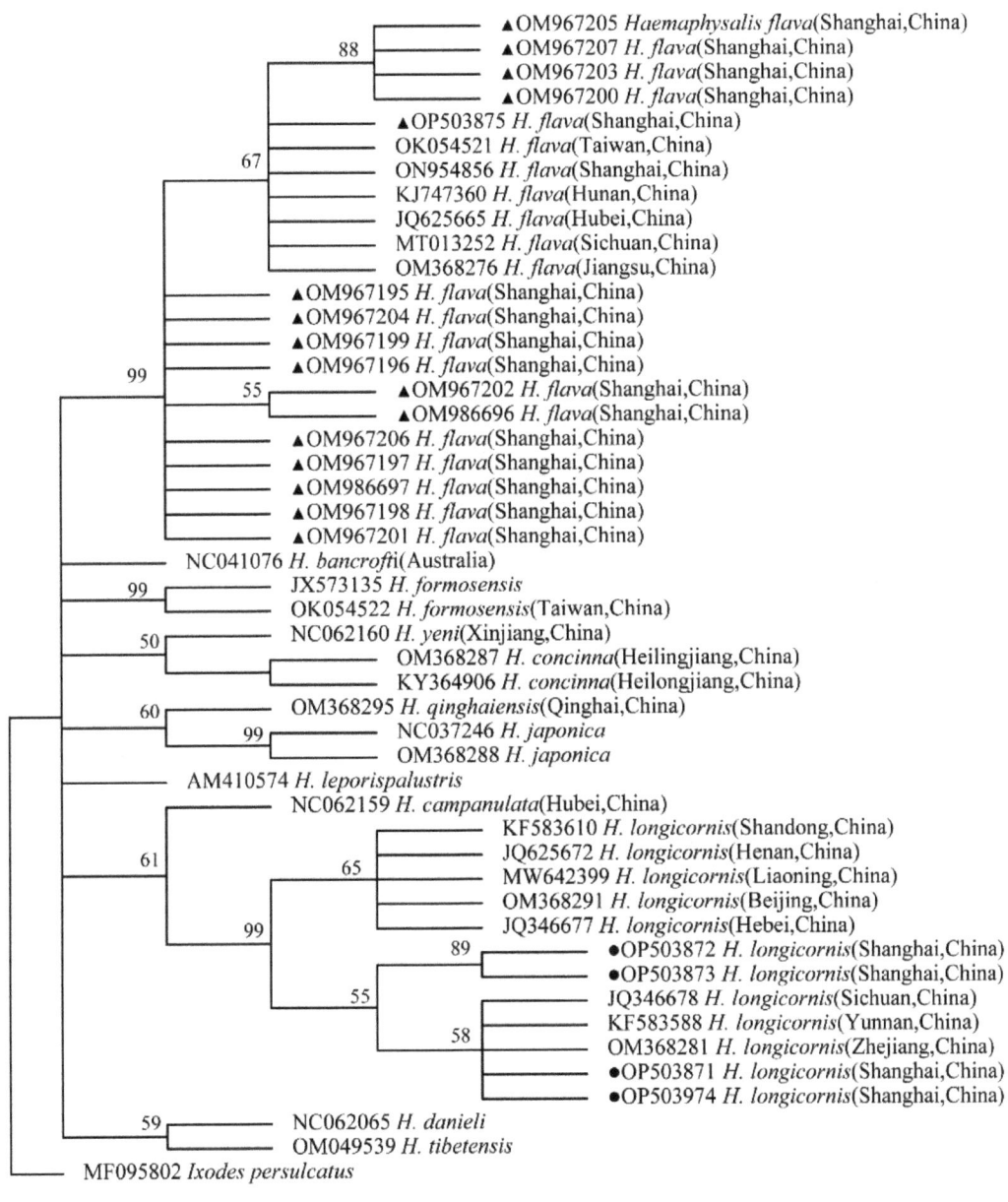

**Figure 9.** Phylogenetic tree of *H. flava* and *H. longicornis* based on partial 12S rDNA gene sequence similarity. The sequence from *H. flava* obtained in this study is indicated with a black triangle, and the sequence from *H. longicornis* obtained in this study is indicated with black dots. Sequences were aligned using the MEGA X (version 10.0) software package. Phylogenetic analysis was performed by the neighbor-joining method (NJ method), and bootstrap values were estimated for 1000 replicates. Kimura's two-parameter model was used as a substitution model for the calculation of the phylogenetic trees.

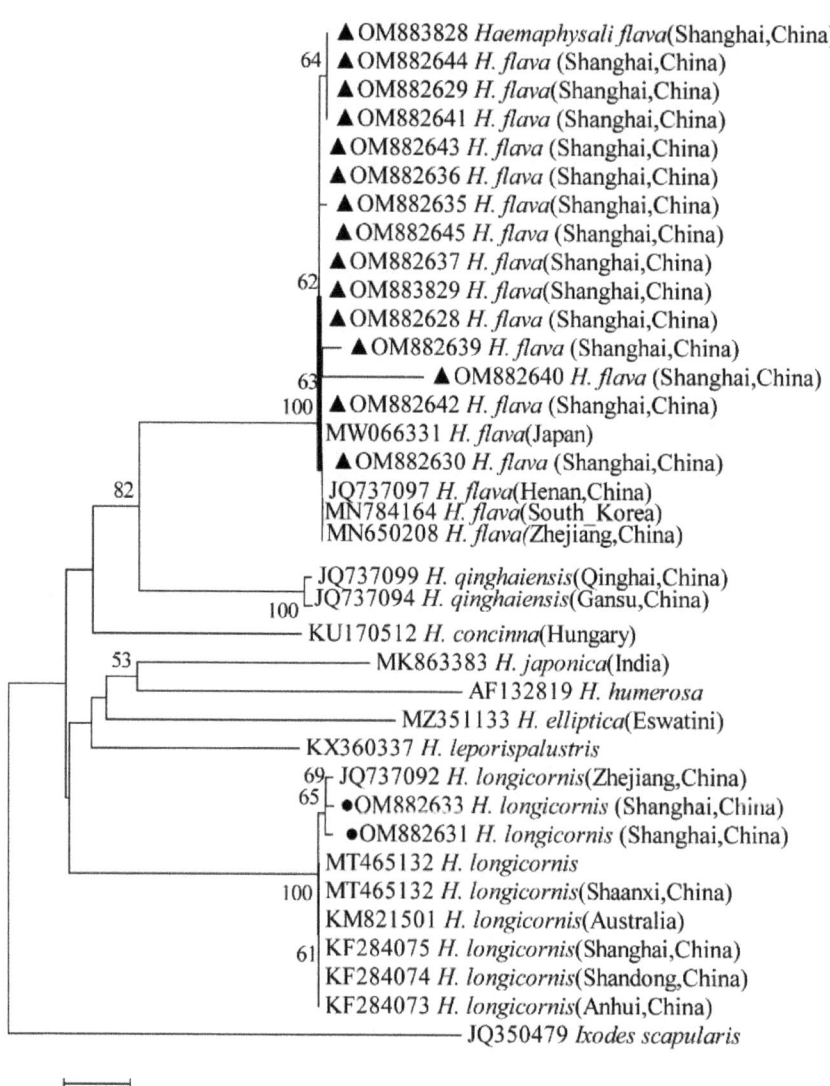

**Figure 10.** Phylogenetic tree of *H. flava* and *H. longicornis* based on partial CO I gene sequence similarity. The sequence from *H. flava* obtained in this study is indicated with a black triangle, and the sequence from *H. longicornis* obtained in this study is indicated with black dots. Sequences were aligned using the MEGA X (version 10.0) software package. Phylogenetic analysis was performed by the neighbor-joining method (NJ method), and bootstrap values were estimated for 1000 replicates. Kimura's two-parameter model was used as a substitution model for the calculation of the phylogenetic trees.

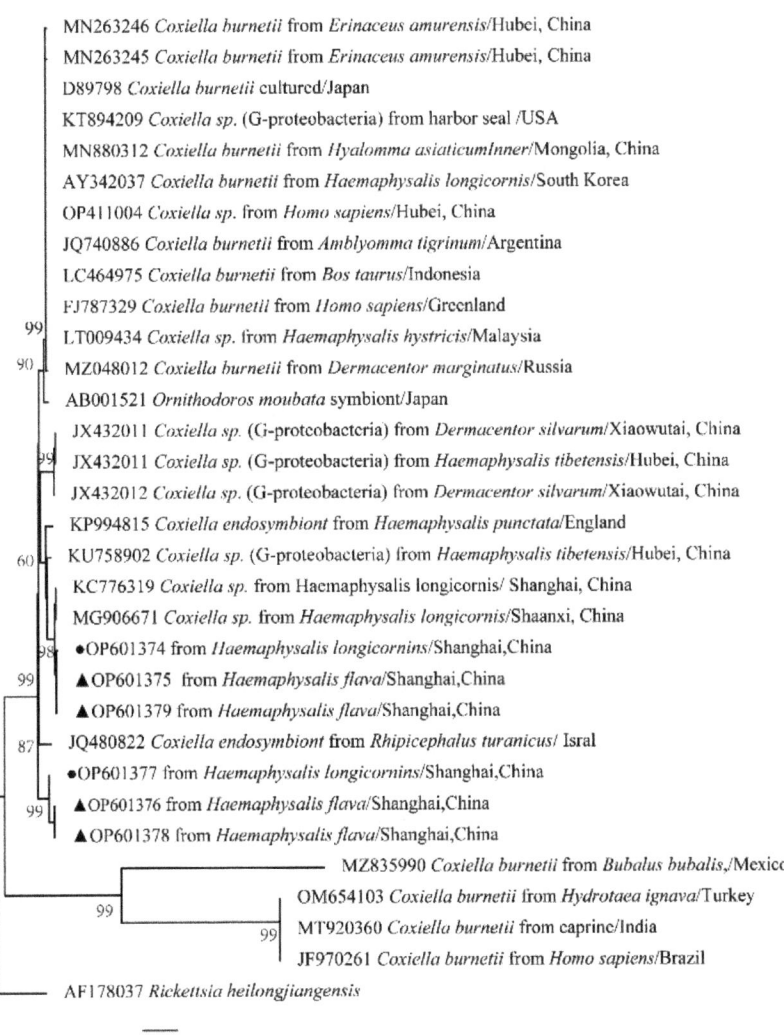

**Figure 11.** Phylogenetic tree of *Coxiella* spp. in ticks based on partial 16S rDNA gene sequence similarity. The sequence from *H. flava* obtained in this study is indicated with a black triangle, and the sequence from *H. longicornis* obtained in this study is indicated with black dots. Sequences were aligned using the MEGA X (version 10.0) software package. Phylogenetic analysis was performed by the neighbor-joining method (NJ method), and bootstrap values were estimated for 1000 replicates. The Kimura two-parameter model was used as a substitution model for the calculation of the phylogenetic trees.

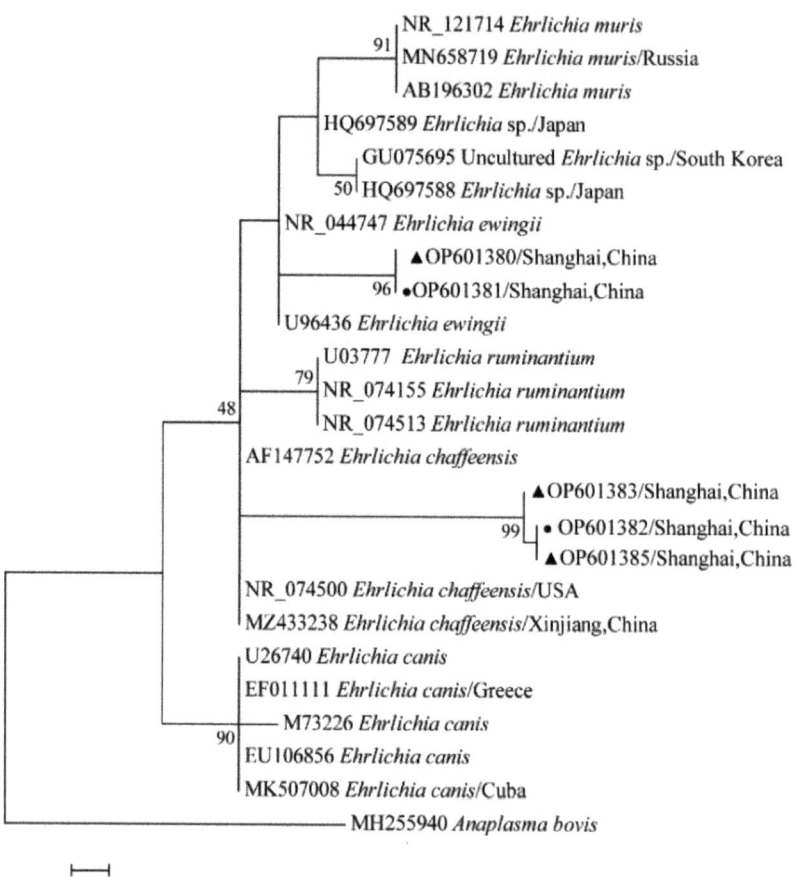

**Figure 12.** Phylogenetic tree of *Ehrlichia* spp. in ticks based on partial 16S rDNA gene sequence similarity. The sequence from *H. flava* obtained in this study is indicated with a black triangle, and the sequence from *H. longicornis* obtained in this study is indicated with black dots. Sequences were aligned by using the MEGA X (version 10.0) software package. Phylogenetic analysis was performed by the neighbor-joining method (NJ method), and bootstrap values were estimated for 1000 replicates. The Kimura two-parameter model was used as a substitution model for the calculation of the phylogenetic trees.

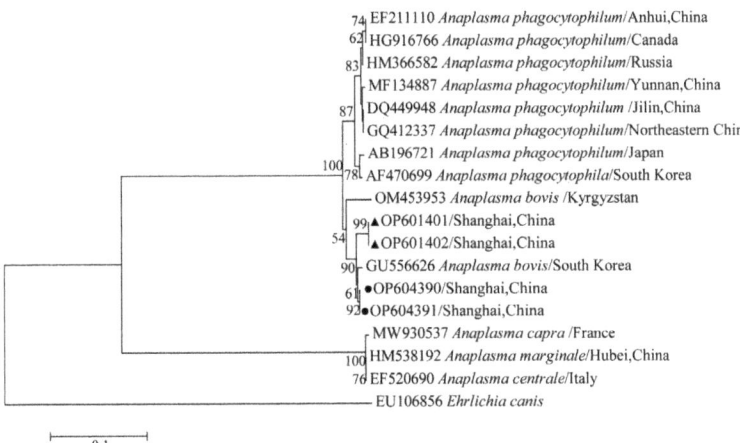

**Figure 13.** Phylogenetic tree of *Anaplasma* spp. in ticks based on partial 16S rDNA gene sequence similarity. The sequence from *H. flava* obtained in this study is indicated with a black triangle, and the sequence from *H. longicornis* obtained in this study is indicated with black dots. Sequences were aligned using the MEGA X (version 10.0) software package. Phylogenetic analysis was performed by the neighbor-joining method (NJ method), and bootstrap values were estimated for 1000 replicates. The Kimura two-parameter model was used as a substitution model for the calculation of the phylogenetic trees.

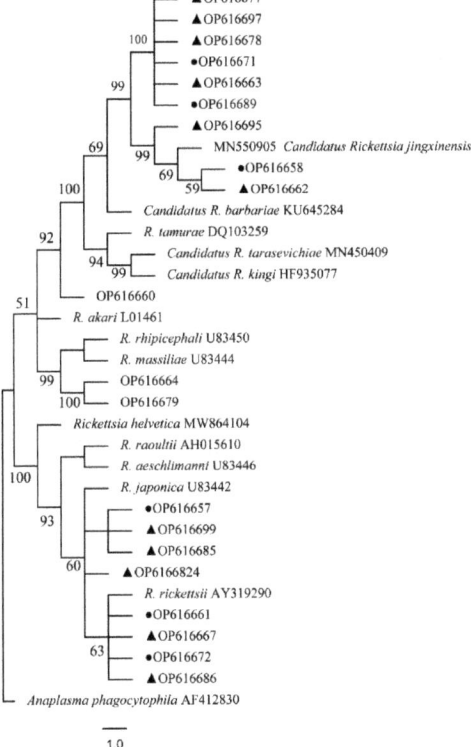

**Figure 14.** Phylogenetic tree of *Rickettsia spp.* in ticks based on partial *ompA* gene sequence similarity.

The sequence from *H. flava* obtained in this study is indicated with a black triangle, and the sequence from *H. longicornis* obtained in this study is indicated with black dots. Sequences were aligned using the MEGA X (version 10.0) software package. Phylogenetic analysis was performed by the neighbor-joining method (NJ method), and bootstrap values were estimated for 1000 replicates. The Kimura two-parameter model was used as a substitution model for the calculation of the phylogenetic trees.

## 4. Discussion

In recent years, more and more attention has focused on emerging TBPs and ticks. Additionally, a wide variety of pathogenic and non-pathogenic bacteria have been identified. In this study, the bacterial community diversity of *Haemaphysalis* spp. in Shanghai was analyzed and compared based on the 16S rDNA high-throughput sequencing technique combined with nested PCR to survey TBPs in *Haemaphysalis* spp. collected from Shanghai, China. It is found that the 16S rDNA V3–V4 variable region sequence of bacteria can effectively detect the bacterial community composition and diversity of *H. flava* and *H. longicornis*. At the same time, sequencing data can also be used to evaluate the relative abundance of bacteria and the differences in flora structure between different groups.

In this study, two species of *Haemaphysalis* ticks: *H. longicornis* and *H. flava*, were collected. *H. flava* often lives in mixed forests and fields, and their hosts are mainly pigs, pig badgers, horses and sheep, while *H. longicornis* mainly live in secondary forests, mountains, or hilly marginal areas, and their hosts are mainly cattle, horses, sheep, goats, bears, hedgehogs, etc. [22]. However, in the past, *H. longicornis* was the main tick species in Shanghai [21], but today, *H. flava*, which has spread all over Shanghai, is the main tick species. In light of the ongoing geographical expansion of ticks caused by climatic change, as well as their increased ability to harbor new pathogens, public health concerns have been raised for both humans and animals [21,30–32]. Many new tick-borne pathogens have been discovered in recent decades, indicating the serious public health threat that tick-borne diseases have imposed on China [30]. The main pathogens reported in *H. flava* are *Ehrlichia*, *Rickettsia japonica*, Crimean–Congo hemorrhagic fever virus (CCHFV), *Pseudomonas aeruginosa* and *Rickettsia raoultii* [9,30]. Additionally, *H. longicornis* carries pathogens such as SFTSV, *Anaplasma*, spotted fever group *Rickettsia* (SFGR), *Babesia*, etc. [33,34]. The number of species of *Haemaphysalis* ticks in Shanghai is small, but its potential harm to human and animal husbandry should not be ignored.

In this study, the diversity of bacterial communities of *H. flava* and *H. longicornis* was different in species and regions. The α diversity analysis of metagenomics also showed that the combinations of tick bacteria were different with different biological factors (such as different developmental stages, age and sex) and differed from the tissue and environmental conditions investigated in other studies [17,35,36]. However, some regional differences were detected in most of the metagenomics β diversity indexes of male and female ticks [17], and any regional and gender differences were also found in the relative abundance of different bacterial groups [35–38]. The core bacterial communities may be influenced by maternal inheritance, the vertebrate animal skin microflora, host blood or the environment on physical contact [39,40]. However, a more specific and long-term association between some blood-feeding arthropods and their bacterial associate is likely mediated by the immune system of the host rather than by their external environment [40–42]. Bacterial taxa such as *Bacillus*, *Clostridium*, *Methylobacterium*, *Mycobacterium*, *Pseudomonas*, *Sphingomonas* and *Staphylococcus*, some of which were found in high abundance in our samples, contain species that may be commonly associated with the environment or as part of the mammalian skin flora [3,40–42]. Therefore, more stringent washing procedures, such as washing with sodium hypochlorite, or limiting sampling to internal organs, such as the salivary glands and mid-gut, may be necessary to determine the internal flora of ticks in further studies [3].

The bacteria in all the arthropod species were dominated by the phylum Proteobacteria, with proportions ranging from 48% to 72%, and their major bacteria phyla that were shared among all the arthropod species included Firmicutes, Bacteroidetes and Actinobacteria [40]. Our results are generally similar to those obtained in previous studies, where arthropod vectors species were dominated by Proteobacteria, including Gammaproteobacteria, Betaproteobacteria, Alphaproteobacteria, and to a lesser extent, Firmicutes, commonly Bacilli and Actinobacteria [40,43–46]. The taxonomic profiles at the genus level confirmed that genera *Rickettsia*, *Anaplasma*, *Ehrlichia* and *Coxiella* existed in the pooled sample, which all predominated in the top six in relative abundance [30]. The mutual connection of symbiotic bacteria hosts exists widely in nature. In recent years, the relationship between symbiotic bacteria and the host has received more and more attention; especially, the mode and mechanism of interaction between symbiotic bacteria and the host have aroused widespread concern. A past study has shown that *Coxiella*-like bacteria are frequently detected in *Haemaphysalis* ticks, although not all species carry them, and *Coxiella*-like endosymbionts have also been reported in other tick species such as *H. shimoga*, *Rhipicephalus sanguineus*, *Amblyomma americanum*, and the soft tick, *Ornithodoros rostratus* [3,47–50]. The significance of *Coxiella* in tick physiology is still unclear. Ticks may depend on bacteria, such as *Coxiella*-like bacteria and *Coxiella*-like endosymbionts (CLE), which play important roles in the processes of food digestion, biosynthesis, growth and development, reproductive regulation and the immune defense of ticks [51]. Studies have confirmed that the CLE genome has complete coding genes of the key coenzyme factor (B vitamins) biosynthesis pathway, which provides a stable source of vitamins for host ticks [52,53]. Removing CLE will significantly reduce the fertility of host ticks [53,54]. The host tick provides CLE with a stable growth environment and nutrition, which makes CLE grow and propagate in ticks and spread to offspring ticks. However, not all individuals of the same tick species will harbor endosymbionts at a similar abundance; some individuals may not carry any *Coxiella*-like endosymbionts at all according to other studies [3,54].

*Coxiella*-like bacteria, *Legionella*, *Sphingomonas* and other strains were detected. *Coxiella*-like bacteria are common in all tick samples, and the content is very high, which indicates that it may be an endosymbiont [55]. So far, in addition to focusing on the study of microbial communities and specific symbionts in ticks, attention has also been paid to bacterial interactions in ticks. There was a negative correlation between symbiotic bacteria and the serous edge of pathogens and a positive correlation among endosymbionts, *Clostridium novyi* and *Corynebacterium cereus* [56]. There also is a repulsion between symbiotic *Rickettsia* and pathogenic *Rickettsia* [35,57]. A detailed understanding of the interaction among microflora in ticks is helpful in developing new strategies for pathogens and tick vector control [17].

After sequencing the DNA fragments amplified by PCR and the sequence comparison, three *Rickettsia* species (*Candidatus R. jingxinnensis*, *R. rickettsii* and *R. japonica*), one *Anaplasma* species (*A. bovis*), two *Coxiella* species (*Coxiella* spp. and *C.*-like endosymbiont) and two *Ehrlichia* species (*E. chaffeensis*, *E. ewingii*) were found in both *H. flava* and *H. longicornis*. In Jiangsu province, China, which is close to Shanghai, Chian, *R. japonica* (81.1%), novel *Rickettsia* spp. (5.1%), *A. bovis* (12%), *A. platys* (6.3%), novel *Ehrlichia* spp. (16.6), *C. burnetii* (10.9%), and a novel *Coxiella*-like endosymbiont (CLE) strain (61.1%), detected in *H. flava* [30], are higher than in Shanghai, China. Especially, *R. japonica* has still been prevalent in China and Japan in recent years and can cause Oriental spotted fever. Interestingly, *H. flava* had a high positive rate (81.1%) of *R. japonica* in Jiangsu province, China [31], compared to the 3.32% detected in this tick species in Shanghai, China, in this study.

At present, there are three known species of *Rickettsia japonica*, *Rickettsia rickettsii* and *Candidatus Rickettsia jingxinensis* in Shanghai, as well as new species of *Rickettsia* that have not been identified or cultivated successfully, which have certain public health risks. Japanese spotted fever (JSF) caused by *Rickettsia japonica* infection is an acute febrile eruptive disease with ticks as the vector. The pathogen can also be detected in *H. longicornis* collected in Shandong, and researchers in Fujian province, China, have also amplified highly similar genes of *Rickettsia japonica*. Japan and South Korea have reported confirmed cases of Japanese spotted fever, and there are reports of *Rickettsia japonica* infection in Hebei, Anhui provinces, China [58]. Rocky Mountain Spotted Fever (RMSF) is caused by *R. rickettsii* infection. It has been observed that *Candidatus R. jingxinensis* can infect humans, showing the clinical features of fever, erythema rash and eschar [59]. Previous studies have shown that the main vectors of *Rickettsia japonica* are *H. flava, H. formosensis, H. longicornis, H. cornigera, Ixodes ovatus, Rhipicephalus haemaphysaloides* and *Dermacentor taiwanensis*. The vectors of RMSF are *Amblyomma sculptum, Amblyomma aureolatum* and *Dermacento anderson*. *Candidatus R. jingxinensis* were also detected in *H. longicornis* in Yunnan, Liaoning, Hebei and Jiangsu provinces, China, and Korea [60,61]. In Shanghai, *Candidatus R. jingxinensis* was detected in not only *H. longicornis* but also *H. flava*. In this study, *Candidatus R. jingxinensis* was detected from two tick species of *Haemaphysalis* spp., especially *H. flava*, which has spread all over Shanghai, China, which indicated that *Candidatus R. jingxinensis* had the characteristics of wide distribution. The deficiency of this study is that all three *Rickettsia* species have been detected in new tick species, but the genotype cannot be further confirmed and isolated by culture.

The two predominant human pathogens within the *Ehrlichia* genus are *E. chaffeensis*, the etiologic agent of human monocytic ehrlichiosis (HME) distributed in the United States, Asia and Europe, and *E. ewingii*, the agent of human *E. ewingii* granulocytic ehrlichiosis [62–64]. In southern and northern China, clues of *E. chaffeensis* were found, which indicated that *E. chaffeensis* might exist in China [65,66]. *E. ewingii*, one of the causative agents of canine granulocytic ehrlichiosis, has been reported in dogs and humans in the USA [67]. However, previous investigations and studies in China have found no clues of *E. ewingii*.

*A. bovis* is mainly distributed in Asia and South America. Cattle and buffalo are considered the main hosts of *A. bovis*, but *A. bovis* has also been found in dogs in China. The intangible disease is a tick-borne disease that is mainly prevalent in tropical and subtropical areas. It is not only healthy for livestock. Additionally, it will also threaten human health. Qin [41] investigated in Jiaonan, Shandong Province, China, the infection rate of the blood of ticks was found to be 0.10% for *A. pagocytophilum*, 1.55% for *A. bovis* and 0.33% for *A. capra* [68].

This study has shown that high-throughput 16S rDNA sequencing analysis can detect multiple pathogens at the same time, which can indicate the main local tick-borne pathogens, but it also has the disadvantage of incomplete detection and is unable to match species. Combined with pathogen-specific detection methods, we can more comprehensively understand the status of local *Haemaphysalis* spp.-carrying pathogens, so we need to combine PCR and metagenomics analysis.

In this study, it is worth noting that *Serratia* was detected in the medical tick group. *Serratia* infection can activate the mosquito's immune system, significantly improve the mosquito's resistance to *Plasmodium berghei* infection and reduce the malaria parasite load in Anopheles. A recent research report showed that *Serratia* isolated in the laboratory could promote insect-borne virus infection in mosquitoes [69,70]. This bacterium secretes a protein called SmEnhancin, which can bind mucin on intestinal mucosa to promote the colonization and spread of the virus in mosquitoes [71]. However, the research on ticks is blank, so we need to further study the interaction between ticks, hosts and the bacterial communities in ticks and pathogens and further explain their interaction mechanism.

## 5. Conclusions

This study reports on the bacterial communities and the prevalence of some TBPs in *Haemaphysalis* spp. from Shanghai, China. The results provide insight into the potential roles of *Haemaphysalis* ticks in the epidemiology of pathogens of veterinary and public health significance. Further studies are needed to elucidate the implications of these findings on animals and humans in Shanghai, China. However, these findings are preliminary. Further studies are required to determine the interaction and roles of some of the bacterial communities in tick survival and vector competence.

**Author Contributions:** Y.Z. and W.Z. designed the study. W.Z., Z.L., T.J., D.C., L.Y., T.H., L.D. and D.Z. collected the tick sample. W.Z. performed all the experiments and analyzed the data, and prepared draft figures. W.Z. and Z.L. prepared the manuscript draft with important intellectual input from Y.F. and Y.Z. All authors have read and agreed to the published version of the manuscript.

**Funding:** This study was financially sponsored by the Fifth Round of the Three-Year Action for Public Health System Construction in Shanghai (No. GWV-10.1-XK13); The Special Foundation of Basic Science and Technology Resources Survey of Ministry of Science and Technology of China (No. 2017FY101203); Shanghai sailing program (No. 21YF1452200).

**Institutional Review Board Statement:** Not applicable.

**Informed Consent Statement:** Not applicable.

**Data Availability Statement:** The DNA sequencing data has been uploaded to GeneBank.

**Acknowledgments:** We are very grateful to the staff from Shanghai Center for Disease Control and Prevention, as well as Fan Mingqiu, Wen Heyi and Lin Chen for the tick sample collection.

**Conflicts of Interest:** The authors declare no conflict of interest.

## References

1. Dantas-Torres, F.; Chomel, B.B.; Otranto, D. Ticks and tick-borne diseases: A One Health perspective. *Trends Parasitol.* **2012**, *28*, 437–446. [CrossRef] [PubMed]
2. Mrzljak, A.; Novak, R.; Pandak, N.; Tabain, I.; Franusic, L.; Barbic, L.; Bogdanic, M.; Savic, V.; Mikulic, D.; Pavicic-Saric, J.; et al. Emerging and neglected zoonoses in transplant population. *World J. Transplant.* **2020**, *10*, 47–63. [CrossRef] [PubMed]
3. Khoo, J.J.; Chen, F.; Kho, K.L.; Shanizza, A.I.A.; Lim, F.S.; Tan, K.K.; Chang, L.Y.; AbuBakar, S. Bacterial community in *Haemaphysalis* ticks of domesticated animals from the Orang Asli communities in Malaysia. *Ticks Tick Borne Dis.* **2016**, *7*, 929–937. [CrossRef] [PubMed]
4. Carmichael, J.R.; Fuerst, P.A. A rickettsial mixed infection in a *Dermacentor variabilis* tick from Ohio. *Ann. N. Y. Acad. Sci.* **2006**, *1078*, 334–337. [CrossRef] [PubMed]
5. Zhao, G.P.; Wang, Y.X.; Fan, Z.W.; Ji, Y.; Liu, M.J.; Zhang, W.H.; Li, X.L.; Zhou, S.X.; Li, H.; Liang, S.; et al. Mapping ticks and tick-borne pathogens in China. *Nat. Commun.* **2021**, *12*, 1075. [CrossRef]
6. Wu, X.B.; Na, R.H.; Wei, S.S.; Zhu, J.S.; Peng, H.J. Distribution of tick-borne diseases in China. *Parasites Vectors* **2013**, *6*, 119. [CrossRef]
7. Fang, L.Q.; Liu, K.; Li, X.L.; Liang, S.; Yang, Y.; Yao, H.W.; Sun, R.X.; Sun, Y.; Chen, W.J.; Zuo, S.Q.; et al. Emerging tick-borne infections in mainland China: An increasing public health threat. *Lancet Infect. Dis.* **2015**, *15*, 1467–1479. [CrossRef]
8. Chen, Z.; Li, H.; Gao, X.; Bian, A.; Yan, H.; Kong, D.; Liu, X. Human Babesiosis in China: A systematic review. *Parasitol. Res.* **2019**, *118*, 1103–1112. [CrossRef]
9. Fang, L.Z.; Lei, S.C.; Yan, Z.J.; Xiao, X.; Liu, J.W.; Gong, X.Q.; Yu, H.; Yu, X.J. Detection of Multiple Intracellular Bacterial Pathogens in *Haemaphysalis flava* Ticks Collected from Hedgehogs in Central China. *Pathogens* **2021**, *10*, 115. [CrossRef]
10. Liu, L.M.; Liu, J.N.; Liu, Z.; Yu, Z.J.; Xu, S.Q.; Yang, X.H.; Li, T.; Li, S.S.; Guo, L.D.; Liu, J.Z. Microbial communities and symbionts in the hard tick *Haemaphysalis longicornis* (Acari: Ixodidae) from north China. *Parasites Vectors* **2013**, *6*, 310. [CrossRef]
11. Tijsse-Klasen, E.; Hansford, K.M.; Jahfari, S.; Phipps, P.; Sprong, H.; Medlock, J.M. Spotted fever group rickettsiae in *Dermacentor reticulatus* and *Haemaphysalis punctata* ticks in the UK. *Parasites Vectors* **2013**, *6*, 212. [CrossRef]
12. Yu, Z.; Wang, H.; Wang, T.; Sun, W.; Yang, X.; Liu, J. Tick-borne pathogens and the vector potential of ticks in China. *Parasites Vectors* **2015**, *8*, 24. [CrossRef]
13. Luo, J.; Ren, Q.; Liu, W.; Li, X.; Hong, Y.; Song, M.; Bo, Z.; Guan, G.; Luo, J.; Liu, G. Micropathogen community identification in ticks (Acari: Ixodidae) using third-generation sequencing. *Int. J. Parasitol. Parasites Wildl.* **2021**, *15*, 238–248. [CrossRef]
14. Zhao, T.; Gong, H.; Shen, X.; Zhang, W.; Shan, T.; Yu, X.; Wang, S.J.; Cui, L. Comparison of Viromes in Ticks from Different Domestic Animals in China. *Virol. Sin.* **2020**, *35*, 398–406. [CrossRef]
15. Ng, T.F.; Willner, D.L.; Lim, Y.W.; Schmieder, R.; Chau, B.; Nilsson, C.; Anthony, S.; Ruan, Y.; Rohwer, F.; Breitbart, M. Broad surveys of DNA viral diversity obtained through viral metagenomics of mosquitoes. *PLoS ONE* **2011**, *6*, e20579. [CrossRef]
16. Jiao, J.; Lu, Z.; Yu, Y.; Ou, Y.; Fu, M.; Zhao, Y.; Wu, N.; Zhao, M.; Liu, Y.; Sun, Y.; et al. Identification of tick-borne pathogens by metagenomic next-generation sequencing in Dermacentor nuttalli and Ixodes persulcatus in Inner Mongolia, China. *Parasites Vectors* **2021**, *14*, 287. [CrossRef]
17. Batool, M.; Blazier, J.C.; Rogovska, Y.V.; Wang, J.; Liu, S.; Nebogatkin, I.V.; Rogovskyy, A.S. Metagenomic analysis of individually analyzed ticks from Eastern Europe demonstrates regional and sex-dependent differences in the microbiota of Ixodes ricinus. *Ticks Tick Borne Dis.* **2021**, *12*, 101768. [CrossRef]
18. Kodama, F.; Yamaguchi, H.; Park, E.; Tatemoto, K.; Sashika, M.; Nakao, R.; Terauchi, Y.; Mizuma, K.; Orba, Y.; Kariwa, H.; et al. A novel nairovirus associated with acute febrile illness in Hokkaido, Japan. *Nat. Commun.* **2021**, *12*, 5539. [CrossRef]

19. Wang, Z.D.; Wang, B.; Wei, F.; Han, S.Z.; Zhang, L.; Yang, Z.T.; Yan, Y.; Lv, X.L.; Li, L.; Wang, S.C.; et al. A New Segmented Virus Associated with Human Febrile Illness in China. *N. Engl. J. Med.* **2019**, *380*, 2116–2125. [CrossRef]
20. Liu, Q.; He, B.; Huang, S.Y.; Wei, F.; Zhu, X.Q. Severe fever with thrombocytopenia syndrome, an emerging tick-borne zoonosis. *Lancet Infect. Dis.* **2014**, *14*, 763–772. [CrossRef]
21. Li, Z.Q.; Li, L.H.; Yin, H.J.; Wei, Z.X.; Guo, Y.H.; Ma, B.; Zhang, Y. Distribution and suitable habitats of ticks in the Yangtze River Delta urban agglomeration. *Chin. J. Schistosomiasis Control* **2021**, *33*, 365–372. [CrossRef]
22. Yamaguti, N.; Tipton, V.J.; Keegan, H.L.; Toshioka, S. Ticks of Japan, Korea and the Ryukyu islands. *Brighan Young Univ. Sci. Bull.* **1971**, *15*, 1–226.
23. Abdullah, H.H.; El-Molla, A.; Salib, F.A.; Allam, N.A.; Ghazy, A.A.; Abdel-Shafy, S. Morphological and molecular identification of the brown dog tick *Rhipicephalus sanguineus* and the camel tick *Hyalomma dromedarii* (Acari: Ixodidae) vectors of Rickettsioses in Egypt. *Vet. World* **2016**, *9*, 1087–1101. [CrossRef] [PubMed]
24. Chitimia, L.; Lin, R.Q.; Cosoroaba, I.; Wu, X.Y.; Song, H.Q.; Yuan, Z.G.; Zhu, X.Q. Genetic characterization of ticks from southwestern Romania by sequences of mitochondrial cox1 and nad5 genes. *Exp. Appl. Acarol.* **2010**, *52*, 305–311. [CrossRef] [PubMed]
25. Nossa, C.W.; Oberdorf, W.E.; Yang, L.; Aas, J.A.; Paster, B.J.; Desantis, T.Z.; Brodie, E.L.; Malamud, D.; Poles, M.A.; Pei, Z. Design of 16S rRNA gene primers for 454 pyrosequencing of the human foregut microbiome. *World J. Gastroenterol.* **2010**, *16*, 4135–4144. [CrossRef]
26. Regnery, R.L.; Spruill, C.L.; Plikaytis, B.D. Genotypic identification of rickettsiae and estimation of intraspecies sequence divergence for portions of two rickettsial genes. *J. Bacteriol.* **1991**, *173*, 1576–1589. [CrossRef]
27. Cicuttin, G.L.; Brambati, D.F.; Rodríguez Eugui, J.I.; Lebrero, C.G.; De Salvo, M.N.; Beltrán, F.J.; Gury Dohmen, F.E.; Jado, I.; Anda, P. Molecular characterization of *Rickettsia massiliae* and *Anaplasma platys* infecting *Rhipicephalus sanguineus* ticks and domestic dogs, Buenos Aires (Argentina). *Ticks Tick Borne Dis.* **2014**, *5*, 484–488. [CrossRef]
28. Callahan, B.J.; McMurdie, P.J.; Rosen, M.J.; Han, A.W.; Johnson, A.J.; Holmes, S.P. DADA2: High-resolution sample inference from Illumina amplicon data. *Nat. Methods* **2016**, *13*, 581–583. [CrossRef]
29. Bolyen, E.; Rideout, J.R.; Dillon, M.R.; Bokulich, N.A.; Abnet, C.C.; Al-Ghalith, G.A.; Alexander, H.; Alm, E.J.; Arumugam, M.; Asnicar, F.; et al. Reproducible, interactive, scalable and extensible microbiome data science using QIIME 2. *Nat. Biotechnol.* **2019**, *37*, 852–857. [CrossRef]
30. Qi, Y.; Ai, L.; Zhu, C.; Ye, F.; Lv, R.; Wang, J.; Mao, Y.; Lu, N.; Tan, W. Wild Hedgehogs and Their Parasitic Ticks Coinfected with Multiple Tick-Borne Pathogens in Jiangsu Province, Eastern China. *Microbiol. Spectr.* **2022**, *10*, e0213822. [CrossRef]
31. Cun, D.J.; Wang, Q.; Yao, X.Y.; Ma, B.; Zhang, Y.; Li, L.H. Potential suitable habitats of Haemaphysalis longicornis in China under different climatic patterns. *Chin. J. Schistosomiasis Control* **2021**, *33*, 359–364. [CrossRef]
32. Zhao, L.; Li, J.; Cui, X.; Jia, N.; Wei, J.; Xia, L.; Wang, H.; Zhou, Y.; Wang, Q.; Liu, X.; et al. Distribution of *Haemaphysalis longicornis* and associated pathogens: Analysis of pooled data from a China field survey and global published data. *Lancet Planet. Health* **2020**, *4*, e320–e329. [CrossRef]
33. Yan, Y.; Wang, K.; Cui, Y.; Zhou, Y.; Zhao, S.; Zhang, Y.; Jian, F.; Wang, R.; Zhang, L.; Ning, C. Molecular detection and phylogenetic analyses of *Anaplasma* spp. in *Haemaphysalis longicornis* from goats in four provinces of China. *Sci. Rep.* **2021**, *11*, 14155. [CrossRef]
34. Jiang, J.; An, H.; Lee, J.S.; O'Guinn, M.L.; Kim, H.C.; Chong, S.T.; Zhang, Y.; Song, D.; Burrus, R.G.; Bao, Y.; et al. Molecular characterization of *Haemaphysalis longicornis*-borne rickettsiae, Republic of Korea and China. *Ticks Tick Borne Dis.* **2018**, *9*, 1606–1613. [CrossRef]
35. Gomard, Y.; Flores, O.; Vittecoq, M.; Blanchon, T.; Toty, C.; Duron, O.; Mavingui, P.; Tortosa, P.; McCoy, K.D. Changes in Bacterial Diversity, Composition and Interactions During the Development of the Seabird Tick *Ornithodoros maritimus* (Argasidae). *Microb. Ecol.* **2021**, *81*, 770–783. [CrossRef]
36. Van Overbeek, L.; Gassner, F.; van der Plas, C.L.; Kastelein, P.; Nunes-da Rocha, U.; Takken, W. Diversity of *Ixodes ricinus* tick-associated bacterial communities from different forests. *FEMS Microbiol. Ecol.* **2008**, *66*, 72–84. [CrossRef]
37. Carpi, G.; Cagnacci, F.; Wittekindt, N.E.; Zhao, F.; Qi, J.; Tomsho, L.P.; Drautz, D.I.; Rizzoli, A.; Schuster, S.C. Metagenomic profile of the bacterial communities associated with *Ixodes ricinus* ticks. *PLoS ONE* **2011**, *6*, e25604. [CrossRef]
38. Thapa, S.; Zhang, Y.; Allen, M.S. Effects of temperature on bacterial microbiome composition in *Ixodes scapularis* ticks. *MicrobiologyOpen* **2019**, *8*, e00719. [CrossRef]
39. Lim, F.S.; Khoo, J.J.; Tan, K.K.; Zainal, N.; Loong, S.K.; Khor, C.S.; AbuBakar, S. Bacterial communities in *Haemaphysalis, Dermacentor* and *Amblyomma* ticks collected from wild boar of an Orang Asli Community in Malaysia. *Ticks Tick Borne Dis.* **2020**, *11*, 101352. [CrossRef]
40. Bennett, K.L.; Almanza, A.; McMillan, W.O.; Saltonstall, K.; Vdovenko, E.L.; Vinda, J.S.; Mejia, L.; Driesse, K.; De León, L.F.; Loaiza, J.R. Habitat disturbance and the organization of bacterial communities in Neotropical hematophagous arthropods. *PLoS ONE* **2019**, *14*, e0222145. [CrossRef]
41. Bonnet, S.I.; Binetruy, F.; Hernández-Jarguín, A.M.; Duron, O. The Tick Microbiome: Why Non-Pathogenic Microorganisms Matter in Tick Biology and Pathogen Transmission. *Front. Cell. Infect. Microbiol.* **2017**, *7*, 236. [CrossRef] [PubMed]
42. Narasimhan, S.; Fikrig, E. Tick microbiome: The force within. *Trends Parasitol.* **2015**, *31*, 315–323. [CrossRef] [PubMed]

43. Duguma, D.; Rugman-Jones, P.; Kaufman, M.G.; Hall, M.W.; Neufeld, J.D.; Stouthamer, R.; Walton, W.E. Bacterial communities associated with culex mosquito larvae and two emergent aquatic plants of bioremediation importance. *PLoS ONE* **2013**, *8*, e72522. [CrossRef] [PubMed]
44. Menchaca, A.C.; Visi, D.K.; Strey, O.F.; Teel, P.D.; Kalinowski, K.; Allen, M.S.; Williamson, P.C. Preliminary assessment of microbiome changes following blood-feeding and survivorship in the *Amblyomma americanum* nymph-to-adult transition using semiconductor sequencing. *PLoS ONE* **2013**, *8*, e67129. [CrossRef]
45. Muturi, E.J.; Ramirez, J.L.; Rooney, A.P.; Kim, C.H. Comparative analysis of gut microbiota of mosquito communities in central Illinois. *PLoS Negl. Trop. Dis.* **2017**, *11*, e0005377. [CrossRef]
46. Osei-Poku, J.; Mbogo, C.M.; Palmer, W.J.; Jiggins, F.M. Deep sequencing reveals extensive variation in the gut microbiota of wild mosquitoes from Kenya. *Mol. Ecol.* **2012**, *21*, 5138–5150. [CrossRef]
47. Ahantarig, A.; Malaisri, P.; Hirunkanokpun, S.; Sumrandee, C.; Trinachartvanit, W.; Baimai, V. Detection of *Rickettsia* and a novel *Haemaphysalis shimoga* symbiont bacterium in ticks in Thailand. *Curr. Microbiol.* **2011**, *62*, 1496–1502. [CrossRef]
48. Noda, H.; Munderloh, U.G.; Kurtti, T.J. Endosymbionts of ticks and their relationship to *Wolbachia* spp. and tick-borne pathogens of humans and animals. *Appl. Environ. Microbiol.* **1997**, *63*, 3926–3932. [CrossRef]
49. Jasinskas, A.; Zhong, J.; Barbour, A.G. Highly prevalent *Coxiella* sp. bacterium in the tick vector *Amblyomma americanum*. *Appl. Environ. Microbiol.* **2007**, *73*, 334–336. [CrossRef]
50. Almeida, A.P.; Marcili, A.; Leite, R.C.; Nieri-Bastos, F.A.; Domingues, L.N.; Martins, J.R.; Labruna, M.B. *Coxiella* symbiont in the tick *Ornithodoros rostratus* (Acari: Argasidae). *Ticks Tick Borne Dis.* **2012**, *3*, 203–206. [CrossRef]
51. Dall'Agnol, B.; McCulloch, J.A.; Mayer, F.Q.; Souza, U.; Webster, A.; Antunes, P.; Doyle, R.L.; Reck, J.; Ferreira, C.A.S. Molecular characterization of bacterial communities of two neotropical tick species (*Amblyomma aureolatum* and *Ornithodoros brasiliensis*) using rDNA 16S sequencing. *Ticks Tick Borne Dis.* **2021**, *12*, 101746. [CrossRef]
52. Klyachko, O.; Stein, B.D.; Grindle, N.; Clay, K.; Fuqua, C. Localization and visualization of a *Coxiella*-type symbiont within the lone star tick, *Amblyomma americanum*. *Appl. Environ. Microbiol.* **2007**, *73*, 6584–6594. [CrossRef]
53. Smith, T.A.; Driscoll, T.; Gillespie, J.J.; Raghavan, R. A *Coxiella*-like endosymbiont is a potential vitamin source for the Lone Star tick. *Genome Biol. Evol.* **2015**, *7*, 831–838. [CrossRef]
54. Tsementzi, D.; Castro Gordillo, J.; Mahagna, M.; Gottlieb, Y.; Konstantinidis, K.T. Comparison of closely related, uncultivated *Coxiella* tick endosymbiont population genomes reveals clues about the mechanisms of symbiosis. *Environ. Microbiol.* **2018**, *20*, 1751–1764. [CrossRef]
55. Tufts, D.M.; Sameroff, S.; Tagliafierro, T.; Jain, K.; Oleynik, A.; VanAcker, M.C.; Diuk-Wasser, M.A.; Lipkin, W.I.; Tokarz, R. A metagenomic examination of the pathobiome of the invasive tick species, *Haemaphysalis longicornis*, collected from a New York City borough, USA. *Ticks Tick Borne Dis.* **2020**, *11*, 101516. [CrossRef]
56. Gall, C.A.; Reif, K.E.; Scoles, G.A.; Mason, K.L.; Mousel, M.; Noh, S.M.; Brayton, K.A. The bacterial microbiome of *Dermacentor andersoni* ticks influences pathogen susceptibility. *ISME J.* **2016**, *10*, 1846–1855. [CrossRef]
57. Macaluso, K.R.; Sonenshine, D.E.; Ceraul, S.M.; Azad, A.F. Rickettsial infection in *Dermacentor variabilis* (Acari: Ixodidae) inhibits transovarial transmission of a second *Rickettsia*. *J. Med. Entomol.* **2002**, *39*, 809–813. [CrossRef]
58. Li, W.; Liu, S.N. *Rickettsia japonica* infections in Huanggang, China, in 2021. *IDCases* **2021**, *26*, e01309. [CrossRef]
59. Kim, Y.S.; Kim, J.; Choi, Y.J.; Park, H.J.; Jang, W.J. Molecular genetic analysis and clinical characterization of *Rickettsia* species isolated from the Republic of Korea in 2017. *Transbound. Emerg. Dis.* **2020**, *67*, 1447–1452. [CrossRef]
60. Qi, Y.; Ai, L.; Jiao, J.; Wang, J.; Wu, D.; Wang, P.; Zhang, G.; Qin, Y.; Hu, C.; Lv, R.; et al. High prevalence of *Rickettsia* spp. in ticks from wild hedgehogs rather than domestic bovine in Jiangsu province, Eastern China. *Front. Cell. Infect. Microbiol.* **2022**, *12*, 954785. [CrossRef]
61. Park, H.J.; Kim, J.; Choi, Y.J.; Kim, H.C.; Klein, T.A.; Chong, S.T.; Jiang, J.; Richards, A.L.; Jang, W.J. Tick-borne *Rickettsiae* in Midwestern region of Republic of Korea. *Acta Trop.* **2021**, *215*, 105794. [CrossRef] [PubMed]
62. Cohen, S.B.; Yabsley, M.J.; Freye, J.D.; Dunlap, B.G.; Rowland, M.E.; Huang, J.; Dunn, J.R.; Jones, T.F.; Moncayo, A.C. Prevalence of *Ehrlichia chaffeensis* and *Ehrlichia ewingii* in ticks from Tennessee. *Vector Borne Zoonotic Dis.* **2010**, *10*, 435–440. [CrossRef] [PubMed]
63. Koh, F.X.; Kho, K.L.; Kisomi, M.G.; Wong, L.P.; Bulgiba, A.; Tan, P.E.; Lim, Y.A.L.; Nizam, Q.N.H.; Panchadcharam, C.; Tay, S.T. *Ehrlichia* and *Anaplasma* Infections: Serological Evidence and Tick Surveillance in Peninsular Malaysia. *J. Med. Entomol.* **2018**, *55*, 269–276. [CrossRef] [PubMed]
64. Shibata, S.; Kawahara, M.; Rikihisa, Y.; Fujita, H.; Watanabe, Y.; Suto, C.; Ito, T. New *Ehrlichia* species closely related to *Ehrlichia chaffeensis* isolated from *Ixodes ovatus* ticks in Japan. *J. Clin. Microbiol.* **2000**, *38*, 1331–1338. [CrossRef] [PubMed]
65. Zhang, X.C.; Zhang, L.X.; Li, W.H.; Wang, S.W.; Sun, Y.L.; Wang, Y.Y.; Guan, Z.Z.; Liu, X.J.; Yang, Y.S.; Zhang, S.G.; et al. Ehrlichiosis and zoonotic anaplasmosis in suburban areas of Beijing, China. *Vector Borne Zoonotic Dis.* **2012**, *12*, 932–937. [CrossRef] [PubMed]
66. Cao, W.C.; Gao, Y.M.; Zhang, P.H.; Zhang, X.T.; Dai, Q.H.; Dumler, J.S.; Fang, L.Q.; Yang, H. Identification of *Ehrlichia chaffeensis* by nested PCR in ticks from Southern China. *J. Clin. Microbiol.* **2000**, *38*, 2778–2780. [CrossRef]
67. Yabsley, M.J.; Varela, A.S.; Tate, C.M.; Dugan, V.G.; Stallknecht, D.E.; Little, S.E.; Davidson, W.R. *Ehrlichia ewingii* infection in white-tailed deer (*Odocoileus virginianus*). *Emerg. Infect. Dis.* **2002**, *8*, 668–671. [CrossRef]
68. Qin, X.R.; Han, F.J.; Luo, L.M.; Zhao, F.M.; Han, H.J.; Zhang, Z.T.; Liu, J.W.; Xue, Z.F.; Liu, M.M.; Ma, D.Q.; et al. Anaplasma species detected in *Haemaphysalis longicornis* tick from China. *Ticks Tick Borne Dis.* **2018**, *9*, 840–843. [CrossRef]

69. Bai, L.; Wang, L.; Vega-Rodríguez, J.; Wang, G.; Wang, S. A Gut Symbiotic Bacterium *Serratia marcescens* Renders Mosquito Resistance to Plasmodium Infection through Activation of Mosquito Immune Responses. *Front. Microbiol.* **2019**, *10*, 1580. [CrossRef]
70. Bando, H.; Okado, K.; Guelbeogo, W.M.; Badolo, A.; Aonuma, H.; Nelson, B.; Fukumoto, S.; Xuan, X.; Sagnon, N.; Kanuka, H. Intra-specific diversity of *Serratia marcescens* in Anopheles mosquito midgut defines Plasmodium transmission capacity. *Sci. Rep.* **2013**, *3*, 1641. [CrossRef]
71. Wu, P.; Sun, P.; Nie, K.; Zhu, Y.; Shi, M.; Xiao, C.; Liu, H.; Liu, Q.; Zhao, T.; Chen, X.; et al. A Gut Commensal Bacterium Promotes Mosquito Permissiveness to Arboviruses. *Cell Host Microbe* **2019**, *25*, 101–112.e105. [CrossRef]

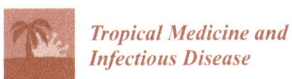

*Tropical Medicine and Infectious Disease*

Article

# The Impact of COVID-19 Quarantine on Tuberculosis and Diabetes Mellitus Cases: A Modelling Study

Nuning Nuraini [1,2,†], Ilham Saiful Fauzi [3,*,†], Bony Wiem Lestari [4,5] and Sila Rizqina [1]

1. Department of Mathematics, Faculty of Mathematics and Natural Sciences, Institut Teknologi Bandung, Bandung 40132, Indonesia
2. Center for Mathematical Modeling and Simulation, Institut Teknologi Bandung, Bandung 40132, Indonesia
3. Department of Accounting, Politeknik Negeri Malang, Malang 65141, Indonesia
4. Department of Public Health, Faculty of Medicine, Universitas Padjadjaran, Bandung 40161, Indonesia
5. Department of Internal Medicine, Radboud Institute for Health Sciences, Radboud University Medical Centre, 6525 GA Nijmegen, The Netherlands
* Correspondence: ilham.fauzi@polinema.ac.id
† These authors contributed equally to this work.

**Abstract:** COVID-19 has currently become a global pandemic and caused a high number of infected people and deaths. To restrain the coronavirus spread, many countries have implemented restrictions on people's movement and outdoor activities. The enforcement of health emergencies such as quarantine has a positive impact on reducing the COVID-19 infection risk, but it also has unwanted influences on health, social, and economic sectors. Here, we developed a compartmental mathematical model for COVID-19 transmission dynamic accommodating quarantine process and including tuberculosis and diabetic people compartments. We highlighted the potential negative impact induced by quarantine implementation on the increasing number of people with tuberculosis and diabetes. The actual COVID-19 data recorded in Indonesia during the Delta and Omicron variant attacks were well-approximated by the model's output. A positive relationship was indicated by a high value of Pearson correlation coefficient, $r = 0.9344$ for Delta and $r = 0.8961$ for Omicron with a significance level of $p < 0.05$. By varying the value of the quarantine parameter, this study obtained that quarantine effectively reduces the number of COVID-19 but induces an increasing number of tuberculosis and diabetic people. In order to minimize these negative impacts, increasing public awareness about the dangers of TB transmission and implementing a healthy lifestyle were considered the most effective strategies based on the simulation. The insights and results presented in this study are potentially useful for relevant authorities to increase public awareness of the potential risk of TB transmission and to promote a healthy lifestyle during the implementation of quarantine.

**Keywords:** COVID-19; tuberculosis; diabetes; mathematical model; quarantine; control strategy

Citation: Nuraini, N.; Fauzi, I.S.; Lestari, B.W.; Rizqina, S. The Impact of COVID-19 Quarantine on Tuberculosis and Diabetes Mellitus Cases: A Modelling Study. *Trop. Med. Infect. Dis.* **2022**, *7*, 407. https://doi.org/10.3390/tropicalmed7120407

Academic Editor: Yannick Simonin

Received: 13 October 2022
Accepted: 23 November 2022
Published: 29 November 2022

**Publisher's Note:** MDPI stays neutral with regard to jurisdictional claims in published maps and institutional affiliations.

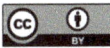

**Copyright:** © 2022 by the authors. Licensee MDPI, Basel, Switzerland. This article is an open access article distributed under the terms and conditions of the Creative Commons Attribution (CC BY) license (https://creativecommons.org/licenses/by/4.0/).

## 1. Introduction

Since 2020, the coronavirus disease 2019 (COVID-19) pandemic has impacted countries globally [1–4]. As of 11 November 2022, about 630 million cases and 6.5 million deaths have been reported [5]. The unprecedented infection and mortality rates have led to the implementation of various public health measures, i.e., lockdowns and social distancing regulations. While these efforts are well-intended to break the chain of transmission, several deleterious health and socioeconomic consequences have been observed [6].

In the field of tuberculosis (TB) management, the COVID-19 pandemic has reversed decades of progress toward TB eradication. Quarantines and stay-at-home measures have increased the risk of TB transmission, particularly among household members [7,8]. This is reflected by the findings from Aznar et al. [9] that observed a significant increase in active TB cases among household contacts in 2020, when compared to 2019. Given that the pandemic also causes a general decrease in healthcare access and increasing poverty rates, both known TB determinants. The number of tuberculosis incidence and mortality are projected to increase by 5–15% within the next five years. This equals hundreds of thousands of additional TB deaths globally [7,8].

The dire situation is potentially exacerbated by comorbidities resulting from quarantine-related lifestyle changes. Several systematic reviews reported that globally, the COVID-19 quarantine measures have led to less physical activity, poorer diet, and a more sedentary lifestyle, all of which are risk factors for many comorbidities, including diabetes [6,10]. In addition, another systematic review reported that lockdowns are associated with deteriorating glycemic control among patients with type-2 diabetes mellitus [11]. Uncontrolled diabetes is a known risk factor for TB infections, poor treatment outcomes, and mortality. In six countries with the highest TB cases, about 10–18% of TB cases can be attributed to diabetes. Overall, diabetes increases the risk of active TB by two- to four-fold [12]. Despite this relationship between TB, diabetes, and COVID-19, however, no study has attempted to model the impact of the pandemic on TB-DM co-occurrence and case management.

This paper aims to investigate the impacts of lockdowns and regional quarantines during the COVID-19 pandemic on TB-DM patients through a modelling study in Indonesia, a country with high burden of TB. Here, we established a mathematical model that divides human population into compartments of three diseases: COVID-19, tuberculosis, and diabetes mellitus. The unobserved parameters were estimated to obtain the best data fitting between the COVID-19 data and the model's output that accommodates the quarantine process. The actual data used in this study is a weekly report of the COVID-19 cases in Indonesia during June 2021-September 2021 and December 2021-April 2022, when Indonesia experienced the Delta and Omicron variant attacks, respectively. The Indonesian government decided to implement the emergency social activity restriction (PPKM darurat) during these periods. In addition, we proposed some strategies that play essential roles in both limiting COVID-19 infection and reducing the negative impacts on TB-DM patients.

## 2. Material and Methods

### 2.1. Mathematical Model

In our mathematical model, we made some modifications to the standard disease transmission model that describes the dynamic of infection. The model includes compartments of three diseases: COVID-19, tuberculosis, and diabetes. TB and diabetes were selected in this model because of the significant impact of the COVID-19 pandemic on TB medical treatment and diabetes progression, especially during the implementation of quarantine and public activity restriction. TB is an infectious disease whose risk of transmission increases during home quarantine among household members. Meanwhile, diabetes is not a contagious disease but it is a co-morbid disease that increases the mortality rate of COVID-19 patients. Public and social measures that restrict residents' activities at home possibly change lifestyles that implicate the development of diabetes.

The actual problem is complex and complicated, so we establish a model that simplifies it by considering only the basic and essential compartments for COVID-19, TB, and diabetes. The human population ($N$) was divided into twelve compartments: susceptible ($S$); quarantined susceptible ($Q_1$); exposed coronavirus ($E_{co}$) i.e., individuals were recently exposed by coronavirus and not infectious; infected coronavirus ($I_{co}$) i.e., individuals were infected and infectious; quarantined infected coronavirus ($Q_2$) i.e., individuals were infected, infectious, and treated; recovered coronavirus ($R_{co}$) i.e., individuals were recovered from coronavirus infection; latent tuberculosis ($L_{tb}$) i.e., individuals were recently exposed tuberculosis and not infectious; infected tuberculosis ($I_{tb}$) i.e., individuals were active TB and infectious; diagnosed tuberculosis ($D_{tb}$) i.e., individuals were active TB and treated; recovered tuberculosis ($R_{tb}$) i.e., individuals were recovered from tuberculosis infection; diabetes without complications ($D_{dm}$); and diabetes with complications ($C_{dm}$). The complete transmission process is shown as transfer diagram in Figure 1.

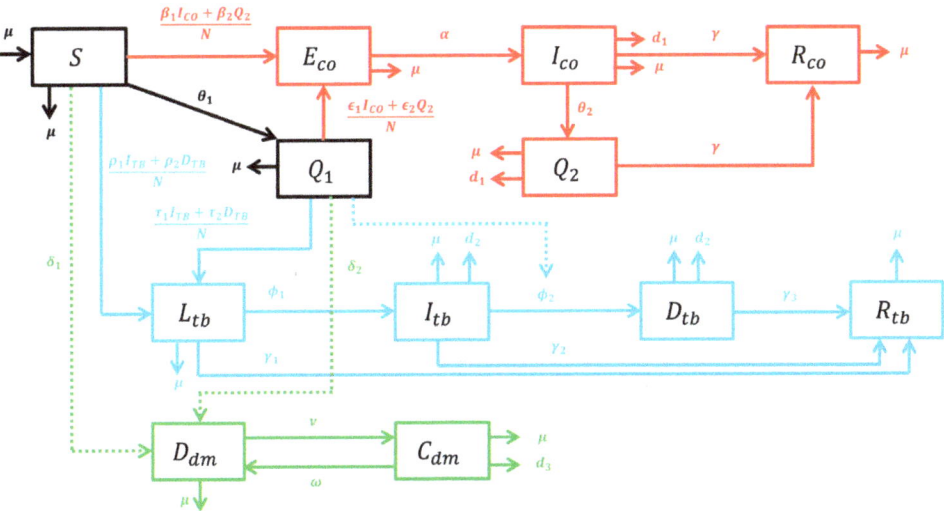

**Figure 1.** A schematic diagram of the disease transmissions including COVID-19, tuberculosis, and diabetes mellitus. The dashed line indicates the indirect effect of the quarantine implementation.

The resulting transmission model is given by the following nonlinear ordinary differential equations system:

$$\begin{aligned}
\frac{dS}{dt} &= \mu N - \left(\frac{\beta_1 I_{co} + \beta_2 Q_2}{N}\right)S - \left(\frac{\rho_1 I_{tb} + \rho_2 D_{tb}}{N}\right)S - (\delta_1 + \theta_1 + \mu)S \\
\frac{dQ_1}{dt} &= \theta_1 S - \left(\frac{\epsilon_1 I_{co} + \epsilon_2 Q_2}{N}\right)Q_1 - \left(\frac{\tau_1 I_{tb} + \tau_2 D_{tb}}{N}\right)Q_1 - (\delta_2 + \mu)Q_1 \\
\frac{dE_{co}}{dt} &= \left(\frac{\beta_1 I_{co} + \beta_2 Q_2}{N}\right)S + \left(\frac{\epsilon_1 I_{co} + \epsilon_2 Q_2}{N}\right)Q_1 - (\alpha + \mu)E_{co} \\
\frac{dI_{co}}{dt} &= \alpha E_{co} - (\theta_2 + \gamma + d_1 + \mu)I_{co} \\
\frac{dR_{co}}{dt} &= \gamma(I_{co} + Q_2) - \mu R_{co} \\
\frac{dQ_2}{dt} &= \theta_2 I_{co} - (\gamma + d_1 + \mu)Q_2 \qquad (1)\\
\frac{dL_{tb}}{dt} &= \left(\frac{\rho_1 I_{tb} + \rho_2 D_{tb}}{N}\right)S + \left(\frac{\tau_1 I_{tb} + \tau_2 D_{tb}}{N}\right)Q_1 - (\phi_1 + \gamma_1 + \mu)L_{tb} \\
\frac{dI_{tb}}{dt} &= \phi_1 L_{tb} - (K\phi_2 + \gamma_2 + d_2 + \mu)I_{tb} \\
\frac{dD_{tb}}{dt} &= K\phi_2 I_{tb} - (\gamma_3 + d_2 + \mu)D_{tb} \\
\frac{dR_{tb}}{dt} &= \gamma_1 L_{tb} + \gamma_2 I_{tb} + \gamma_3 D_{tb} - \mu R_{tb} \\
\frac{dD_{dm}}{dt} &= \delta_1 S + \delta_2 Q_1 + \omega C_{dm} - (\nu + \mu)D_{dm} \\
\frac{dC_{dm}}{dt} &= \nu D_{dm} - (\omega + d_3 + \mu)C_{dm}
\end{aligned}$$

The recruitment rate of susceptible is equal to human average life expectancy, $\mu_h$. Compartments $Q_1$ and $Q_2$ are the additional compartments to accommodate the implementation of the COVID-19 quarantine. Persons in compartment $S$ are transferred into $Q_1$ with quarantine rate $\theta_1$ and persons in compartment $I_{co}$ are transferred into $Q_2$ with quarantine rate $\theta_2$. Quarantined susceptibles $Q_1$ are still possible to be infected by coronavirus when they have a contact with $I_{co}$ and $Q_2$, but at a different infection rate with susceptible $S$. Persons in compartment $Q_1$ can be transferred into latent tuberculosis $L_{tb}$ when they are in a close contact with infectious and active TB individuals, $I_{tb}$ or $D_{tb}$, during the quarantine at home. The portion of susceptibles ($S$) who develop diabetes without complication is $\delta_1$ which is shown by green dashed lines in Figure 1 considering that diabetes is not an infectious disease. Persons in compartment $Q_1$ also can develop diabetes as an indirect effect of quarantine through lifestyle changes and be transferred into compartment $D_{dm}$ with portion $\delta_2$. In addition, people with diabetes who initially do not expose a complication can progress into diabetes with complications ($C_{dm}$) at rate $\nu$, and diabetic people who recover from complications are assumed to still suffer from diabetes with rate $\omega$.

There are disease-related deaths caused by the COVID-19 with rate $d_1$, tuberculosis with rate $d_2$, and diabetes with rate $d_3$, then we assumed that the total population $N$ is not constant. The dynamic of the total population $N$ is given by the following equation:

$$\frac{dN}{dt} = \mu(N - X) - d_1(I_{co} + Q_2) - d_2(I_{tb} + D_{tb}) - d_3 C_{dm}$$

where $X = S + Q_1 + E_{co} + I_{co} + R_{co} + Q_2 + L_{tb} + I_{tb} + D_{tb} + R_{tb} + D_{dm} + C_{dm}$.

Furthermore, to accommodate the inability of health center to optimally diagnose and treat the infected tuberculosis during the implementation of quarantine, we defined a constant $K$ influencing the diagnosis rate $\phi_2$ as follow:

$$K = \begin{cases} 1 & \text{if } \theta_1 = 0 \\ 0.5 & \text{if } 0 < \theta_1 \leq 1 \end{cases}$$

In this model, the population change proportion for each compartment is described by the dynamic of equation system (1). The descriptions and values of each parameter are shown in Table A1 for the fixed parameter values.

## 2.2. Data Fitting

The raw data used in the present study is a weekly recorded COVID-19 cases. The mathematical model will be fitted to a data recorded by Indonesian Health Ministry during the Delta variant and Omicron variant attacks. The Delta variant of the coronavirus has been detected in Indonesia since early June 2021 and the high cases were reported in July 2021 to August 2021, followed by high number of deaths. Indonesia experienced the third wave of the COVID-19 infection with the Omicron variant of the coronavirus in mid-December 2021 to April 2022. The Indonesian government announced a plan to implement the emergency social activity restriction (PPKM darurat) in early July 2021 and mid-January 2022 to anticipate the worst possible consequences caused by the infection of these two variants. Infected corona patients become the priority to get medical treatment during the implementation of quarantine to reduce the number of viral transmission as soon as possible. The inability of health centers to provide optimal services during quarantine induces the other acute health threats to not be handled and treated properly.

The values of unobserved parameter, $(\beta_1, \beta_2, \epsilon_1, \epsilon_2, \rho_1, \rho_2, \tau_1, \tau_2, \delta_1, \delta_2, \phi_2)$, were estimated by minimizing error between the result of numerical simulation and the actual data. We used Spiral Dynamics Optimization (SDO) method developed by Tamura and Yasuda [13] to minimize root-mean-square error (RMSE) between the data of infected COVID-19 and the model output ($I_{co} + Q_2$). Further, we implemented 100 bootsrap realizations to obtain the values of parameter with 95% confidence interval. The values of the remaining parameters were obtained from the literature and the references were cited therein (see Table 1 for the value of the fixed parameters).

The initial value of the total population, $N(0)$, approximates the total population in Indonesia at 270 million people. The initial values of COVID-19 compartments were obtained from data retrieved from https://www.covid19.go.id (accessed on 10 July 2022) [14] in the first week of June 2021 for Delta period and third week of December 2021 for Omicron period. In early June 2021, the number of infected was approximately 40 thousand and the number of recovered was 1.7 million, while in mid-December 2021, there were 1287 infected people and around 4.1 milion people recovered from the coronavirus infection. We assumed that only 25% of infected people are quarantined in hospital to receive medical treatment. The number of people exposed by coronavirus but not infectious were considered to be 100 thousand in first week of June 2021 and 50 thousand in third week of December 2021. Using the information obtained from https://www.tbindonesia.or.id (accessed on 10 July 2022) [15], we set the initial value $I_{tb}(0) = 200,000$ and $D_{tb}(0) = 150,000$ at the beginning of Delta period. In the numerical simulation, we also used the initial value $L_{tb}(0) = 500,000$ and $R_{tb}(0) = 2,000,000$. The number of people with diabetes in Indonesia is about 10.8 million, and we assumed that about 25 percent of diabetics have complications. For the Omicron period in mid-December 2021, the initial values were adjusted with some increases from the Delta period.

Furthermore, to accomodate the implementation of quarantine by government, we defined parameter $\theta_1$ that denotes the quarantine rate of susceptible who stay at home to restrict social interaction, and parameter $\theta_2$ that represents the quarantine rate of coronavirus infected people who get medical treatment from health services during the pandemic. In this research, the quarantine refers to public and social measures that restrict people's movements and isolate them at home. The implementation of emergency social activity restriction (PPKM darurat) by Indonesian government was considered as the macro quarantine, because it restricted most of non-critical public activities. We assumed that the higher the quarantine level, the lower the ability of health services to accommodate and provide medical treatment for infected people due to the increased number of hospital visits during the COVID-19 pandemic. Further, the value of parameter $\theta_2$ decreases when the quarantine was implemented. Table 1 shows the value of quarantine parameters used in numerical simulation for three quarantine scenarios.

**Table 1.** The variations of quarantine rate value based on the level of quarantine.

| Parameter | Description | Level of Quarantine | | |
|---|---|---|---|---|
| | | No | Micro | Macro |
| $\theta_1$ | Quarantine rate from susceptible to quarantined susceptible | 0.00 | 0.30 | 0.75 |
| $\theta_2$ | Quarantine rate from infected coronavirus to quarantined infected | 0.95 | 0.85 | 0.75 |

*2.3. Control Strategies*

Some continuous controls were modelled by adding a reduction or addition, $u_i(t)$ where $t$ represents time in weekly unit, in the differential equation of state related to the controls. The proposed control strategies in this work help to reduce the risk of tuberculosis infection and the risk of diabetes developement during the implementation of quarantine. We added to the mathematical model three control functions $(u_1(t), u_2(t), u_3(t))$ associated to tuberculosis interventions and two control functions $(u_4(t), u_5(t))$ related to diabetes interventions. The interpretation of each control is given as follow:

1. Control $u_1(t)$: proportion of awareness program for quarantined susceptible to restrict the interaction with tuberculosis suspects in the environment.
2. Control $u_2(t)$: proportion of awareness program for latent tuberculosis by intensifying the latent identification and putting under treatment.
3. Control $u_3(t)$: proportion of diagnosis program for infected tuberculosis by managing a specific team for diagnosis or optimizing the use of telemedicine.
4. Control $u_4(t)$: proportion of awareness program for quarantined susceptible by implementing healthy lifestyle and exercising inside the house.
5. Control $u_5(t)$: proportion of awareness program for diabetic people without complications by applying healthy diet and diet tracking in quarantine period.

The resulting states completed by the controls for each compartment are given by the equations shown in Appendix A.2. In the numerical simulation, we also combined controls $(u_1, u_2, u_3)$ to reduce the risk of tuberculosis and controls $(u_4, u_5)$ to minimize the risk of diabetes. We measured the efficacy of each control strategy by calculating the percentage of reduced cases for some noticed compartments during the time observation.

## 3. Results

In this section, we present the result of numerical simulation using the estimated parameter values that minimize error between the actual COVID-19 data during the Delta and Omicron variant outbreaks with the model's output. The actual COVID-19 data is data that indicates the weekly number of people infected with COVID-19 recorded by Indonesian government. The output of mathematical model refers to the result of numerical simulation that shows the number of COVID-19 infected people, $I_{co} + Q_2$, in a week. We examined the effect of quarantine implementation by comparing the dynamic of TB and diabetes compartments in three scenarios: no quarantine, micro quarantine, and macro quarantine. In addition, we suggested the implementation of some control strategies to reduce the risk of tuberculosis transmission and diabetes development in quarantine period. We considered the variations of control parameter separately, and interpreted the simulation's result for each proposed control.

### 3.1. Numerical Simulation of Mathematical Model Accomodating Quarantine Process

The weekly data of COVID-19 cases during the observation time was fitted with the output of mathematical model to obtain the estimated parameters. Table 2 displays the estimated values for each unobserved parameter with 95% confidence interval obtained from 100 bootstrap realizations. As can be seen in Figure 2a,b, the results of simulation produced a good data fitting in both of Delta period and Omicron period. In order to assess the goodness of fit, we calculated the Pearson correlation coefficient between the actual data and the model's output, denoted by coefficient $r_d$ for Delta and $r_o$ for Omicron. The calculation yielded $r_d = 0.9343$ and $r_o = 0.8961$ with significance level $p < 0.05$, indicating a strong positive relationship between data and simulation result.

Table 2. Description of parameters used in mathematical model with estimated value.

| Parameter | Description | Delta (95% CI) | Omicron (95% CI) |
|---|---|---|---|
| $\beta_1$ | Infection rate of susceptible by contact with infected | 4.411 (4.077, 4.745) | 5.569 (5.313, 5.825) |
| $\beta_2$ | Infection rate of susceptible by contact with quarantined infected | 6.125 (5.671, 6.580) | 6.371 (6.001, 6.742) |
| $\epsilon_1$ | Infection rate of quarantined susceptible by contact with infected | 3.595 (3.414, 3.776) | 4.429 (4.372, 4.486) |
| $\epsilon_2$ | Infection rate of quarantined susceptible by contact with quarantined infected | 5.985 (5.528, 6.442) | 5.129 (4.763, 5.494) |
| $\rho_1$ | Infection rate of susceptible by contact with infected TB | 0.335 (0.291, 0.378) | 1.884 (1.624, 2.144) |
| $\rho_2$ | Infection rate of susceptible by contact with diagnosed TB | 0.349 (0.307, 0.391) | 1.628 (1.302, 1.954) |
| $\tau_1$ | Infection rate of quarantined susceptible by contact with infected TB | 0.486 (0.426, 0.545) | 2.101 (1.869, 2.333) |
| $\tau_2$ | Infection rate of quarantined susceptible by contact with diagnosed TB | 0.492 (0.436, 0.548) | 2.839 (2.672, 3.007) |
| $\phi_2$ | Diagnosis rate of infected TB | 0.497 (0.438, 0.555) | 2.237 (1.905, 2.569) |
| $\delta_1$ | Probability of susceptible developing diabetes | 0.091 (0.084, 0.098) | 0.067 (0.062, 0.072) |
| $\delta_2$ | Probability of quarantined susceptible developing diabetes | 0.129 (0.121, 0.136) | 0.085 (0.076, 0.093) |

For the Delta period, the actual data and model's output indicate same period of infection peak, the second week of July 2021. The highest number of COVID-19 cases shown in the recorded data was 341,749, while the model resulted 288,169 cases at the peak of infection. The number of COVID-19 cases started to decline significantly in the subsequent weeks. For the Omicron period, the peak of infection shown by data and model's output is in the third week of February 2022. The number of infected people on this infection peak that recorded in actual data is 385,769 cases, whereas the simulation result indicates that the potential highest case number is only 286,566 cases.

We used the estimated parameter values in Table 2 to simulate the dynamic of TB and diabetes compartments in three scenarios. In Figure 2c,d, we observed that the number of COVID-19 infected people, $(I_{co} + Q_2)$, decreased when the quarantine was implemented during the Delta and Omicron variant outbreaks. The implementation of quarantine not only reduced positive cases but also led to the early occurrence of infection peak; thereby, the emergency period lasted shorter. The summary of simulation results without or with accomodating the implementation of quarantine was given in Table 3. The implementation of micro quarantine reduced 51.48 percent of COVID-19 cases in the Delta period and 69.76 percent in the Omicron period. As expected, a higher decrease in the number of COVID-19 cases was resulted from the implementation of macro quarantine that is 64.17% and 79.60% for the Delta and Omicron period, respectively. When micro and macro quarantine were implemented in Delta period, the number of infected individuals on the peak of infection were 47.40% and 60.76%, respectively, lower than no quarantine scenario. In Omicron period, the percentages of case reduction in the infection peak affected by micro and macro quarantine implementation were 69.19% and 79.27%. The peak of infection shifted two weeks later when the quarantine was not implemented. These implied that quarantine enforced by the government could significantly limiting the spread of COVID-19 infection, particularly during the Delta and Omicron variant outbreaks.

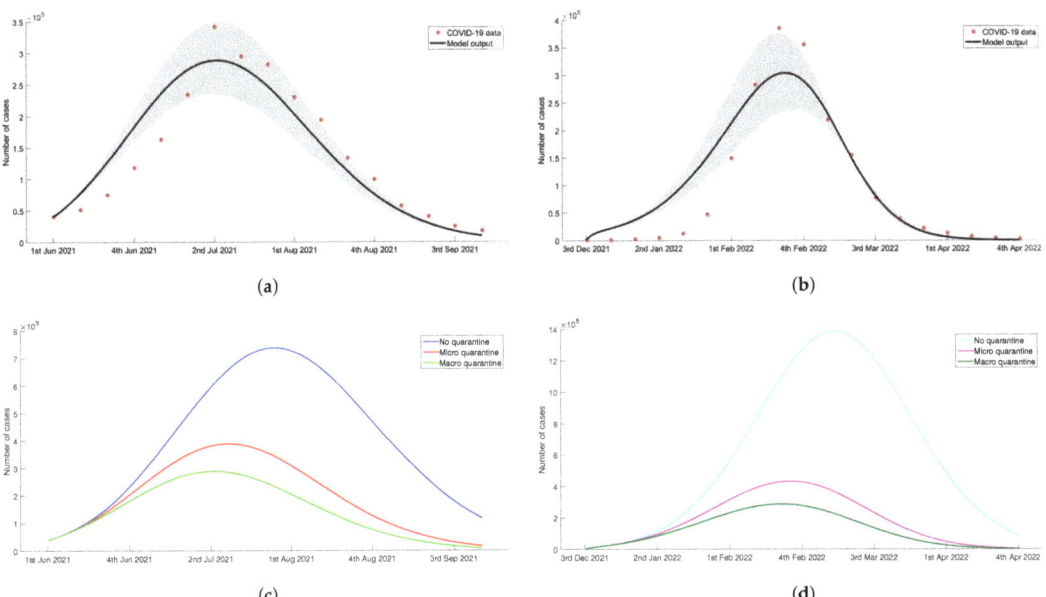

**Figure 2.** The results of data fitting between the actual COVID-19 data in Indonesia and the output of model during the period of Delta and Omicron variant were shown in (**a,b**), respectively. Further, figure (**c,d**) show the number of COVID-19 infected people, $I_{co} + Q_2$, based on the simulation results of some quarantine scenarios when Indonesia experienced Delta and Omicron variant attacks. (**a**) Data fitting during Delta period. (**b**) Data fitting during Omicron period. (**c**) The number of COVID-19 infected people for each quarantine scenario during Delta period. (**d**) The number of COVID-19 infected people for each quarantine scenario during Omicron period.

In Table 2, we observed that infection rate parameters of quarantined susceptible by contact with infected and diagnosed TB, $\tau_1$ and $\tau_2$, were higher than the infection rates of susceptible, $\rho_1$ and $\rho_2$, in both the Delta and Omicron periods. This implied a higher number of tuberculosis cases during the quarantine. Figure 3 illustrates how micro and macro quarantine increase the number of TB cases, $I_{tb}$ and $D_{tb}$. We considered three values for $\theta_1$ : 0, 0.3, and 0.75. We noticed that as the quarantine rate ($\theta_1$) increases, the number of $I_{tb}$ and $D_{tb}$ increase. When micro and macro quarantine were implemented during Delta variant outbreak, the number of active infected TB were 13.24% and 14.09%, respectively, higher than the number $I_{tb}$ of no quarantine scenario at the end of observation time. Similar results were also seen in the Omicron period where $I_{tb}$ during micro and macro quarantine scenarios were 36.18% and 37.5% higher than no quarantine. The significant increase in the number of compartment $I_{tb}$ led to the increment in the number of tuberculosis diagnosed individuals despite the diagnosis ability of health services decreased during pandemic. In the last week of September 2021, the number of diagnosed TB of micro and macro quarantine were 8.04% and 9.91%, respectively, higher than the scenario of no implementation of quarantine. In the last week of April 2022, there were 47.10% and 55.21% higher potential diagnosed TB for micro and macro quarantine, respectively. Table 4 displays the summary of quarantine effect on the increasing number of people with tuberculosis and diabetes during the observation time, the Delta and Omicron periods.

**Table 3.** The summary of COVID-19 infected people, $I_{co} + Q_2$, in three scenarios of quarantine.

| Variant | Indicator | No Quarantine | Micro Quarantine | Macro Quarantine |
|---|---|---|---|---|
| Delta (B.1.617.2) | Total infected individuals in 17 weeks | 6,691,270 | 3,246,557 | 2,397,179 |
| | Peak of infection | 4th week of July 2021 | 3rd week of July 2021 | 2nd week of July 2021 |
| | Highest potential number of cases | 734,323 | 386,249 | 288,169 |
| | Number of cases at the end of observation | 117,673 | 16,968 | 9201 |
| | Percentage of reduced cases | - | 51.48% | 64.17% |
| Omicron (B.1.1.529) | Total infected individuals in 19 weeks | 11,188,961 | 3,383,183 | 2,282,320 |
| | Peak of infection | 1st week of March 2022 | 4th week of February 2022 | 3th week of February 2022 |
| | Highest potential number of cases | 1,382,465 | 426,239 | 286,566 |
| | Number of cases at the end of observation | 88,804 | 4155 | 2021 |
| | Percentage of reduced cases | - | 69.76% | 79.60% |

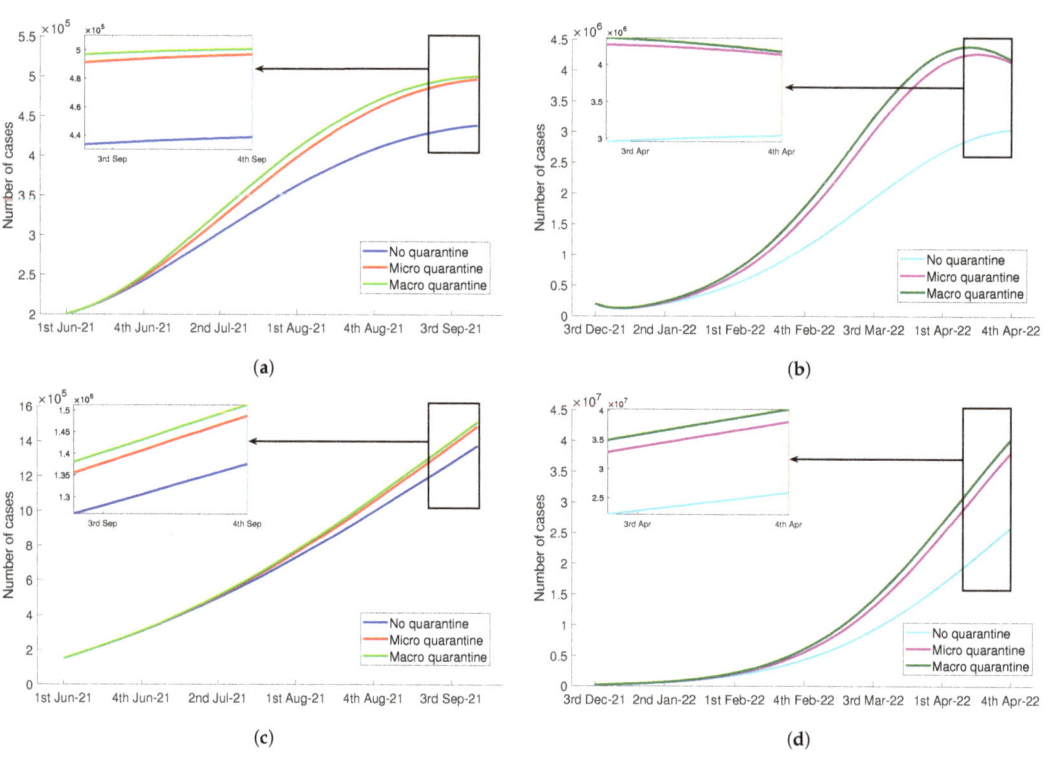

**Figure 3.** The negative impact of quarantine during Delta variant and Omicron variant of the COVID-19 pandemic to the increasing number of tuberculosis infected people, $I_{tb}$ and $D_{tb}$. (**a**) The number of $I_{tb}$ during Delta period. (**b**) The number of $I_{tb}$ during Omicron period. (**c**) The number of $D_{tb}$ during Delta period. (**d**) The number of $D_{tb}$ during Omicron period.

Table 4. The number of infected tuberculosis and diabetic people in the end of observation time.

| Variant | Compartment | No Quarantine | Micro Quarantine | Macro Quarantine |
|---|---|---|---|---|
| Delta (B.1.617.2) | Infected tuberculosis ($I_{tb}$) | $4.39 \times 10^5$ | $4.97 \times 10^5$ | $5.01 \times 10^5$ |
| | Diagnosed tuberculosis ($D_{tb}$) | $1.38 \times 10^6$ | $1.49 \times 10^6$ | $1.51 \times 10^6$ |
| | Diabetes without complications ($D_{dm}$) | $1.77 \times 10^8$ | $1.93 \times 10^8$ | $1.96 \times 10^8$ |
| | Diabetes with complications ($C_{dm}$) | $2.72 \times 10^7$ | $2.96 \times 10^7$ | $3.03 \times 10^7$ |
| Omicron (B.1.1.529) | Infected tuberculosis ($I_{tb}$) | $3.04 \times 10^6$ | $4.14 \times 10^6$ | $4.18 \times 10^6$ |
| | Diagnosed tuberculosis ($D_{tb}$) | $2.59 \times 10^7$ | $3.81 \times 10^7$ | $4.02 \times 10^7$ |
| | Diabetes without complications ($D_{dm}$) | $1.35 \times 10^8$ | $1.38 \times 10^8$ | $1.39 \times 10^8$ |
| | Diabetes with complications ($C_{dm}$) | $2.50 \times 10^7$ | $2.63 \times 10^7$ | $2.66 \times 10^7$ |

In Table 2, the probability of quarantined susceptible developing diabetes, $\delta_2$, was higher than the probability of susceptible developing diabetes, $\delta_1$. This indicated that the implementation of quarantine possibly caused the increase in the number of people with diabetes. We presented the effect of quarantine rate $\theta_1$ to the number of diabetic without complication ($D_{dm}$) and diabetic with complications ($C_{dm}$) in Figure 4. Here, we also considered three values of susceptible quarantine rate: $\theta_1 = 0$ (no quarantine), $\theta_1 = 0.3$ (micro quarantine), and $\theta_1 = 0.75$ (macro quarantine). We observed that the stricter quarantine implementation, that was, greater values for $\theta_1$, the higher number of individuals developing diabetes (see Table 4 for the number of people with diabetes without and with complications). More precisely, at the end of Delta variant observation time, micro quarantine increased the number of diabetes without complications 9.53% higher than no quarantine scenario, and macro quarantine led 10.93% increased cases. On the other hand, the number of diabetes with complications in the last week of September 2021 increased 8.94% and 11.62% in case the government decided to enforce micro and macro quarantine. For the Omicron period, micro quarantine resulted 2.22% and 5.20% higher number of $D_{dm}$ and $C_{dm}$, respectively. When the macro quarantine option was selected, it was possible that the number of diabetic without complications increases 2.96% and the number of diabetic with complications increases 6.40% in the end of observation.

### 3.2. Effect of Tuberculosis and Diabetes Control Strategies during COVID-19 Quarantine

We proposed some control strategies in this work to reduce the risk of tuberculosis and diabetes during the implementation of quarantine that focus at mitigating the COVID-19 disease transmission. We added three control functions ($u_1, u_2, u_3$) related to the reduction of infected tuberculosis, and two controls ($u_4, u_5$) intended to minimize the probability of developing diabetes. We assumed that the controls were continuous defined by a constant rate. Each control simulated both separately and combined. Here, the percentage of reduction in the total number of cases during observation time compared to no quarantine scenario was chosen to illustrate the efficacy of each control strategy.

For the first scenario, we used merely the control $u_1(t)$. This control intended to increase public awareness to protect them from tuberculosis risk during quarantine at home. The awareness program were carried out by direct campaigns or by using mass media and social media to inform the citizens about the dangers of TB transmission in the close environment when they stayed at home. Using constant rate $u_1 = 0.5$, Figure 5a,b display significant reduction of latent TB during Delta and Omicron period. The variations in the value of control $u_1$, ranging $0 \leq u_1 \leq 1$, showed the efficacy in reducing latent TB up to 72.28% for Delta variant and 98.01% for Omicron variant (see Figure 5c,d). Also, reduced cases can be seen in the number infected TB ($I_{tb}$) during both Delta and Omicron variant outbreaks (see Figure 6a,b). In Figure 6c,d, we can see that the efficacy of control $u_1(t)$ to reduce the number of active infected TB during the pandemic of Delta and Omicron variant was up to 58.64% and 97.19%, respectively.

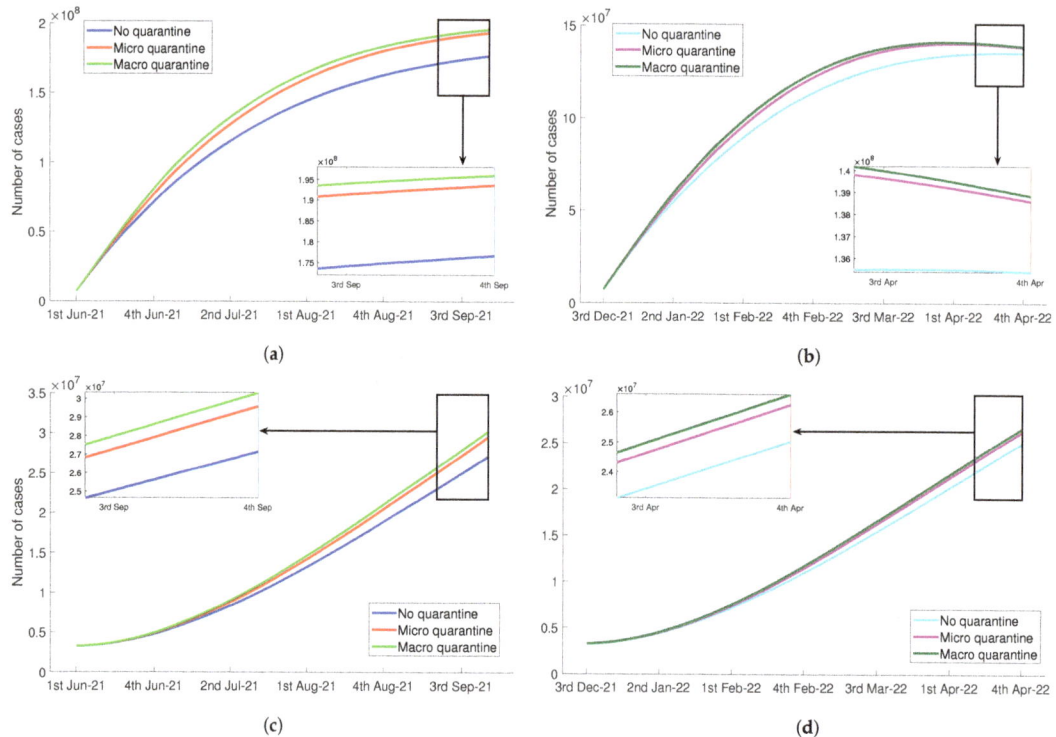

**Figure 4.** The negative impact of quarantine during Delta variant and Omicron variant of the COVID-19 pandemic to the increasing number of people with diabetes, $D_{dm}$ and $C_{dm}$. (**a**) The number of $D_{dm}$ during Delta period. (**b**) The number of $D_{dm}$ during Omicron period. (**c**) The number of $C_{dm}$ during Delta period. (**d**) The number of $C_{dm}$ during Omicron period.

Next, we used only the control $u_2(t)$ for the second scenario. This control represented the proportion of latent individuals $L_{tb}$ that was identified and received medical treatment. The expansion of the screening test and diagnosis for latent TB or people at high infection risk could be adopted. In Figure 5a,b, using constant rate $u_2 = 0.5$, we observed that the decrease in the number of latent $L_{tb}$ in both periods were less significant than the first proposed TB control strategy. Now, by varying control rate value, $0 \leq u_2 \leq 1$, the percentage of reduced cases were only up to 6.519% for Delta and only up to 4.463% for Omicron, as can be seen in Figure 5b,d. In addition, control $u_2$ also was not more effective than $u_1$ in reducing the number of infected TB ($I_{tb}$). In Figure 6c,d, the effectiveness measurement showed that the efficacy of this type of control was only up to 4.938% during Delta period and 6.301% during Omicron period.

The third control proposed to reduce tuberculosis risk was $u_3(t)$. In this strategy, the diagnosis program for the infected individuals was intensified. A specific team could be formed to continue TB diagnosis and treatment program even though COVID-19 was a priority during the pandemic. This control was focused on the diagnosis of infected, so the latent was not significantly reduced. Even, in the Omicron period there was no decrease in the number of latent TB. In Figure 5c, we observed that the number of latent decreased only up to 0.115%. Although control $u_3$ was not significantly affecting latent TB, this control has potential to reduce the number of infected TB quite notably. The efficacy of this control in reducing $I_{tb}$ was up to 41.17% for Delta period and 48.62% for Omicron period as shown in Figure 6, with the values of control $u_3$ ranging $[0,1]$.

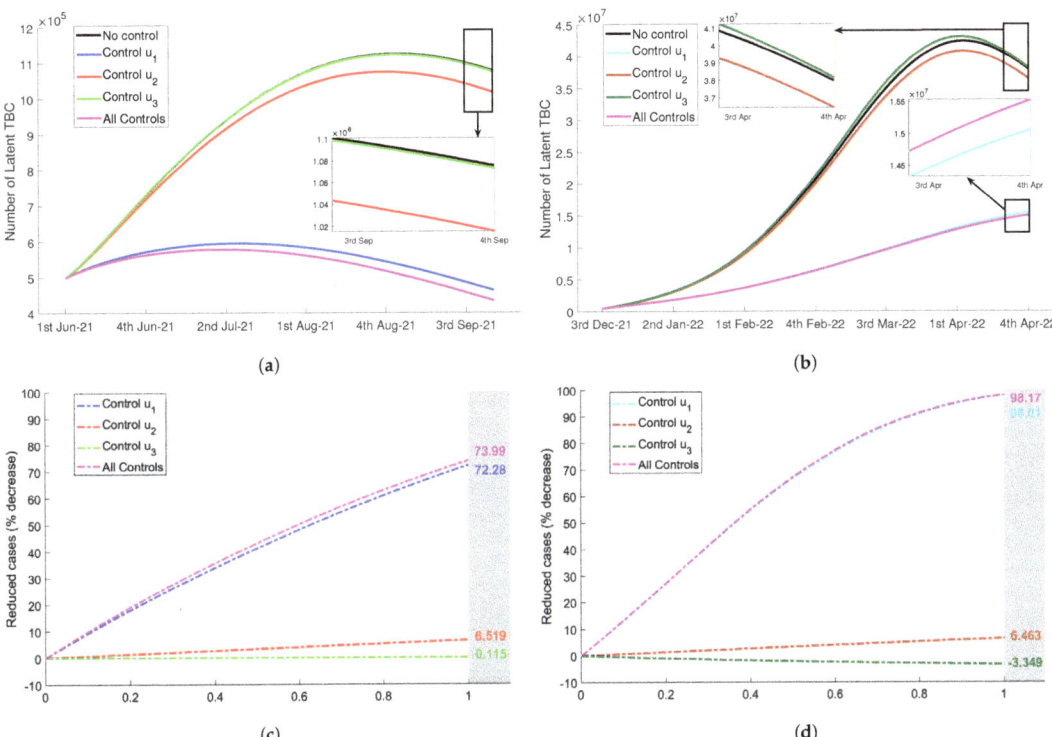

**Figure 5.** The impact of TB controls implementation ($u_i = 0.5$) to the number of latent people $L_{tb}$ during Delta period (**a**), and Omicron period (**b**). Next, the efficacy of tuberculosis controls with the variations of control value, $0 \leq u_1, u_2, u_3 \leq 1$ to reduce the number of latent $L_{tb}$ were shown in figure (**c**) for Delta and in figure (**d**) for Omicron. (**a**) The number of $L_{tb}$ during Delta period. (**b**) The number of $L_{tb}$ during Omicron period. (**c**) Controls efficacy reducing $L_{tb}$ during Delta period. (**d**) Controls efficacy reducing $L_{tb}$ during Omicron period.

For the last scenario of tuberculosis control strategy, we combined all proposed control, $u_1$, $u_2$, and $u_3$. We assumed that all controls were implemented with equal rate, that was, $u_1 = u_2 = u_3$. As expected, Figures 5 and 6 show that this combination decreased the number of $L_{tb}$ and $I_{tb}$ more significant than three previous single controls. More precisely, the latent individuals decreased up to 73.99% and 98.17% during Delta and Omicron period. For the infected individuals, there were reductions by 77.93% and 98.48% during the observation time starting from June 2021 to September 2021 for Delta variant and from December 2021 to April 2022 for Omicron variant, respectively.

One of the important indicators that need to be considered regarding the effectiveness of a TB control strategy was the ratio between $D_{tb}$ and $I_{tb}$. The high ratio of diagnosed who receive medical treatment from health services over the infected indicated that the strategy was more effective. In Appendix A, Figure A1 shows the number of $D_{tb}$ during the observation time, and we observed that the highest ratio of $D_{tb}$ over $I_{tb}$ was shown by the combination of all controls. The control $u_3$ significantly increased the ratio because it was focused on the increase of diagnosis rate. The control $u_2$, aimed to reduce the number of latent, showed low value of $D_{tb}/I_{tb}$ and did not significantly influence the diagnosis rate.

For the first diabetes reduction scenario, we compared the number of diabetic with complications ($C_{dm}$), with and without control $u_4(t)$. The goal of this strategy was to increase public awareness to implement healthy lifestyle, set a good diet, and exercise at home regularly in quarantine period. The implementation of constant control $u_4 = 0.5$

reduced the number of $C_{dm}$ as shown in Figure 7a,b. Figure 7c,d show that the upper bound of this control efficacy was equal to 61.28% and 59.04% for Delta and Omicron period, respectively. This implied a reduction in the number of people with diabetes of more than half of the total cases when control $u_4$ was not considered.

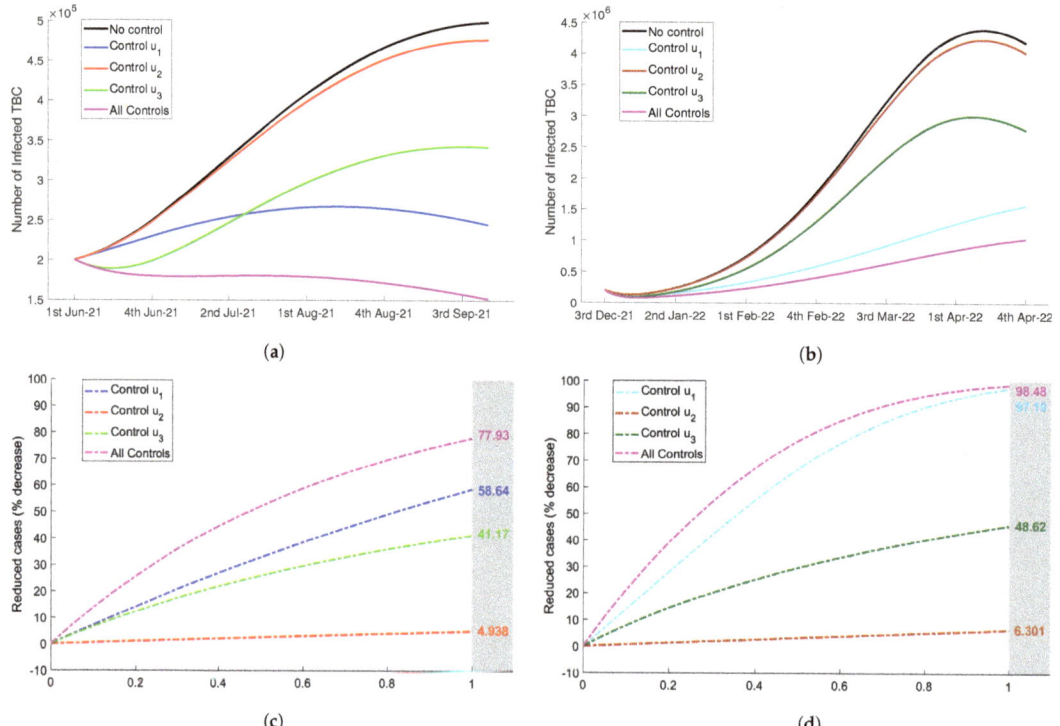

**Figure 6.** The impact of TB controls implementation ($u_i = 0.5$) to the number of infected people $I_{tb}$ during Delta period (**a**), and Omicron period (**b**). Next, the efficacy of tuberculosis controls with the variations of control value, $0 \leq u_1, u_2, u_3 \leq 1$ to reduce the number of infected $I_{tb}$ were shown in figure (**c**) for Delta and in figure (**d**) for Omicron. (**a**) The number of $I_{tb}$ during Delta period. (**b**) The number of $I_{tb}$ during Omicron period. (**c**) Controls efficacy reducing $I_{tb}$ during Delta period. (**d**) Controls efficacy reducing $I_{tb}$ during Omicron period.

Next, we used only the control $u_5(t)$ to reduce the probability of diabetics developing complications during the implementation of quarantine. Diet tracking, regular diet, and healthy lifestyle in the quarantine period could be adopted to prevent the emergence of complications. In Figure 7a,b, we observed that the number of $C_{dm}$ reduced more significant than control $u_4$. By using constant rate $0 \leq u_5 \leq 1$ shown in Figure 7c,d, the percentage of reduced cases was up to 78.11% for Delta and 76.08% for Omicron.

In addition, we combined control $u_4$ and control $u_5$. In this strategy, the two controls were applied at the same time in order to obtain better numerical results. We assumed that the controls had equal rate, $u_4 = u_5$. In Figure 7a,b, we used controls $u_4 = u_5 = 0.5$ in the numerical simulation. The uppper bound of the efficacy of this control combination was equal to the upper bound of single control $u_5$, but lower values of this combination yielded higher efficacy than control $u_5$ as shown in Figure 7c,d.

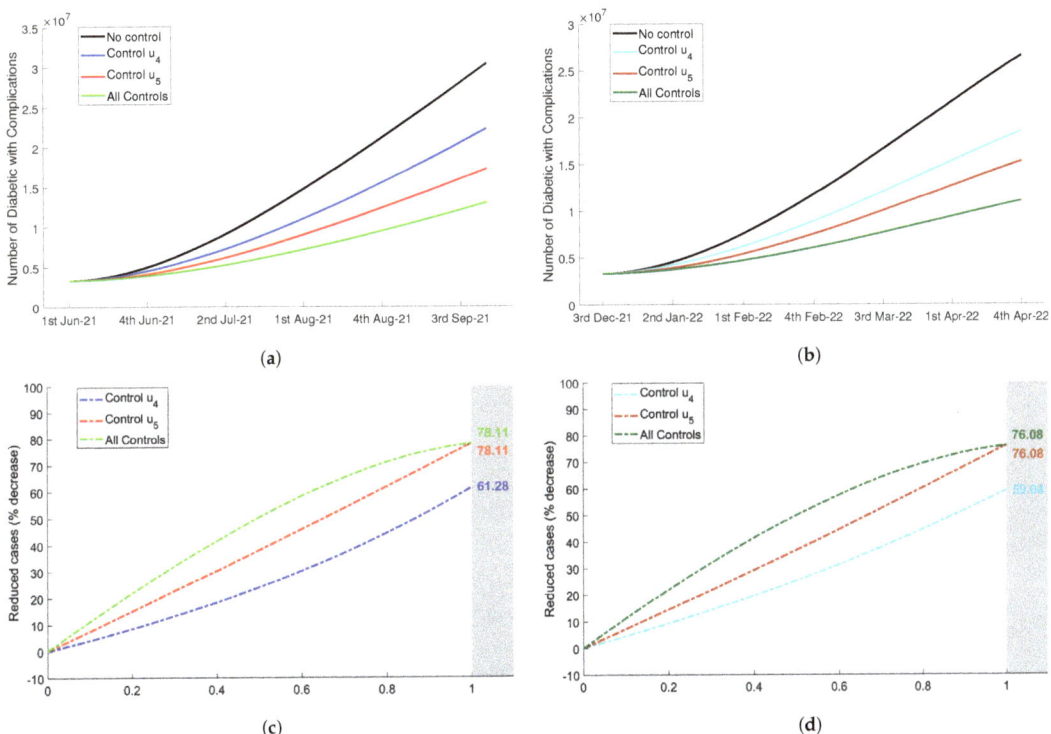

**Figure 7.** The impact of diabetes controls implementation to the number of diabetic people with complications $C_{dm}$, figure (**a**) for Delta period and figure (**b**) for Omicron period. The efficacy of diabetes controls to reduce the number of diabetics $C_{dm}$ with the variations of control value, $0 \leq u_4, u_5 \leq 1$ were shown in figure (**c**) and (**d**) for Delta variant and Omicron variant, respectively. (**a**) The number of $C_{dm}$ during Delta period. (**b**) The number of $C_{dm}$ during Omicron period. (**c**) Controls efficacy reducing $C_{dm}$ during Delta period. (**d**) Controls efficacy reducing $C_{dm}$ during Omicron period.

In Appendix A, Figure A2 shows that control $u_4$ significantly reduced the number of diabetic without complications but this control did not detain the progression from $D_{dm}$ to diabetic with complications, $C_{dm}$. The implementation of control $u_5$, that was aimed to reduce the probability of developing complications, showed the low percentage of $D_{dm}$ becoming $C_{dm}$. The fatal impact of diabetes with complications could be minimized by implementing strategy $u_5$ during quarantine period. On the other hand, control $u_5$ was not effective to decline the number of diabetic without complications $D_{dm}$. The combination of control $u_4$ and $u_5$ could be considered as the best strategy to reduce the risk of diabetes development during quarantine implementation. These strategies decreased the number of $D_{dm}$ and $C_{dm}$, and reduced the possibility of $D_{dm}$ developing complications.

## 4. Discussion

In order to control the COVID-19 transmission during pandemic, numerous countries have decided to adopt lockdown and regional quarantine policies. It had been a considerable time since such strategies were last introduced, and currently they were implemented on global scale. Despite the fact that quarantines have been implemented relatively recently, some contributions have already appeared in the literature, aimed at evaluating how this policies work, along with its efficacy in terms of controlling virus infection. Lau et al. [16] have analysed the Wuhan case and have highlighted the significance of these measures to reduce the contagion probability by significantly decrease the growth rate and increase the doubling time of cases. Guzzetta et al. [17] have reported that national lockdown in Italy brought net reproduction ratio ($R_t$) below 1 within 2 weeks and the epidemic was brought under control only after the implementation of lockdown. A similar finding was reported by Megarbane et al. [18] that lockdown and quarantine were considered as an effective intervention to halt coronavirus epidemic progression in nine different countries (UK, USA, Germany, Spain, New Zealand, Italy, France, Netherlands, and Sweden).

Delta (B.1.617.2) and Omicron (B.1.1.529) are two variants of SARS-CoV-2 that causes high infection during COVID-19 pandemic. The Delta variant was originally found in India in December 2020 and the Omicron variant was firstly observed in South Africa in the early days of November 2021 [19,20]. The Delta variant has spread over very fast because of its capability to invade the host's immune system, but the Omicron variant has been reported to be more infectious than previous variants with a short doubling time. In this work, we found that the infection rates of Omicron variant, $(\beta_1, \beta_2, \epsilon_1, \epsilon_2)$, were approximately 1.04–1.26 times higher than the infection rates of Delta variant. This finding is in accordance with the results of research conducted by Lyngse et al. [21] in Denmark that the rate of Omicron virus infection was 1.17 times higher than Delta variant, especially for unvaccinated people. Chaguza et al. [22] also reported that Omicron variant is 1.3 times more infectious than Delta due to the increased transmission acquired from the mutation.

The implementation of lockdown and regional quarantine to control COVID-19 pandemic have influenced tuberculosis clinical management and health services related to TB. In the countries and territories where healthcare personnel assigned in TB programs have been diverted to handle COVID-19 patients, the impact of pandemic on tuberculosis treatments is estimated to be severe. Numerous countries have ruled out TB programs because COVID-19 control programs are priority and urgently needed. Health facilities throughout the country become the battleground for COVID-19. To decrease the potential risk of viral transmission to either health care workers or patients during their visits, hospitals are minimizing the number of daily outpatient visits. Several health services are prepared to meet the demands of the overwhelming number of COVID-19 patients.

Migliori et al. [23] have reported that COVID-19 pandemic has interfered TB-related services globally. Data from 33 TB centers in 16 countries indicated the reductions in the diagnosis of newly active TB and total outpatient visits of active or latent TB during lockdown and regional quarantine in the first 4 months of 2020. The study by Lange et al. [24] showed a significant decline in emergency department visits such as TB centers, suggesting that patients may be avoiding care or unable to access care during the pandemic. The reduction in the number of outpatient visits may be due to the patient's fear of exposure severe acute respiratory syndrome COVID-19 [25]. Because of lockdown and quarantine, progression to active TB from latent TB who did not obtain preventive measure and medical treatment was possibly occurred [26]. Despite the number of outpatient TB visits decreased, the implementation of lockdown and regional quarantine have increased the interest to use telemedicine. TB programs offered new service called telehealth. The use of telehealth services in the United Kingdom, India, Russia, and Australia was considerably higher in 2020, driven by social distancing policies and in accordance with the innovation program to answer challenges during the pandemic [27,28]. In Indonesia, some examples of telehealth services are https://www.temenin.kemkes.go.id (accessed on 14 November 2022) provided by Indonesian Health Ministry and Halodoc, an application developed by PT Media Dokter Investama. These services bring together patients with expert doctors for online consultations, diagnosing the patient's condition, and providing medicine recommendations or other medical treatments.

In tuberculosis epidemiology, the duration and proximity of exposure to an active TB as the source of infection led to an increased risk of TB infection. It should be noticed that the implementation of lockdown and regional quarantine may possibly increase the risk of TB infection during COVID-19 pandemic. The government enforced stay-at-home policies and confined the citizens in their family environment. In the family-household setting, a persistent close contact with family members suffering from active TB and still undiagnosed increased the transmission risk to susceptible persons [29]. The prevention method and awareness program should be adopted, through the campaign of awareness directly or indirectly using mass media or social media to inform the citizens about the dangers of TB transmission in the close environment when they stay at home. By taking preventive measures such as applying health lifestyle, covering coughs and sneezes, and keeping hands clean, the risk of TB infection could be reduced. Family members who show TB symptoms should immediately visit the health service or contact the health care by using telehealth facility to avoid wider transmission caused by undetected case.

The change in nutritional habits and lifestyle are unavoidable negative consequences of lockdown and quarantine. Limited access to food and reduced availability of goods caused by restricted opening hours of store lead to the changing in nutritional habits and the switching to unhealthy food. A recent review by Brooks et al. [30] reported negative psychological effects of quarantine including stress and anxiety. Mental health issues such as stress and anxiety are considered to be associated with unhealthy lifestyle that drive people to eat and drink in an attempt to get better feeling. Eating unhealthy foods regularly such as snacks, chocolates, junk foods, fast foods, and soda cola, and drinking spirits and wine more frequently are more likely to be new habits of these stress-driven eaters and drinkers. This leads to weight gain that may possibly contributes to development of diabetes. In order to reduce diabetes risk as the side effect of the implementation of lockdown and quarantine, a healthy diet should be applied. Vegetarian diet and Mediteranian diet are the examples of healthy diet that give important metabolic advantages for preventing and treating diabetes and its complications [31,32].

Other than the unhealthy eating habits, the reduction of physical activity also contributes the weight gain in quarantine period. Pandemic-related closure of public exercise facilities such as sports centers, gymnasiums, and swimming pools may disproportionately influence active individuals. Notwithstanding the guidances to exercise at home, only few citizens comply. Regular physical activity is mandatory to maintain health status. The human body's metabolism is strongly influenced by physical activity. Doing more physical activity is one important factor to lowering the risk of diabetes because it decreases the glucose level in blood circulation by increasing glucose uptake [33,34]. Promotion of physical activity in home needs to be intensified during the implementation of lockdown and regional quarantine. In addition, wherever and whenever possible and allowed, while following the government rules, people should be suggested to be more active outdoors, preferably in green open space. As in all other situations, regulations of wearing mask and social distancing are also essential in outdoors to reduce the COVID-19 infection risk.

## 5. Conclusions

In this paper, we proposed a mathematical model and used numerical simulation to describe the impact of quarantine on tuberculosis and diabetic people during COVID-19 pandemic. A compartmental nonlinear deterministic epidemic model, including three diseases: COVID-19, tuberculosis, and diabetes, was formulated. We aimed to point out the potential negative effects, particularly on tuberculosis and diabetic people, when the government implemented isolation measures such as lockdown and regional quarantine. The mathematical model fitted with the actual data of COVID-19 cases in Indonesia when the Delta and Omicron variants were identified. We also suggested some control strategies to reduce the negative impact in both tuberculosis and diabetic people during quarantine. The results of numerical simulation indicate different effectiveness and efficacy of each control strategy. By increasing public awareness about the dangers of TB transmission in environment when they stayed at home, the number of newly infected TB during quarantine can be reduced significantly. In addition, in order to minimize the risk of diabetes progression with or without complications, the implementation of healthy lifestyle and exercise inside the house are considered as the most effective strategy.

This study has several limitations that can be developed for future research. The actual problem is complex and this study aims to simplify it. Therefore, the mathematical model that we developed only consists of the basic compartments and variables of the COVID-19 disease that we consider essential. Immunity level due to vaccination, time between infection and the acute phase of disease, symptomatic or asymptomatic infected individuals, and other important variables can be taken into account in further studies. The second limitation is the realtionship between TB and diabetes mellitus is not accommodated in the mathematical model, even though diabetes is an important factor and a comorbid of TB. Thirdly, the availability of TB and diabetes data during the COVID-19 pandemic is potentially improve the output of model, where the results of the data fitting are not only in accordance with the COVID-19 data but also the TB and diabetes data. In our study, we were unable to obtain the proper TB and diabetes due to the lack of data recording.

**Author Contributions:** Conceptualization, N.N. and I.S.F.; methodology, N.N. and I.S.F.; software, I.S.F; formal analysis, N.N. and B.W.L.; investigation, N.N., I.S.F., B.W.L. and S.R.; resources, I.S.F. and S.R.; data curation, N.N. and S.R.; writing—original draft preparation, I.S.F. and S.R.; writing—review and editing, N.N. and B.W.L.; visualization, I.S.F.; supervision, N.N. and B.W.L. All authors have read and agreed to the published version of the manuscript.

**Funding:** This research was supported by Ministry of Education and Culture Republic of Indonesia: UKICIS LPDP Scheme 2022 No. 4345/E4/AL.04/2022.

**Data Availability Statement:** The data presented in this study are available on request from the corresponding author.

**Acknowledgments:** The authors would like to thank those individuals who participated in this research for their contribution.

**Conflicts of Interest:** The authors declare no conflict of interest.

## Appendix A

*Appendix A.1*

**Table A1.** Description of parameters used in mathematical model with fixed value.

| Parameter | Description | Value | Unit | References |
|---|---|---|---|---|
| $\mu_h$ | Human natural birth or mortality rate | $1/(65 \times 52)$ | week$^{-1}$ | [35–37] |
| $\alpha$ | Rate of progression to infected from exposed | 7/6.5 | week$^{-1}$ | [38–40] |
| $d_1$ | Mortality rate caused by COVID-19 infection | 0.00039 | week$^{-1}$ | data |
| $\gamma$ | Recovery rate of infected and quarantined of COVID-19 | 7/3.6 | week$^{-1}$ | [40–42] |
| $\phi_1$ | Rate of progression to infected from latent | 7/60 | week$^{-1}$ | [43,44] |
| $\gamma_1$ | Recovery rate of latent tuberculosis | 0.01285 | week$^{-1}$ | [43,44] |
| $\gamma_2$ | Recovery rate of infected tuberculosis | 0.00122 | week$^{-1}$ | [43] |
| $\gamma_3$ | Recovery rate of diagnosed tuberculosis | 0.00764 | week$^{-1}$ | [43] |
| $d_2$ | Mortality rate caused by tuberculosis infection | 0.00111 | week$^{-1}$ | [45] |
| $\nu$ | Probability of diabetic people developing complications | 0.01303 | week$^{-1}$ | [46] |
| $\omega$ | Probability of diabetic people recovered from complications | 0.00714 | week$^{-1}$ | [46] |
| $d_3$ | Mortality rate caused by diabetes mellitus | 0.00013 | week$^{-1}$ | [46] |

*Appendix A.2*

The resulting states completed by the controls for each compartment are given by the following equations:

$$\frac{dQ_1}{dt} = \theta_1 S - \left(\frac{\epsilon_1 I_{co} + \epsilon_2 Q_2}{N}\right)Q_1 - (1 - u_1(t))\left(\frac{\tau_1 I_{tb} + \tau_2 D_{tb}}{N}\right)Q_1 - ((1 - u_4(t))\delta_2 + \mu)Q_1$$

$$\frac{dL_{tb}}{dt} = \left(\frac{\rho_1 I_{tb} + \rho_2 D_{tb}}{N}\right)S + (1 - u_1(t))\left(\frac{\tau_1 I_{tb} + \tau_2 D_{tb}}{N}\right)Q_1 - (\phi_1 + (1 + u_2(t))\gamma_1 + \mu)L_{tb}$$

$$\frac{dI_{tb}}{dt} = \phi_1 L_{tb} - ((1+u_3(t))K\phi_2 + \gamma_2 + d_2 + \mu)I_{tb}$$

$$\frac{dD_{tb}}{dt} = (1+u_3(t))K\phi_2 I_{tb} - (\gamma_3 + d_2 + \mu)D_{tb}$$

$$\frac{dR_{tb}}{dt} = (1+u_2(t))\gamma_1 L_{tb} + \gamma_2 I_{tb} + \gamma_3 D_{tb} - \mu R_{tb}$$

$$\frac{dD_{dm}}{dt} = \delta_1 S + (1-u_4(t))\delta_2 Q_1 + \omega C_{dm} - ((1-u_5(t))\nu + \mu)D_{dm}$$

$$\frac{dC_{dm}}{dt} = (1-u_5(t))\nu D_{dm} - (\omega + d_3 + \mu)C_{dm}$$

where the remaining states did not change.

*Appendix A.3*

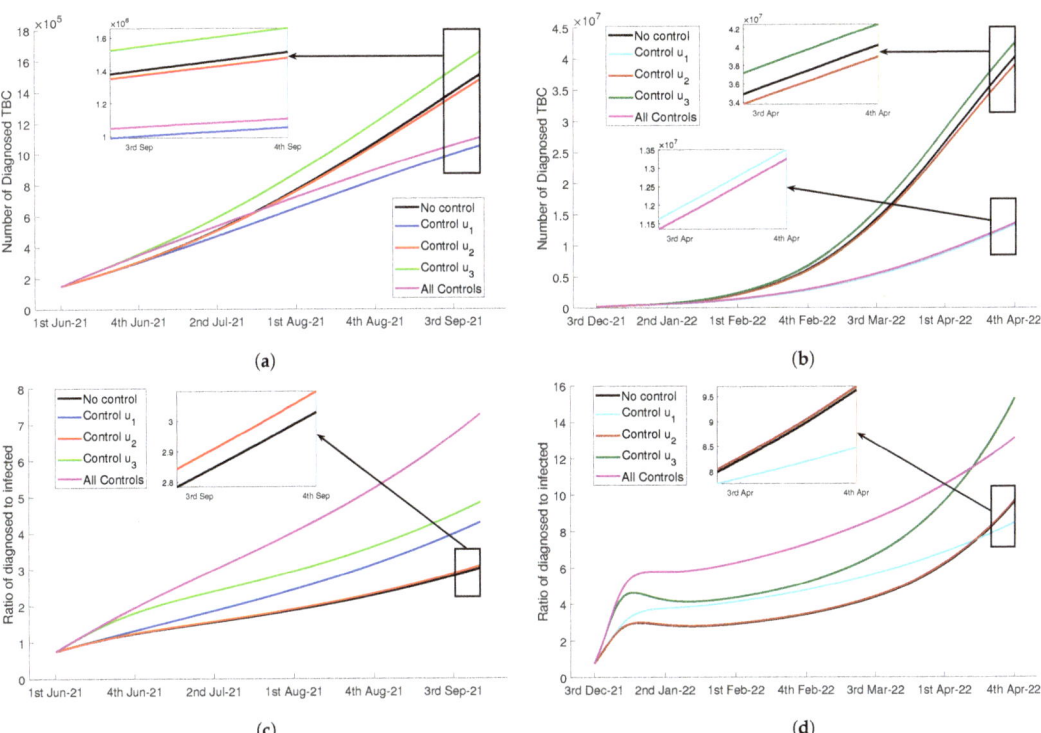

**Figure A1.** The impact of tuberculosis controls implementation to the number of diagnosed people $D_{tb}$ for Delta period (**a**), and Omicron period (**b**). The ratios of diagnosed people $D_{tb}$ over infected people $I_{tb}$ during quarantine during Delta and Omicron variant attacks were shown in figure (**c**) and (**d**), respectively. (**a**) The number of $D_{tb}$ during Delta period. (**b**) The number of $D_{tb}$ during Omicron period. (**c**) The ratio of $D_{tb}$ to $I_t b$ during Delta period. (**d**) The ratio of $D_{tb}$ to $I_t b$ during Omicron period.

*Appendix A.4*

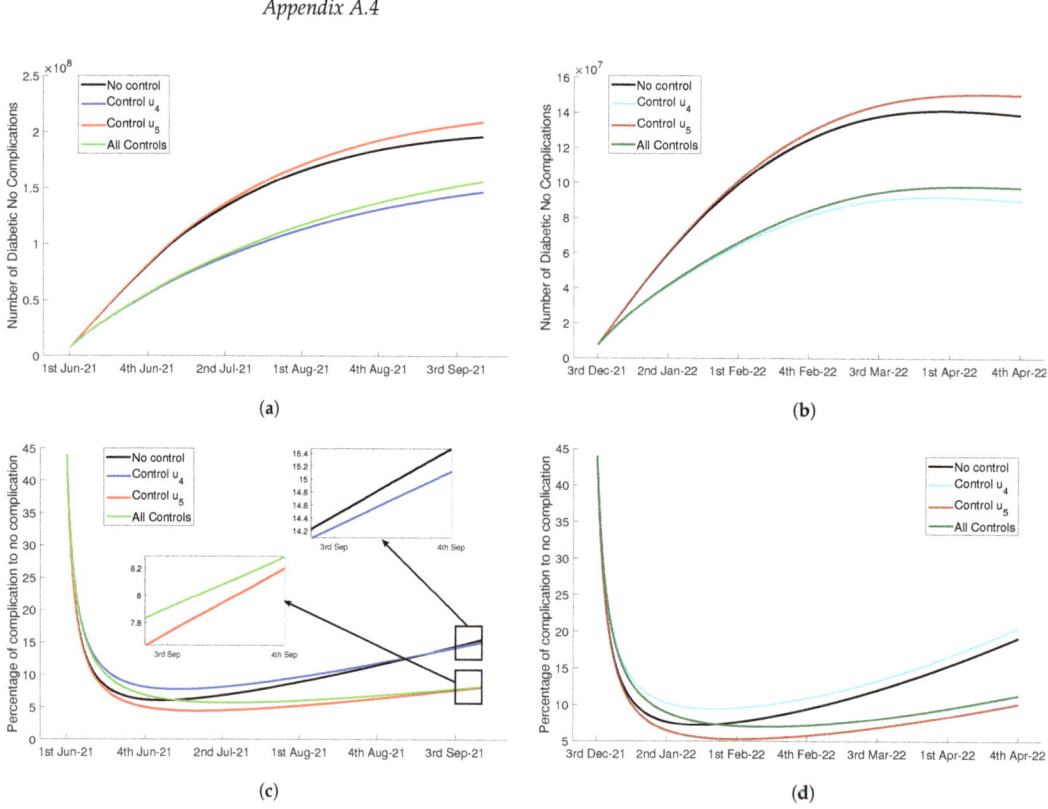

**Figure A2.** The impact of diabetes controls implementation to the number of diabetic people without complications $D_{dm}$ during Delta period shown in (**a**) and during Omicron period shown in (**b**). The percentage of diabetic people with complications $C_{dm}$ over the diabetic without complications $D_{dm}$ on Delta and Omicron quarantine were shown in figure (**c**) and (**d**), respectively. (**a**) The number of $D_{dm}$ during Delta period. (**b**) The number of $D_{dm}$ during Omicron period. (**c**) Percentage of $C_{dm}$ to $D_{dm}$ during Delta period. (**d**) Percentage of $C_{dm}$ to $D_{dm}$ during Omicron period.

## References

1. Anderson, D.E.; Sivalingam, V.; Kang, A.E.Z.; Ananthanarayanan, A.; Arumugam, H.; Jenkins, T.M.; Hadjiat, Y.; Eggers, M. Povidone-Iodine demonstrates rapid in vitro virucidal activity against SARS-CoV-2, the virus causing COVID-19 disease. *Infect. Dis. Ther.* **2020**, *9*, 669–675. [CrossRef] [PubMed]
2. Pedersen, S.F.; Ho, Y.C. SARS-CoV-2: A storm is raging. *J. Clin. Investig.* **2020**, *130*, 2202–2205. [CrossRef] [PubMed]
3. Sukandar, K.K.; Louismono, A.L.; Volisa, M.; Kusdiantara, R.; Fakhruddin, M.; Nuraini, N.; Soewono, E. A Prospective Method for Generating COVID-19 Dynamics. *Computation* **2022**, *10*, 107. [CrossRef]
4. Watson, O.J.; Barnsley, G.; Toor, J.; Hogan, A.B.; Winskill, P.; Ghani, A.C. Global impact of the first year of COVID-19 vaccination: A mathematical modelling study. *Lancet Infect. Dis.* **2022**, *22*, 1293–1302. [CrossRef]
5. World Health Organization. WHO Coronavirus (COVID-19) Dashboard. Available online: https://covid19.who.int (accessed on 14 November 2022).
6. Chiesa, V.; Antony, G.; Wismar, M.; Rechel, B. COVID-19 pandemic: Health impact of staying at home, social distancing and 'lockdown' measures-a systematic review of systematic reviews. *J. Public Health* **2021**, *43*, e462–e481. [CrossRef] [PubMed]
7. McQuaid, C.F.; Vassall, A.; Cohen, T.; Fiekert, K.; White, R.G. The impact of COVID-19 on TB: A review of the data. *Int. J. Tuberc. Lung Dis.* **2021**, *25*, 436–446. [CrossRef] [PubMed]
8. World Health Organization. *Global Tuberculosis Report 2022*; World Health Organization: Geneva, Switzerland, 2022.

9. Aznar, M.L.; Espinosa-Pereiro, J.; Saborit, N.; Jové, N.; Sánchez-Martinez, F.; Pérez-Recio, S.; Vitoria, A.; Sanjoaquin, I.; Gallardo, E.; Llenas-García, J.; et al. Impact of the COVID-19 pandemic on tuberculosis management in Spain. *Int. J. Infect. Dis.* **2021**, *108*, 300–305. [CrossRef]
10. Runacres, A.; Mackintosh, K.A.; Knight, R.L.; Sheeran, L.; Thatcher, R.; Shelley, J.; McNarry, M.A. Impact of the COVID-19 pandemic on sedentary time and behaviour in children and adults: A systematic review and meta-analysis. *Int. J. Environ. Res. Public Health* **2021**, *18*, 11286. [CrossRef]
11. Eberle, C.; Stichling, S. Impact of COVID-19 lockdown on glycemic control in patients with type 1 and type 2 diabetes mellitus: A systematic review. *Diabetol. Metab. Syndr.* **2021**, *13*, 95. [CrossRef] [PubMed]
12. Al-Rifai, R.H.; Pearson, F.; Critchley, J.A.; Abu-Raddad, L.J. Association between diabetes mellitus and active tuberculosis: A systematic review and meta-analysis. *PLoS ONE* **2017**, *12*, e0187967. [CrossRef] [PubMed]
13. Tamura, K.; Yasuda, K. Spiral dynamics inspired optimization. *J. Adv. Comput. Intell. Intell. Inform.* **2011**, *15*, 1116–1122. [CrossRef]
14. Satuan Tugas Penanganan COVID-19. Available online: https://www.covid19.go.id/ (accessed on 10 July 2022).
15. TB Indonesia Kementerian Kesehatan. Available online: https://www.tbindonesia.id/ (accessed on 10 July 2022).
16. Lau, H.; Khosrawipour, V.; Kocbach, P.; Mikolajczyk, A.; Schubert, J.; Bania, J.; Khosrawipour, T. The positive impact of lockdown in Wuhan on containing the COVID-19 outbreak in China. *J. Travel Med.* **2020**, *27*, taaa037. [CrossRef] [PubMed]
17. Guzzetta, G.; Riccardo, F.; Marziano, V.; Poletti, P.; Trentini, F.; Bella, A.; Andrianou, X.; Del Manso, M.; Fabiani, M.; Bellino, S.; et al. Impact of a nationwide lockdown on SARS-CoV-2 transmissibility, Italy. *Emerg. Infect. Dis.* **2021**, *27*, 267–270. [CrossRef] [PubMed]
18. Megarbane, B.; Bourasset, F.; Scherrmann, J.M. Is lockdown effective in limiting SARS-CoV-2 epidemic progression? A cross-country comparative evaluation using epidemiokinetic tools. *J. Gen. Intern. Med.* **2021**, *36*, 746–752. [CrossRef] [PubMed]
19. Novelli, G.; Colona, V.L.; Pandolfi, P.P. A focus on the spread of the delta variant of SARS-CoV-2 in India. *Indian J. Med. Res.* **2021**, *153*, 537–541. [CrossRef] [PubMed]
20. Gowrisankar, A.; Priyanka, T.M.C.; Banerjee, S. Omicron: A mysterious variant of concern. *Eur. Phys. J. Plus* **2022**, *137*, 100. [CrossRef] [PubMed]
21. Lyngse, F.P.; Mortensen, L.H.; Denwoood, M.J.; Christiansen, L.E.; Moller, C.H.; Skov, R.L.; Spiess, K.; Fomsgaard, A.; Lassauniere, R.; Rasmussen, M.; et al. SARS-CoV-2 Omicron VOC Transmission in Danish Households. *medRxiv* **2021**, 21268278.
22. Chaguza, C.; Coppi, A.; Earnest, R.; Ferguson, D.; Kerantzas, N.; Warner, F.; Young, H.P.; Breban, M.I.; Billig, K.; Koch, R.T.; et al. Rapid emergence of SARS-CoV-2 Omicron variant is associated with an infection advantage over Delta in vaccinated persons. *Med* **2022**, *3*, 325–334.e4. [CrossRef] [PubMed]
23. Migliori, G.B.; Thong, P.M.; Akkerman, O.; Alffenaar, J.W.; Alvarez-Navascues, F.; Assao-Neino, M.M.; Bernard, P.V.; Biala, J.S.; Blanc, F.X.; Bogorodskaya, E.M.; et al. Worldwide effects of coronavirus disease pandemic on tuberculosis services, January-April 2020. *Emerg. Infect. Dis.* **2020**, *26*, 2709–2712. [CrossRef] [PubMed]
24. Lange, S.J.; Ritchey, M.D.; Goodman, A.B.; Dias, T.; Twentyman, E.; Fuld, J.; Schieve, L.A.; Imperatore, G.; Benoit, S.R.; Kite-Powell, A.; et al. Potential indirect effects of the COVID-19 pandemic on use of emergency departments for acute life-threatening conditions—United States, January–May 2020. *Am. J. Transpl.* **2020**, *20*, 2612–2617. [CrossRef] [PubMed]
25. Ong, C.W.M.; Migliori, G.B.; Ravligione, M.; MacGregor-Skinner, G.; Sotgiu, G.; Alffenaar, J.W.; Tiberi, S.; Adlhoch, C.; Alonzi, T.; Archuleta, S.; et al. Epidemic and pandemic viral infections: Impact on tuberculosis and the lung. *Eur. Respir. J.* **2020**, *56*, 2001727. [CrossRef] [PubMed]
26. Esmail, H.; Cobelens, F.; Goletti, D. Transcriptional biomarkers for predicting development of tuberculosis: Progress and clinical considerations. *Eur. Respir. J.* **2020**, *55*, 1901957. [CrossRef]
27. Migliori, G.B.; Thong, P.M.; Alffenaar, J.W.; Denholm, J.; Tadolini, M.; Alyaquobi, F.; Blanc, F.X.; Buonsenso, D.; Cho, J.G.; Codecasa, L.R.; et al. Gauging the impact of the COVID-19 pandemic on tuberculosis services: A global study. *Eur. Respir. J.* **2021**, *58*, 2101786. [CrossRef]
28. Programmatic Innovations to Address Challenges in Tuberculosis Prevention and Care during the COVID-19 Pandemic. Available online: https://apps.who.int/iris/handle/10665/341307 (accessed on 10 July 2022)
29. Augustynowicz-Kopec, E.; Jagielski, T.; Kozinska, M.; Kremer, K.; Soolingen, D.V.; Bielecki, J.; Zwolska, Z. Transmission of tuberculosis within family-households. *J. Infect.* **2012**, *64*, 596–608. [CrossRef] [PubMed]
30. Brooks, S.K.; Webster, R.K.; Smith, L.E.; Woodland, L.; Wessely, S.; Greenberg, N.; Rubin, G.J. The psychological impact of quarantine and how to reduce it: Rapid review of the evidence. *Lancet* **2020**, *395*, 912–920. [CrossRef] [PubMed]
31. Jenkins, D.J.; Kendall, C.W.; Marchie, A.; Jenkins, A.L.; Kendall, C.W.; Augustin, L.S.A.; Ludwig, D.S.; Barnard, N.D.; Anderson, J.W. Type 2 diabetes and the vegetarian diet. *Am. J. Clin. Nutr.* **2003**, *78*, 610S–616S. [CrossRef]
32. Bendall, C.L.; Mayr, H.L.; Opie, R.S.; Bes-Rastrollo, M.; Itsiopoulos, C.; Thomas, C.J. Central obesity and the Mediterranean diet: A systematic review of intervention trials. *Crit. Rev. Food Sci. Nutr.* **2018**, *58*, 3070–3084. [CrossRef] [PubMed]
33. Colberg, S.R.; Sigal, R.J.; Yardley, J.E.; Riddell, M.C.; Dunstan, D.W.; Dempsey, P.C.; Horton, E.S.; Castorino, K.; Tate, D.F. Physical activity/exercise and diabetes: A position statement of the American diabetes association. *Diabetes Care* **2016**, *39*, 2065–2079. [CrossRef] [PubMed]
34. Riddell, M.C.; Iscoe, K.E. Physical activity, sport, and pediatric diabetes. *Pediatr. Diabetes* **2006**, *7*, 60–70. [CrossRef] [PubMed]
35. Silva, C.J.; Torres, D.F.M. Optimal control for a tuberculosis model with reinfection and post-exposure interventions. *Math. Biosci.* **2013**, *244*, 154–164. [CrossRef]

36. Fauzi, I.S.; Fakhruddin, M.; Nuraini, N.; Wijaya, K.P. Comparison of dengue transmission in lowland and highland area: Case study in Semarang and Malang, Indonesia. *Commun. Biomath. Sci.* **2019**, *2*, 23–37. [CrossRef]
37. Nuraini, N.; Fauzi, I.S.; Fakhruddin, M.; Sopaheluwakan, A.; Soewono, E. Climate-based dengue model in Semarang, Indonesia: Predictions and descriptive analysis. *Infect. Dis. Model.* **2021**, *6*, 598–611. [CrossRef]
38. Gill, B.S.; Jayaraj, V.J.; Singh, S.; Ghazali, S.M.; Cheong, Y.L.; Md Iderus, N.H.; Sundram, B.M.; Aris, T.B.; Mohd Ibrahim, H.; Hong, B.H.; et al. Modelling the effectiveness of epidemic control measures in preventing the transmission of COVID-19 in Malaysia. *Int. J. Environ. Res. Public Health* **2020**, *17*, 5509. [CrossRef]
39. Fauzi, I.S.; Nuraini, N.; Ayu, R.W.S.; Lestari, B.W. Temporal trend and spatial clustering of the dengue fever prevalence in West Java, Indonesia. *Heliyon* **2022**, *8*, e10350. [CrossRef] [PubMed]
40. Backer, J.A.; Klinkenberg, D.; Wallinga, J. The incubation period of 2019-nCoV infections among travellers from Wuhan, China. *Eurosurveillance* **2020**, *25*, 2000062. [PubMed]
41. Read, J.M.; Bridgen, J.R.; Cumming, D.A.; Ho, A.; Jewell, C.P. Novel coronavirus 2019-nCoV: Early estimation of epidemiological parameters and epidemic forecasts. *Philosopical Trans. R. Soc. Biol. Sci.* **2021**, *376*, 20200265. [CrossRef]
42. Fuady, A.; Nuraini, N.; Sukandar, K.K.; Lestari, B.W. Targeted vaccine allocation could increase the COVID-19 vaccine benefits amidst its lack of availability: A mathematical modeling study in Indonesia. *Vaccines* **2021**, *9*, 462. [CrossRef] [PubMed]
43. Liu, S.; Bi, Y.; Liu, Y. Modeling and dynamic analysis of tuberculosis in mainland China from 1998 to 2017: The effect of DOTS strategy and further control. *Theor. Biol. Med. Model.* **2020**, *17*, 1–10. [CrossRef]
44. Li, J. The spread and prevention of tuberculosis. *Chin. Remedies Clin.* **2013**, *13*, 482–483.
45. Tewa, J.J.; Bowong, S.; Mewoli, B. Mathematical analysis of two-patch model for the dynamical transmission of tuberculosis. *Appl. Math. Model.* **2012**, *36*, 2466–2485. [CrossRef]
46. Widyaningsih, P.; Affan, R.C.; Saputro, D.R.S. A mathematical model for the epidemiology of diabetes mellitus with lifestyle and genetic factors. *J. Phys. Conf. Ser.* **2018**, *1028*, 012110. [CrossRef]

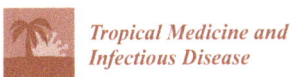 

Article

# Arbovirus Seroprevalence Study in Bangphae District, Ratchaburi Province, Thailand: Comparison between ELISA and a Multiplex Rapid Diagnostic Test (Chembio DPP® ZCD IgG)

Ruba Chakma [1], Pimolpachr Sriburin [1], Pichamon Sittikul [1], Jittraporn Rattanamahaphoom [1], Warisa Nuprasert [1], Nipa Thammasonthijarern [2], Pannamas Maneekan [3], Janjira Thaipadungpanit [4,5], Watcharee Arunsodsai [1], Chukiat Sirivichayakul [1], Kriengsak Limkittikul [1] and Supawat Chatchen [1,*]

[1] Department of Tropical Pediatrics, Faculty of Tropical Medicine, Mahidol University, Bangkok 10400, Thailand
[2] Department of Parasitology, Faculty of Veterinary Medicine, Kasetsart University, Bangkok 10900, Thailand
[3] Department of Tropical Hygiene, Faculty of Tropical Medicine, Mahidol University, Bangkok 10400, Thailand
[4] Department of Clinical Tropical Medicine, Faculty of Tropical Medicine, Mahidol University, Bangkok 10400, Thailand
[5] Mahidol-Oxford Tropical Medicine Research Unit, Faculty of Tropical Medicine, Mahidol University, Bangkok 10400, Thailand
* Correspondence: supawat.cht@mahidol.ac.th; Tel.: +66-2354-9161

**Abstract:** Arboviruses, particularly dengue virus (DENV), Zika virus (ZIKV), and Chikungunya virus (CHIKV), pose a growing threat to global public health. For disease burden estimation and disease control, seroprevalence studies are paramount. This study was performed to determine the prevalence of DENV, ZIKV, and CHIKV on healthy individuals aged from 1–55 years old in Bangphae district, Ratchaburi province, Thailand. Enzyme-linked immunosorbent assays (ELISAs) and rapid diagnostic tests (RDTs) were performed on archived samples from a dengue serological survey conducted from 2012–2015. All 2012 samples had been previously tested using an anti-DENV immunoglobulin (Ig)G ELISA, and 400 randomly selected samples stratified by age, sex, and residential area were assessed by an in-house anti-ZIKV IgG ELISA and a commercial anti-CHIKV IgG ELISA to determine virus-specific antibody levels. An RDT (Chembio DPP® ZCD IgM/IgG System) was also used to investigate the presence of antibodies against DENV, ZIKV, or CHIKV. The ELISA results indicate that the seroprevalences of DENV, ZIKV, and CHIKV were 84.3%, 58.0%, and 22.5%, respectively. The youngest age group had the lowest seroprevalence for all three arboviruses, and the seroprevalences for these viruses were progressively higher with increasing participant age. The DPP® IgG sensitivities, as compared with ELISAs, for DENV, ZIKV, and CHIKV were relatively low, only 43.92%, 25.86%, and 37.78%, respectively. The ELISA results indicate that 16% of the study population was seropositive for all three viruses. DENV had the highest seroprevalence. ZIKV and CHIKV were also circulating in Bangphae district, Ratchaburi province, Thailand. The DPP® ZCD rapid test is not sensitive enough for use in seroprevalence studies.

**Keywords:** dengue virus; zika virus; chikungunya virus; seroprevalence; ELISA; RDT; Thailand

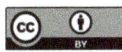

## 1. Introduction

Arboviruses are maintained in nature principally through their biological transmission between susceptible vertebrate hosts by blood-sucking arthropod vectors. These viruses are found worldwide but are more common in tropical and subtropical countries. There are ~500 known arboviruses, of which ~100 cause disease in humans and ~40 cause disease in domestic animals [1]. Although they are predominant in tropical and subtropical regions, owing to population growth and urbanization, international travel and trade, vector adaption, and global warming in recent decades, arbovirus infections have spread worldwide. Travelers have played a particularly important role in the worldwide transmission of mosquito-borne viruses [2,3]. Three major arthropod-borne viruses, dengue virus (DENV), Zika virus (ZIKV), and Chikungunya virus (CHIKV), are becoming public health concerns because of the growing threat they pose to global health and socioeconomic development.

DENV and ZIKV are mosquito-borne single-stranded RNA viruses in the genus *Flavivirus*, family *Flaviviridae*. Dengue, an infection caused by four antigenically distinct DENVs, has caused a huge disease burden in tropical and subtropical regions [4,5]. Due to a dramatic increase in DENV incidence over recent decades, it is estimated that there are now approximately 390 million DENV infections each year worldwide, with 500,000 cases of severe dengue requiring hospitalization and 20,000 deaths [6–8]. ZIKV was first isolated from a rhesus monkey in the Zika forest in 1947 [9], and the first case of human infection was reported from Nigeria in 1954 [10]. The first outbreak of ZIKV infection was reported from the Yap islands and Federal states of Micronesia in 2007 [11]. The pandemic of ZIKV in Brazil began in Bahia, a northeastern state, and became a large outbreak throughout the Americas [12]. More than 3000 cases of microcephaly were identified, and ZIKV was isolated from the autopsy brain tissue from a ZIKV infected infant [13]. On February 2016, the World Health Organization declared ZIKV infection a public health emergency of international concern [14].

CHIKV belongs to the genus *Alphavirus* in the family *Togaviridae*. The primary vectors of this virus are the *Ades aegypti* and *Aedes albopictus* mosquitoes, the same vectors that spread DENV and ZIKV. The main symptoms of CHIKV infection are high fever and joint pain in the acute phase, often accompanied by headache, diffuse back pain, myalgia, nausea, vomiting, polyarthritis, rash, and conjunctivitis; these symptoms are similar to those observed in dengue fever, especially in the acute phase. The first clinical report of CHIKV fever was as early as the 1770s, and the first CHIKV outbreak in Asia was reported from Bangkok in 1958 [15]. CHIKV epidemics later occurred in Cambodia, Vietnam, Malaysia, and Taiwan. In the 2005–2006 outbreak of CHIKV in La Reunion Island in the Indian Ocean, infected patients presented with severe complicated manifestations, primarily associated with encephalopathy and hemorrhagic fever [16]. Owing to challenges in accurately diagnosing the disease, there is no accurate estimate for the number of people affected by this virus. Because of the severe debilitating nature of the disease and the discovery of a new mutant in Caribbean countries and territories in 2013, CHIKV has become a global threat [17].

In Thailand, which has a well-established national dengue surveillance system, the prevalence and incidence rates of dengue are documented. However, similar to other countries in Southeast Asia, information regarding the periodic outbreaks of other mosquito-borne viral infections, such as those caused by ZIKV or CHIKV, is scarce [18,19]. Moreover, the acute stages of arboviral infections usually cause undifferentiated clinical manifestations, ranging from asymptomatic to severe illness, such that these diseases cannot be accurately differentiated from each other [20,21]. Despite the evidence that the arboviral diseases caused by DENV, ZIKV, and CHIKV contribute substantially to morbidity in Thailand, there are only a few studies that investigated the seroprevalence of these three major arboviruses [22]. A regular confirmatory laboratory test for arbovirus infection is generally not performed in healthy or mildly ill individuals. Consequently, the actual disease burdens and their spreading natures cannot be accurately estimated and the distributions of these viruses in Thailand remain uncertain.

A seroprevalence study can provide important information for disease control, and the development of a rapid diagnostic test (RDT) for use in such studies would ensure that low- and middle-income countries have a diagnostic tool for clinical management and surveillance, providing early alert against future outbreaks. The Chembio Dual Path Platform (DPP) ZCD (Zika/Chikungunya/Dengue) immunoglobulin (Ig)M/IgG system is a rapid immunochromatographic test for the separation and detection of IgM and IgG antibodies against DENV, ZIKV, and CHIKV in 10 µL of whole blood, serum, or plasma. Its results are read 10–15 min after adding buffer. Here, we investigated the seroprevalences of DENV, ZIKV, and CHIKV by testing archived samples from a dengue cohort study conducted in children and adults of central Thailand from 2012 to 2015 [23]. The present work aimed to explore the seroprevalence of DENV, ZIKV, and CHIKV by using ELISAs and the DPP® ZCD IgM/IgG System to detect antibodies against DENV, ZIKV, and CHIKV in archived samples from a dengue cohort study of children and adults in Bangphae district, Ratchaburi province, Thailand.

## 2. Materials and Methods

### 2.1. Study Site and Serum Samples

This seroprevalence study was performed by using archived data and serum samples collected (stored at −80 °C) from a cohort study of DENV conducted in Bangphae district, Ratchaburi province, Thailand from 2012 to 2015 (Figure 1). This previous study enrolled 2012 healthy children and adults aged between 1 and 55 years in 2012. The subjects were prospectively followed for six visits during the period from 2012–2015. The longitudinal serosurvey study of DENV was performed using an indirect IgG ELISA against DENV as described previously [23]. It was found that the overall prevalence of past DENV infection as measured by IgG ELISA was 74.3% in 2012 and had increased to 79.4% by 2015. Because DENV, ZIKV, and CHIKV can be transmitted by the same mosquito vector and co-circulate in the same area, we selected the serum samples from the first visit in this Bangphae study for use in our research. The minimum sample size for the present arbovirus seroprevalence study was calculated from an estimated prevalence of 50% for ZIKV and CHIKV, with a 95% confidence level and 5% absolute precision. The estimated minimum sample size was then adjusted by 4% to allow for possible error, resulting in an estimated necessary sample size of approximately 400 samples. The DENV ELISA results were taken from the previous cohort study. All selected samples were assessed using ZIKV and CHIKV IgG ELISAs. The samples were also tested with the RDT (DPP® ZCD IgM/IgG System).

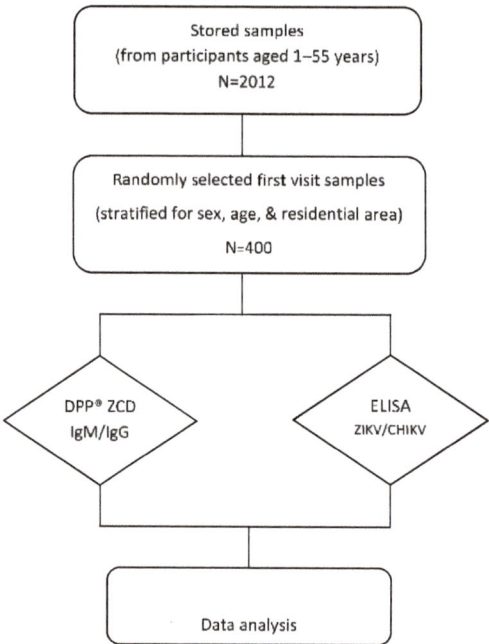

**Figure 1.** Schematic diagram of the study design and procedures. Four hundred serum samples were selected and used to perform ZIKV and CHIKV immunoglobulin (Ig) G enzyme-linked immunosorbent assay (ELISA) tests (DENV ELISA results were used from previous study) and the DPP® ZCD IgM/IgG system.

The protocol for this study was reviewed and approved by the Ethics Committee of the Faculty of Tropical Medicine, Mahidol University (protocol TMEC 22-016). Procedures conducted in this study were in accordance with the standard criteria of the Human Ethical Research committee of Faculty of Tropical Medicine, Mahidol University.

*2.2. In-House DENV IgG ELISA*

The present study used the in-house indirect sandwich DENV IgG ELISA using a dengue monoclonal antibody 2H2 and an equal mixture of inactivated DENV 1–4 antigen. The data from a previous report, in which the method used to acquire these data is described [23,24].

*2.3. In-House ZIKV NS1 IgG ELISA*

An in-house ZIKV NS1 IgG ELISA was performed using the ZIKV NS1 protein, a recombinant protein produced in *E. coli* BL21(DE3), to evaluate the immune status against ZIKV of the study participants [25,26]. Briefly, 96-well ELISA plates were sensitized with 60 µL/well of ZIKV NS1 protein (500 ng) in 0.018 M carbonate buffer. After an overnight incubation at 4 °C, the plates were washed six times with 300 µL/well of phosphate-buffered saline (PBS) containing 1% Tween 20 (PBS-T) and then blocked with assay buffer (5% skim milk in PBS-T) for 1 h at 37 °C. After additional washing procedures were conducted, 50 µL/well of the tested serum diluted 1:100 with assay buffer and controls were added in duplicate and then the plates were incubated at 37 °C for 1.5 h. After being washed again, the plates were filled with 50 µL/well of a goat anti-human IgG antibody conjugated to horse radish peroxidase (KPL Inc., Gaithersburg, MD, USA), diluted at 1:5000 in assay buffer. After being incubated at 37 °C for 90 min, the plates were washed six times, and the substrate SureBlue™ TMP (KPL Inc., Gaithersburg, MD, USA) was added for 30 min incubation at room temperature. The colorimetric reaction was stopped by the addition of 50 µL of 0.2 M sulfuric acid to each well, and the optical density (OD) at 450 nm was read using an ELISA plate reader.

### 2.4. CHIKV IgG ELISA

The EUROIMMUN CHIKV ELISA test kit (EUROIMMUN Co., Lubeck, Germany) is a semi-quantitative in vitro assay for the detection of human IgG-class antibodies against CHIKV in serum. The kits contain microtiter strips, each with eight break-off reagent wells coated with CHIKV antigens. First, 10 µL of the sample was diluted into 1.0 mL of sample buffer. The Euroimmun anti-CHIKV IgG ELISA was performed as following the manufacturer's instructions. The results were evaluated by calculating the ratio of the extinction value of the control or sample divided by the extinction value of the calibrator. This assay was evaluated on an ELISA plate reader.

### 2.5. Chembio DPP® ZCD IgM/IgG System

The DPP® ZCD IgM/IgG System employs Chembio's patented DPP technology (Dual membrane Path Platform), consisting of a sample path that distributes samples onto two test strips. The upper test strip (window labelled "1, 2, 3") is for detecting IgM antibodies against DENV, ZIKV, and CHIKV, respectively, and the bottom test strip (window also labelled "1, 2, 3") is for the detection of IgG antibodies against DENV, ZIKV, and CHIKV, respectively. To initiate the test, a 10-µL specimen is diluted with a buffer and applied to the SAMPLE + BUFFER well located in the middle of the sample transfer strip of the DPP® ZCD IgM/IgG Test Device. The DPP® ZCD IgM/IgG System was performed according to manufacturer's instructions. At the time of reading the results, the DPP® Micro reader and cassette adapter must be used to obtain the test results.

### 2.6. Criteria for Seropositivity

For DENV and ZIKV IgG ELISA results, the criterion for seropositivity was the sample OD greater than or equal to twice over the OD from the negative control [23,25]. For the CHIKV ELISA results, a sample was classified as seropositive when the sample OD greater than or equal to 1.1 times over the OD from the calibrator. In accordance with the DPP® ZCD IgM/IgG system protocol, a sample was classified as positive when the level of the sample from the reader was greater than or equal 22. The DPP® ZCD IgG levels were used to compare with the ELISA results.

### 2.7. Statistical Analysis

A descriptive summary of study participant characteristics is presented stratified by sex, location, and age group; participant age was divided into five age groups for comparative purposes. The Mann-Whitney U-test was performed to compare continuous variables between study groups. The correlation coefficient was used to compare the DPP® and ELISA results. Sensitivity, specificity, and predictive values were calculated for the DPP® using the corresponding ELISA as a standard. Differences were considered statistically significant if the $p$-value was less than 0.05. All analyses were performed using SPSS software version 18.0 (SPSS Inc., Chicago, IL, USA).

## 3. Results

### 3.1. Demographic Data

The demographic data for our study participants were described previously [23]. The serosurvey of dengue in Bangphae district, Ratchaburi province, Thailand from 2012 to 2015 was conducted by performing an indirect DENV IgG ELISA. Over that study period, approximately 2000 children and adults were enrolled in the dengue serosurvey. Archived serum samples from visit 1 (Y2012) and the associated demographic data were used for the present study. From each of the five age groups, a group of 80 serum samples with an equal sex and location distribution was randomly selected (total: 400 serum samples) for use in this study (Table 1).

**Table 1.** Demographic characteristic of subjects [n (%)].

|  | Visit 1 | Selected |
|---|---|---|
| number/samples | 2012 | 400 |
| Male:Female | 903:1109 | 200:200 |
|  | 0.81:1 | 1:1 |
| **Sub-district** |  |  |
| Wang-Yen | 348 (17.30) | 57 |
| Bang-Phae | 301 (15.00) | 58 |
| Wat-Kaew | 250 (12.40) | 57 |
| Hau-Pho | 254 (12.60) | 57 |
| Don-Kha | 152 (7.60) | 57 |
| Don-Yai | 203 (10.00) | 57 |
| Pho-Hak | 504 (25.00) | 57 |
| **Age group** |  |  |
| 1–10 | 695 (34.54) | 80 |
| 11–20 | 733 (36.43) | 80 |
| 21–30 | 180 (8.95) | 80 |
| 31–40 | 170 (8.45) | 80 |
| 41–55 | 234 (11.63) | 80 |

### 3.2. Arbovirus Seroprevalences

The seroprevalence of DENV, ZIKV, and CHIKV according to the ELISA results and a descriptive summary of participant characteristics are presented in Table 2. The IgG ELISA results show that the arbovirus with the highest seroprevalence was DENV (84.25%), followed by ZIKV (58.00%) and CHIKV (22.50%). According to the ELISA results, the DENV seroprevalence was very high in all tested areas (77.19–92.98%).

**Table 2.** Seropositivity to three arboviruses according to ELISA [n (%)].

|  | DENV | ZIKV | CHIKV |
|---|---|---|---|
| number/samples | 337 (84.25) | 232 (58.00) | 90 (22.50) |
| Male:Female | 163:174 | 117:115 | 39:51 |
|  | 0.94:1 | 1.02:1 | 0.76:1 |
| **Sub-district** |  |  |  |
| Wang-Yen | 53 (92.98) | 45 (78.95) | 12 (21.05) |
| Bang-Phae | 49 (84.48) | 31 (53.45) | 13 (22.41) |
| Wat-Kaew | 49 (85.96) | 24 (42.11) | 8 (14.04) |
| Hau-Pho | 45 (78.95) | 40 (70.18) | 20 (35.09) |
| Don-Kha | 45 (78.95) | 23 (40.35) | 10 (17.54) |
| Don-Yai | 44 (77.19) | 23 (40.35) | 15 (26.32) |
| Pho-Hak | 52 (91.23) | 46 (80.70) | 12 (21.05) |
| **Age group** |  |  |  |
| 1–10 | 37 (46.25) | 25 (31.25) | 4 (5.00) |
| 11–20 | 65 (81.25) | 51 (63.75) | 5 (6.25) |
| 21–30 | 76 (95.00) | 40 (50.00) | 6 (7.50) |
| 31–40 | 80 (100.00) | 57 (71.25) | 26 (32.50) |
| 41–55 | 79 (98.75) | 59 (73.75) | 49 (61.25) |

Among the three arboviruses, DENV had the highest seroprevalence, according to the ELISA results, in all sub-districts (77.19–92.98%), while CHIKV had the lowest seroprevalence, particularly in the youngest three age groups. The pattern of seroprevalence for the three tested arboviruses varied in different areas. Wang-Yen sub-district had the highest percentage of DENV seropositivity (92.98%), Pho-Hak had the highest percentage of ZIKV seropositivity (80.70%), and Hau-Pho had the highest percentage of CHIKV seropositivity

(35.09%). Don-Kha and Don-Yai had the lowest percentage of ZIKV seropositivity (40.35%), and Wat-Kaew had the lowest percentage of CHIKV seropositivity (14.04%).

Overall, the seroprevalence for each of the three arboviruses was progressively higher with increasing age. The age-specific seroprevalence of DENV reached its peak level in those aged 31–40 years old. For ZIKV, the seroprevalence dropped from 63.75% in the 11–20 years old age group to 50% in the 21–30 years old age group, but trended upward again in the remaining older age groups (Figure 2). For CHIKV, the seroprevalence was 5% in the 1–10 years old age group, 6.25% in the 11–20 years old age group, and 7.50% in the 21–30 years old age group. The seroprevalence of CHIKV was dramatically higher in the 31–40 years old age group (32.5%) and higher again in the 40–55 years old age group (61.25%).

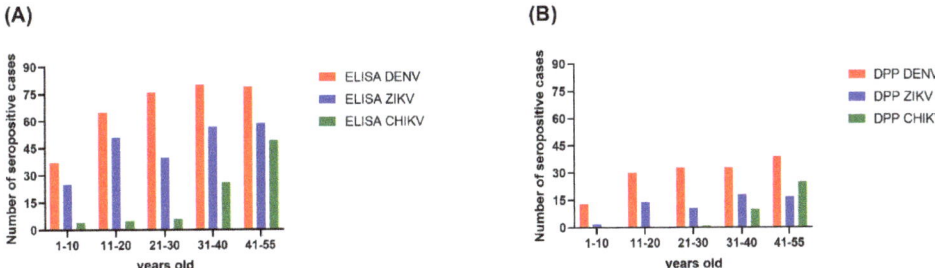

**Figure 2.** Seroprevalence of three arboviruses by age group. (**A**) The ELISA results; (**B**) The DPP® ZCD IgG results. The x-axes describe the DENV (red), ZIKV (blue), and CHIKV (green) distributions for five age groups in Bangphae district, Ratchaburi province, Thailand. The y-axes represent the seroprevalence, as shown by the number of cases.

The Chembio DPP® ZCD results indicate overall DENV, ZIKV, and CHIKV seroprevalences lower than those estimated from the ELISA results. There were 160, 64, and 37 cases determined by the Chembio DPP® ZCD as being seropositive for anti-DENV, -ZIKV, and -CHIKV IgM or IgG, respectively; the numbers of cases seropositive for only virus-specific IgG were 148, 62, and 36, respectively (Table 3). When judging the seroprevalence by the DPP data instead of the ELISA data, the areas with the highest seroprevalence of DENV and ZIKV were Don-Yai instead of Wang-Yen and Don-Kha instead of Pho-Hak, respectively, but the area with the highest seroprevalence of CHIKV (Hau-Pho) remained the same (Figure 3). The pattern of age-specific seroprevalence for these arboviruses in children and adults according to the DPP data was similar to those estimated from the ELISA data but with lower seroprevalences (Table 3, Figure 2).

Table 3. Seropositivity for three arboviruses according to DPP® ZCD system [n (%)].

| | DENV IgM | DENV IgG | ZIKV IgM | ZIKV IgG | CHIKV IgM | CHIKV IgG |
|---|---|---|---|---|---|---|
| number/samples | 28 (7.00) | 148 (37.00) | 5 (1.25) | 62 (15.50) | 14 (3.50) | 35 (8.75) |
| Male:Female | 17:11 1.55:1 | 72:76 0.95:1 | 3:2 1.50:1 | 30:32 0.94:1 | 6:8 0.75:1 | 14:21 0.67:1 |
| **Sub-district** | | | | | | |
| Wang-Yen | 4 (7.02) | 21 (36.84) | 1 (1.75) | 9 (15.79) | 2 (3.51) | 6 (12.53) |
| Bang-Phae | 2 (3.45) | 22 (37.93) | 0 (0.00) | 10 (17.24) | 2 (3.45) | 4 (6.90) |
| Wat-Kaew | 1 (1.75) | 8 (14.04) | 1 (1.75) | 2 (3.51) | 3 (5.26) | 2 (3.51) |
| Hau-Pho | 1 (1.75) | 17 (29.82) | 1 (1.75) | 7 (12.28) | 2 (3.51) | 9 (15.79) |
| Don-Kha | 3 (5.26) | 26 (45.61) | 1 (1.75) | 10 (17.54) | 1 (1.75) | 5 (8.77) |
| Don-Yai | 11 (19.30) | 30 (52.63) | 1 (1.75) | 7 (12.28) | 2 (3.51) | 6 (10.53) |
| Pho-Hak | 6 (10.53) | 24 (42.11) | 0 (0.00) | 7 (12.28) | 2 (3.51) | 3 (5.26) |
| **Age group** | | | | | | |
| 1–10 | 3 (3.75) | 13 (16.25) | 1 (1.25) | 2 (2.50) | 4 (5.00) | 0 (0.00) |
| 11–20 | 6 (7.50) | 30 (37.50) | 2 (2.50) | 14 (17.50) | 2 (2.50) | 0 (0.00) |
| 21–30 | 8 (10.00) | 33 (41.25) | 1 (1.25) | 11 (13.75) | 3 (3.75) | 1 (1.25) |
| 31–40 | 5 (6.25) | 33 (41.25) | 1 (1.25) | 18 (22.50) | 2 (2.50) | 10 (12.50) |
| 41–55 | 6 (7.50) | 39 (48.75) | 0 (0.00) | 17 (21.25) | 3 (3.75) | 24 (30.00) |

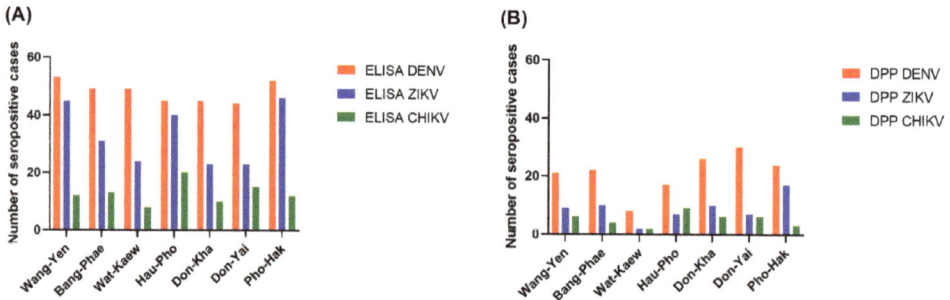

**Figure 3.** Seroprevalence of three arboviruses by residential area. (**A**) The ELISA results; (**B**) The DPP® ZCD IgG results. The x-axes describe the DENV (red), ZIKV (blue), and CHIKV (green) distributions for the seven sub-districts of Bangphae district, Ratchaburi province, Thailand. The y-axes represent the seroprevalence, as shown by the number of cases.

*3.3. Co-Seropositivity for DENV, ZIKV, and CHIKV*

According to the ELISA results, 115 (38.75%) individuals were jointly positive for DENV- and ZIKV-specific IgG antibodies, and 64 (16.00%) were jointly positive for DENV-, ZIKV-, and CHIKV-specific IgG antibodies (Figure 4). The prevalence of IgG antibodies against all three arboviruses (DENV, ZIKV, and CHIKV) was highest in Hau-Pho sub-district (18 cases), followed by Bang-Phae sub-district (12 cases), and Pho-Hak sub-district (9 cases). The age group with the highest joint seroprevalence of DENV and ZIKV was the 11–20-years-old group at 52.50%, whereas the highest joint seropositivity for DENV-specific and CHIKV-specific antibodies was 15.00% in the 41–55-years-old age group. The prevalence of IgG antibodies against all three arboviruses showed a gradual rise with age during early life (i.e., slightly higher prevalence in young adults than in children); however, the prevalence of these antibodies rapidly became higher with increasing ages above 30 years (Table 4). The highest co-seropositivity (38.75%) was seen for DENV-specific and ZIKV-specific antibodies. In contrast, only 25 (6.25%) of study participants were jointly seropositive for DENV-specific and CHIKV-specific antibodies. The Chembio DPP® IgG revealed 87 (21.75%) individuals as seropositive for DENV-specific IgG, 14 (3.50%) for ZIKV-specific IgG, and 10 (2.50%) for CHIKV-specific IgG. Moreover, the co-seropositive for both DENV and ZIKV IgG, and for DENV, ZIKV, and CHIKV IgG were 35 (8.75%) and 13 (3.25%), respectively.

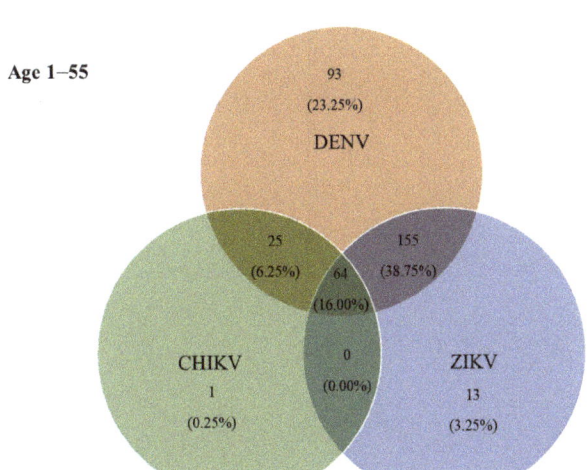

**Figure 4.** Co-circulation of three ELISA-positive arboviruses in Bangphae district, Ratchaburi province, Thailand. Number and percentage (%) of samples found to be positive by ELISA for immunoglobulin G (IgG) antibodies to single or multiple exposures of DENV, ZIKV, and CHIKV.

**Table 4.** Co-circulation of three arboviruses according to ELISA [n (%)].

|  | DENV | ZIKV | CHIKV | D + Z | D + C | Z + C | D + Z + C |
|---|---|---|---|---|---|---|---|
| number/samples | 93 (23.25) | 13 (3.25) | 1 (0.25) | 155 (38.75) | 25 (6.25) | 0 (0.00) | 64 (16.00) |
| Age group |  |  |  |  |  |  |  |
| 1–10 | 17 (21.25) | 6 (7.50) | 1 (1.25) | 17 (21.25) | 1 (1.25) | 0 (0.00) | 2 (2.50) |
| 11–20 | 18 (22.50) | 6 (7.50) | 0 (0.00) | 42 (52.50) | 2 (2.50) | 0 (0.00) | 3 (3.75) |
| 21–30 | 33 (41.25) | 0 (0.00) | 0 (0.00) | 37 (46.25) | 3 (3.75) | 0 (0.00) | 3 (3.75) |
| 31–40 | 16 (20.00) | 0 (0.00) | 0 (0.00) | 38 (47.50) | 7 (8.75) | 0 (0.00) | 19 (23.75) |
| 41–55 | 9 (11.25) | 1 (1.25) | 0 (0.00) | 21 (26.25) | 12 (15.00) | 0 (0.00) | 37 (46.25) |

*3.4. Comparison of ELISA and Chembio DPP® ZCD IgG*

Among the three arboviruses, DENV had the highest seroprevalence, according to both the ELISA and Chembio DPP® ZCD system results. Comparing the ELISA and Chembio DPP® ZCD IgG results revealed that the sensitivity of the Chembio DPP® IgG for DENV was relatively low, only 43.92% (95% confidence interval (CI): 38.54–49.40%). Additionally, although the specificity was 100% (95% CI: 94.31–100.00%), the accuracy was only 52.75% (95% CI: 47.73–57.73%). The sensitivity and specificity of the Chembio DPP® IgG for ZIKV as compared with ELISA were 25.86% (95% CI 20.35–32.00%) and 98.81% (95% CI: 95.77–99.86%), respectively; the accuracy was only 56.50% (95% CI: 51.48–61.42%). The accuracy for CHIKV rapid tests (85.50%, 95% CI: 81.66–88.80%) was relatively higher compared with the rapid tests for DENV and ZIKV; however, the sensitivity was only 37.78% (95% CI: 27.77–48.62%), and the specificity was 99.35% (95% CI: 97.69–99.92%).

Overall, the immunochromatographic test of the Chembio DPP® ZCD system showed a low sensitivity when compared with ELISA. Figure 5 shows the average values of the Chembio DPP® ZCD IgG in the ELISA-based seropositive and seronegative groups. All Chembio DPP® ZCD systems for the three arboviruses produced a statistically significant difference in antibody levels between the ELISA-based seropositive and seronegative groups.

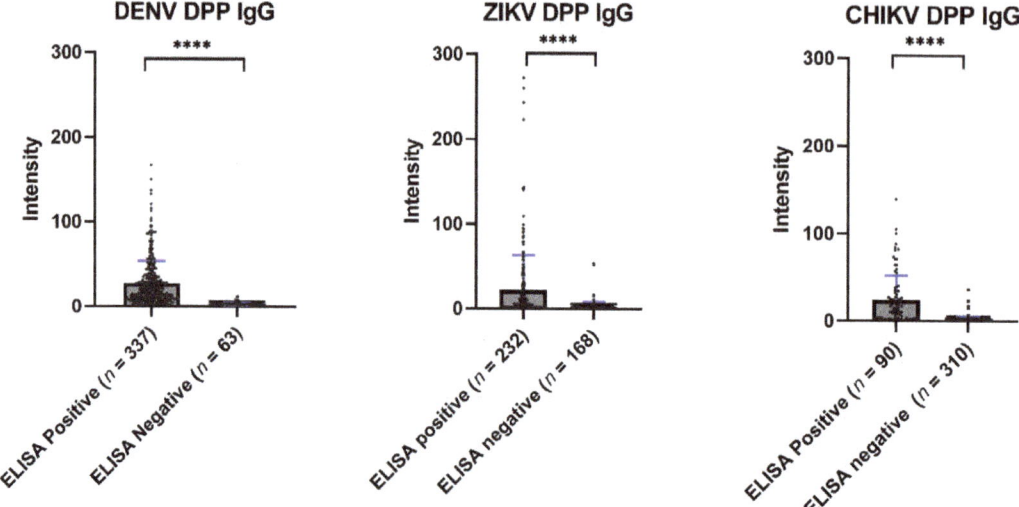

**Figure 5.** Scatter plot of the DPP® ZCD system results by ELISA-positive and ELISA-negative samples. The median DENV DPP® results from ELISA-positive and -negative samples were 18.00 and 2.50, respectively (**** $p < 0.0001$). The median ZIKV DPP® results from ELISA-positive and -negative samples were 5.90 and 1.30, respectively (**** $p < 0.0001$). The median CHIKV DPP® results from ELISA-positive and -negative samples were 14.50 and 2.10, respectively (**** $p < 0.0001$).

## 4. Discussion

The primary purpose of this study was to assess the seroprevalence status of three important arboviruses, i.e., DENV, ZIKV, and CHIKV. In addition, this study also aimed to evaluate the sensitivity and specificity of the DPP® ZCD IgG rapid test as compared with ELISA and assess the prevalence of exposure to multiple arboviruses in the population. To this end, 400 serum samples, from healthy participants without febrile illness evenly split across five age groups with equal male:female ratios and equal representation of seven sub-districts of the Bangphae district, Ratchaburi province, Thailand, were selected from archived serum samples collected by the previous study, "Dengue virus seroprevalence study in Bangphae district, Ratchaburi, Thailand: A cohort study in 2012–2015" [23].

The seroprevalence of exposure to all three major arboviruses was progressively higher with advancing age, i.e., the younger age groups had lower seroprevalences compared with the older age groups. This occurrence in endemic areas may be due to older people having a higher cumulative exposure to these arboviruses. From the ELISA results, the highest percentage of co-seropositivity was for the combination of DENV and ZIKV (38.75%). DENV and ZIKV are closely related flaviviruses that share a high degree of structural and sequence homology. Moreover, the cross-reactivity between DENV and ZIKV is a challenging serological diagnostic problem. The cross-reactivity of antibodies between these two closely related viruses could explain this finding. A previous study on the seroprevalence of Zika in pregnant women in Thailand also noticed a cross-reaction between DENV and ZIKV [27]. According to past studies, the sensitivity and specificity of in-house DENV IgG ELISA were 94.37% and 87.33%, respectively, when comparing with PRNT [24]. Comparison with PRNT results revealed that the sensitivity and the specificity of the in-house ZIKV NS1 IgG ELISA were 100% and 70.27%, respectively [26]. Furthermore, this low specificity in the ZIKV NS1 IgG ELISA mainly caused by the secondary DENV infection samples. Additionally, the trend of ZIKV seroprevalence differed across age groups, which could be the result of susceptibility variation, as suggested by a previous study on ZIKV that also proposed variable susceptibility to ZIKV [28]. Other related work found that age and sex had roles in susceptibility to ZIKV infection [29]. In the present study, the arbovirus with the highest seroprevalence was found to be DENV in all seven sub-districts, followed by ZIKV and CHIKV. Compared with other sub-districts, Wang-Yen and Pho-Hak had the highest seroprevalence of DENV and ZIKV, respectively, and Hua-Pho had the highest seroprevalence of CHIKV. A previous CHIKV study in Vietnam found a different scenario for CHIKV seroprevalence, reporting that different areas had different patterns [15]. Here, the younger age group had little exposure to CHIKV, and the seroprevalence of this virus was progressively higher among the middle and older age groups but varied among different locations. This study result is similar to that of a 2017 study on CHIKV seroprevalence in India, in which the younger age group had a lower seroprevalence compared with the older age group, and the seroprevalence was progressively higher in increasingly older groups [30].

Our work reveals the co-circulation of three important arboviruses in the study area. DENV had the highest seroprevalence among the tested arboviruses. The ELISA result indicates that there was no statistically significant difference in seropositivity for DENV, ZIKV, or CHIKV between males and females, although the percentages of seropositivity for DENV and CHIKV trended higher in the group of female participants and the percentage of seropositivity for ZIKV trended higher in the group of male participants. The similarity of the DENV seroprevalence found in our work to that reported by a previous study confirms the appropriate sampling of serum samples in this research [23]. Regarding ZIKV, our finding that the seroprevalence trended slightly higher in male participants than in female participants is inconsistent with the report by a previous ZIKV study in Thailand showing 61% of confirmed ZIKA cases occurring in female patients [31,32]. As ZIKV infection can impact pregnancy outcome, infection of female individuals with this virus remains a major concern. Regarding CHIKV, the observed trend of a higher seroprevalence in female participants than in male participants in our study is similar to the reported higher percentage of CHIKV-confirmed cases in female patients than in male patients (57.8% vs. 42.2%) during a large-scale outbreak of CHIKV infection in Thailand in 2018–2019 [33]. However, an opposite scenario was seen in a previous study of CHIKV conducted in southern and central Vietnam [15]. Regarding the secondary study objective of comparing DPP® ZCD with ELISA, we found that although the specificity of DPP® ZCD was high, its sensitivity and accuracy were relatively low; a Kappa test showed a positive correlation between the ELISA and DPP® rapid test results. Higher ELISA values were positively correlated with higher DPP® values. The previous study on the evaluation of Zika rapid tests found that these tests had relatively higher sensitivity for clinical diagnosis of ZIKV [34]. However, the sensitivity of the ZIKV rapid test from the present serosurvey study was low compared with the sensitivity results for DENV and CHIKV rapid tests. The accuracy of the CHIKV rapid test was 85.50%, which is the highest accuracy value among all three rapid tests in the DPP® ZCD system.

The limitations of the study were also considered. The study samples were selected from previously archived (10 years ago) serum collected in a dengue endemic area, which lacked information regarding ZIKV and CHIKV infections. Moreover, the ELISAs for the DENV-specific and ZIKV-specific antibody were performed with in-house ELISAs, whereas a commercial ELISA was used for the detection of the CHIKV-specific antibody.

## 5. Conclusions

This study shows that, among DENV, ZIKV, and CHIKV, DENV had the highest seroprevalence; however, ZIKV and CHIKV are still important co-circulating arboviruses in Bangphae district, Ratchaburi province, Thailand. The DPP® ZCD rapid test alone may not be practical for use in a seroprevalence study, owing to its low sensitivity compared with ELISAs. Further study to determine the true scenario of arbovirus disease burden and their spreading nature is needed in other endemic areas for informing future disease prevention and control.

**Author Contributions:** Conceptualization, S.C. and R.C.; methodology, S.C.; formal analysis, S.C. and R.C.; investigation, R.C., P.S. (Pimolpachr Sriburin), P.S. (Pichamon Sittikul), J.R. and W.N.; writing—original draft preparation, S.C. and R.C.; writing—review and editing, N.T., P.M., J.T., W.A., C.S. and K.L.; supervision, N.T., P.M., J.T., W.A., C.S. and K.L.; funding acquisition, S.C. All authors have read and agreed to the published version of the manuscript.

**Funding:** This study was supported by the Department of Tropical Pediatrics, Faculty of Tropical Medicine, Mahidol University. The APC was funded by Mahidol University and the Faculty of Tropical Medicine, Mahidol University, Thailand.

**Institutional Review Board Statement:** The study was conducted according to the guidelines of the Declaration of Helsinki and approved by the Ethics Committee of Faculty of Tropical Medicine, Mahidol University, Thailand (No. TMEC 22-016).

**Informed Consent Statement:** Not applicable.

**Data Availability Statement:** Not applicable.

**Acknowledgments:** The authors thank May C. Chu from the Department of Epidemiology, Colorado School of Public Health, University of Colorado, CO, USA for providing the DPP® ZCD IgM/IgG system in this study. They also thank Katie Oakley.

**Conflicts of Interest:** The authors declare no conflict of interest.

## References

1. Bassett, M. The Emergence and History of Arboviruses, Microbiology Society. Available online: https://microbiologysociety.org/blog/the-emergence-and-history-of-arboviruses.html (accessed on 10 January 2022).
2. Girard, M.; Nelson, C.B.; Picot, V.; Gubler, D.J. Arboviruses: A global public health threat. *Vaccine* **2020**, *38*, 3989–3994. [CrossRef] [PubMed]
3. Yuan, B.; Lee, H.; Nishiura, H. Analysis of international traveler mobility patterns in Tokyo to identify geographic foci of dengue fever risk. *Theor. Biol. Med. Model.* **2021**, *18*, 17. [CrossRef]
4. Endy, T.P.; Chunsuttiwat, S.; Nisalak, A.; Libraty, D.H.; Green, S.; Rothman, A.L.; Vaughn, D.W.; Ennis, F.A. Epidemiology of inapparent and symptomatic acute dengue virus infection: A prospective study of primary school children in Kamphaeng Phet, Thailand. *Am. J. Epidemiol.* **2002**, *156*, 40–51. [CrossRef] [PubMed]
5. Guzman, M.G.; Fuentes, O.; Martinez, E.; Perez, A.B. Dengue. In *International Encyclopedia of Public Health*, 2nd ed.; Quah, S.R., Ed.; Academic Press: Oxford, UK, 2017; pp. 233–257.
6. Gubler, D.J. Dengue/dengue haemorrhagic fever: History and current status. *Novartis Found. Symp.* **2006**, *277*, 3–16; discussion 16–22, 71–73, 251–253. [CrossRef]
7. Singhi, S.; Kissoon, N.; Bansal, A. Dengue and dengue hemorrhagic fever: Management issues in an intensive care unit. *J. Pediatr.* **2007**, *83*, S22–S35. [CrossRef]
8. World Health Organization. Global Strategy for Dengue Prevention and Control 2012–2020. Available online: https://apps.who.int/iris/bitstream/handle/10665/75303/9789241504034_eng.pdf (accessed on 10 January 2022).
9. Dick, G.W.; Kitchen, S.F.; Haddow, A.J. Zika virus. I. Isolations and serological specificity. *Trans. R. Soc. Trop. Med. Hyg.* **1952**, *46*, 509–520. [CrossRef]
10. Macnamara, F.N. Zika virus: A report on three cases of human infection during an epidemic of jaundice in Nigeria. *Trans. R. Soc. Trop. Med. Hyg.* **1954**, *48*, 139–145. [CrossRef]
11. Lanciotti, R.S.; Kosoy, O.L.; Laven, J.J.; Velez, J.O.; Lambert, A.J.; Johnson, A.J.; Stanfield, S.M.; Duffy, M.R. Genetic and serologic properties of Zika virus associated with an epidemic, Yap State, Micronesia, 2007. *Emerg. Infect. Dis.* **2008**, *14*, 1232–1239. [CrossRef]
12. Hennessey, M.; Fischer, M.; Staples, J.E. Zika Virus Spreads to New Areas—Region of the Americas, May 2015–January 2016. *MMWR Morb. Mortal. Wkly. Rep.* **2016**, *65*, 55–58. [CrossRef]
13. Schuler-Faccini, L.; Ribeiro, E.M.; Feitosa, I.M.; Horovitz, D.D.; Cavalcanti, D.P.; Pessoa, A.; Doriqui, M.J.; Neri, J.I.; Neto, J.M.; Wanderley, H.Y.; et al. Possible Association Between Zika Virus Infection and Microcephaly—Brazil, 2015. *MMWR Morb. Mortal. Wkly. Rep.* **2016**, *65*, 59–62. [CrossRef]
14. Pillinger, M. WHO Declared a Public Health Emergency about Zika's Effects. Here Are Three Takeaways. Available online: https://www.washingtonpost.com/news/monkey-cage/wp/2016/02/02/who-declared-a-public-health-emergency-about-zikas-effects-here-are-three-takeaways/ (accessed on 10 January 2022).
15. Quan, T.M.; Phuong, H.T.; Vy, N.H.T.; Thanh, N.T.L.; Lien, N.T.N.; Hong, T.T.K.; Dung, P.N.; Chau, N.V.V.; Boni, M.F.; Clapham, H.E. Evidence of previous but not current transmission of chikungunya virus in southern and central Vietnam: Results from a systematic review and a seroprevalence study in four locations. *PLOS Negl. Trop. Dis.* **2018**, *12*, e0006246. [CrossRef] [PubMed]

16. Soumahoro, M.-K.; Boelle, P.-Y.; Gaüzere, B.-A.; Atsou, K.; Pelat, C.; Lambert, B.; La Ruche, G.; Gastellu-Etchegorry, M.; Renault, P.; Sarazin, M.; et al. The Chikungunya Epidemic on La Réunion Island in 2005–2006: A Cost-of-Illness Study. *PLOS Negl. Trop. Dis.* **2011**, *5*, e1197. [CrossRef] [PubMed]
17. Van Bortel, W.; Dorleans, F.; Rosine, J.; Blateau, A.; Rousset, D.; Matheus, S.; Leparc-Goffart, I.; Flusin, O.; Prat, C.; Cesaire, R.; et al. Chikungunya outbreak in the Caribbean region, December 2013 to March 2014, and the significance for Europe. *Eur. Surveill. Bull. Eur. Sur Les Mal. Transm. Eur. Commun. Dis. Bull.* **2014**, *19*, 20759. [CrossRef] [PubMed]
18. Hapuarachchi, H.C.; Bandara, K.B.; Sumanadasa, S.D.; Hapugoda, M.D.; Lai, Y.L.; Lee, K.S.; Tan, L.K.; Lin, R.T.; Ng, L.F.; Bucht, G.; et al. Re-emergence of Chikungunya virus in South-east Asia: Virological evidence from Sri Lanka and Singapore. *J. Gen. Virol.* **2010**, *91*, 1067–1076. [CrossRef] [PubMed]
19. Wiwanitkit, V. The current status of Zika virus in Southeast Asia. *Epidemiol. Health* **2016**, *38*, e2016026. [CrossRef]
20. Forshey, B.M.; Guevara, C.; Laguna-Torres, V.A.; Cespedes, M.; Vargas, J.; Gianella, A.; Vallejo, E.; Madrid, C.; Aguayo, N.; Gotuzzo, E.; et al. Arboviral etiologies of acute febrile illnesses in Western South America, 2000–2007. *PLoS Negl. Trop. Dis.* **2010**, *4*, e787. [CrossRef]
21. Labeaud, A.D.; Bashir, F.; King, C.H. Measuring the burden of arboviral diseases: The spectrum of morbidity and mortality from four prevalent infections. *Popul. Health Metr.* **2011**, *9*, 1. [CrossRef] [PubMed]
22. Tongthainan, D.; Mongkol, N.; Jiamsomboon, K.; Suthisawat, S.; Sanyathitiseree, P.; Sukmak, M.; Wajjwalku, W.; Poovorawan, Y.; Ieamsaard, G.; Sangkharak, B.; et al. Seroprevalence of Dengue, Zika, and Chikungunya Viruses in Wild Monkeys in Thailand. *Am. J. Trop. Med. Hyg.* **2020**, *103*, 1228–1233. [CrossRef]
23. Limkittikul, K.; Chanthavanich, P.; Lee, K.S.; Lee, J.S.; Chatchen, S.; Lim, S.K.; Arunsodsai, W.; Yoon, I.K.; Lim, J.K. Dengue virus seroprevalence study in Bangphae district, Ratchaburi, Thailand: A cohort study in 2012–2015. *PLoS Negl. Trop. Dis.* **2022**, *16*, e0010021. [CrossRef] [PubMed]
24. Sirivichayakul, C.; Limkittikul, K.; Chanthavanich, P.; Yoksan, S.; Ratchatatat, A.; Lim, J.K.; Arunsodsai, W.; Sabcharoen, A. Monoclonal antibody-based capture ELISA in the diagnosis of previous dengue infection. *Virol. J.* **2019**, *16*, 125. [CrossRef]
25. Sriburin, P.; Sittikul, P.; Kosoltanapiwat, N.; Sirinam, S.; Arunsodsai, W.; Sirivichayakul, C.; Limkittikul, K.; Chatchen, S. Incidence of Zika Virus Infection from a Dengue Epidemiological Study of Children in Ratchaburi Province, Thailand. *Viruses* **2021**, *13*, 1802. [CrossRef] [PubMed]
26. Sittikul, P.; Sriburin, P.; Rattanamahaphoom, J.; Limkittikul, K.; Sirivichayakul, C.; Chatchen, S. Combining Immunoassays to Identify Zika Virus Infection in Dengue-Endemic Areas. *Trop. Med. Infect. Dis.* **2022**, *7*, 254. [CrossRef] [PubMed]
27. Phatihattakorn, C.; Wongsa, A.; Pongpan, K.; Anuwuthinawin, S.; Mungmanthong, S.; Wongprasert, M.; Tassaneetrithep, B. Seroprevalence of Zika virus in pregnant women from central Thailand. *PLoS ONE* **2021**, *16*, e0257205. [CrossRef] [PubMed]
28. Legros, V.; Jeannin, P.; Burlaud-Gaillard, J.; Chaze, T.; Gianetto, Q.G.; Butler-Browne, G.; Mouly, V.; Zoladek, J.; Afonso, P.V.; Gonzàlez, M.N.; et al. Differentiation-dependent susceptibility of human muscle cells to Zika virus infection. *PLoS Negl. Trop. Dis.* **2020**, *14*, e0008282. [CrossRef] [PubMed]
29. Coelho, F.C.; Durovni, B.; Saraceni, V.; Lemos, C.; Codeco, C.T.; Camargo, S.; de Carvalho, L.M.; Bastos, L.; Arduini, D.; Villela, D.A.; et al. Higher incidence of Zika in adult women than adult men in Rio de Janeiro suggests a significant contribution of sexual transmission from men to women. *Int. J. Infect. Dis. IJID Off. Publ. Int. Soc. Infect. Dis.* **2016**, *51*, 128–132. [CrossRef] [PubMed]
30. Kumar, M.S.; Kamaraj, P.; Khan, S.A.; Allam, R.R.; Barde, P.V.; Dwibedi, B.; Kanungo, S.; Mohan, U.; Mohanty, S.S.; Roy, S.; et al. Seroprevalence of chikungunya virus infection in India, 2017: A cross-sectional population-based serosurvey. *Lancet Microbe* **2021**, *2*, e41–e47. [CrossRef]
31. Ruchusatsawat, K.; Wongjaroen, P.; Posanacharoen, A.; Rodriguez-Barraquer, I.; Sangkitporn, S.; Cummings, D.A.T.; Salje, H. Long-term circulation of Zika virus in Thailand: An observational study. *Lancet Infect. Dis.* **2019**, *19*, 439–446. [CrossRef]
32. Sirinam, S.; Chatchen, S.; Arunsodsai, W.; Guharat, S.; Limkittikul, K. Seroprevalence of Zika Virus in Amphawa District, Thailand, after the 2016 Pandemic. *Viruses* **2022**, *14*, 476. [CrossRef]
33. Khongwichit, S.; Chansaenroj, J.; Thongmee, T.; Benjamanukul, S.; Wanlapakorn, N.; Chirathaworn, C.; Poovorawan, Y. Large-scale outbreak of Chikungunya virus infection in Thailand, 2018–2019. *PLoS ONE* **2021**, *16*, e0247314. [CrossRef]
34. Boeras, D.; Diagne, C.T.; Pelegrino, J.L.; Grandadam, M.; Duong, V.; Dussart, P.; Brey, P.; Ruiz, D.; Adati, M.; Wilder-Smith, A.; et al. Evaluation of Zika rapid tests as aids for clinical diagnosis and epidemic preparedness. *EClinicalMedicine* **2022**, *49*, 101478. [CrossRef]

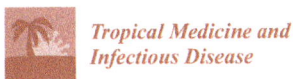 *Tropical Medicine and Infectious Disease*

Article

# Recombinant Vaccinia Virus Expressing *Plasmodium berghei* Apical Membrane Antigen 1 or Microneme Protein Enhances Protection against *P. berghei* Infection in Mice

Min-Ju Kim [1,†], Ki-Back Chu [2,†], Su-Hwa Lee [3], Hae-Ji Kang [1], Keon-Woong Yoon [1], Md Atique Ahmed [4] and Fu-Shi Quan [2,3,*]

1. Department of Biomedical Science, Graduate School, Kyung Hee University, Seoul 02447, Korea
2. Medical Research Center for Bioreaction to Reactive Oxygen Species and Biomedical Science Institute, School of Medicine, Graduate School, Kyung Hee University, Seoul 02447, Korea
3. Department of Medical Zoology, School of Medicine, Kyung Hee University, Seoul 02447, Korea
4. ICMR-Regional Medical Research Centre, NE Region, Dibrugarh 786010, Assam, India
\* Correspondence: fsquan@khu.ac.kr
† These authors contributed equally to this work.

**Abstract:** Recombinant vaccinia viruses (rVV) are effective antigen delivery vectors and are researched widely as vaccine platforms against numerous diseases. Apical membrane antigen 1 (AMA1) is one of the candidate antigens for malaria vaccines but rising concerns regarding its genetic diversity and polymorphism have necessitated the need to search for an alternative antigen. Here, we compare the efficacies of the rVV vaccines expressing either AMA1 or microneme protein (MIC) of *Plasmodium berghei* in mice. Mice (BALB/c) were immunized with either rVV-AMA1 or rVV-MIC and subsequently challenge-infected with *P. berghei*. Compared to the control group, both antigens elicited elevated levels of parasite-specific antibody responses. Immunization with either one of the two vaccines induced high levels of T cells and germinal center B cell responses. Interestingly, rVV-MIC immunization elicited higher levels of cellular immune response compared to rVV-AMA1 immunization, and significantly reduced pro-inflammatory cytokine productions were observed from the former vaccine. While differences in parasitemia and bodyweight changes were negligible between rVV-AMA1 and rVV-MIC immunization groups, prolonged survival was observed for the latter of the two. Based on these results, our findings suggest that the rVV expressing the *P. berghei* MIC could be a vaccine-candidate antigen.

**Keywords:** *Plasmodium berghei*; recombinant vaccinia virus (rVV); vaccine; apical membrane antigen 1; microneme protein

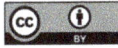

## 1. Introduction

Malaria is one of the diseases that account for a large proportion of disease-related mortality worldwide, particularly in Africa. Statistically, on a global scale, approximately 241 million malaria cases and 627,000 malaria-related deaths were reported in 2020 [1]. However, despite decades of research, commercialized vaccines are unavailable. RTS,S/AS01 vaccine based on the *P. falciparum* circumsporozoite protein (CSP) is the most advanced malaria vaccine reported to date, but its recent phase 3 clinical trial results were disappointing. Specifically, the vaccines were initially protective, but their efficacies drastically waned over 7 years of follow-up [2]. Given this circumstance, additional efforts using different methods of approach are required. One such approach is the use of modified vaccinia virus Ankara (MVA) vectors.

Historically, vaccinia viruses were used as smallpox vaccines in the 20th century and were integral to eradicating smallpox [3]. The MVA is a replication-deficient attenuated form of the vaccinia virus that is capable of expressing recombinant genes, thus highlighting their use as potent viral vector vaccines. The MVA vaccine platform is highly regarded as being safe and immunogenic, with the latter of the two aspects being subjected to change depending on the immunization dose and immunization regimen [4]. As such, a large number of studies involving MVA vaccines were conducted in an attempt to develop an efficacious malaria vaccine, and positive findings were confirmed through numerous clinical trials. A prime-boost regimen using the recombinant chimpanzee adenovirus 63 (ChAd63) and MVA vaccines encoding the *P. falciparum* CSP were confirmed to be safe and immunogenic in a clinical trial [5]. Using the same approach, ChAD63-MVA vaccines encoding the apical membrane antigen 1 (AMA1) induced potent T cell and antibody responses in vaccinees [6]. Another clinical study reported that heterologous immunization with ChAD63-MVA vectors expressing either the merozoite surface protein 1 (MSP1) or AMA1 elicited an increase in antigen-specific seroreactivity in vaccinees, even after controlled human malaria infection [7]. Despite these promising findings, many of the surface proteins of *Plasmodium* spp. are highly polymorphic and often result in vaccine-induced immune responses being allele-specific. This genetic diversity, in turn, compromises the vaccine efficacy by exerting selection pressure towards escape mutation [8]., Other antigen candidates must be explored to address these issues.

Microneme (MIC) is a secretory organelle commonly found in Apicomplexan parasites, and several studies have reported the immunogenicity of these micronemal antigens. Antibodies raised against the *Eimeria tenella* microneme protein 2 (MIC2) inhibited the parasitic invasion of host cells, and immunizing chickens with the MIC2-expressing DNA vaccines lessened the severity of infection [9]. Similarly, antibodies raised against the micronemal protein 1 of another Apicomplexan parasite, *Babesia bigemina* neutralized merozoite invasion when tested in vitro [10]. Chimeric antigen prepared by fusing the microneme and rhoptry proteins of *Neospora caninum* significantly reduced the cerebral parasite burden and protected mice against neosporosis [11]. In the case of *Plasmodium* spp., only a handful of malaria vaccine studies have evaluated the immunogenicity of micronemal antigens. Antibodies raised against the *P. falciparum* glycosylphosphatidylinositol-anchored micronemal antigen (GAMA) were capable of inhibiting parasitic invasion [12]. Similarly, the *P. vivax* GAMA protein vaccine induced both cellular and humoral immune responses in individuals naturally infected with *P. vivax*, thus highlighting their further development as blood-stage vaccine candidates [13]. To date, a *P. berghei* microneme antigen-based vaccine study has yet to be conducted. Furthermore, the rodent malaria *P. berghei* shares multiple features resembling those of the human malaria *P. falciparum* [14], making them highly desirable for vaccine studies. Here, we evaluate the efficacy of recombinant vaccinia virus vaccines expressing the micronemal antigen. We also compare the efficacy of this vaccine to that of a vaccinia-based vaccine expressing the AMA1 antigen reported in our previous study [15], which conferred suboptimal protection.

## 2. Materials and Methods

### 2.1. Animals, Parasites, Cells, and Antibodies

To maintain the *Plasmodium berghei* ANKA strain and immunization vaccines, female seven-week-old BALB/c mice were purchased from NARA Biotech (Seoul, Korea). Mice were housed in an institute-approved facility with a 12 h day and night cycle, with easy access to food and water. Nesting material and enrichment were also provided to prevent the development of abnormal behaviors. The *P. berghei* ANKA strain was used for challenge infection and antigen preparation. CV1 cells (CCL-70) and Vero cells (CCL-81) were purchased from the American Type Culture Collection (Manassas, VA, USA). Both cell lines were cultured using Dulbecco's Modified Eagle Media, supplemented with fetal bovine serum and penicillin/streptomycin at 37 °C, 5% $CO_2$ for production and characterization of rVVs. Sera of *P. berghei*-infected mice polyclonal antibodies were collected through retro-orbital plexus puncture. Horseradish peroxidase (HRP)-conjugated goat anti-mouse immunoglobulin G (IgG) was purchased from Southern Biotech (Birmingham, AL, USA).

## 2.2. P. berghei Antigen Preparation

The *P. berghei* ANKA strain antigen was prepared as described previously [16]. Briefly, red blood cells (RBCs) were collected from the whole blood of *P. berghei*-infected mice with parasitemia exceeding 20% by low-speed centrifugation. Pelleted RBCs were lysed with an equal volume of 0.15% saponin in PBS, and the released parasites were pelleted and washed 3 times with PBS. Parasites were sonicated at 30 s, at 40% amplitude, for two cycles on ice and stored at −20 °C until used. The *P. berghei* antigen was used as coating antigens for enzyme-linked immunosorbent assay (ELISA) and as the stimulant for flow cytometric analysis.

## 2.3. Generation of Recombinant Vaccinia Virus

To generate the *P. berghei* recombinant vaccinia virus, codon-optimized *P. berghei* AMA1 or MIC genes containing *EcoR*I and *Hind*III restriction enzyme sites were purchased from GenScript (Piscataway, NJ, USA). The codon-optimized AMA1 and MIC genes were cloned into the green fluorescent protein (GFP)-expressing pRB21 vaccinia virus vectors, which were kindly provided by Dr. Sang-Moo Kang at Georgia State University (Atlanta, GA, USA). CV-1 cells were cultured in DMEM supplemented with 10% inactivated FBS and 1% penicillin/streptomycin antibiotics. Confluent monolayers of CV-1 cells initially infected vRB12 using DMEM media without antibiotics for 1 h at 37 °C. Afterward, cells were transfected with pRB21-AMA1, pRB21-MIC, or GFP-expressing pRB21 vector control using the Lipofectamine LTX/PLUS™ (Thermo Fisher, Waltham, MA, USA) transfection reagent and incubated for 2–3 days at 37 °C. Cells were monitored under a fluorescent microscope to evaluate successful transfection. After 3 days, recombinant vaccinia virus was harvested and centrifuged at 2000 rpm for 10 min. Cell culture supernatants were discarded, and pelleted cells were resuspended in DMEM media, and stored at −80 °C. Frozen cells were repeatedly thawed in a 37 °C water bath and re-frozen at −80 °C. Recombinant vaccinia viruses were released from CV-1 cells via sonication and stored at −80 °C until use. To confirm the presence of AMA1 and MIC in the recombinant vaccinia virus, Western blots were performed, and membranes were sequentially probed with a primary antibody (anti-*P. berghei* polyclonal antibody) and then a secondary antibody (HRP-conjugated anti-mouse IgG). As a loading control for Western blots, membranes were probed with monoclonal beta-actin antibody (SC-47778; Santa Cruz Biotechnology, Dallas, TX, USA). Bands were developed using the enhanced chemiluminescence (ECL) purchased from Bio-Rad (Bio-Rad #1705061; Hercules, CA, USA) and visualized using ChemiDoc (Bio-Rad, Hercules, CA, USA).

## 2.4. Recombinant Vaccinia Virus Plaque Assay

Recombinant vaccinia virus titers were determined using Vero cells. Confluent monolayers of Vero cells cultured in 12-well plates were infected with the vaccinia virus diluted in serum-free DMEM media for 1 h at 37 °C. Overlay media was made with DMEM media containing 2% FBS and 1% agarose. After 1 h, the virus inoculum in each well was aspirated, and 1 mL of overlay media was added to each well. Plates were incubated at 37 °C, 5% $CO_2$, until noticeable plaque development occurred, which enables quantification.

## 2.5. Immunization and Challenge

Seven-week-old female BALB/c mice were randomly divided into four experimental groups (naïve, naïve challenge, AMA1 rVV, MIC rVV; $n = 8$ per group) to evaluate the protective efficacies of PbAMA1 and PbMIC rVV vaccines. Mice were intramuscularly immunized with AMA1 (Prime: $1.8 \times 10^7$, 1st boost: $6.8 \times 10^7$, 2nd boost: $1.3 \times 10^8$ PFU/mouse) or MIC (Prime: $1.8 \times 10^7$, 1st boost: $6 \times 10^7$, 2nd boost: $1 \times 10^8$ PFU/mouse) rVV at weeks 0, 4, and 8. Four weeks after the 2nd boost immunization, mice were challenged with 0.5%/100 uL in PBS ($0.5 \times 10^4$) of *P. berghei* by intraperitoneal (IP) injection, as described previously [15]. Four mice from each group were euthanized at 6 days post-infection (dpi) for blood, spleen, and inguinal lymph node sample collection. The remaining four mice were observed daily to monitor changes in body weight and parasitemia in blood. The human intervention point was set as 20% of initial body weight loss, and mice that reached this point were humanely euthanized using $CO_2$.

*2.6. Antibody Responses in Sera*

Mice sera were collected from all groups 4 weeks after prime, 1st boost immunization, and 2nd boost immunization using a retro-orbital plexus puncture. Sera from naïve mice were used as a negative control. Antibody responses against *P. berghei* antigen, AMA1 rVV, and MIC rVV were determined by enzyme-linked immunosorbent assay (ELISA), as described previously [17]. Briefly, 96-well immunoplates were coated with 100 µL of *P. berghei* antigen, AMA1 rVV, or MIC rVV at a final concentration of 2, 0.5, and 0.5 µg/mL, each respectively in 0.05 M, pH 9.6 carbonate bicarbonate buffer per well at 4 °C overnight. Afterwards, 100 µL of serially diluted serum samples were added into the respective wells and incubated at 37 °C for 1.5 h. HRP-conjugated goat anti-mouse IgG (100 µL/well, diluted 1:2000 in PBS) was used to determine the *P. berghei*-specific IgG antibody response. O-phenylenediamine was dissolved in citrate substrate buffer, and $OD_{492}$ was measured using an EZ Read 400 microplate reader (Biochrom Ltd., Cambridge, UK).

*2.7. Immune Cell Responses by Flow Cytometry*

To determine the immune cell responses, the levels of T and B cell populations from the blood and inguinal lymph nodes (ILN) of mice were evaluated by flow cytometry. The ILNs of mice were aseptically removed, and lymphocytes were acquired as previously described [18], and placed on top of a cell strainer. The cell strainer containing the ILNs was placed on a Petri plate and immersed in 1 mL PBS. Lymph nodes were thoroughly homogenized using the plunger portion of a syringe, and the resulting homogenates were carefully collected. $CD4^+$ and $CD8^+$ T cells from the blood were detected at 6 dpi. The levels of $CD8^+$ T cells and germinal center (GC) B cell proliferation were measured from ILN cells at 6 dpi. Immune cell populations ($1 \times 10^6$ cells per sample) were resuspended in PBS and stimulated with 0.05 µg of *P. berghei* antigen for 2 h at 37 °C before staining with surface antigen antibodies. Cells were incubated in FACS staining buffer (2% bovine serum albumin and 0.1% sodium azide in 0.1 M PBS) for 15 min at 4 °C with Fc Block antibody (clone 2.4G2; BD Biosciences, San Jose, CA, USA). Afterwards, cells were incubated with the fluorophore-conjugated cell surface antigen antibodies (CD3e-PE-Cy5, CD4-FITC, CD8a-PE, B220-FITC, GL7-PE; BD Biosciences, CA, USA) at 4 °C for 30 min. Stained cells were acquired using a BD Accuri C6 Flow Cytometer (BD Biosciences, CA, USA), and the data were analyzed using C6 Analysis software (BD Biosciences, CA, USA).

*2.8. Inflammatory Cytokine Production in the Spleen*

At 6 dpi, the mice were euthanized, and spleens were harvested. Single cell suspensions of splenocytes were prepared from individual spleens by homogenization. Briefly, spleens were firmly pressed using two frosted glass slides in RPMI media. Homogenates were carefully collected into 15 mL conical tubes and centrifuged at 2000 rpm for 5 min. The resulting supernatants were collected to detect inflammatory cytokines interferon-gamma (IFN-γ) and tumor necrosis factor-alpha (TNF-α). The levels of splenic cytokine expressions were detected using the BD OptEIA IFN-γ, TNF-α ELISA kits (BD Biosciences, San Jose, CA, USA). Cytokine concentrations were quantified following the manufacturer's instructions.

*2.9. Parasitemia*

Infected mouse blood samples were collected via retro-orbital plexus puncture. After resuspending 2 µL of the blood samples into microcentrifuge tubes containing 500 U/mL of heparin premixed in 100 µL of PBS, RBCs were stained using 1 µL SYBR Green I (Invitrogen, Carlsbad, CA, USA). Samples were incubated at 37 °C for 30 min in the dark. After incubation, 0.1 M PBS was added to each sample and flow cytometry was performed [19].

*2.10. Statistics*

All parameters were recorded for individuals in all the groups. The data were presented as mean ± SD, and statistical significances between groups. They were analyzed by one-way analysis of variance (ANOVA) and Student's *t*-test using GraphPad Prism version 6.0 (GraphPad Software, San Diego, CA, USA). *p* values (* $p < 0.05$) were considered statistically significant.

## 3. Results

*3.1. Gene Cloning and Recombinant Vaccinia Virus Generation*

An illustration depicting the location of the AMA1 and MIC antigens within the *Plasmodium* parasites was provided (Figure A1). To generate recombinant vaccinia viruses expressing the *P. berghei* AMA1 or MIC, the AMA1 or MIC in the pRB21 vector were designed (Figure 1A,B). AMA1 (1621 bp) or MIC (901 bp) DNAs were PCR amplified and cloned into a pRB21 vector. Successful clones were confirmed by restriction enzyme digestion (Figure 1C,D). Clones PbAMA1 and PbMIC DNAs were transfected into CV-1 cells for rVV-AMA1 and rVV-MIC production. Representative brightfield and fluorescence images for transfection were provided. Cellular lysis, identified by the empty regions in the cell monolayer, was not observed in the non-transfected control. Lysed cells were detectable at 1 dpi onward and a noticeable increase in cellular lysis was observed as time progressed (Figure 2A). Cells were also monitored daily under a fluorescent microscope, to confirm successful transfection of rVV-AMA1 and rVV-MIC. As expected, on day 0, non-transfected cells did not emit fluorescence. Low levels of green fluorescence emission were observed from cells at 1 dpi, thereby indicating successful transfection. By 2 dpi, a drastic increase in transfected cell populations was observed. The irregularly shaped dark regions indicate areas of cellular lysis. At 3 dpi, a substantial increase in cellular lysis was observable, consistent with the brightfield images (Figure 2B). A western blot was performed to confirm the presence of AMA1 and MIC in the recombinant vaccinia virus. Polyclonal *P. berghei* antibody was used to determine AMA1 and MIC expressions at molecular weights of 61 and 35 kDa, respectively (Figure 2C).

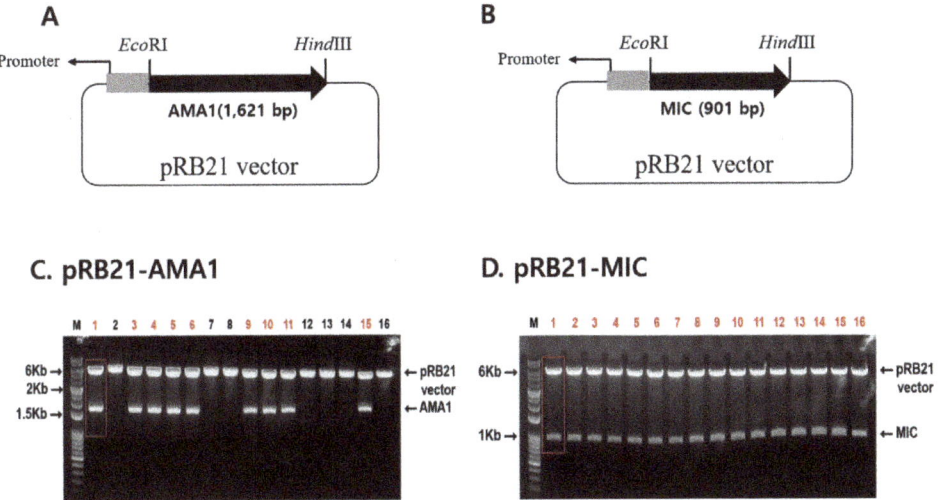

**Figure 1.** Gene cloning. To generate *P. berghei* AMA1 and MIC recombinant vaccinia virus (rVV), gene cassettes with promoters and recombination sites were designed, shown as a schematic diagram (**A**,**B**). PbAMA1 or PbMIC genes were cloned into the pRB21 vector, and clones pRB21-AMA1 (**C**) and pRB21-MIC (**D**) were confirmed by restrictive enzyme digestion with *Eco*RI and *Hind*III. The red color font denotes successful clones.

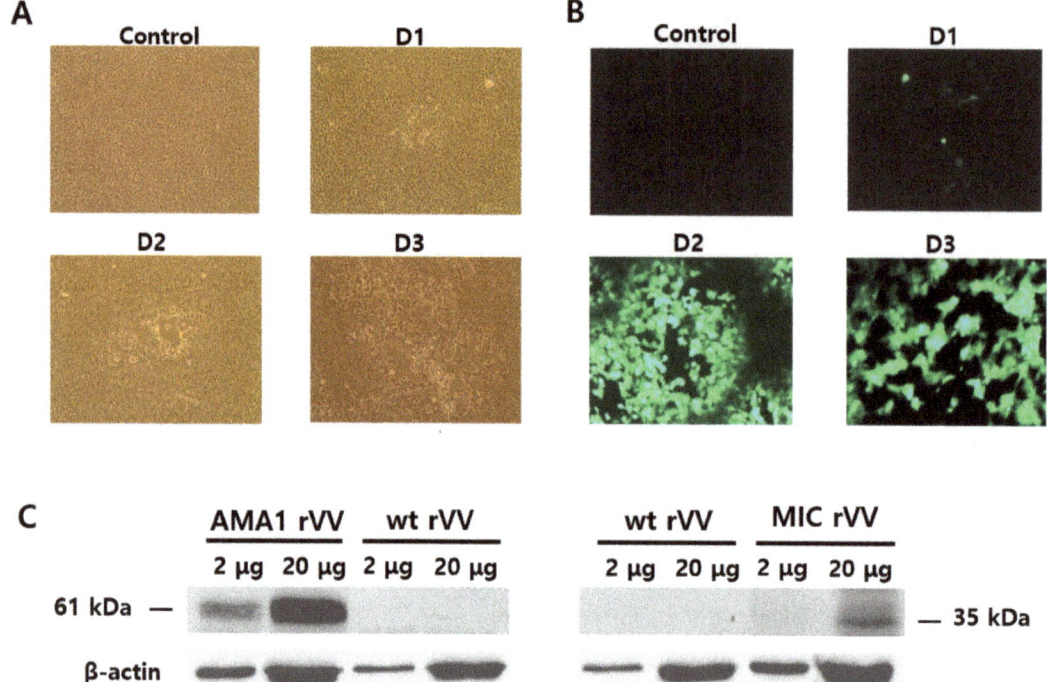

**Figure 2.** Transfection of CV-1 and confirming the production of rVV. The pRB21-PbAMA1 and pRB21-PbMIC DNA constructs were transfected into CV-1 cells, along with the vaccinia virus, to generate rVV-AMA1 and rVV-MIC. Representative images of rVV transfection under brightfield (**A**) and fluorescent microscope (**B**) are illustrated over the course of 3 days. AMA1 and MIC rVVs were identified by a Western blot using a *P. berghei* polyclonal antibody and a wild-type vaccinia virus (wt VV) control (**C**).

*3.2. IgG Antibody Responses*

A schematic diagram depicting immunization and challenge infection schedules was provided (Figure A2). Sera were regularly collected from mice 4 weeks after prime, 1st boost, and 2nd boost immunizations to assess parasite-specific IgG antibody responses against *P. berghei* antigen. Differences in antibody responses elicited by the two vaccines after prime immunizations were negligible. At 4 weeks after the 1st boost immunization, antibody responses were slightly enhanced, with significantly greater levels induced by rVV-AMA1. However, after the 2nd boost immunization, the trend was reversed. Immunization with the rVV-MIC elicited a stronger antibody response reacting to the malaria antigen than rVV-AMA1 (Figure 3A). To determine the levels of IgG antibody responses that are reactive to the recombinant vaccinia virus, sera were collected at 4 weeks after the 1st boost immunization, and ELISA was performed (Figure 3B,C). As seen in Figure 3B,C, higher levels of IgG antibody responses were observed using rVV-AMA1 (Figure 3B) or rVV-MIC as coating antigens (Figure 3C) compared to naïve control.

*3.3. $CD4^+$, $CD8^+$ T Cells and Germinal Center B Cell Response in the Blood and ILN*

At 6 dpi, the blood and ILN samples were collected from mice, and the single cell populations were prepared to analyze the $CD4^+$, $CD8^+$ T cell, and germinal center B cell frequencies by flow cytometry. A sample gating strategy for flow cytometric analysis of T cells has been provided (Figure A3). Both rVV-AMA1 and rVV-MIC immunization elicited significantly enhanced CD4⁺ T cell frequencies compared to naïve challenge groups (Figure 4A, * $p < 0.05$). However, blood CD8⁺ T cell populations were negligibly changed (Figure 4B). In the ILN, significant differences in CD8⁺ T cell proliferation were observed across the groups. While enhanced CD8⁺ T cell frequencies were detected from both AMA1 and MIC rVV vaccines, induction was significantly greater in the latter of the two (Figure 4C; * $p < 0.05$, ** $p < 0.01$, *** $p < 0.001$). A similar trend was observed for the GC B cells. Recombinant vaccinia virus vaccines significantly elevated the expression of GC B cells, with higher induction occurring in the ILNs of the rVV-MIC immunization group (Figure 4D; * $p < 0.05$, ** $p < 0.01$, *** $p < 0.001$).

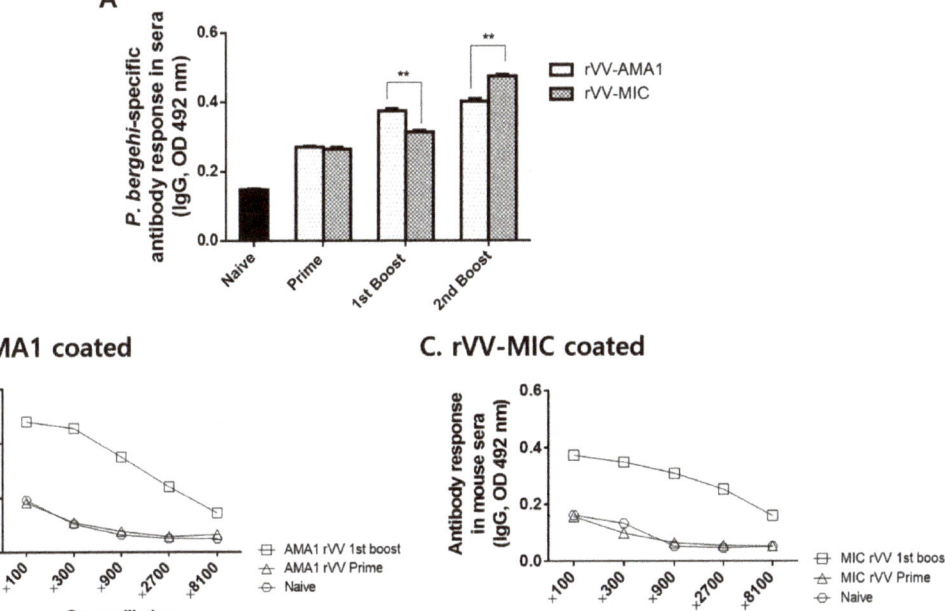

**Figure 3.** IgG antibody response in sera. On week 4 after prime, 1st boost, and 2nd boost immunization, the sera of mice were collected to investigate the levels of IgG antibody response. The 96-well immunoplates coated with *P. berghei* antigen (**A**), rVV-AMA1 (**B**), or rVV-MIC (**C**) were used to verify IgG antibody response by ELISA. Data are expressed as mean ± SD (** $p < 0.01$).

### 3.4. Inflammatory Cytokine Production in Splenocytes

Individual spleens were collected and homogenized to determine the levels of inflammatory cytokines IFN-γ and TNF-α. Production of the two inflammatory cytokines was assessed using the spleen homogenate supernatant. Significantly reduced splenic IFN-γ levels were observed in the rVV-MIC immunization group. While a marginal reduction in IFN-γ was observed from the rVV-AMA1 immunized mice, the vaccine-induced changes were negligible (Figure 5A, * $p < 0.05$). Contrary to this finding, statistical significance between the groups was not observed for the splenic TNF-α levels (Figure 5B).

### 3.5. Parasitemia, Bodyweight Reduction, and Survival Rate

As seen in Figure 6, kinetic changes for parasitemia (A), body weight changes (B), and survival rate (C) between immunized mice and non-immunized control (Naïve + challenge) from days 0 to day 65 post-challenge were monitored. On day three post-challenge, 2–3% of parasitemia with 1.2% of this value corresponding to the fluorescence background as demonstrated from naïve mice (D-H). On day 45 post-challenge, parasitemia in the naïve + cha, rVV-MIC, and rVV-AMA1 were 73.4%, 26.7%, and 37.5% each, respectively (Figure 6D–H). Interestingly, lower levels of parasitemia were observed from rVV-MIC compared to rVV-AMA1 immunization. Compared to the naïve + cha group, rVV-AMA1 and rVV-MIC immunization prolonged the survival of mice by 12 and 17 days, respectively (Figure 6C). The highest differences in parasitemia (H) and body weight (I) between immunized mice and non-immunized naïve control were observed at days 45 and 48 post-challenge infections, respectively, thus indicating that protections were induced in both AMA1 and MIC groups.

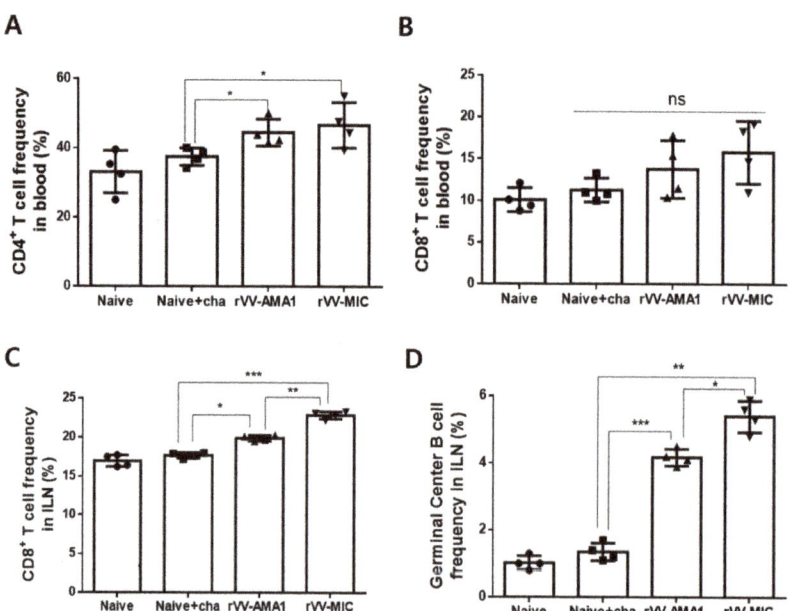

**Figure 4.** T cell and germinal center B cell response in blood and inguinal lymph nodes (ILN). Immunized mice (*n* = 8) were challenge-infected with *P. berghei*, and blood samples were collected at 6 dpi. Inguinal lymph nodes (ILN) from mice were collected at 6 dpi. After surface marker staining with the fluorophore-conjugated antibodies, CD4$^+$ (**A**) and CD8$^+$ (**B**) T cell responses in the blood and CD8$^+$ (**C**) T cell, germinal center B cell (**D**) responses in ILN were assessed by flow cytometry. Data are expressed as mean ± SD (* $p < 0.05$, ** $p < 0.01$, *** $p < 0.001$; ns: no statistical significance).

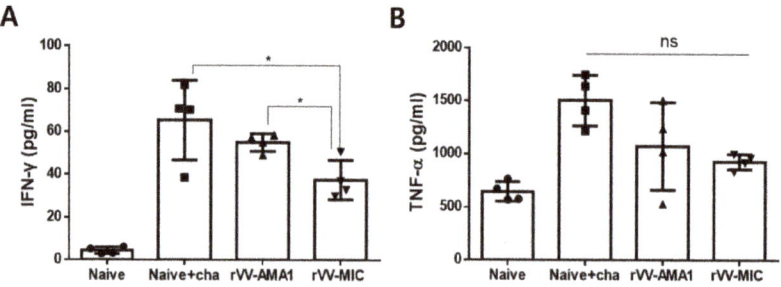

**Figure 5.** Inflammatory cytokine production in the spleen. Inflammatory cytokine productions were assessed from the spleens of mice at 6 dpi with *P. berghei*. Splenic IFN-γ (**A**) and TNF-α (**B**) cytokines were investigated using the BD OptEIA IFN-γ, TNF-α ELISA kits. Data are expressed as mean ± SD (* $p < 0.05$; ns: no statistical significance).

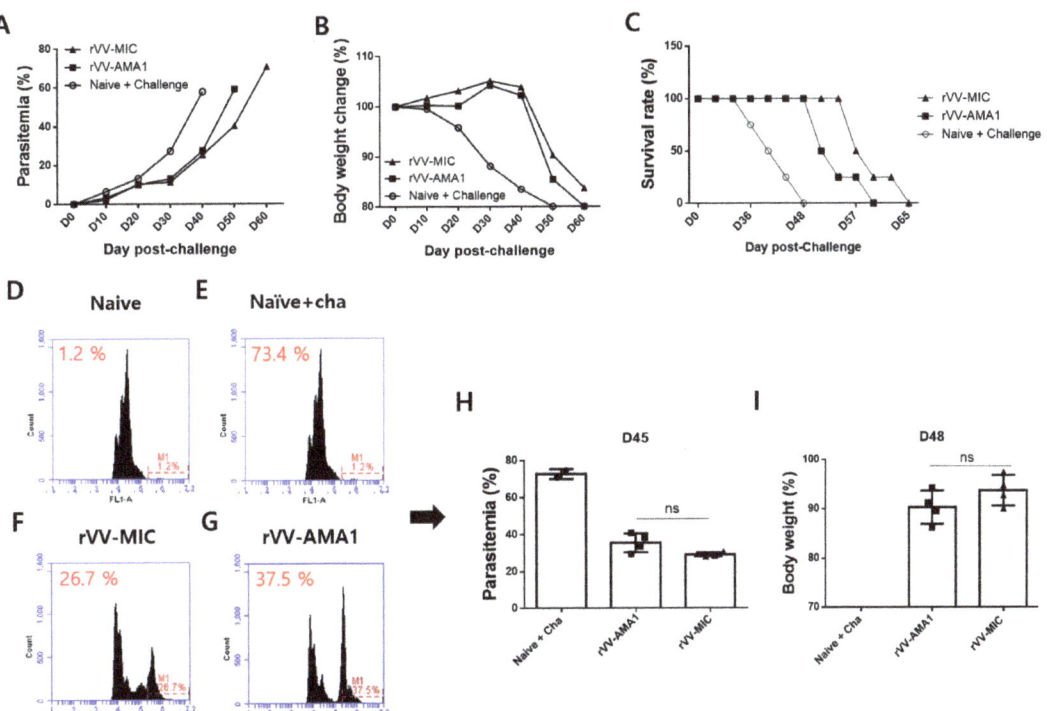

**Figure 6.** Parasitemia, body weight, and survival rate. After immunization with the rVV-AMA1 or rVV-MIC vaccines, mice ($n$ = 8) were infected intraperitoneally with 0.05% of *P. berghei* and monitored at regular intervals to assess changes in parasitemia, body weight, and survival. Parasitemia (**A**), body weight changes (**B**), and survival rate (**C**) from days 0 to 65 post-challenge infections have been monitored. The highest differences in parasitemia (**D–H**) and body weight (**I**) between immunized mice and non-immunized naïve control were observed at days 45 and 48 post-challenge infections, respectively. ns: no statistical significance.

## 4. Discussion

The complex life cycle of *Plasmodium* spp. continues to hinder the development of an efficacious malaria vaccine; a monumental task that remains unresolved. Currently, many of the blood-stage vaccines are designed based on the surface antigens of *Plasmodium* spp., such as the AMA1. A major drawback of the AMA1 antigen is its highly polymorphic nature, resulting in allele-specific immune protection [8,20]. Consequently, AMA1-based vaccines failed to demonstrate protective efficacies in controlled clinical trials [21]. To address these recurring issues with the antigens, we explored the potential of MIC antigen as a vaccine candidate. Our findings revealed that rVV-MIC immunization elicited stronger antibody responses after 2nd boost immunization. Although CD4$^+$ and CD8$^+$ T cell responses from the blood were comparable between rVV-AMA1 and rVV-MIC immunized mice, ILN CD8$^+$ T cell and GC B cell inductions were significantly greater for the rVV-MIC. This fact, paired with reduced splenic inflammatory cytokine production, contributed to enhanced survival and lessened parasitemia in the blood of rVV-MIC immunized mice.

The majority of the findings presented here are consistent with the literature, especially those of our previous studies. In our previous study, immunization of *P. berghei* MSP-8 and MSP-9 virus-like particles (VLPs) significantly lessened pro-inflammatory cytokine IFN-γ [22,23]. Consistent with these previous results, the rVV vaccines used in our study elicited a significant reduction of the inflammatory cytokine IFN-γ while changes to TNF-α were negligible. Germinal center B cells are an integral component of the humoral immune response, with their roles in memory B cell and long-lived plasma cell production [24]. In our study, antigen-specific GC B cells in inguinal lymph nodes were higher in the immunized group, contributing to increasingly high levels of parasite-specific IgG antibody response. These effects combined led to reduced parasitemia, marginal bodyweight change, and prolonged survival of immunized mice. Differences in TNF-α were also observed compared to results from others that assessed the efficacies of vaccines against *P. berghei* ANKA. Immunizing mice with the macrophage migration inhibitory factor ortholog produced in *Plasmodium* spp. reduced the production of TNF-α cytokines [25]. Similar to this finding, while the vaccinia virus-vectored vaccines used in the present study reduced the production of TNF-α, the changes were not statistically significant.

There were some striking differences in survival compared to our previous studies, but the underlying cause of this discrepancy can be attributed to the challenge infection dose and immunization schedule. In both of our previous studies, mice were challenge-infected with $1 \times 10^5$ or $1 \times 10^4$ *P. berghei* via IP routes following a prime-boost regimen [15,22]. Here, we used $5 \times 10^4$ *P. berghei* for challenge infection dose with three vaccine immunizations for mice, which may have led to longer survival duration for both control and immunized mice. GC B cell responses from the MVA-based vaccines were much weaker than the findings presented in our VLP vaccine study [15]. A possible explanation for this phenomenon could be the vaccine platform used in the study. One study reported that MVA-induced antigen-specific GC B cell and antibody responses were much weaker than adenovirus vectored vaccines or the protein subunit vaccines [26]. Another possibility is due to the parasitic nature of *Plasmodium* spp, particularly during the blood stage of its life cycle. It has been reported that the blood stage infection by *Plasmodium* spp. can interfere with the differentiation of CSP-specific GC B cells, consequently leading to aberrant humoral response [27]. Given that high levels of type I inflammatory cytokines such as IFN-γ can inhibit GC B cell response in *P. berghei* ANKA infection, this is another possibility [28].

RTS, S vaccine is the most advanced malaria vaccine to date, and its development served as a giant step forward for malaria vaccines. Unfortunately, the clinical endpoint results indicated that this vaccine failed to confer durable protection [2]. Several factors are thought to be associated with the low efficacy of the RTS,S vaccine, including the intensity of malaria transmission in the region and the reduced levels of circulating antibodies in vaccinees [29]. In our study, high levels of parasite-specific antibodies were detected. Yet, the durability of these antibody responses and the extent of their contribution to protection against rodent malaria requires further elucidation prior to evaluation using human malaria. Similar to the RTS, S vaccine, the protection conferred by the vaccine used in the present study was incomplete as all of the immunized mice eventually succumbed to death, thus signifying the need for additional improvements.

It is noteworthy to mention that genomic databases are not well-characterized for *P. berghei*. Evidently, the MIC protein used in our experiment was a putative protein with an unknown function. Nevertheless, immunization with the *P. berghei* MIC resulted in protection exceeding that of the rVV-AMA1 vaccine. For this reason, an actual immunoproteomic study elucidating the function of the protein used in this study must be performed for further development. Notably, the microneme organelle contains numerous proteins involved in various parasitic functions and surprisingly, many of these proteins were reported to be conserved between *P. falciparum* and *P. berghei* [30]. Surprisingly, some multiple microneme-derived proteins, such as the AMA1, were also highly conserved across the phylum Apicomplexa. These interesting findings suggest microneme antigen-based vaccines targeting other apicomplexan parasites could also be employed as an antimalarial vaccine. For instance, multiple microneme proteins are highly conserved and functionally interchangeable between *T. gondii* and *Plasmodium* spp., despite the large differences in their sequence identities [31,32]. Several microneme antigen-based experimental vaccines have been reported for *T. gondii*. DNA vaccines constructed using the *T. gondii* microneme antigen fragments conferred protection in mice, indicated by an 84% brain cyst burden reduction [33]. In our previous study, VLP vaccines expressing the *T. gondii* microneme protein eight protected mice against the virulent *T. gondii* RH strain [17]. Based on these reports, applying the *T. gondii* MIC-based vaccines to target malaria could prove to be useful and investigating the feasibility of this vaccination approach would be interesting.

## 5. Conclusions

The rVV vaccines expressing the *P. berghei* AMA1 or MIC antigens induced humoral and cellular immune responses, which aided in lessening pro-inflammatory cytokine production and parasitemia of immunized mice to prolong their survival. Further studies investigating methods to enhance their efficacies, such as incorporating heterologous immunization strategies, should be conducted to develop successful antimalarial blood-stage vaccines.

**Author Contributions:** Conceptualization, F.-S.Q.; methodology, M.-J.K. and F.-S.Q.; validation, M.-J.K.; formal analysis, M.-J.K.; investigation, M.-J.K., S.-H.L., H.-J.K., K.-W.Y. and M.A.A.; resources, M.A.A., data curation, M.-J.K.; writing—original draft preparation, M.-J.K., K.-B.C. and F.-S.Q.; writing—review and editing, K.-B.C., F.-S.Q.; visualization, M.-J.K. and K.-B.C.; supervision, F.-S.Q.; project administration, F.-S.Q.; funding acquisition, F.-S.Q. All authors have read and agreed to the published version of the manuscript.

**Funding:** This research was funded by the National Research Foundation of Korea (NRF) (2018R1A6A1A03025124); the Ministry of Health & Welfare, Korea (HV20C0085, HV20C0142).

**Institutional Review Board Statement:** This study was conducted according to the guidelines set by Kyung Hee University Institutional Animal Care and Use Committee (IACUC), and all experimental protocols involving animals have been approved (Permit number: KHUIBC (SE) 19-034).

**Informed Consent Statement:** Not applicable.

**Data Availability Statement:** The original contributions presented in this study are included in the article. Further inquiries can be directed to the corresponding author.

**Conflicts of Interest:** The authors declare no conflict of interest.

## Appendix A

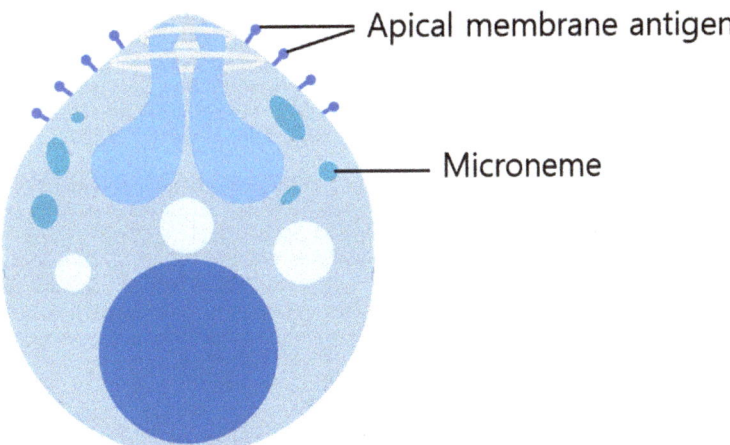

**Figure A1.** The diagram of the *Plasmodium* organism. The diagram describes the Plasmodium organism and the specified target gene (AMA1, MIC).

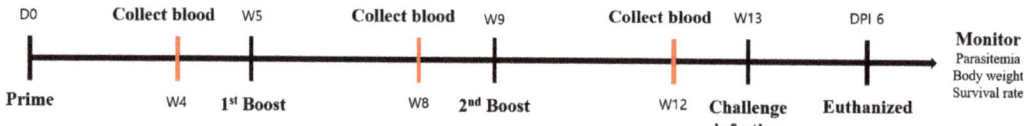

**Figure A2.** A schematic diagram depicting animal experimental schedule. Immunization intervals, blood collection, challenge infection, and euthanasia time points are indicated.

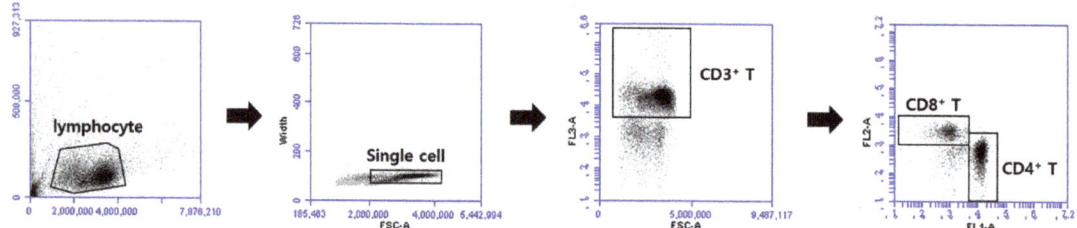

**Figure A3.** The gating strategy for CD4$^+$ and CD8$^+$ T cells. Lymphocytes were gated as indicated to analyze the frequencies of CD4$^+$ and CD8$^+$ T cells by flow cytometry.

## References

1. WHO. *World Malaria Report 2021*; World Health Organization: Geneva, Switzerland, 2021.
2. Olotu, A.; Fegan, G.; Wambua, J.; Nyangweso, G.; Leach, A.; Lievens, M.; Kaslow, D.C.; Njuguna, P.; Marsh, K.; Bejon, P. Seven-Year Efficacy of RTS,S/AS01 Malaria Vaccine among Young African Children. *N. Engl. J. Med.* **2016**, *374*, 2519–2529. [CrossRef] [PubMed]
3. Price, P.J.; Torres-Domínguez, L.E.; Brandmüller, C.; Sutter, G.; Lehmann, M.H. Modified Vaccinia virus Ankara: Innate immune activation and induction of cellular signalling. *Vaccine* **2013**, *31*, 4231–4234. [CrossRef] [PubMed]
4. Gilbert, S.C. Clinical development of Modified Vaccinia virus Ankara vaccines. *Vaccine* **2013**, *31*, 4241–4246. [CrossRef]
5. de Barra, E.; Hodgson, S.H.; Ewer, K.J.; Bliss, C.M.; Hennigan, K.; Collins, A.; Berrie, E.; Lawrie, A.M.; Gilbert, S.C.; Nicosia, A.; et al. A phase Ia study to assess the safety and immunogenicity of new malaria vaccine candidates ChAd63 CS administered alone and with MVA CS. *PLoS ONE* **2014**, *9*, e115161. [CrossRef]
6. Sheehy, S.H.; Duncan, C.J.; Elias, S.C.; Biswas, S.; Collins, K.A.; O'Hara, G.A.; Halstead, F.D.; Ewer, K.J.; Mahungu, T.; Spencer, A.J.; et al. Phase Ia clinical evaluation of the safety and immunogenicity of the Plasmodium falciparum blood-stage antigen AMA1 in ChAd63 and MVA vaccine vectors. *PLoS ONE* **2012**, *7*, e31208. [CrossRef]
7. Biswas, S.; Choudhary, P.; Elias, S.C.; Miura, K.; Milne, K.H.; de Cassan, S.C.; Collins, K.A.; Halstead, F.D.; Bliss, C.M.; Ewer, K.J.; et al. Assessment of humoral immune responses to blood-stage malaria antigens following ChAd63-MVA immunization, controlled human malaria infection and natural exposure. *PLoS ONE* **2014**, *9*, e107903. [CrossRef] [PubMed]
8. Takala, S.L.; Coulibaly, D.; Thera, M.A.; Batchelor, A.H.; Cummings, M.P.; Escalante, A.A.; Ouattara, A.; Traoré, K.; Niangaly, A.; Djimdé, A.A.; et al. Extreme polymorphism in a vaccine antigen and risk of clinical malaria: Implications for vaccine development. *Sci. Transl. Med.* **2009**, *1*, 2ra5. [CrossRef] [PubMed]
9. Yan, M.; Cui, X.; Zhao, Q.; Zhu, S.; Huang, B.; Wang, L.; Zhao, H.; Liu, G.; Li, Z.; Han, H.; et al. Molecular characterization and protective efficacy of the microneme 2 protein from Eimeria tenella. *Parasite* **2018**, *25*, 60. [CrossRef]
10. Hernández-Silva, D.J.; Valdez-Espinoza, U.M.; Mercado-Uriostegui, M.A.; Aguilar-Tipacamú, G.; Ramos-Aragón, J.A.; Hernández-Ortiz, R.; Ueti, M.; Mosqueda, J. Immunomolecular Characterization of MIC-1, a Novel Antigen in Babesia bigemina, Which Contains Conserved and Immunodominant B-Cell Epitopes that Induce Neutralizing Antibodies. *Vet. Sci.* **2018**, *5*, 32. [CrossRef]
11. Monney, T.; Rütti, D.; Schorer, M.; Debache, K.; Grandgirard, D.; Leib, S.L.; Hemphill, A. RecNcMIC3-1-R is a microneme- and rhoptry-based chimeric antigen that protects against acute neosporosis and limits cerebral parasite load in the mouse model for Neospora caninum infection. *Vaccine* **2011**, *29*, 6967–6975. [CrossRef]
12. Arumugam, T.U.; Takeo, S.; Yamasaki, T.; Thonkukiatkul, A.; Miura, K.; Otsuki, H.; Zhou, H.; Long, C.A.; Sattabongkot, J.; Thompson, J.; et al. Discovery of GAMA, a Plasmodium falciparum merozoite micronemal protein, as a novel blood-stage vaccine candidate antigen. *Infect. Immun.* **2011**, *79*, 4523–4532. [CrossRef] [PubMed]
13. Changrob, S.; Han, J.H.; Ha, K.S.; Park, W.S.; Hong, S.H.; Chootong, P.; Han, E.T. Immunogenicity of glycosylphosphatidylinositol-anchored micronemal antigen in natural Plasmodium vivax exposure. *Malar. J.* **2017**, *16*, 348. [CrossRef] [PubMed]
14. De Niz, M.; Heussler, V.T. Rodent malaria models: Insights into human disease and parasite biology. *Curr. Opin. Microbiol.* **2018**, *46*, 93–101. [CrossRef] [PubMed]
15. Lee, D.H.; Chu, K.B.; Kang, H.J.; Lee, S.H.; Chopra, M.; Choi, H.J.; Moon, E.K.; Inn, K.S.; Quan, F.S. Protection induced by malaria virus-like particles containing codon-optimized AMA-1 of Plasmodium berghei. *Malar. J.* **2019**, *18*, 394. [CrossRef]

16. Cao, Y.; Zhang, D.; Pan, W. Construction of transgenic Plasmodium berghei as a model for evaluation of blood-stage vaccine candidate of Plasmodium falciparum chimeric protein 2.9. *PLoS ONE* **2009**, *4*, e6894. [CrossRef] [PubMed]
17. Lee, S.H.; Kim, A.R.; Lee, D.H.; Rubino, I.; Choi, H.J.; Quan, F.S. Protection induced by virus-like particles containing Toxoplasma gondii microneme protein 8 against highly virulent RH strain of Toxoplasma gondii infection. *PLoS ONE* **2017**, *12*, e0175644. [CrossRef] [PubMed]
18. Lim, J.F.; Berger, H.; Su, I.H. Isolation and Activation of Murine Lymphocytes. *J. Vis. Exp. JoVE* **2016**, *116*, e54596. [CrossRef]
19. Somsak, V.; Srichairatanakool, S.; Yuthavong, Y.; Kamchonwongpaisan, S.; Uthaipibull, C. Flow cytometric enumeration of Plasmodium berghei-infected red blood cells stained with SYBR Green I. *Acta Trop.* **2012**, *122*, 113–118. [CrossRef]
20. Duan, J.; Mu, J.; Thera, M.A.; Joy, D.; Kosakovsky Pond, S.L.; Diemert, D.; Long, C.; Zhou, H.; Miura, K.; Ouattara, A.; et al. Population structure of the genes encoding the polymorphic Plasmodium falciparum apical membrane antigen 1: Implications for vaccine design. *Proc. Natl. Acad. Sci. USA* **2008**, *105*, 7857–7862. [CrossRef]
21. Payne, R.O.; Milne, K.H.; Elias, S.C.; Edwards, N.J.; Douglas, A.D.; Brown, R.E.; Silk, S.E.; Biswas, S.; Miura, K.; Roberts, R.; et al. Demonstration of the Blood-Stage Plasmodium falciparum Controlled Human Malaria Infection Model to Assess Efficacy of the P. falciparum Apical Membrane Antigen 1 Vaccine, FMP2.1/AS01. *J. Infect. Dis.* **2016**, *213*, 1743–1751. [CrossRef]
22. Lee, S.H.; Kang, H.J.; Chu, K.B.; Basak, S.; Lee, D.H.; Moon, E.K.; Quan, F.S. Protective Immunity Induced by Virus-Like Particle Containing Merozoite Surface Protein 9 of Plasmodium berghei. *Vaccines* **2020**, *8*, 428. [CrossRef] [PubMed]
23. Lee, S.H.; Chu, K.B.; Kang, H.J.; Basak, S.; Kim, M.J.; Park, H.; Jin, H.; Moon, E.K.; Quan, F.S. Virus-like particles expressing Plasmodium berghei MSP-8 induce protection against P. berghei infection. *Parasite Immunol.* **2020**, *42*, e12781. [CrossRef] [PubMed]
24. Shlomchik, M.J.; Weisel, F. Germinal center selection and the development of memory B and plasma cells. *Immunol. Rev.* **2012**, *247*, 52–63. [CrossRef]
25. Baeza Garcia, A.; Siu, E.; Sun, T.; Exler, V.; Brito, L.; Hekele, A.; Otten, G.; Augustijn, K.; Janse, C.J.; Ulmer, J.B.; et al. Neutralization of the Plasmodium-encoded MIF ortholog confers protective immunity against malaria infection. *Nat. Commun.* **2018**, *9*, 2714. [CrossRef] [PubMed]
26. Wang, C.; Hart, M.; Chui, C.; Ajuogu, A.; Brian, I.J.; de Cassan, S.C.; Borrow, P.; Draper, S.J.; Douglas, A.D. Germinal Center B Cell and T Follicular Helper Cell Responses to Viral Vector and Protein-in-Adjuvant Vaccines. *J. Immunol.* **2016**, *197*, 1242–1251. [CrossRef] [PubMed]
27. Keitany, G.J.; Kim, K.S.; Krishnamurty, A.T.; Hondowicz, B.D.; Hahn, W.O.; Dambrauskas, N.; Sather, D.N.; Vaughan, A.M.; Kappe, S.H.I.; Pepper, M. Blood Stage Malaria Disrupts Humoral Immunity to the Pre-erythrocytic Stage Circumsporozoite Protein. *Cell. Rep.* **2016**, *17*, 3193–3205. [CrossRef]
28. Ryg-Cornejo, V.; Ioannidis, L.J.; Ly, A.; Chiu, C.Y.; Tellier, J.; Hill, D.L.; Preston, S.P.; Pellegrini, M.; Yu, D.; Nutt, S.L.; et al. Severe Malaria Infections Impair Germinal Center Responses by Inhibiting T Follicular Helper Cell Differentiation. *Cell. Rep.* **2016**, *14*, 68–81. [CrossRef]
29. White, M.T.; Verity, R.; Griffin, J.T.; Asante, K.P.; Owusu-Agyei, S.; Greenwood, B.; Drakeley, C.; Gesase, S.; Lusingu, J.; Ansong, D.; et al. Immunogenicity of the RTS,S/AS01 malaria vaccine and implications for duration of vaccine efficacy: Secondary analysis of data from a phase 3 randomised controlled trial. *Lancet Infect. Dis.* **2015**, *15*, 1450–1458. [CrossRef]
30. Dubois, D.J.; Soldati-Favre, D. Biogenesis and secretion of micronemes in Toxoplasma gondii. *Cell. Microbiol.* **2019**, *21*, e13018. [CrossRef]
31. Carruthers, V.B.; Tomley, F.M. Microneme Proteins in Apicomplexans. In *Molecular Mechanisms of Parasite Invasion: Subcellular Biochemistry*; Burleigh, B.A., Soldati-Favre, D., Eds.; Springer: New York, NY, USA, 2008; pp. 33–45.
32. Kappe, S.; Bruderer, T.; Gantt, S.; Fujioka, H.; Nussenzweig, V.; Ménard, R. Conservation of a gliding motility and cell invasion machinery in Apicomplexan parasites. *J. Cell. Biol.* **1999**, *147*, 937–944. [CrossRef]
33. Beghetto, E.; Nielsen, H.V.; Del Porto, P.; Buffolano, W.; Guglietta, S.; Felici, F.; Petersen, E.; Gargano, N. A combination of antigenic regions of Toxoplasma gondii microneme proteins induces protective immunity against oral infection with parasite cysts. *J. Infect. Dis.* **2005**, *191*, 637–645. [CrossRef] [PubMed]

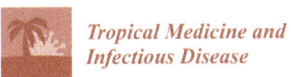

*Tropical Medicine and Infectious Disease*

Article

# Surveillance of Tahyna Orthobunyavirus in Urban Areas in Croatia—The "One Health" Approach

Vladimir Stevanovic [1,*,†], Tatjana Vilibic-Cavlek [2,3,*,†], Vladimir Savic [4], Ana Klobucar [5], Snjezana Kovac [1], Marcela Curman Posavec [5], Suncica Petrinic [5], Maja Bogdanic [2], Marija Santini [6], Vanja Tesic [5,7], Nathalia de Albuquerque Soares [1] and Ljubo Barbic [1]

1. Department of Microbiology and Infectious Diseases with Clinic, Faculty of Veterinary Medicine, University of Zagreb, 10000 Zagreb, Croatia
2. Department of Virology, Croatian Institute of Public Health, 10000 Zagreb, Croatia
3. Department of Microbiology, School of Medicine, University of Zagreb, 10000 Zagreb, Croatia
4. Poultry Center, Croatian Veterinary Institute, 10000 Zagreb, Croatia
5. Department of Epidemiology, Andrija Stampar Teaching Institute of Public Health, 10000 Zagreb, Croatia
6. Department for Adult Intensive Care and Neuroinfections, University Hospital for Infectious Diseases "Dr. Fran Mihaljevic", 10000 Zagreb, Croatia
7. Department of Social Medicine and Epidemiology, Medical Faculty, University of Rijeka, 51000 Rijeka, Croatia
* Correspondence: vladimir.stevanovic@vef.unizg.hr (V.S.); tatjana.vilibic-cavlek@hzjz.hr (T.V.-C.)
† These authors contributed equally to this work.

**Abstract:** Background: Tahyna orthobunyavirus (TAHV) is a neglected mosquito-borne bunyavirus. Although the virus is widespread in continental Europe, TAHV infections are rarely reported. We analyzed the prevalence of TAHV in humans and different animal species as well as mosquitoes collected in urban areas of Zagreb and its surroundings in the period from 2020 to 2022. Methods: The study included 32 patients with neuroinvasive disease (NID), 218 asymptomatic individuals, 98 horses, 94 pet animals (dogs and cats), and 4456 *Aedes vexans* mosquitoes. Cerebrospinal fluid (CSF) and urine samples of patients with NID were tested for the TAHV RNA using a real-time reverse transcription-polymerase chain reaction (RT-qPCR). Human and animal serum samples were tested for TAHV-neutralizing (NT) antibodies using a virus-neutralization test (VNT). Mosquito pools were tested for TAHV RNA using an RT-qPCR. Results: TAHV NT antibodies were detected in 3/9.4% of patients with NID, 8/3.7% of asymptomatic individuals, 29/29.6% of horses, and 11/11.7% of pet animals. There was no difference in the seroprevalence according to age, sex, and area of residence in asymptomatic individuals. In addition, TAHV seropositivity did not differ according to age and sex in pet animals. None of the tested mosquito pools was TAHV RNA-positive. Conclusions: The presented results highlight the importance of interdisciplinary surveillance ("One Health") of this neglected viral zoonosis.

**Keywords:** Tahyna orthobunyavirus; humans; horses; pet animals; mosquitoes; Croatia; One Health

## 1. Introduction

Tahyna orthobunyavirus (TAHV) is an arthropod-borne virus of the family *Peribunyaviridae*, genus *Orthobunyavirus*, California encephalitis serogroup [1]. Hares, rabbits, hedgehogs, and rodents are vertebrate hosts for TAHV in a natural cycle, while floodwater mosquitoes *Aedes vexans* are the primary arthropod vectors. Humans represent only incidental or dead-end hosts for TAHV [2].

In humans, TAHV infections are typically asymptomatic. Symptomatic disease is usually presented as an influenza-like illness occurring in late summer and early autumn, mainly in children [3]. Fever, gastrointestinal disorders, atypical pneumonia, or myocarditis are the most common symptoms of TAHV infection [4]. Despite its association with neurovirulence (meningitis), TAHV infection is still an underdiagnosed disease, with only a few human clinical cases reported in recent decades [5].

TAHV is widespread throughout continental Europe, as evidenced by the virus detection and isolation from mosquitoes as well as the detection of antibodies in humans and animals [6–8]. High seroprevalence rates of up to 60–80% have been consistently observed among adult human populations of endemic foci, such as in the Czech Republic [9].

In addition, although transmission is focal and not uniform, seroprevalence studies conducted in wild ungulates in Austria, Hungary, and Romania have revealed that TAHV transmission to animals is widespread in Europe, particularly among wild boars, with a mean seroconversion rate of 15% [8]. In some high-endemic countries, such as the Czech Republic, TAHV antibodies were detected in various animal species with different seroprevalence rates: horses 34.4%, pigs 55%, cattle 5.6%, songbirds 14.0%, cormorants 22.6%, ducks 13.2%, mouflons 33.8%, deer 36.4–40.0%, wild boar 70.0%, and European hares 42.5% [9–14].

The presence of TAHV in mosquitoes (virus isolation or RNA detection) was confirmed in many countries including the Czech Republic [15], Slovakia [16], Italy [17], Austria [5,18], Russia [19], and China [20]. After the first isolation in Slovakia in 1958, TAHV was detected in several mosquito species, including *Ae. caspius, Ae. cinereus, Ae. dorsalis, Ae. cantans, Anopheles hyrcanus, Ae. punctor, Ae. communis, Ae. flavescens, Ae. excrucians, Oc. detritus* and *Culex pipiens, Cx. modestus,* and *Culiseta annulata* [5,7,20–22].

In Croatia, serologic evidence of TAHV dates back to the 1970s. Very rare seroprevalence studies showed TAHV antibodies in 7.9% of inhabitants of northeast Croatia and 0.2–1.47% of inhabitants of the Croatian littoral [23,24]. Only one study (1984–1988) detected TAHV hemagglutination-inhibiting antibodies in the serum samples of free-ranging European brown bears (*Ursus arctos*) collected within the Plitvice Lakes and Risnjak National Parks [25]. A more recently conducted Croatian study detected TAHV neutralizing (NT) antibodies in 10.1% of patients with unsolved neuroinvasive disease (NID) tested from 2017 to 2021, who developed symptoms during the arbovirus transmission season. In two patients presenting with meningitis, NT antibodies were also confirmed in the cerebrospinal fluid (CSF), suggesting a recent TAHV infection. The majority of seropositive patients (90.9%) were residents of floodplains along the rivers in continental Croatia; however, sporadic infections were also confirmed in the coastal region [26].

The aim of this study was to analyze the prevalence of TAHV in humans and different animal species as well as the virus detection in mosquitoes collected from urban areas of Zagreb and its surroundings.

## 2. Materials and Methods

### 2.1. Study Area

The study was conducted during a three-year period (May 2020–July 2022) and included patients with NID, asymptomatic individuals (seroprevalence investigation), pet animals (dogs, cats), horses, and mosquitoes. The sampling area included Zagreb, the capital of Croatia, and its surroundings. Zagreb is located in the northwest of the country on the banks of the river Sava (GPS coordinates 45°48′55.43″ N, 15°57′59.64″ E) at an elevation of approximately 112 m above sea level. The city is subdivided into 17 districts, of which the majority are located in the River Sava valley, at a low level. The city's core region is densely built, while the northern part is situated on the Medvednica mountain's slopes, with forest vegetation and smaller urban settlements. Agricultural lands dominate the eastern, southern, and western parts of the city area. The surface waterways abound in the city's vicinity. Seven artificial lakes and several artificial watercourses are located in the city area.

Thirty-two mosquito species have been detected in the city of Zagreb. The species *Cx. pipiens* form molestus predominates in indoor breeding sites. Natural mosquito breeding sites in forested and flooded areas are active only in the spring (March–June), and the most common species are *Ae. sticticus, Ae. cantans, Ae. vexans,* and *Ae. geniculatus. Culex pipiens* is the most frequent mosquito species found in streams, while *Ae. albopictus* and *Cx. pipiens* are the most common mosquito species in artificial breeding sites [27,28].

The sampling area (human and animal sampling) in northwestern Croatia is presented in Figure 1.

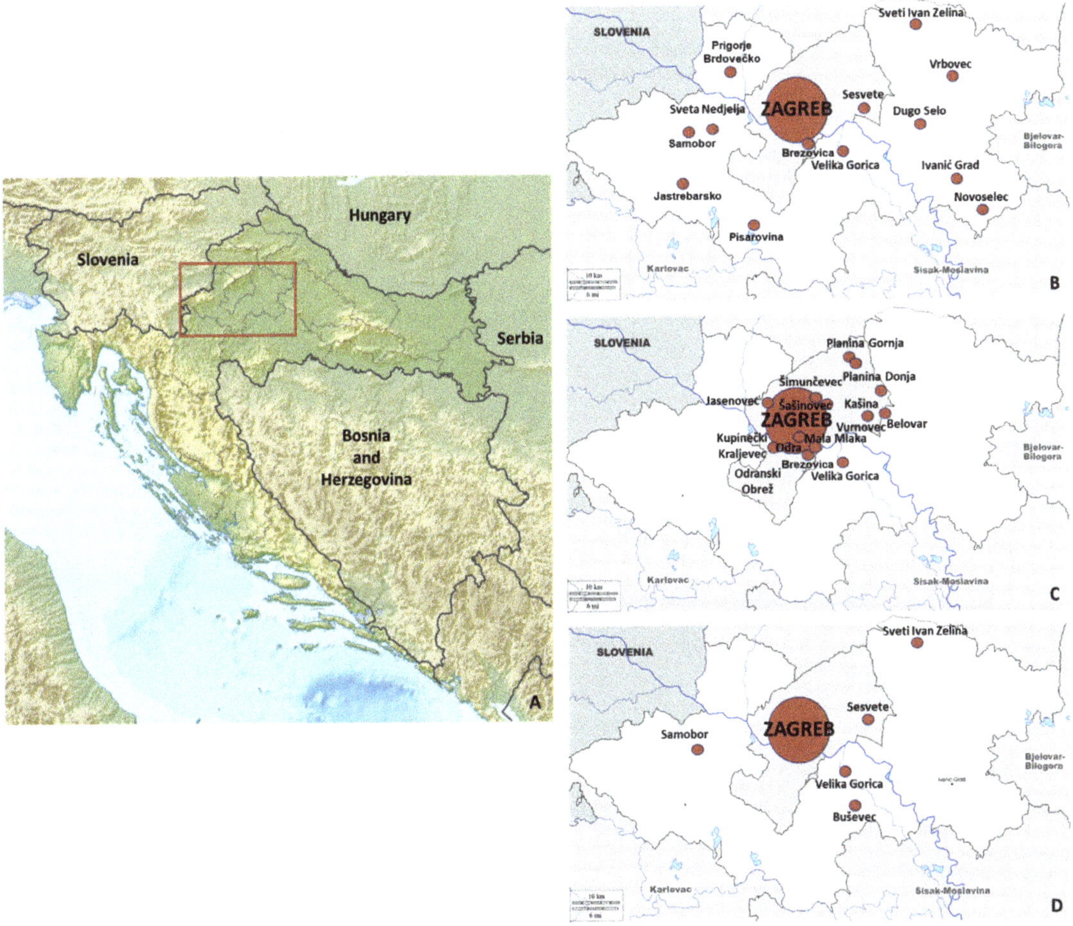

**Figure 1.** Sampling area in continental Croatia (**A**): human (**B**), horse (**C**), and pet animals (**D**) sampling areas.

*2.2. Human Sampling and Testing*

A total of 32 hospitalized patients presented with NID (febrile headache, meningitis, meningoencephalitis) were tested. Serum, CSF, and urine samples were collected from all patients. In addition, to determine the seroprevalence, a total of 218 serum samples from asymptomatic individuals were tested for the presence of TAHV NT antibodies. Samples were collected from patients during a routine check-up (part of physical examination, prior to surgery, prenatal testing, couples undergoing medically assisted reproduction). No participant reported a recent febrile disease.

CSF and urine samples of patients with NID were tested for the presence of TAHV RNA using a real-time reverse transcription polymerase chain reaction (RT-qPCR). The following primers and probes were used: forward primer: 5′-CCATTCCGTTAGGATCTTCTTCCT-3′, reverse primer 5′-CCTTCCTCTCCGGCTTACG-3′ and probe: FAM-5′-AATGCCGCAAAAG-CCAAAGCTGC-3′-TAMRA [29].

TAHV antibodies were detected using a virus-neutralization test (VNT). UVE/TAHV/1958/CS/92 virus strain grown in Vero E6 cells was used as an antigen for the VNT. Virus titer (median tissue culture infectious dose; $TCID_{50}$) was calculated using the Reed and Muench formula. Serum samples were heat-inactivated (30 min/56 °C) and diluted two-fold starting at 1:5. An equal amount of inactivated serum dilutions and 100 $TCID_{50}$ of TAHV (25 µL) were mixed and incubated for one hour at 37 °C with $CO_2$. Finally, 50 µL of $2 \times 10^5$ Vero E6 cells/mL were added to each well. The plates were incubated at 37 °C with $CO_2$ and inspected for the cytopathic effect after incubation for three days. NT antibody titer was defined as the reciprocal value of the highest serum dilution that showed at least 50% neutralization. Serum samples with neutralizing activity at dilutions $\geq$ 1:10 were considered seropositive [26].

### 2.3. Animal Sampling and Testing

Horses and pet animals (cats and dogs) were the animal species included in the study. Animal samples included 98 horse serum samples, 70 dog serum samples, and 24 cat serum samples from Zagreb and its surroundings. Sex and age were available for pet animals, while for horses, data were missing. TAHV VNT was performed as described above.

### 2.4. Mosquito Sampling and Testing

Mosquitoes were collected by two methods: CDC Mini Light traps (BioQuip, Products, Rancho Dominguez, CA, USA), and aspirator collection (human landing collection). CDC Mini Light traps were equipped with dry ice ($CO_2$) as an attractant and used to collect adult mosquitoes. Traps were placed in the late afternoon before sunset, left overnight, and removed after sunrise (07:00–10:00). Over three years (2020–2022), the traps were set at the same eight collection sites (Figure 2, yellow marks) every 14 days, from May to October in 2020 and 2021 and from May to July in 2022. A total of 248 sampling occasions were gathered (2020: $n$ = 96; 2021: $n$ = 88; 2022: $n$ = 64). Additionally, the sampling occasions using the CDC Mini Light trap were conducted once at three collection sites (Figure 2, green marks). During the same period, mosquito individuals were collected by aspirator as well as using the human landing collection method (Figure 2, blue dots). A total of 30 sampling occasions with *Ae. vexans* mosquitoes were gathered (2020: $n$ = 18; 2021: $n$ = 11; 2022: $n$ = 1). Various habitats were selected for mosquito sampling: woods and gardens in the urban part of the city and populated areas close to the green belt.

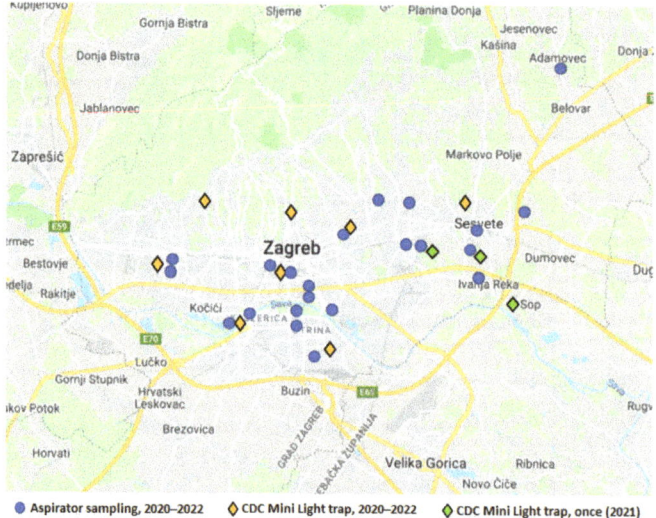

**Figure 2.** Distribution of mosquito sampling locations.

The mosquitoes sampled by CDC Mini Light traps were transported to the laboratory in containers with dry ice, transferred to plastic tubes, and stored on dry ice until identification. Mosquitoes collected by the aspirator were transported alive to the laboratory in the aspirator, placed briefly in a freezer at −18 °C, and identified. Female mosquitoes were morphologically identified by species on a chilling surface under a stereomicroscope, using the determination keys by Becker et al. (2010) [30] and Schaffner et al. (2001) [31]. Specimens belonging to the same species collected on the same day and at the same sampling site were pooled, with up to 60 individuals per pool, and stored at −80 °C until virological testing. Only *Ae. vexans* individuals were tested.

Mosquito pools were tested for the presence of TAHV RNA as described above.

*2.5. Statistical Analysis*

The differences in seropositivity rates according to sex, age, and area of residence were compared using a chi-square or Fisher's exact test. The strength of the association between dependent (VNT positivity) and independent variables was assessed by logistic regression. $p < 0.05$ was considered statistically significant. Statistical analysis was performed using Stata version 16 software.

## 3. Results

TAHV seroprevalence results are presented in Table 1. In humans, TAHV NT antibodies were detected in 3/32 (9.4%) patients with the neuroinvasive disease and 8/218 (3.7%) asymptomatic individuals. In addition, 29/98 (29.6%) of horses and 11/94 (11.7%) of pet animals were found to be TAHV-seropositive.

**Table 1.** Tahyna virus seroprevalence in Zagreb and the surrounding area.

|  | Study Population | N Tested | N (%) VNT-Positive | 95% CI |
|---|---|---|---|---|
| Humans | Patients with neuroinvasive disease | 32 | 3 (9.4) | 1.9–25.0 |
|  | Asymptomatic individuals | 218 | 8 (3.7) | 1.6–7.1 |
| Animals | Horses | 98 | 29 (29.6) | 20.8–39.6 |
|  | Pet animals | 94 | 11 (11.7) | 5.9–19.9 |

VNT, virus-neutralization test; CI, confidence interval.

In asymptomatic persons, the seroprevalence rate was highest in 70+ year-olds (7.7%) compared to 2.5–3.8% in other age groups; however, this difference was not significant. No significant difference in seropositivity was found between males and females (3.7% vs. 3.6%) as well as among residents of urban and suburban areas (4.2% vs. 0%) (Table 2).

**Table 2.** Tahyna virus seroprevalence in asymptomatic individuals according to demographic characteristics.

| Characteristic |  | N (%) Tested | N (%) Positive | 95% CI | p |
|---|---|---|---|---|---|
| Sex | Male | 108 (49.5) | 4 (3.7) | 1.0–9.2 | 0.978 |
|  | Female | 110 (50.5) | 4 (3.6) | 1.0–9.1 |  |
| Age | <30 years | 33 (15.1) | 1 (3.0) | 0.1–15.7 | 0.677 |
|  | 30–49 years | 79 (36.3) | 2 (2.5) | 0.3–8.8 |  |
|  | 50–69 years | 80 (36.7) | 3 (3.8) | 0.8–10.6 |  |
|  | 70+ years | 26 (11.9) | 2 (7.7) | 0.9–25.1 |  |
| Area of residence | Urban | 192 (88.1) | 8 (4.2) | 1.8–8.0 | 0.288 |
|  | Suburban | 26 (11.9) | 0 (0) | 0–13.2 * |  |

* One-sided 97.5% confidence interval; CI, confidence interval.

Results of the risk analysis in asymptomatic humans showed no association of TAHV seroprevalence with age, sex, and area of residence (Table 3).

**Table 3.** Risk analysis for Tahyna virus seropositivity.

| Characteristic | OR | 95% CI OR | p | RR | 95% CI RR | p |
|---|---|---|---|---|---|---|
| Male (Ref.) vs. female sex | 1.019 | 0.248–4.013 | 0.978 | 1.018 | 0.261–3.969 | 0.978 |
| Age | | | | | | |
| <30 years | Ref. | | | Ref. | | |
| 30–49 years | 0.831 | 0.072–9.494 | 0.881 | 0.835 | 0.078–8.900 | 0.881 |
| 50–69 years | 1.246 | 0.124–12.441 | 0.851 | 1.237 | 0.133–11.469 | 0.851 |
| 70+ years | 2.666 | 0.228–45.547 | 0.782 | 2.538 | 0.243–26.480 | 0.436 |
| Suburban (Ref.) vs. urban area of residence | 2.441 | 0.136–4.183 | 0.543 | 2.378 | 0.141–40.045 | 0.547 |

OR, odds ratio; CI, confidence interval; RR, relative risk.

In pet animals, there was no difference in the prevalence of TAHV NT antibodies according to age and sex (Table 4).

**Table 4.** Seroprevalence of Tahyna virus in pet animals according to sex and age.

| Characteristic | Dogs | | | | Cats | | | |
|---|---|---|---|---|---|---|---|---|
| | N (%) Tested | N (%) Positive | 95% CI | p | N (%) Tested | N (%) Positive | 95% CI | p |
| Sex | | | | | | | | |
| Male | 37 (52.8) | 5 (13.5) | 4.5–28.7 | 0.713 | 15 (62.5) | 1 (6.7) | 0.2–31.9 | 0.533 |
| Female | 33 (47.2) | 3 (9.1) | 1.9–24.3 | | 9 (37.5) | 2 (22.2) | 2.8–60.0 | |
| Age | | | | 0.675 | | | | 0.115 |
| <5 years | 19 (27.5) | 3 (15.8) | 3.4–39.6 | | 9 (40.9) | 2 (22.2) | 2.8–60.0 | |
| >5 years | 50 (72.5) | 5 (10.0) | 3.3–21.8 | | 13 (59.1) | 1 (7.7) | 0.2–36.0 | |

The geographic distribution of seropositive humans and animals is presented in Figure 3. All seropositive humans were residents of urban areas. Among seropositive horses, 9 were from Zagreb city, and 20 were from suburban areas of Zagreb surroundings. In a group of pet animals, only one dog was from a suburban area.

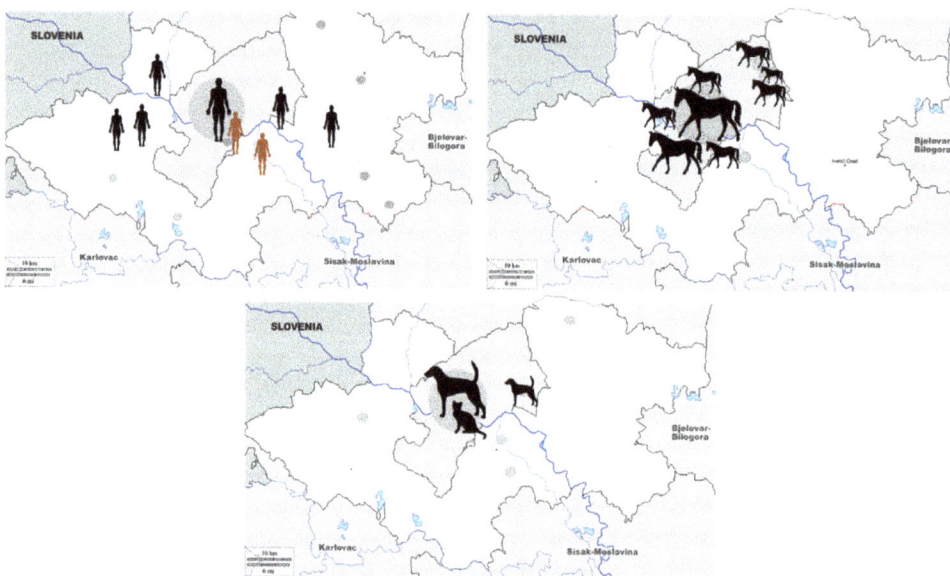

**Figure 3.** Geographic distribution of Tahyna virus seropositive humans, horses, and pet animals. (symbol size represents the number of cases).

Comparing the TAHV NT antibody titers, a substantially higher titer was observed in horses (median 80, IQR = 40–160) compared to humans (median 10, IQR = 10–40) and pet animals (median 10, IQR = 10–10) (Figure 4).

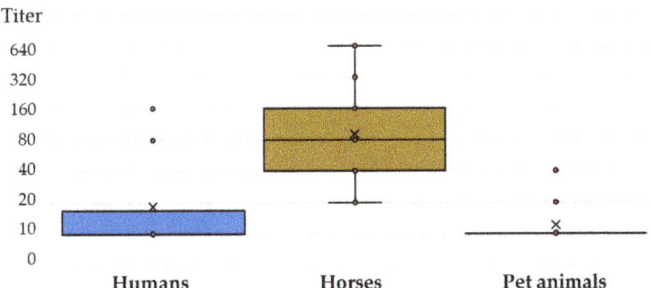

**Figure 4.** Tahyna virus-neutralizing antibody titers in humans and animals.

A total of 4456 *Ae. vexans* mosquitoes were collected and identified in the Zagreb area, of which 4053/90.9% mosquitoes were sampled by traps with $CO_2$, while 403/9.1% were sampled by the aspirator. Mosquito specimens were sorted in 159 pools and tested for the presence of TAHV (Table 5). All tested pools were negative for TAHV.

**Table 5.** Number of collected *Aedes vexans* mosquitoes/pools tested for Tahyna virus.

| Sampling Method | N Collected Specimens/N Pools Tested for the Presence of TAHV | | | |
|---|---|---|---|---|
| Year | 2020 | 2021 | 2022 | Total |
| CDC Mini Light trap | 1414/44 | 2215/66 | 424/18 | 4053/128 |
| Aspirator | 266/18 | 119/12 | 18/1 | 403/31 |
| Total | 1680/62 | 2334/78 | 442/19 | 4456/159 |

## 4. Discussion

Although TAHV is widely distributed in Europe, the number of clinical cases as well as the seroprevalence rates are probably underreported due to the lack of commercially available testing.

The frequency of TAHV NT antibody detection among patients with neuroinvasive disease from Zagreb and its surroundings was similar (9.4%) to a previous Croatian study (10.1%) conducted in patients from both continental and coastal regions. Only one published study, which was from the Sverdlovsk region (Russia) in 1994, analyzed the prevalence of TAHV in patients with encephalitis and found that up to 60% of patients had TAHV antibodies [32]. Therefore, the true prevalence and clinical significance of this neglected virus remain to be determined.

The TAHV seroprevalence rate in asymptomatic Croatian individuals was 3.7%, which was lower than the reported seroprevalence of 7.9% in the eastern region in the 1970s [23]. This difference should be explained at least in part by the studied population. This study included only inhabitants of a restricted urban area in northwest Croatia, while in the 1970s, individuals from a broad geographic area (northeastern continental and middle and south coastal area) were tested. However, the reported seroprevalence in this study was similar to the seroprevalence reported in some urban areas in Europe and Asia. In 2002, residents of an area in the Czech Republic affected by the flood were tested for the presence of antibodies to TAHV. While the highest seroprevalence rates of up to 28% were detected in rural and suburban populations of the forested floodplain along the Labe and Vltava Rivers, low seropositivity of 5% was found in the urban Prague area [33]. Two more recent studies showed lower TAHV seropositivity rates. A seroprevalence of 2% was recorded in Nasiriyah, the capital of the Dhi Qar Governorate in Southern Iraq, in 2012–2013 [34] In addition, TAHV NT antibodies were detected in 0.3% of blood donors from the Alpine Central European region of the Tyrol (North and East Tyrol, Austria, and South Tyrol, northern Italy) [18].

Outside Europe, very high TAHV NT seroprevalence rates ranging from 25% to 52% were recorded in the rural adult population of Cameroon in 2002–2003 [35]. In addition, epidemiological investigations showed high TAHV endemicity in both urban and rural areas in the Lao PDR. Several studies carried out in the communities of the Nakai plateau revealed a TAHV seropositivity of 30.45% in 2007 and 29.06% in 2010 using ELISA [36]. In patients presenting with fever with or without rash, the prevalence of TAHV antibodies was 13% using indirect immunofluorescence in an urban Kashi region, Xinjiang Province, China (2007) [37]. In the Lao PDR, TAHV antibodies were found in 37.7% of young patients under the age of 18 in 2015 [36].

The older age groups had a higher probability of infection and a higher prevalence of antibodies, and such a trend is usually seen in people and animals living in long-term enzootic regions [33]. Interestingly, in a Chinese study conducted at three locations in the Qinghai-Tibet Plateau, all seropositive individuals were under the 30-age group, with seroprevalence ranging from 1.1% to 4.3%. The authors supposed that higher seroprevalence in young age groups may suggest that TAHV was recently imported into the Qinghai-Tibet Plateau [21]. In the present study, no significant difference in seropositivity was found among age groups (2.5–7.7%).

Several studies have shown that TAHV circulates in wildlife in Central and Eastern Europe although seroconversion rates may vary by location and year. Several studies from the Czech Republic showed a declining trend in the TAHV seroprevalence among wild boars. The hemagglutination-inhibiting antibodies were found in 41.7% and 46.7% of wild boars in 1990 and 1993–1997, respectively [13,14]. A lower seropositivity rate of 19.4% was detected in the wild boars sampled at 24 hunting grounds of the Břeclav District (South Moravia) from 2000 to 2002. All these regions are characterized by the presence of wetland/fishpond ecosystems or floodplain forests as well as large mosquito populations [38]. In addition, TAHV NT antibodies were found in 28.9% of examined wild boars in Záhorská Lowland, western Slovakia, in the 1970s [39]. During 2016 and 2017, serum samples from wild boar (*Sus scrofa*), roe deer (*Capreolus capreolus*), and red deer (*Cervus elaphus*) were collected from Austria, Hungary, and Romania. In the wild boar population, TAHV NT seroprevalence rates were reported to be 25.9–27.5% in Austria, 0–55.6% in Romania, and 0–50.0% in Hungary. In addition, the seroprevalence in Austria was highest in wild boar (26.7%) compared to red deer (9.8%), while no roe deer were found seropositive [8].

TAHV seroprevalence in horses from urban areas of Zagreb and its surroundings tested in this study was 29.6%. This high seropositivity rate was similar to those detected in some endemic areas in the Czech Republic. In South Moravia (Břeclav District), a seroprevalence of 34.4% was reported in 1980. In addition, a very high seroprevalence rate of 55% was observed in pigs, while it was low in cattle (5.6%) [9]. In 2007, serum samples were collected from livestock (cows, sheep, and swine) at the abattoirs in Geermu City, Xining City, and Minhe County, China. In addition to IgG seropositivity of 6.7% in cows, 10.0% in sheep, and 3.3% in swine, IgM antibodies were detected in 3.3% of cows, 7.8% of sheep, and 5.0% of swine [21].

In this study, the TAHV seroprevalence rate in dogs and cats was 11.7%, with no difference according to sex and age. To our knowledge, there are no published data on the prevalence of TAHV in pet animals. In addition, there is no research on the clinical impact of TAHV infection in horses and pet animals. The results of this study clearly show that TAHV is circulating in selected animal species. There was additional reasoning for serosurvey of pet animals and horses. Compared to wildlife, serum samples are easier to collect. Moreover, unlike wildlife and other farm animals, these species are living in urban areas. Dogs and cats may live in close proximity to their owners and therefore have shared exposure to household and recreational risk factors. Finally, dogs and cats are scavengers, and pathogens bioaccumulate in them. The listed attributes make animal species selected for this study potential sentinel animals to monitor TAHV activity in cities. In analyzing the NT titers in humans and animals, substantially higher titers were observed in horses compared to humans and pet animals. Although there are no data regarding the longevity of TAHV antibody response in horses, it is still to be determined if higher titer makes them more sensitive tools for TAHV surveillance.

Many studies reported the detection of TAHV in mosquitoes. In 2006, TAHV was isolated from *Culex* spp. mosquitoes collected in Xinjiang, China [37]. Subsequently, in 2007–2008), TAHV was isolated from *Ae. dorsalis* and *Cx. modestus* pools in Inner Mongolia [20]. In 2013, the virus was isolated from *An. hyrcanus* mosquitoes collected on the fishponds in South Moravia (Czech Republic), a finding that represents the first isolation of TAHV from *An. hyrcanus* in Europe [7]. In a more recent study (2019), mosquitoes collected at floodplain habitats along three major rivers in eastern Austria, i.e., the Danube River, the Morava River, and the Leitha River, were tested. TAHV RNA was detected in two pools of *Ae. vexans* collected on the Leitha River. Phylogenetic analysis showed that the sequences obtained were remarkably similar to earlier TAHV isolates from the area, dating back to the initial TAHV isolate in 1958 [5]. In a very recently conducted study (2021), TAHV was detected in *Ae. caspius* and *Cx. pipiens* pools collected in the Emilia Romagna Region, Northern Italy. In addition, one isolated strain was obtained from one of the *Ae. caspius* pool collected in the municipality of Comacchio. Furthermore, TAHV was detected in 10 mosquito pools sampled in 2009, 2010, and 2020, confirming the continuous presence of the virus in this region [22]. In the present study, all tested *Ae. vexans* pools collected in the Zagreb area were negative for TAHV RNA.

When comparing the seropositivity rates between countries, it is important to keep in mind that the different serological methods (ELISA, IFA, and VNT) used to detect TAHV antibodies may have an impact on the seroprevalence results. In addition, there are some limitations of this study that should be noted. Since a small number of animals were included in the study, the seroprevalence results should be interpreted with caution. In addition, data on the sex and age of the horses were missing.

## 5. Conclusions

The presented results indicate the circulation of TAHV in northwestern Croatia. Further studies on large samples of humans, animals, and mosquitoes are needed to determine the prevalence of this neglected viral zoonosis.

**Author Contributions:** Conceptualization, V.S. (Vladimir Stevanovic) and T.V.-C.; methodology, V.S. (Vladimir Stevanovic), V.S. (Vladimir Savic), A.K. and S.K.; formal analysis, A.K., N.d.A.S. and S.K.; investigation, A.K., M.C.P., S.P., M.B., M.S. and V.T.; writing—original draft preparation, V.S., T.V.-C. and A.K.; writing—review and editing, V.S. (Vladimir Stevanovic); visualization, T.V.-C.; supervision, L.B.; funding acquisition, T.V.-C. All authors have read and agreed to the published version of the manuscript.

**Funding:** This research was funded by the Croatian Science Foundation, grant number IP-2016-06-7456: Prevalence and molecular epidemiology of emerging and re-emerging neuroinvasive arboviral infections in Croatia; CRONEUROARBO (to T.V.-C.) and the European Virus Archive goes Global (EVAg) project that has received funding from the European Union's Horizon 2020 research and innovation program under grant agreement No. 653316.

**Institutional Review Board Statement:** The study was conducted according to the guidelines of the Declaration of Helsinki and approved by the Ethics Committees of the Croatian Institute of Public Health (protocol code 80-1092/1-16, approved on 3 June 2016) and the University Hospital for Infectious Diseases, "Dr. Fran Mihaljevic", Zagreb (protocol code 01-1347-5-2018, approved on 13 September 2018). The animal study protocol was approved by the Ethics Committee of the Faculty of Veterinary Medicine, University of Zagreb (decision number: 640-01/20-02/12, approved on 18 December 2020).

**Informed Consent Statement:** Informed consent was obtained from all subjects involved in the study.

**Data Availability Statement:** Not applicable.

**Conflicts of Interest:** The authors declare no conflict of interest. The funders had no role in the design of the study; in the collection, analyses, or interpretation of data; in the writing of the manuscript; or in the decision to publish the results.

## References

1. ICTV. Genus: Orthobunyavirus. Available online: https://talk.ictvonline.org/ictv-reports/ictv_online_report/negative-sense-rna-viruses/w/peribunyaviridae/1238/genus-orthobunyavirus (accessed on 10 September 2022).
2. Hubálek, Z. Mosquito-borne viruses in Europe. *Parasitol. Res.* **2008**, *103* (Suppl. S1), S29–S43. [CrossRef] [PubMed]
3. Bárdos, V.; Medek, M.; Kania, V.; Hubálek, Z.; Juricova, Z. Das klinische Bild der Tahyna-Virus (California-Gruppe)–Infektionen bei Kindern [The clinical picture in Tahyna virus (California group) infections in children]. *Padiatr. Grenzgeb.* **1980**, *19*, 11–23. [PubMed]
4. Xia, H.; Wang, Y.; Atoni, E.; Zhang, B.; Yuan, Z. Mosquito-Associated Viruses in China. *Virol. Sin.* **2018**, *33*, 5–20. [CrossRef] [PubMed]
5. Camp, J.V.; Kniha, E.; Obwaller, A.; Walochnik, J.; Nowotny, N. The transmission ecology of Tahyna orthobunyavirus in Austria as revealed by longitudinal mosquito sampling and blood meal analysis in floodplain habitats. *Parasit. Vectors* **2021**, *14*, 561. [CrossRef] [PubMed]
6. Hubalek, Z.; Zeman, P.; Halouzka, J.; Juricova, Z.; Bálková, H.; Sikutová, S.; Rudolf, I. Antibodies against mosquito-borne viruses in human population of an area of Central Bohemia affected by the flood of 2002. *Epidemiol. Mikrobiol. Imunol.* **2004**, *53*, 112–120.
7. Hubalek, Z.; Sebesta, O.; Pesko, J.; Betasova, L.; Blazejova, H.; Venclikova, K.; Rudolf, I. Isolation of Tahyna Virus (California Encephalitis Group) From Anopheles hyrcanus (Diptera, Culicidae), a Mosquito Species New to, and Expanding in, Central Europe. *J. Med. Entomol.* **2014**, *51*, 1264–1267. [CrossRef]
8. Camp, J.V.; Haider, R.; Porea, D.; Oslobanu, L.E.; Forgách, P.; Nowotny, N. Serological surveillance for Tahyna virus (California encephalitis orthobunyavirus, Peribunyaviridae) neutralizing antibodies in wild ungulates in Austria, Hungary and Romania. *Zoonoses Public Health* **2018**, *65*, 459–463. [CrossRef]
9. Hubálek, Z. History of Arbovirus Research in the Czech Republic. *Viruses* **2021**, *13*, 2334. [CrossRef]
10. Juricová, Z.; Hubálek, Z.; Halouzka, J.; Sikutová, S. Serological examination of songbirds (Passeriformes) for mosquito-borne viruses Sindbis, Tahyna, and Batai in a south Moravian wetland (Czech Republic). *Vector Borne Zoonotic Dis.* **2009**, *9*, 295–299. [CrossRef]
11. Ernek, E.; Kozuch, O.; Nosek, J.; Hudec, K.; Folk, C. Virus neutralizing antibodies to arboviruses in birds of the order Anseriformes in Czechoslovakia. *Acta Virol.* **1975**, *19*, 349–353.
12. Juricová, Z.; Hubálek, Z.; Halouzka, J.; Machácek, P. Virologic detection of arboviruses in greater cormorants. *Vet. Med.* **1993**, *38*, 3759.
13. Juricová, Z.; Hubálek, Z. Serological surveys for arboviruses in the game animals of southern Moravia (Czech Republic). *Folia Zool.* **1999**, *48*, 185–189.
14. Juricova, Z. Antibodies to arboviruses in game animals in South Moravia (in Czech). *Vet. Med.* **1992**, *37*, 633–636.
15. Hubálek, Z.; Rudolf, I.; Bakonyi, T.; Kazdová, K.; Halouzka, J.; Sebesta, O.; Sikutová, S.; Juricová, Z.; Nowotny, N. Mosquito (Diptera: Culicidae) surveillance for arboviruses in an area endemic for West Nile (Lineage Rabensburg) and Tahyna viruses in Central Europe. *J. Med. Entomol.* **2010**, *47*, 466–472. [CrossRef] [PubMed]
16. Danielová, V.; Málková, D.; Minár, J.; Rehse-Küpper, B.; Hájková, Z.; Halgos, J.; Jedlicka, L. Arbovirus isolations from mosquitoes in South Slovakia. *Folia Parasitol.* **1978**, *25*, 187–190.
17. Calzolari, M.; Bonilauri, P.; Bellini, R.; Caimi, M.; Defilippo, F.; Maioli, G.; Albieri, A.; Medici, A.; Veronesi, R.; Pilani, R.; et al. Arboviral survey of mosquitoes in two northern Italian regions in 2007 and 2008. *Vector Borne Zoonotic Dis.* **2010**, *10*, 875–884. [CrossRef]
18. Sonnleitner, S.T.; Lundström, J.; Baumgartner, R.; Simeoni, J.; Schennach, H.; Zelger, R.; Prader, A.; Schmutzhard, E.; Nowotny, N.; Walder, G. Investigations on California serogroup orthobunyaviruses in the Tyrols: First description of Tahyna virus in the Alps. *Vector Borne Zoonotic Dis.* **2014**, *14*, 272–277. [CrossRef]
19. Nikiforova, M.A.; Kuznetsova, N.A.; Shchetinin, A.M.; Butenko, A.M.; Kozlova, A.A.; Larichev, V.P.; Vakalova, E.V.; Azarian, A.R.; Rubalsky, O.V.; Bashkina, O.A.; et al. Arboviruses in the Astrakhan region of Russia for 2018 season: The development of multiplex PCR assays and analysis of mosquitoes, ticks, and human blood sera. *Infect. Genet. Evol.* **2021**, *88*, 104711. [CrossRef]
20. Cao, Y.; Fu, S.; Tian, Z.; Lu, Z.; He, Y.; Wang, H.; Wang, J.; Guo, W.; Tao, B.; Liang, G. Distribution of mosquitoes and mosquito-borne arboviruses in Inner Mongolia, China. *Vector Borne Zoonotic Dis.* **2011**, *11*, 157–781. [CrossRef]
21. Li, W.J.; Wang, J.L.; Li, M.H.; Fu, S.H.; Wang, H.Y.; Wang, Z.Y.; Jiang, S.Y.; Wang, X.W.; Guo, P.; Zhao, S.C.; et al. Mosquitoes and mosquito-borne arboviruses in the Qinghai-Tibet Plateau–focused on the Qinghai area, China. *Am. J. Trop. Med. Hyg.* **2010**, *82*, 705–711. [CrossRef]

22. Calzolari, M.; Bonilauri, P.; Grisendi, A.; Dalmonte, G.; Vismarra, A.; Lelli, D.; Chiapponi, C.; Bellini, R.; Lavazza, A.; Dottori, M. Arbovirus Screening in Mosquitoes in Emilia-Romagna (Italy, 2021) and Isolation of Tahyna Virus. *Microbiol. Spectr.* **2022**, *27*, e0158722. [CrossRef] [PubMed]
23. Vesenjak-Hirjan, J.; Galinović-Weisglass, M.; Urlić, V.; Bendiš, M.; Miović, P.; Vujošević, N.; Vuksanović, P. Occurrence of arboviruses in the Middle and the South Adriatic (Yugoslavia). In *Arboviruses in the Mediterranean Countries*; Vesenjak-Hirjan, J., Ed.; Gustav Fischer Verlag: Stuttgart, Germany; New York, NY, USA, 1980; pp. 303–310.
24. Turković, B.; Brudnjak, Z. Arboviruses in Croatia. *Acta Med. Croat.* **1998**, *52*, 87–89.
25. Madić, J.; Huber, D.; Lugović, B. Serologic survey for selected viral and rickettsial agents of brown bears (*Ursus arctos*) in Croatia. *J. Wildl. Dis.* **1993**, *29*, 572–576. [CrossRef]
26. Vilibic-Cavlek, T.; Stevanovic, V.; Savic, V.; Markelic, D.; Sabadi, D.; Bogdanic, M.; Kovac, S.; Santini, M.; Tabain, I.; Potocnik-Hunjadi, T.; et al. Detection of Tahyna Orthobunyavirus-Neutralizing Antibodies in Patients with Neuroinvasive Disease in Croatia. *Microorganisms* **2022**, *10*, 1443. [CrossRef] [PubMed]
27. Klobucar, A.; Benic, N.; Krajcar, D.; Kosanovic-Licina, M.L.; Tesic, V.; Merdic, E.; Vrucina, I.; Savic, V.; Barbic, L.; Stevanovic, V.; et al. An overview of mosquitoes and emerging arboviral infections in the Zagreb area, Croatia. *J. Infect. Dev. Ctries.* **2016**, *10*, 1286–1293. [CrossRef]
28. Klobučar, A.; Lipovac, I.; Žagar, N.; Mitrović-Hamzić, S.; Tešić, V.; Vilibić-Čavlek, T.; Merdić, E. First record and spreading of the invasive mosquito *Aedes japonicus japonicus* (Theobald, 1901) in Croatia. *Med. Vet. Entomol.* **2019**, *33*, 171–176. [CrossRef] [PubMed]
29. Li, H.; Cao, Y.X.; He, X.X.; Fu, S.H.; Lyu, Z.; He, Y.; Gao, X.Y.; Liang, G.D.; Wang, H.Y. Real-time RT-PCR Assay for the detection of Tahyna Virus. *Biomed. Environ. Sci.* **2015**, *28*, 374–377. [CrossRef]
30. Becker, N.; Petric, D.; Zgomba, M.; Boase, C.; Dahl, C.; Madon, M.; Kaiser, A. *Mosquito and Their Control*, 2nd ed.; Springer: Berlin/Heidelberg, Germany, 2010; p. 577.
31. Schaffner, F.; Angel, G.; Geoffroy, B.; Hervy, J.P.; Rhaiem, A.; Brunhes, J. *The Mosquitoes of Europe—An Identification and Training Programme*; CD Rom, IRD Editions & EID Méditerranée: Montpellier, France, 2001.
32. Glinskikh, N.P.; Fedotova, T.T.; Pereskokova, I.G.; Melnikov, V.G.; Volkova, L.I. The potentials for the comprehensive diagnosis of viral encephalitis in Sverdlovsk Province. *Vopr. Virusol.* **1994**, *39*, 190–191.
33. Hubálek, Z.; Zeman, P.; Halouzka, J.; Juricová, Z.; Stovicková, E.; Bálková, H.; Sikutová, S.; Rudolf, I. Mosquitoborne viruses, Czech Republic, 2002. *Emerg. Infect. Dis.* **2005**, *11*, 116–118. [CrossRef] [PubMed]
34. Barakat, A.M.; Smura, T.; Kuivanen, S.; Huhtamo, E.; Kurkela, S.; Putkuri, N.; Hasony, H.J.; Al-Hello, H.; Vapalahti, O. The Presence and Seroprevalence of Arthropod-Borne Viruses in Nasiriyah Governorate, Southern Iraq: A Cross-Sectional Study. *Am. J. Trop. Med. Hyg.* **2016**, *94*, 794–799. [CrossRef] [PubMed]
35. Kuniholm, M.H.; Wolfe, N.D.; Huang, C.Y.; Mpoudi-Ngole, E.; Tamoufe, U.; LeBreton, M.; Burke, D.S.; Gubler, D.J. Seroprevalence and distribution of Flaviviridae, Togaviridae, and Bunyaviridae arboviral infections in rural Cameroonian adults. *Am. J. Trop. Med. Hyg.* **2006**, *74*, 1078–1083. [CrossRef] [PubMed]
36. Arbovirus Surveillance Project. Institut Pasteur du Laos. Available online: https://www.pasteur.la/project-carried-on-in-thelab-2016-2017-lao-fr1/research-and-development/ (accessed on 30 July 2022).
37. Lu, Z.; Lu, X.J.; Fu, S.H.; Zhang, S.; Li, Z.X.; Yao, X.H.; Feng, Y.P.; Lambert, A.J.; Ni, D.X.; Wang, F.T.; et al. Tahyna virus and human infection, China. *Emerg. Infect. Dis.* **2009**, *15*, 306–309. [CrossRef] [PubMed]
38. Halouzka, J.; Juricová, Z.; Jankova, J.; Hubalek, Z. Serologic survey of wild boars for mosquito-borne viruses in South Moravia (Czech Republic). *Vet. Med.* **2008**, *53*, 266–271. [CrossRef]
39. Kozuch, O.; Nosek, J.; Gresikova, M.; Ernek, E. Surveillance of mosquito-borne natural focus in Zahorska Lowland, 115–118. In *2nd International Arbeitskolloquium Uber Die Naturherde von Infektionskrankheiten in Zentraleuropa*; Sixl, W., Ed.; Hygiene Institut der Universitat: Graz, Austria, 1976.

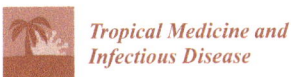

*Tropical Medicine and Infectious Disease*

Article

# Infant HIV Testing Amid the COVID-19 Pandemic and Evolving PMTCT Guidelines in Johannesburg, South Africa

Coceka N. Mnyani [1,*], Andomei Smit [1] and Gayle G. Sherman [2,3]

1. Department of Obstetrics and Gynaecology, School of Clinical Medicine, University of the Witwatersrand, Johannesburg 2193, South Africa
2. Centre for HIV and STIs, National Institute for Communicable Diseases, Division of the National Health Laboratory Service, Johannesburg 2192, South Africa
3. Department of Paediatrics and Child Health, School of Clinical Medicine, University of the Witwatersrand, Johannesburg 2193, South Africa
* Correspondence: coceka.mnyani@wits.ac.za

**Abstract: Background:** The COVID-19 pandemic impacted HIV programmes with the diversion of resources and lockdown measures. We assessed the impact of COVID-19 on infant HIV diagnosis in the context of updated 2019 prevention of mother-to-child transmission of HIV (PMTCT) guidelines in Johannesburg, South Africa. **Methods:** HIV PCR data for children <2 years were extracted from the National Health Laboratory Service database from October 2018 to September 2021, inclusive. Trends in the total number of tests performed and the total number of children with HIV diagnosed, stratified by age, were determined to assess the effect of different COVID-19 lockdown levels and updated guidelines. **Results:** When comparing three 12-month periods ending September 2019–2021, respectively, the total number of HIV PCR tests performed increased (from 41 879 to 47 265 to 56 813), and the total number of children with HIV decreased (from 659 to 640 to 620), year-on-year. There was a substantial increase in 6-month testing in response to updated guidelines. Excluding 6-month testing, the year-on-year increase in total tests was maintained with birth and 10-week testing closely approximating total live births to women living with HIV. A decrease in the total number of children with HIV diagnosed was noted in Q2 2020, coinciding with the most restrictive lockdown, followed by a rebound in cases. **Conclusions:** Despite the restrictions and diversion of resources associated with COVID-19, there was a successful implementation of PMTCT guideline updates and minimal disruption to infant HIV testing. However, much work remains in order to achieve the elimination of mother-to-child transmission of HIV.

**Keywords:** PMTCT; HIV; COVID-19

## 1. Introduction

COVID-19, which was declared a pandemic in March 2020, has had a devastating impact globally, not only in terms of morbidity and mortality associated with infections but also impact on health programmes, including the provision of HIV care. Various commentaries and modelling studies predicted the negative impact the pandemic would have on HIV programmes, as resources were diverted and various lockdown measures implemented in a bid to curb the spread of infections [1–4]. In a model-based analysis of the potential impact of COVID-19-associated interruptions in the UNAIDS 21 priority countries, there were projected interruptions in paediatric HIV prevention and care [4]. The projections included a decline in pregnant women accessing prevention of mother-to-child transmission of HIV (PMTCT) services, with a subsequent increase in new paediatric HIV infections and disruptions in care for children living with HIV. The analysis could not project the impact on infant HIV testing as a result of insufficient pre-COVID-19 data from the countries [4].

The published data have subsequently shown the impact of COVID-19 throughout the HIV care cascade, and the impact is likely to be felt for years to come. Early in the pandemic, the Global Fund reported that several countries reported high or very high-level disruptions in HIV care, with the prevention, testing and support of people living with HIV the most impacted [5]. South Africa, where the first case of COVID-19 was identified on 5 March 2020, and a stringent national lockdown subsequently implemented on 27 March 2020, has not been spared from the effects of the pandemic [6]. At the time, the country was implementing revised PMTCT guidelines, which included the introduction of dolutegravir-based antiretroviral therapy (ART) and changes in maternal monitoring and infant HIV testing [7]. A July 2020 UNICEF report showed limited implementation of the guidelines [8]. Hence, the aim of this study was to assess the impact of COVID-19 on infant HIV diagnosis in the context of updated 2019 PMTCT guidelines in the Johannesburg Health District, South Africa.

## 2. Materials and Methods

### 2.1. Study Setting

The Johannesburg Health District has seven subdistricts, A–G, and had a population of over five million people in 2021 [9]. The HIV prevalence in pregnant women in the district was estimated to be around 25% in 2019, with high ART coverage of over 90% during pregnancy [10]. The revised PMTCT guidelines were signed off for implementation in November 2019. The revisions included the introduction of dolutegravir-based ART for first-line treatment, initially with caution for use in the first trimester because of the then-reported increased risk of neural tube defects with periconception use [11,12]. This caution was later removed in July 2021 from the South African PMTCT guidelines as accumulating data showed no increased risk of neural tube defects with dolutegravir use compared to other ART regimens [13].

Several updates related to routine infant HIV testing were made [7]. In addition to the birth and 10-weeks HIV PCR testing that was already in place, a 6-months PCR test was added for all HIV-exposed infants who had previously tested HIV-negative. The rationale for choosing the 6-month instead of the 9-month screening recommended by the World Health Organization (WHO) was based on the decreased testing coverage with increasing infant age experienced in early infant diagnosis (EID). Moreover, the findings from a nationally representative South African cohort demonstrated that 82% of cumulative MTCT occurred by 6 months of age, at which time breastfeeding prevalence is less than 30% [14]. Universal HIV testing at 18 months for all infants was also introduced, with a rapid HIV antibody test used for screening and a PCR test used for confirmation of a positive result. Confirmatory PCR testing was recommended for up to two years of age. Age-appropriate HIV testing for symptoms consistent with HIV infection and 6 weeks post cessation of breastfeeding remained in place in the revised guidelines [7].

### 2.2. Study Design

HIV PCR data for children aged less than two years who were tested in the Johannesburg Health District in the period 01 October 2018 to 30 September 2021 were extracted from the Surveillance Data Warehouse (DW) at the National Institute for Communicable Diseases (NICD), a division of the National Health Laboratory Service (NHLS). NHLS performs all pathology tests for the public health sector nationally, serving more than 80% of the South African population, and captures these records in a laboratory information system. In order to facilitate the monitoring of HIV programs such as EID of HIV, test data are transferred to the NICD DW. In the absence of a unique health identifier, the DW utilises a probabilistic linking algorithm to link multiple HIV tests belonging to the same patient, employing predominantly the variables name, surname and date of birth to allocate a DW unique identifier. The accuracy of this algorithm is compromised by the use of poor demographic details provided at the time of birth testing that is updated for testing at later time points, precluding accurate longitudinal monitoring from birth [15]. However, where infants test HIV PCR positive, and a confirmatory test follows shortly thereafter, similar demographic details generally allow for linkage facilitating de-duplication of HIV PCR positive tests to infants with HIV. Other variables used include the facility where the specimen was collected, facility GPS coordinates, date of specimen registration and age at testing, HIV PCR test result and the DW unique identifier.

Data from the DW were compared to EID indicators collected by the District Health Information System (DHIS), which reports on birth and around 10-week HIV PCR tests by counting the total number of tests performed and the total number of positive tests in these two age groups, respectively. DHIS is the South African Department of Health system used to collect aggregate routine data from public healthcare facilities. Birth HIV PCR test is defined by DHIS as tests performed from birth to less than 6 weeks of infant age, and 10-week HIV PCR test as tests performed from 6 weeks to less than 14 weeks of age. As there was no 6-month testing reported on DHIS at the time of the study, the NICD definition of a 6-month HIV PCR test was used and refers to testing performed from 14 weeks of infant age to less than 9 months. Other DHIS indicators used included total live births and total live births to women living with HIV (WLHIV).

*2.3. Data Analysis*

An analysis was performed using RStudio Version 1.3.1056 on a 64-bit Windows device to generate the total number of tests performed, the total number of children with HIV diagnosed and the geospatial maps. Trends in the total number of tests performed and the total number of HIV PCR-positive tests, stratified by age, were determined to assess the effects of the introduction of revised PMTCT guidelines and different COVID-19 lockdown levels. Testing coverage was calculated as the total number of HIV PCR tests performed divided by the total number of live births to WLHIV reported by DHIS. Case rates were calculated using the total number of first HIV PCR-positive tests at an age less than 2 years as a proxy for newly diagnosed children with HIV, divided by the DHIS indicator of total live births and expressed per 100,000. In the study, a year was defined as the period from the beginning of the fourth quarter, i.e., 01 October to 31 December, to the end of the third quarter, i.e., 01 July to 30 September. There were five COVID-19 lockdown levels that were introduced at various times in South Africa, with level 5 being the most restrictive, severely limiting people's movements and economic activity [6]. Healthcare facilities remained open throughout the different lockdown levels.

*2.4. Ethics*

Ethics approval for the study was obtained from the University of the Witwatersrand Human Research Ethics committee (Protocol numbers M201186 and M210752). De-identified data were analysed on a secure share point folder hosted by the NICD.

## 3. Results

A total of 153,723 HIV PCR tests were analysed, belonging to 127,515 unique patients as allocated by the probabilistic linking algorithm in the NICD DW. Total HIV PCR tests performed increased over the study period from 10,179 to 14,538 per quarter, attributable to an increase in tests performed in all age groups but predominantly a consequence of a three-fold increase in testing around 6 months of age in line with new PMTCT guideline recommendations (Figure 1).

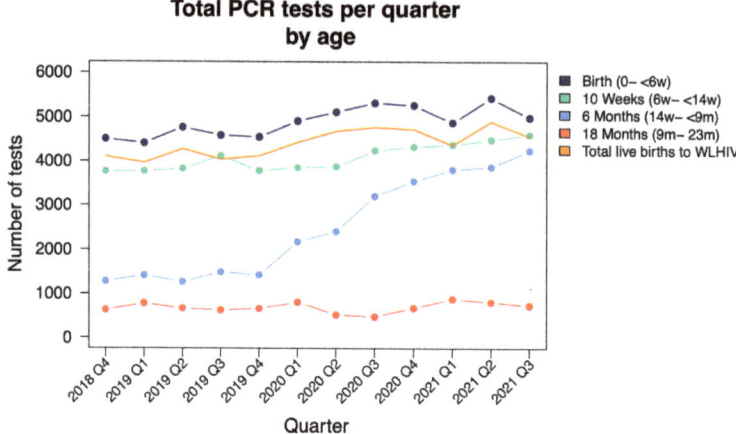

**Figure 1.** HIV PCR tests performed quarterly from October 2018 to September 2021, stratified by age; NICD data (d = days; w = weeks; m = months; WLHIV = women living with HIV).

* Total birth tests performed are higher than the total live births to WLHIV, likely due to a combination of under-reporting of the DHIS indicator and repeat HIV PCR tests performed in the first 6 weeks of life.

Deduplicated HIV PCR-positive test results decreased year on year from 659 to 620, with a total of 1919 newly diagnosed infants and children with HIV identified during the study period (Figure 2; Table 1).

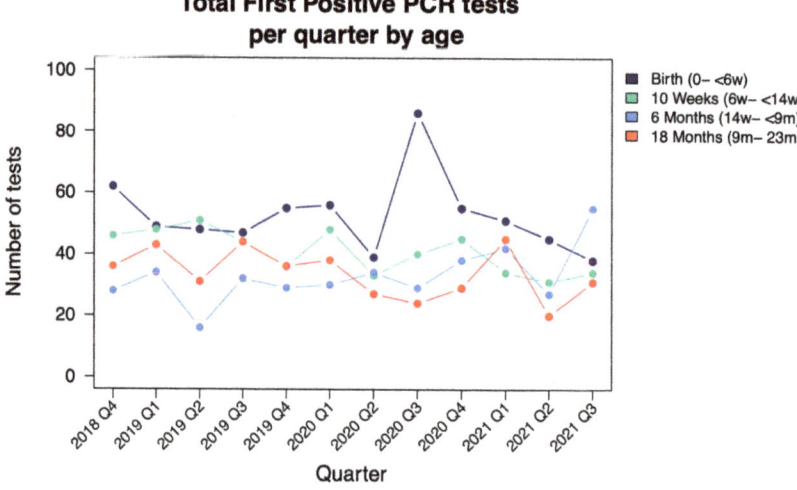

**Figure 2.** Children testing HIV PCR positive performed quarterly from October 2018 to September 2021, stratified by age; NICD data (d = days; w = weeks; m = months).

Table 1. Comparison of NICD and DHIS HIV PCR tests performed and positive tests identified, October 2018–September 2021.

| Year | NICD Data | | | | | | DHIS | | | |
|---|---|---|---|---|---|---|---|---|---|---|
| | <2 Years | | Birth | | 10 Weeks | | Birth | | 10 Weeks | |
| | Total Tests | Positive Tests | Total Tests | Positive Tests | Total Tests | Positive Tests | Total Tests | Positive Tests | Total Tests | Positive Tests |
| Year 1 | 41 879 | 659 | 18 254 | 206 | 15 478 | 189 | 16 884 | 98 | 14 997 | 76 |
| Year 2 | 47 265 | 640 | 19 869 | 236 | 15 738 | 157 | 17 639 | 108 | 16 137 | 108 |
| Year 3 | 56 813 | 620 | 20 533 | 189 | 17 766 | 144 | 17 292 | 120 | 19 201 | 80 |
| Total | 145 957 | 1 919 | 58 656 | 631 | 48 982 | 490 | 51 815 | 326 | 50 335 | 264 |

NICD = National Institute for Communicable Disease; DHIS = District Health Information System; Year 1 = 1 October 2018 to 30 September 2019; Year 2 = 01 October 2019 to 30 September 2020; Year 3 = 01 October 2020 to 30 September 2021.

According to the DHIS data, there was a total of 51,334 live births to WLHIV during the study period, with an average of 4278 live births to WLHIV per quarter. The decrease in positive HIV PCR tests translates to a declining annual case rate of newly diagnosed less than two-year-old infants and children of 905 to 804 per 100,000 live births. During the most stringent COVID-19 lockdown period viz. Q2 2020, there appears to be a decrease in the number of newly diagnosed children with HIV at birth and around 10 weeks of age, followed by a rebound when restrictions were eased in Q3 2020. A decrease in total PCR testing at these time periods is less obvious.

Birth testing coverage remained around 100% throughout the study period whilst 10-week testing coverage averaged 85%, with a mild decrease to 79.5% during Q2 and Q3 of 2020. Coverage of 6-month testing increased steadily from 36% to 90% during the study period. Birth testing was the time point that yielded the highest number of first HIV PCR-positive tests in comparison to 10-week and 6-month testing, with a total of 631 cases during the study period in comparison to 490 at 10 weeks and 394 at 6 months. A total of 1515/1919 (79%) first HIV PCR-positive tests were detected in the first eight months of life. The increased tests performed at 6 months of age demonstrated an annual increase in first HIV PCR-positive cases from 110 to 122 to 162, year-on-year.

During the study period, the total number of HIV PCR tests performed correlated fairly well between DHIS and NICD data—Table 1. Total birth and 10-week tests were recorded by DHIS as 51,815 and 50,335 in comparison to NICD 58,656 and 48,982, respectively. Thus, NICD recorded 5488 more PCR tests being performed at birth and 10 weeks of age. Triangulation of first HIV PCR-positive tests correlates less well with newly diagnosed children at birth and 10-week tests reported by DHIS as 326 and 264 in comparison to NICD 631 and 490, respectively. DHIS reports a total of 590 newly diagnosed infants to 1121 reported by NICD. In order to reduce the effect of NICD data overcounting newly diagnosed infants because of the inability to link patient tests accurately, the age ranges for birth and 10-week testing for NICD data were narrowed from 0–<6 weeks to <7 days of age and from 6 weeks–<14 weeks to 8–12 weeks of age, respectively, which again yielded higher numbers of infected infants than DHIS reports at 441 and 341 newly diagnosed infants at birth and 10 weeks, respectively.

A third of all HIV PCR tests performed in the Johannesburg Health District is performed in subdistrict D ($n$ = 46,896), with the least by subdistrict C ($n$ = 9 831), a reflection of where the large delivery units, including hospitals, are situated (Figure 3). Unsurprisingly, subdistrict D also yields the first HIV PCR-positive results at 608 over the study period, followed by subdistrict F ($n$ = 301) and subdistrict A ($n$ = 279).

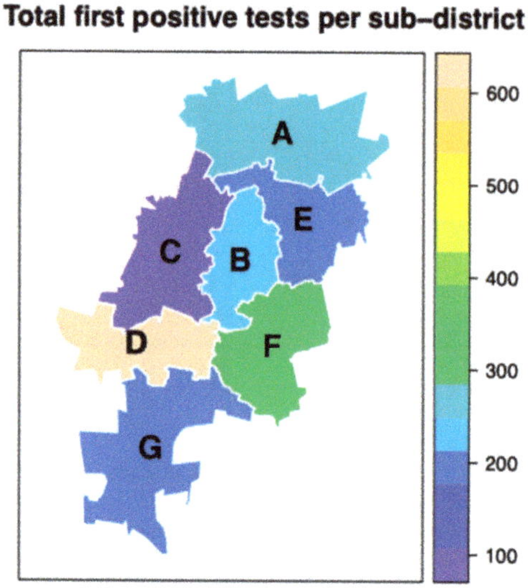

**Figure 3.** Total first HIV PCR positive tests per subdistrict in the Johannesburg Health District, October 2018–September 2021.

## 4. Discussion

In this 3-year review of HIV PCR data of children less than two years of age tested in the Johannesburg Health District, there was an increase in tests performed across all age groups. The increase was more pronounced in testing around six months of age, where there was a three-fold increase in HIV PCR testing during the study period, in line with revised PMTCT guidelines. There was an overall decrease in positive HIV PCR tests, translating to a declining annual case rate of newly diagnosed children less than two years of age. The period associated with stringent COVID-19 regulations early in the pandemic in South Africa showed a decrease in positive HIV PCR tests identified with birth and 10-week testing, with a subsequent rebound when restrictions were eased. The majority (79%) of first HIV PCR-positive tests were detected in the first eight months of life.

The finding of minimal interruptions to infant HIV testing during the peak of the COVID-19 pandemic and associated restrictions in South Africa, and interruptions in health services, is reassuring and shows the robustness of the PMTCT program in the Johannesburg Health District. This finding is similar to that of a retrospective review of routinely collected data in KwaZulu-Natal province, South Africa, where there was evidence of a significant decline in birth PCR testing in the period March to May 2020—the period coinciding with the most restrictive COVID-19 regulations—with recovery in testing rates seen in June 2020 [16]. While there was no obvious decrease in the total number of PCR tests performed during the stringent lockdown period in our study, the rebound in positive HIV PCR tests following the easing of restrictions was evident for birth (0–<6 weeks) testing. This is likely to represent a combination of increased and duplicate testing across different facilities where there would have been concerns of reduced testing and/or less access to laboratory records to check results. The algorithm deduplicating laboratory test records perform less accurately across different facilities. In another review of programmatic data from 65 primary care facilities also in KwaZulu Natal, there was an almost 50% decline in HIV testing and ART initiation during the early stages of the COVID-19 lockdown [17]. There were, however, no details on early infant diagnosis.

The increase in testing at around six months of age reflects the successful implementation of a component of the revised 2019 PMTCT guidelines. This is reassuring given the reported interruptions in HIV care with the COVID-19 pandemic and the 2020 UNICEF report that showed the limited implementation of the revised guidelines [8]. While our study did not assess dolutegravir use in PWLHIV and interruptions in accessing ART during the lockdowns, the decrease in positive HIV PCR tests in children less than two years of age could be attributable to the transition to dolutegravir-based first-line ART regimens. Dolutegravir-based ART has been shown to achieve a faster rate of viral load suppression compared to non-nucleoside reverse transcriptase-based ART [18]. While there was a decrease in cases of children with HIV, the decrease might be smaller than anticipated with dolutegravir-based ART due to interruptions in accessing ART.

In our study, 79% of first HIV PCR-positive tests were identified in infants aged eight months or less, a finding similar to that reported by Goga et al. [14]. In their review of a nationally representative sample of 9120 HIV-exposed infants, 81% of cumulative MTCT cases had occurred by six months. While there was a good correlation in total HIV PCR tests performed between the NICD and DHIS data in our study, there was a large disparity in the number of first HIV PCR-positive tests for birth and 10-weeks testing. This has important implications as DHIS data are used for modelling, planning and tracking progress toward eMTCT. The data are also important in ensuring that children that test HIV positive are linked to care. The spatial analysis in our study on where the HIV PCR-positive cases are is important for the allocation of resources for PMTCT and HIV care for children who test positive.

While the large NICD infant HIV PCR testing database is a strength of our study, there are several limitations. The absence of a unique patient identifier and thus eliminating duplication of tests is an important limitation. The NICD DW probabilistic linking algorithm, while intended to minimise this duplication, is not without limitations as it relies on demographic data provided by clinicians. The mobility of patients may also contribute to the duplication of tests. Despite the limitations, our study contributes important data on the robustness of an established PMTCT programme and how there were minimal interruptions in the implementation of guidelines despite the devastating impact of COVID-19 on health services. While there has been a decline in the number of children under the age of two years testing HIV PCR positive, much work remains in ensuring that the number decreases further as the case rates in our study are far above what is required for eMTCT, which is <50 HIV PCR positive cases per 100 000 live births [19,20]. We also need to ensure that those children who test positive are linked to and remain in care.

**Author Contributions:** Conceptualisation, G.G.S. and C.N.M.; methodology, G.G.S. and C.N.M.; formal analysis, A.S. and G.G.S.; writing—original draft preparation, review and editing, C.N.M. and G.G.S.; funding acquisition, C.N.M. All authors have read and agreed to the published version of the manuscript.

**Funding:** This research was funded by the Carnegie Corporation of New York Post-Doctoral Clinician Fellowship (Grant number: G17-55194).

**Institutional Review Board Statement:** The study was conducted in accordance with the Declaration of Helsinki and approved by the University of the Witwatersrand Human Research Ethics committee (Protocol numbers M201186 and M210752). De-identified data were analysed on a secure share point folder hosted by the NICD.

**Informed Consent Statement:** Patient consent was waived due to the fact that routinely collected, de-identified data were used.

**Data Availability Statement:** De-identified data available on request.

**Acknowledgments:** The authors thank the NHLS and the South African National Department of Health for the data used.

**Conflicts of Interest:** The authors declare no conflict of interest. The funders had no role in the design of the study; in the collection, analyses, or interpretation of data; in the writing of the manuscript, or in the decision to publish the results.

## References

1. The Lancet. Maintaining the HIV response in a world shaped by COVID-19. *Lancet Glob Health* **2020**, *8*, e1132-41. [CrossRef]
2. Jewell, B.L.; Mudimu, E.; Stover, J.; Ten Brink, D.; Phillips, A.N.; Smith, J.A.; Martin-Hughes, R.; Teng, Y.; Glaubius, R.; Mahiane, S.G.; et al. for the HIV Modelling Consortium. Potential effects of disruption to HIV programmes in sub-Saharan Africa caused by COVID-19: Results from multiple mathematical models. *Lancet HIV* **2020**, *7*, e629-40. [CrossRef]
3. Stover, J.; Kelly, S.L.; Mudimu, E.; Green, D.; Smith, T.; Taramusi, I.; Bansi-Matharu, L.; Martin-Hughes, R.; Phillips, A.N.; Bershteyn, A. The risks and benefits of providing HIV services during the COVID-19 pandemic. *PLoS ONE* **2021**, *16*, e0260820. [CrossRef] [PubMed]
4. Flanagan, C.F.; McCann, N.; Strover, J.; Freedberg, K.A.; Ciaranello, A.L. Do not forget the children: A model-based analysis on the potential impact of COVID-19-associated interruptions in paediatric HIV prevention and care. *J. Int. AIDS Soc.* **2022**, *25*, e25864. [CrossRef] [PubMed]
5. Global Fund COVID-19 Situational Report #32. Reporting Period 28 October–11 November 2020. Available online: https://www.theglobalfund.org/media/10304/covid19_2020-11-11-situation_report_en.pdf (accessed on 13 August 2022).
6. South African Government. COVID-19/Novel Coronavirus. Available online: https://www.gov.za/Coronavirus#:~{}:text=The%20National%20State%20of%20Disaster,13%20to%2030%20September%202021 (accessed on 17 September 2022).
7. The South African National Department of Health. *ART Clinical Guidelines for the Management of HIV in Adults, Pregnancy, Adolescents, Children, Infants and Neonates*; The South African National Department of Health: Pretoria, South Africa, 2019. Available online: https://www.health.gov.za/wp-content/uploads/2020/11/2019-art-guideline.pdf (accessed on 17 September 2022).
8. UNICEF's HIV Programming in the Context of COVID-19: Sustaining the Gains and Reimagining the Future for Children, Adolescents and Women. Compendium of Innovative Approaches in Eastern and Southern Africa; UNICEF: 2020. Available online: https://www.unicef.org/esa/media/6621/file/HIV%20COVID-19%20Compendium%20-July%202020.pdf (accessed on 10 August 2022).
9. Johannesburg, South Africa Metro Area Population 1950–2022. Available online: https://macrotrends.net/cities/22486/johannesburg/population (accessed on 17 September 2022).
10. *District Health Barometer 2019/20*; Massyn, N.; Day, C.; Ndlovu, N.; Padayachee, T. (Eds.) Health Systems Trust: Durban, South Africa, 2020. Available online: https://www.hst.org.za/publications/District%20Health%20Barometers/18%20(Section%20B)%20Gauteng%20Province.pdf (accessed on 15 August 2022).
11. Zash, R.; Makhema, J.; Shapiro, R.L. Neural-tube defects with dolutegravir treatment from the time of conception. *N. Engl. J. Med.* **2018**, *379*, 979–981. [CrossRef] [PubMed]
12. Zash, R.; Holmes, L.; Diseko, M.; Jacobson, D.L.; Brummel, S.; Mayondi, G.; Isaacson, A.; Davey, S.; Mabuta, J.; Mmalane, M.; et al. Neural-tube defects and antiretroviral treatment regimens in Botswana. *N. Engl. J. Med.* **2019**, *381*, 827–840. [CrossRef] [PubMed]
13. Zash, R.; Holmes, L.B.; Diseko, M.; Jacobson, D.; Mayondi, G.; Mabuta, J.; Mmalane, M.; Gaolathe, T.; Lockman, S.; Makhema, J.; et al. Update on neural tube defects with antiretroviral exposure in the Tsepamo study, Botswana. In Proceedings of the 24th International AIDS Conference, Montreal, Canada, 29 July–2 August 2022; abstract PELBB02. Available online: https://programme.aids2022.org/Abstract/Abstract/?abstractid=12759 (accessed on 17 September 2022).
14. Goga, A.E.; Lombard, C.; Jackson, D.; Ramokolo, V.; Ngandu, N.K.; Sherman, G.; Puren, A.; Chirinda, W.; Bhardwaj, S.; Makhari, N.; et al. Impact of breastfeeding, maternal antiretroviral treatment and health service factors on 18-month vertical transmission of HIV and HIV-free survival: Results from a nationally representative HIV-exposed infant cohort, South Africa. *J. Epidemiol. Community Heal.* **2020**, *74*, 1069–1077. [CrossRef]
15. Radebe, L.; Haeri Mazanderani, A.; Sherman, G.G. Evaluating patient data quality in South Africa's National Health Laboratory Service Data Warehouse, 2017–2020: Implications for monitoring child health programmes. *BMC Public Health* **2022**, *22*, 1266. [CrossRef] [PubMed]
16. Jensen, C.; McKerrow, N.H. Child health services during a COVID-19 outbreak in KwaZulu-Natal Province, South Africa. *South Afr. Med J.* **2021**, *111*, 114–119. [CrossRef] [PubMed]
17. Dorward, J.; Khubone, T.; Gate, K.; Ngobese, H.; Sookrajh, Y.; Mkhize, S.; Jeewa, A.; Bottomley, C.; Lewis, L.; Baisley, K.; et al. The impact of the COVID-19 lockdown on HIV care in 65 South African primary care clinics: An interrupted time series analysis. *Lancet HIV* **2021**, *8*, e158–e165. [CrossRef]
18. WHO Recommends Dolutegravir as Preferred HIV Treatment Option in All Populations; World Health Organization: 2019. Available online: https://www.who.int/news/item/22-07-2019-who-recommends-dolutegravir-as-preferred-hiv-treatment-option-in-all-populations (accessed on 17 September 2022).
19. World Health Organization. Global Guidance on Criteria and Processes for Validation: Elimination of Mother-to-Child Transmission of HIV and Syphilis; World Health Organization: 2014. Available online: https://apps.who.int/iris/handle/10665/112858 (accessed on 17 September 2022).
20. World Health Organization. Global Guidance on Criteria and Processes for Validation: Elimination of Mother-to-Child Transmission of HIV, Syphilis and Hepatitis B Virus; World Health Organization: 2022. Available online: https://www.who.int/publications/i/item/9789240039360 (accessed on 17 September 2022).

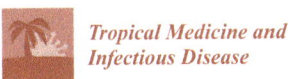 *Tropical Medicine and Infectious Disease*

Article

# Association between Chlamydial Infection with Ectopic and Full-Term Pregnancies: A Case-Control Study

Valliammai Jayanthi Thirunavuk Arasoo [1,*], Mariyammah Masalamani [1], Amutha Ramadas [1], Nisha Angela Dominic [1], Darien Daojuin Liew [1], Robin Wai Jen Sia [1], Anuradha Wanigaratne [1], Keshawa Weerawarna [1], William Lik Loong Wong [1] and Ravichandran Jeganathan [2]

[1] Jeffrey Cheah School of Medicine and Health Sciences, Monash University Malaysia, Bandar Sunway 47500, Selangor, Malaysia
[2] Department of Obstetrics and Gynaecology, Hospital Sultanah Aminah Johor Bahru, Johor Bahru 81200, Johor, Malaysia
* Correspondence: t.jayanthi@monash.edu

**Abstract:** Ectopic pregnancies (EPs) are potentially fatal if not recognized early. Evidence of an association with chlamydial infection in South East Asia is lacking. This case-control study aims to (i) compare chlamydial infection in women with EP to women who delivered a full-term pregnancy, (ii) investigate classical factors associated with EP, and (iii) investigate rupture status in EP. Seventy-two women with a confirmed diagnosis of EP and sixty-nine who delivered a full-term pregnancy in a tertiary hospital in Malaysia were recruited from November 2019 to January 2022. Demographic and relevant clinical data and intraoperative findings were documented. Blood samples for testing IgG levels of chlamydia were obtained. Women with EP were more likely to have tested positive for chlamydia than those with a full-term delivery (34.7% vs. 13.0%, AOR = 4.18, 95% CI = 1.67–10.48, $p$ = 0.002). The majority did not have the classic risk factors associated with EP. An amount of 52.8% presented with a ruptured EP, with 84.2% of ruptures occurring after six weeks of gestation. An amount of 44.2% had an estimated blood loss of more than 500 cc, with 20% losing more than 1500 cc of blood. The prevalence of prior chlamydial infection in women with EP is significant enough to necessitate a review of early pregnancy care.

**Keywords:** ectopic pregnancy; chlamydia infection

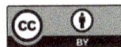

## 1. Introduction

Ectopic pregnancy (EP) was the fourth leading cause of maternal mortality in Malaysia in the years 2019 and 2020 [1]. Common risk factors include infections, surgery, smoking, in vitro fertilization, previous EP, previous pelvic surgery, and intrauterine device use [2–4]. Although the exact pathogenesis of EP is unknown, it is hypothesized that impaired embryo tubal transportation and alterations in the tubal environment result in embryo retention within the fallopian tubes [2,3].

The tubal environment is governed by sex hormones, cytokines, growth factors, expression proteins, and the surveillance of immune cells. Infection-stimulated cytokines are involved in the development of EP. There is an increased interleukin-6 (IL-6) level and leukemia inhibitory factor (LIF) in the fallopian tubes of women with EP [3]. Epithelial shedding due to chronic salpingitis is thought to result in the exposure of the stromal surface in the fallopian tube, producing high levels of the LIF, facilitating the implantation of the arrested embryo [2]. Prior studies postulate that EP could be linked to chronic pelvic inflammation [2,5,6].

*Chlamydia trachomatis* (*C. trachomatis*) has been reported as the most common pathogen that leads to sexually transmitted infections (STIs) [3,7]. The World Health Organization estimates that in 2016, there were 376 million new infections, with one in four being STIs: chlamydia (127 million), gonorrhea (87 million), syphilis (6.3 million), and trichomoniasis

(156 million). *C. trachomatis* is associated with pelvic inflammatory disease, infertility, and EP [8]. Other common bacterial infections include *Neisseria gonorrhoea* and *Mycoplasma genitalium* [3]. In healthy women, the expression of intrauterine integrins is associated with successful intrauterine implantation. However, a prior *C. trachomatis* infection results in increased integrin expression in the tubal epithelial cells, which likely promotes trophoblast attachment leading to EP [9].

A recent meta-analysis concluded that EP was more likely in pregnant women who tested positive than those who did not [6]. Although this meta-analysis categorized eight studies as Asian, only two studies were from South East Asia, namely, Thailand [10] and Vietnam [11], which reported relatively smaller sample sizes. Additionally, studies exploring the prevalence of chlamydia infection in Malaysia were targeted at specific populations such as the urban population [12], prostitutes [13], and those seen at the infertility clinic [14,15]. As there is a scarcity of regional data on the prevalence of *C. trachomatis* infection, presenting features, and intraoperative findings in patients with EP, this study could provide some insight.

Hence, we aimed (i) to compare the prevalence of prior chlamydial infection in women with EP and women who delivered from 37 weeks onwards, (ii) to assess the contribution of chlamydial infection and associated risk factors to EP, and (iii) to document the period of gestation when an EP is more likely to rupture.

## 2. Materials and Methods

### 2.1. Study Design

This was an unmatched case-control study conducted in Hospital Sultanah Aminah Johor Bahru, Malaysia, among adult women (>18 years) with a confirmed diagnosis of EP (case) or admitted for delivery from 37 weeks onwards (control). We obtained ethical approval from the Malaysian Research Ethics Committee (MREC) (NMMR: 18-3214-44797) and the Monash University Human Research Ethics Committee (MUHREC) (ID: 18558) prior to the commencement of the study.

### 2.2. Recruitment and Data Collection

Consenting patients aged 18 and above admitted for management of a confirmed diagnosis of EP were recruited with informed consent. Patients who were clinically stable either pre- or post-operative were recruited. Controls were those aged 18 and above admitted for delivery from 37 weeks onwards. Only those in the latent phase of labor or admitted for labor induction were recruited as controls. Patients above 18 who had impairments such as hearing impairment were excluded.

Demographic data that were collected included age, ethnicity, marital status and education level. Relevant clinical data recorded included the number of sexual partners, parity status, risk factors for EP, and clinical findings. These are tabulated in Tables 1 and 2. Blood samples totaling 5 mL were obtained for testing IgG levels of chlamydia. Detection of chlamydia IgG was performed by an independent external lab using CHLG-chlamydia IgG (immunoblot), and a result, >1.00 was considered positive.

The study recruitment and primary data collection took place at Hospital Sultanah Aminah Johor Bahru, Malaysia, between November 2019 and January 2022. Although an average of two patients with EP were treated per week, data collection was paused during the COVID-19 pandemic due to the government's implementation of the movement control order (MCO). At this center, the primary method of treatment employed for EP was the surgical approach (either laparoscopic or laparotomy). Patients who were clinically stable underwent the laparoscopic approach. However, if there were significant challenges intraoperatively or if the patient had significant hemoperitoneum, the approach was converted to laparotomy.

**Table 1.** Demographic characteristics of the study patients (N = 141).

|  |  | All Patients | Ectopic Pregnancy (Case) | Non-Ectopic Full-Term Pregnancy (Control) | $p$ Value |
|---|---|---|---|---|---|
|  |  | (N = 141) | (n = 72) | (n = 69) |  |
| Age (years) | Mean (SD) | 30.16 (5.07) | 30.44 (4.68) | 29.87 (5.47) | 0.503 |
| Ethnicity | Malay | 112 (79.2) | 59 (81.9) | 53 (76.8) | 0.718 |
|  | Chinese | 10 (7.1) | 4 (5.6) | 6 (8.7) |  |
|  | Indian | 18 (12.8) | 9 (12.5) | 9 (13.0) |  |
|  | East Malaysian Native | 1 (0.7) | 0 (0.0) | 1 (1.4) |  |
| Education | Primary | 4 (2.8) | 2 (2.8) | 2 (2.9) | 0.512 |
|  | Secondary | 72 (51.1) | 40 (55.6) | 32 (46.4) |  |
|  | Tertiary | 65 (46.1) | 30 (41.7) | 35 (50.7) |  |
| Employment | Yes | 93 (66.0) | 49 (68.1) | 44 (63.8) | 0.591 |
|  | No | 48 (34.0) | 23 (31.9) | 25 (36.2) |  |
| Patient's marital status | Single | 4 (2.8) | 2 (2.8) | 2 (2.9) |  |
|  | First marriage | 118 (83.7) | 60 (83.3) | 58 (84.1) |  |
|  | Second marriage or more | 19 (13.5) | 10 (13.9) | 9 (13.0) |  |
| Partner's marital status | Single | 5 (3.5) | 2 (2.8) | 3 (4.3) | 0.816 |
|  | First marriage | 118 (83.7) | 60 (83.3) | 58 (84.1) |  |
|  | Second marriage or more | 18 (12.8) | 10 (13.9) | 8 (11.6) |  |
| Number of partners | 0 | 1 (0.7) | 1 (1.4) | 0 (0.0) | 0.155 |
|  | 1 | 114 (82.0) | 60 (85.7) | 54 (78.3) |  |
|  | 2 | 23 (16.5) | 8 (11.4) | 15 (21.7) |  |
|  | 3 | 1 (0.7) | 1 (1.4) | 0 (0.0) |  |

**Table 2.** Clinical characteristics of the study patients (N = 141).

|  |  | All Patients | Ectopic Pregnancy (Case) | Non-Ectopic Full-Term Pregnancy (Control) | $p$ Value |
|---|---|---|---|---|---|
|  |  | (N = 141) | (n = 72) | (n = 69) |  |
| Gravida | 1 | 49 (34.8) | 30 (41.7) | 19 (27.5) | 0.193 |
|  | 2–3 | 58 (41.1) | 25 (34.7) | 33 (47.8) |  |
|  | 4–5 | 23 (16.3) | 13 (18.1) | 10 (14.5) |  |
|  | More than 5 | 11 (7.8) | 4 (5.6) | 7 (10.1) |  |
| Parity | 0 | 58 (41.1) | 36 (50.0) | 22 (31.9) | 0.088 |
|  | 1–2 | 64 (45.4) | 28 (38.9) | 36 (52.2) |  |
|  | 3–4 | 17 (12.1) | 8 (11.1) | 9 (13.0) |  |
|  | More than 4 | 2 (1.4) | 0 (0.0) | 2 (2.9) |  |
| History of EP | Yes | 5 (3.5) | 4 (5.6) | 1 (1.4) | 0.367 |
|  | No | 136 (96.5) | 68 (94.4) | 68 (98.6) |  |
| History of PID | Yes | 5 (3.5) | 4 (5.6) | 1 (1.4) | 0.367 |
|  | No | 136 (96.5) | 68 (94.4) | 68 (98.6) |  |
| History of pelvic surgery | Yes | 9 (6.4) | 4 (5.8) | 5 (6.9) | 1.000 |
|  | No | 132 (93.6) | 65 (94.2) | 67 (93.1) |  |
| History of smoking | Yes | 8 (5.7) | 5 (6.9) | 3 (4.3) | 0.719 |
|  | No | 133 (94.3) | 67 (93.1) | 66 (95.7) |  |
| Duration of smoking (years) | Mean (SD) | 10.23 (7.90) | 14.60 (6.02) | 2.97 (4.36) | 0.028 * |

Table 2. Cont.

|  |  | All Patients | Ectopic Pregnancy (Case) | Non-Ectopic Full-Term Pregnancy (Control) | p Value |
|---|---|---|---|---|---|
|  |  | (N = 141) | (n = 72) | (n = 69) |  |
| Prior use of copper IUD | Yes | 3 (2.1) | 1 (1.4) | 2 (2.9) | 0.614 |
|  | No | 138 (97.9) | 71 (98.6) | 67 (97.1) |  |
| Purulent per vaginal discharge | Yes | 13 (9.2) | 9 (12.5) | 4 (5.8) | 0.169 |
|  | No | 128 (90.8) | 63 (87.5) | 65 (94.2) |  |
| Abdominal pain with fever | Yes | 6 (4.3) | 4 (5.6) | 2 (2.9) | 0.681 |
|  | No | 135 (95.7) | 68 (94.4) | 67 (97.1) |  |
| Pelvic pain with fever | Yes | 1 (0.7) | 1 (1.4) | 0 (0.0) | 1.000 |
|  | No | 140 (99.3) | 71 (98.6) | 69 (100.0) |  |

EP = ectopic pregnancy, PID = pelvic inflammatory disease. * Significant at $p < 0.05$.

### 2.3. Sample Size Justification

The minimal sample size was estimated using OpenEPI [16] based on the difference in the proportion of outcome (EP) according to parity (1 vs. >3) as reported by Mpiima et al. [17] The authors reported the prevalence of ectopic pregnancy among those in parity of 1 (unexposed) to be 2.38% as opposed to those with parity >3 (exposed) which was 18.75%. A minimum sample size of 66 was required in each group to give the study 80% power at $\alpha = 0.05$ (two-sided).

### 2.4. Statistical Analysis

Data collected were tabulated and analyzed using IBM® SPSS® Statistics Ver.26.0. Descriptive statistics such as frequencies, percentages, means, and standard deviations were used to describe the study participants' characteristics. Associations between categorical variables and study groups were determined with Pearson's chi-square or Fisher's exact tests. Mean values of continuous variables were compared between the study groups using independent t-tests. Multivariable logistic regression (enter method) was used to determine the relationship between chlamydia infection and EP. Variables with a $p$ value >0.25 in the bivariate analysis were adjusted for in the multivariate model. The model's goodness-of-fit was determined using the Hosmer–Lemeshow test. The adjusted model was also assessed for multicollinearity and interactions between variables. Statistical significance was set at $p < 0.05$.

## 3. Results

Seventy-two patients with EP and sixty-nine women with a non-ectopic full-term pregnancy between 37 and 40 weeks of gestation were recruited for the study. The mean age of the study patients was 30.16 years (SD = 5.07 years). The majority of them were of Malay ethnicity (79.1%), were Muslim (80.1%), had at least a secondary level of education (97.2%), and were employed (66%). More than 80% of the patients and their partners were married for the first time and had only one partner. None of the demographic characteristics differed between the study groups (Table 1).

Nine study patients had pelvic surgery performed within the past year. Three patients underwent lower segment caesarean section (LSCS); others underwent one of the following surgeries: appendectomy, dilatation and curettage (D and C), endometrial polypectomy, laparoscopic myomectomy, laparoscopic salpingectomy, and salpingectomy. Although only eight patients had a smoking history, those with EP had been smoking for significantly longer than controls (14.60 ± 6.02 years vs. 2.97 ± 4.36 years, $p = 0.028$). The remaining clinical characteristics did not differ between study groups (Table 2).

Almost a quarter of all pregnancies were also infected with chlamydia, as observed with the presence of chlamydia IgG antibodies (Table 3). Chlamydia infection was more prevalent in EP patients compared to non-ectopic pregnancy patients (34.7% vs. 13.0%). After adjusting for potential confounding factors, the odds for chlamydia infection were higher than four-fold in EP patients than in the control group (aOR = 4.18, 95% CI = 1.67–10.48, $p$ = 0.002).

**Table 3.** Association between chlamydia IgG antibodies and ectopic pregnancies (N = 141).

|  |  | All Patients | Ectopic Pregnancy (Case) | Non-Ectopic Full-Term Pregnancy (Control) |
|---|---|---|---|---|
|  |  | (N = 141) | (n = 72) | (n = 69) |
| Chlamydia IgG antibodies | Positive | 34 (24.1) | 25 (34.7) | 9 (13.0) |
|  | Negative | 107 (75.9) | 47 (65.3) | 60 (87.0) |
| OR [a] (95% CI) $p$ value |  |  | 3.55 (1.51–8.31) 0.004 * | 1.000 |
| aOR [b] (95% CI) $p$ value |  |  | 4.18 (1.67–10.48) 0.002 * | 1.000 |

[a] Unadjusted logistic regression model; [b] Adjusted for number of partners, gravidity, and purulent per vaginal discharge. Model fulfilled Hosmer–Lemeshow test ($p$ = 0.211), multicollinearity, and interaction assumptions. * Significant at $p < 0.05$.

In subsequent analysis, we explored the association between EP-related characteristics and chlamydia IgG antibodies (Table 4). Per vaginal bleeding was twice more common in chlamydia-infected EP cases compared to EP cases negative for the infection (50.0% vs. 24.0%, $p$ = 0.033). The choice of management options also differed between those with and without infection ($p$ = 0.002). Laparotomy salpingectomy was the most common management choice among all patients (47.9%), especially those infected with chlamydia (60.0%). However, laparoscopic salpingectomy was more common among those without the infection (56.5%). Other variables were not found to be associated with chlamydia infection.

**Table 4.** Association between ectopic pregnancy-related characteristics and chlamydia IgG antibodies (n = 72).

|  |  | All EP Patients | Chlamydia IgG Antibodies | | $p$ Value |
|---|---|---|---|---|---|
|  |  |  | Positive | Negative |  |
|  |  | (N = 72) | (n = 25) | (n = 47) |  |
| History of EP | Yes | 4 (5.6) | 1 (4.0) | 3 (6.4) | 1.000 |
|  | No | 68 (94.4) | 24 (96.0) | 44 (93.6) |  |
| History of PID | Yes | 4 (5.6) | 1 (4.0) | 3 (6.4) | 1.000 |
|  | No | 68 (94.4) | 24 (96.0) | 44 (93.6) |  |
| History of pelvic surgery | Yes | 5 (6.9) | 0 (0.0) | 5 (10.6) | 0.156 |
|  | No | 67 (93.1) | 25 (100.0) | 42 (89.4) |  |
| History of smoking | Yes | 5 (6.9) | 1 (4.0) | 4 (8.5) | 0.652 |
|  | No | 67 (93.1) | 24 (96.0) | 43 (91.5) |  |
| Number of partners | 0 | 1 (2.9) | 0 (0.0) | 1 (0.7) | 0.071 |
|  | 1 | 25 (73.5) | 91 (85.0) | 116 (82.3) |  |
|  | 2 | 7 (20.6) | 16 (15.0) | 23 (16.3) |  |
|  | 3 | 1 (2.9) | 0 (0.0) | 1 (0.7) |  |
| Prior use of copper IUD | Yes | 1 (98.6) | 0 (0.0) | 1 (2.1) | 1.000 |
|  | No | 71 (1.4) | 25 (100.0) | 46 (97.9) |  |

Table 4. Cont.

|  |  | All EP Patients | Chlamydia IgG Antibodies | | p Value |
|---|---|---|---|---|---|
|  |  |  | Positive | Negative |  |
|  |  | (N = 72) | (n = 25) | (n = 47) |  |
| Period of gestation (weeks) | Unsure/<5 | 6 (8.5) | 2 98.0) | 4 (8.7) | 0.714 |
|  | 5–5+6 | 4 (5.6) | 0 (0.0) | 4 (8.7) |  |
|  | 6–6+6 | 19 (26.8) | 9 (36.0) | 10 (21.7) |  |
|  | 7–7+6 | 11 (15.5) | 3 (12.0) | 8 (17.4) |  |
|  | 8–8+6 | 23 (32.4) | 7 (28.0) | 16 (34.8) |  |
|  | ≥9 | 8 (11.3) | 4 (16.0) | 4 (8.7) |  |
| Purulent per vaginal discharge | Yes | 9 (12.5) | 4 (16.0) | 5 (10.6) | 0.710 |
|  | No | 63 (84.0) | 21 (84.0) | 42 (89.4) |  |
| Abdominal pain with fever | Yes | 4 (5.6) | 1 (4.0) | 3 (6.4) | 1.000 |
|  | No | 68 (94.4) | 24 (96.0) | 44 (93.6) |  |
| Pelvic pain with fever | Yes | 1 (1.4) | 1 (4.0) | 0 (0.0) | 0.347 |
|  | No | 71 (98.6) | 24 (96.0) | 47 (100.0) |  |
| Ectopic status | Not ruptured | 34 (47.2) | 9 (36.0) | 25 (53.2) | 0.164 |
|  | Ruptured | 38 (52.8) | 16 (64.0) | 22 (46.8) |  |
| Per vaginal bleeding [a] | Yes | 42 (59.2) | 23 (50.0) | 6 (24.0) | 0.033 * |
|  | No | 29 (40.8) | 23 (50.0) | 19 (76.0) |  |
| Abdominal pain [a] | Yes | 60 (84.5) | 20 (80.0) | 40 (87.0) | 0.501 |
|  | No | 11 (15.5) | 5 (20.0) | 6 (13.0) |  |
| Management options [a] | Laparoscopy salpingostomy | 2 (2.8) | 1 (4.0) | 1 (2.2) | 0.002 * |
|  | Laparoscopy salpingectomy | 31 (43.7) | 5 (20.0) | 26 (56.5) |  |
|  | Laparotomy salpingostomy | 2 (2.8) | 2 (8.0) | 0 (0.0) |  |
|  | Laparotomy salpingectomy | 34 (47.9) | 15 (60.0) | 19 (41.3) |  |
|  | Laparotomy cornual resection | 2 (2.8) | 2 (8.0) | 0 (0.0) |  |
| Uterus [b] | Uniformly enlarged | 23 (32.9) | 5 (20.0) | 18 (40.0) | 0.106 |
|  | Fibroids | 1 (1.4) | 1 (4.0) | 0 (0.0) |  |
|  | Normal | 46 (65.7) | 19 (76.0) | 27 (60.0) |  |
| Peritubal adhesions at least one side [b] | Yes | 6 (8.6) | 4 (16.0) | 2 (4.4) | 0.177 |
|  | No | 64 (91.4) | 21 (84.0) | 43 (95.6) |  |
| Peritubal adhesions at both sides [b] | Yes | 2 (2.9) | 2 (8.0) | 0 (0.0) | 0.124 |
|  | No | 68 (97.1) | 23 (92.0) | 45 (100.0) |  |
| Blood loss (ml) [b] | <500 | 39 (55.7) | 11 (44.0) | 28 (62.2) | 0.457 |
|  | 500–999 | 12 (17.1) | 5 (20.0) | 7 (15.6) |  |
|  | 1000–1499 | 5 (7.1) | 2 (8.0) | 3 (6.7) |  |
|  | ≥1500 | 14 (20.0) | 7 (28.0) | 7 (15.6) |  |

[a] n = 71; [b] n = 70. * Significant at p < 0.05.

No association between EP rupture status and gestation period was found (Table 5).

Table 5. Association between gestation period (weeks) and rupture status in ectopic pregnancies.

| Period of Gestation (weeks) | All EP Patients | Rupture Status | | p Value |
| --- | --- | --- | --- | --- |
| | | Ruptured | Not Ruptured | |
| | (N = 71) | (n = 38) | (n = 33) | |
| <5/unsure | 6 (8.5) | 4 (10.5) | 2 (6.1) | 0.517 |
| 5–5+6 | 4 (5.6) | 2 (5.3) | 2 (6.1) | |
| 6–6+6 | 19 (26.8) | 13 (34.2) | 6 (18.2) | |
| 7–7+6 | 11 (15.5) | 4 (10.5) | 7 (21.2) | |
| 8–8+6 | 23 (32.4) | 12 (31.6) | 11 (33.3) | |
| ≥9 | 8 (11.3) | 3 (7.9) | 5 (15.2) | |

## 4. Discussion

In our study, 34.7% of women with EP and 13.0% who delivered full term were IgG positive for chlamydia. Very few studies in South East Asia report the prevalence of chlamydia infection in women with EP. An analysis of 177 women with EP in Vietnam reported that only 24.9% tested IgG positive for chlamydia [11]. In a small study of 32 Thai women with EP, although 34.38% had chlamydia DNA in the fallopian tube, only 21.88% had serum-specific IgG for chlamydia. However, no strong independent association between EP risk and chlamydia antibodies was demonstrated [10]. Detecting chlamydial antibodies decreases with time since the initial infection. However, a higher proportion of women with more than one diagnosed chlamydial infection have detectable antibody levels beyond six months [18]. Based on these two studies [10,18], it can be postulated that our sample of women with EP had chlamydial infections much earlier and tested negative for the antibodies. It could also suggest that the women in our study who tested positive were possibly in the first six months of initial infection or had more than one episode of infection.

Although we reported a higher prevalence of chlamydia antibodies in our participants compared to others from the region, a study conducted in Uganda reported double our figures, where 60% of women with EP and 26.32% of those with an intrauterine pregnancy had chlamydia antibodies [17]. This may be attributed to differences in the prevalence of chlamydia in the general population. Malaysia currently does not have data on the prevalence of chlamydia infection in the general population.

Intraoperatively, only 16.0% of those who were IgG positive and 4.4% who were negative had peri tubal adhesions on at least one side. A developed mathematical model estimated that 10% of untreated chlamydial infections could result in PID [19]. Our findings were not that far off from the estimate of the mathematical model. Peri tubal adhesions in our study were not classified according to any validated scoring system. It should be noted and included in patient counselling that a higher revised American Fertility Society score is associated with a higher occurrence of repeat EPs [20].

Traditional risk factors associated with EP include a history of PID, smoking, history of pelvic surgery, and use of copper IUCD. In our study, none of these factors were significantly associated with EP. Similar findings were reported by another study [21]. Hence, a meta-analysis should be conducted to understand the usefulness of traditional risk factors in current times.

Although there were twenty-five women with EP and nine women with a full-term pregnancy who tested positive, they largely did not report symptoms to suggest PID. This finding is not unique to our study, as other studies have also reported that chlamydia seropositivity was more common than a documented or reported history of infection [22,23].

Other microorganisms such as *Mycoplasma genitalium* [24] and *Neisseria gonorrhoea* [25] also cause PID that can damage the tubes resulting in EP. Although we did not test for these microorganisms, it is known that *C. trachomatis* infection occurs more frequently than *M. genitalium* or *N. gonorrhoea* infection.

A prospective cohort study of 5704 Dutch women (29.5% chlamydia positive) reported an EP incidence rate of 0.8 per 1000 person-years (0.4 to 1.5) in those who had prior chlamydia infection and 0.6 per 1000 person-years (0.4 to 0.6) for women who were chlamydia negative [26]. The incidence of EP in both groups was approximately the same. This, combined with our findings that 65.5% of women with EP tested negative for chlamydia and had no association with traditional risk factors, leads to the question of whether another factor facilitates blastocyst implantation in the fallopian tube before it reaches the uterine cavity. There is also the possibility of undetected microbes colonizing the tubes or even dysbiosis.

Our study aims included documenting the period of gestation (POG) that tubal EP ruptured. Ruptures were seen in 38 (52.8%) women with EP. Although there was no statistically significant specific POG that rupture occurred in our study, 84.2% of EPs ruptured after a six-week POG. Patient factors that led to a delay in seeking early pregnancy care were not explored in our study. This suggests that early self-tests and seeking pregnancy care earlier should be encouraged. A study of 48 women with ruptured EP and 51 women with unruptured EP, reported that the POG for a ruptured EP was $8.0 \pm 0.9$ weeks and $7.3 \pm 1.0$ weeks for an unruptured EP. However, these values were statistically insignificant [27]. In another study of 144 women with ruptured EP and 79 women with unruptured EP, a rupture occurred at $53.9 \pm 4.7$ days ($7.7 \pm 0.7$ weeks). This finding was reported as borderline significant [21]. The plausible reason we failed to document any significant POG for tubal rupture is that the POGs recorded in our study were largely calculated based on the self-reported first day of the last menstrual period, thus, making them less objective.

Approximately 44% ($n = 31$) of the EPs had significant blood loss of more than 500 mls, with approximately half of them having a massive hemorrhage, likely requiring blood transfusion. Approximately 45% ($n = 14$) of this group were IgG positive for chlamydia, while the remainder were negative, which was not statistically significant. However, this degree of hemorrhage remains a contributing factor to maternal morbidity and mortality, as reflected by our recent statistics [1].

Our study is one of the very few studies from South East Asia that documented the presence of chlamydial infection in women with EP compared to women who delivered full term. We found an alarmingly high presence of prior chlamydial infection in women with EP and an unexpected presence of prior infection in women who delivered full term.

A limitation of this study is that we tested only for chlamydial infection and not for other microorganisms such as *M. genitalium* and *N. gonorrhoea*. Another limitation is that the test kit did not discern the type of chlamydia infection. However, *Chlamydia psitacci* infection is uncommon in our population.

## 5. Conclusions

EP continues to be a significant cause of maternal mortality in Malaysia. Early diagnosis and prompt management are crucial as ruptures tend to occur after a six-week POG. Although chlamydial infection is significantly associated with EP, almost two-thirds of the women with EP in our study did not have the infection. Relying on traditional textbook risk factors to formulate a diagnosis is not helpful as our study reported no significant risk factors. A meta-analysis could be conducted to understand the usefulness of traditional risk factors in current times. The authors believe that further research should explore the role of female reproductive tract dysbiosis and the role of passive smoking as causative factors of EP. Research into the duration from which infection occurs until the time EP results could explain why some women with prior chlamydial infection delivered a full-term pregnancy.

**Author Contributions:** Conceptualization, V.J.T.A., D.D.L., R.W.J.S., A.W. and R.J.; Data curation, M.M. and A.R.; Formal analysis, A.R.; Funding acquisition, V.J.T.A.; Investigation, M.M., K.W. and W.L.L.W.; Methodology, V.J.T.A., D.D.L., R.W.J.S. and A.W.; Project administration, V.J.T.A. and N.A.D.; Resources, V.J.T.A. and N.A.D.; Software, A.R.; Supervision, V.J.T.A., N.A.D. and R.J.; Validation, A.R.; Writing—original draft, V.J.T.A., M.M., A.R., D.D.L., R.W.J.S., A.W., K.W. and W.L.L.W.; Writing—review and editing, V.J.T.A., M.M., A.R., N.A.D., D.D.L., R.W.J.S., A.W., K.W., W.L.L.W. and R.J. All authors have read and agreed to the published version of the manuscript.

**Funding:** This study was funded by the Tropical Medicine and Biology Platform Seed grant (TMB-2022-CR3185140918) and the Monash University Malaysia Internal Seed grant (SCH SEED/2020/002).

**Institutional Review Board Statement:** The study was conducted in accordance with the Declaration of Helsinki and approved by the Malaysian Research Ethics Committee (MREC) (NMMR: 18-3214-44797) and the Monash University Human Research Ethics Committee (MUHREC) (ID: 18558).

**Informed Consent Statement:** Informed consent was obtained from all subjects involved in the study.

**Data Availability Statement:** The data presented in this study are available on request from the corresponding author. The data are not publicly available due to informed consent conditions.

**Conflicts of Interest:** The authors declare no conflict of interest.

## References

1. Department of Statistics, Malaysia. *Population and Demography*; Department of Statistics: Putrajaya, Malaysia, 2021.
2. Shaw, J.L.V.; Dey, S.K.; Critchley, H.O.D.; Horne, A.W. Current knowledge of the aetiology of human tubal ectopic pregnancy. *Hum. Reprod. Update* **2010**, *16*, 432–444. [CrossRef] [PubMed]
3. Refaat, B.; Ashshi, A.M.; Batwa, S.A.; Ahmad, J.; Idris, S.; Kutbi, S.Y.; Malibary, F.A.; Kamfar, F.F. The prevalence of *Chlamydia trachomatis* and *Mycoplasma genitalium* tubal infections and their effects on the expression of IL-6 and leukaemia inhibitory factor in Fallopian tubes with and without an ectopic pregnancy. *Innate Immun.* **2016**, *22*, 534–545. [CrossRef] [PubMed]
4. Li, C.; Zhao, W.-H.; Zhu, Q.; Cao, S.J.; Ping, H.; Xi, X.; Qin, G.-J.; Yan, M.-Y.; Zhang, D.; Qiu, J.; et al. Risk factors for ectopic pregnancy: A multi-center case-control study. *BMC Pregnancy Childbirth* **2015**, *15*, 187. [CrossRef] [PubMed]
5. Shaw, J.L.V.; Wills, G.S.; Lee, K.-F.; Horner, P.J.; McClure, M.O.; Abrahams, V.M.; Wheelhouse, N.; Jabbour, H.N.; Critchley, H.O.D.; Entrican, G.; et al. Chlamydia trachomatis Infection increases fallopian tube PROKR2 via TLR2 and NFκB activation resulting in a microenvironment predisposed to ectopic pregnancy. *Am. J. Pathol.* **2011**, *178*, 253–260. [CrossRef] [PubMed]
6. Xia, Q.; Wang, T.; Xian, J.; Song, J.; Qiao, Y.; Mu, Z.; Liu, H.; Sun, Z. Relation of *Chlamydia trachomatis* infections to ectopic pregnancy: A meta-analysis and systematic review. *Medicine* **2020**, *99*, e18489. [CrossRef] [PubMed]
7. Keegan, M.B.; Diedrich, J.T.; Peipert, J.F. *Chlamydia trachomatis* infection: Screening and management. *J. Clin. Outcomes Manag.* **2014**, *21*, 30–38. [PubMed]
8. Rowley, J.; Vander Hoorn, S.; Korenromp, E.; Low, N.; Unemo, M.; Abu-Raddad, L.J.; Chico, R.M.; Smolak, A.; Newman, L.; Gottlieb, S.; et al. Chlamydia, gonorrhoea, trichomoniasis and syphilis: Global prevalence and incidence estimates, 2016. *Bull. World Health Organ.* **2019**, *97*, 548–562. [CrossRef]
9. Ahmad, S.F.; Brown, J.K.; Campbell, L.L.; Koscielniak, M.; Oliver, C.; Wheelhouse, N.; Entrican, G.; McFee, S.; Wills, G.S.; McClure, M.O.; et al. Pelvic chlamydial infection predisposes to ectopic pregnancy by upregulating integrin β1 to promote embryo-tubal attachment. *EBioMedicine* **2018**, *29*, 159–165. [CrossRef]
10. Pientong, C.; Ekalaksananan, T.; Wonglikitpanya, N.; Swadpanich, U.; Kongyingyoes, B.; Kleebkaow, P. *Chlamydia trachomatis* infections and the risk of ectopic pregnancy in Khon Kaen women. *J. Obstet. Gynaecol. Res.* **2009**, *35*, 775–781. [CrossRef]
11. Hornung, S.; Thuong, B.C.; Gyger, J.; Kebbi-Beghdadi, C.; Vasilevsky, S.; Greub, G.; Baud, D. Role of *Chlamydia trachomatis* and emerging Chlamydia-related bacteria in ectopic pregnancy in Vietnam. *Epidemiol. Infect.* **2015**, *143*, 2635–2638. [CrossRef]
12. Ngeow, Y.F.; Rachagan, S.P.; Ramachandran, S. Prevalence of chlamydial antibody in Malaysians. *J. Clin. Pathol.* **1990**, *43*, 400–402. [CrossRef]
13. Ramachandran, S.; Ngeow, Y.F. The prevalence of sexually transmitted diseases among prostitutes in Malaysia. *Genitourin Med.* **1990**, *66*, 334–336. [CrossRef] [PubMed]
14. Yeow, T.C.; Wong, W.F.; Sabet, N.S.; Sulaiman, S.; Shahhosseini, F.; Tan, G.M.Y.; Movahed, F.; Looi, C.Y.; Shankar, E.M.; Gupta, R.; et al. Prevalence of plasmid-bearing and plasmid-free Chlamydia trachomatis infection among women who visited obstetrics and gynecology clinics in Malaysia. *BMC Microbiol.* **2016**, *16*, 45. [CrossRef] [PubMed]
15. Suvra, B.; Zainul, R.; Zalina, I.; Anita, S. Prevalence rates of *Chlamydia Trachomatis* and other sexually transmitted organisms in infertile couples attending a tertiary medical centre in Malaysia. *IIUM Med. J. Malays.* **2020**, *19*, 61–74. [CrossRef]
16. Sullivan, K.M.; Dean, A.; Minn Minn, S.O.E. OpenEpi: A web-based epidemiologic and statistical calculator for public health. *Public Health Rep.* **2009**, *124*, 471–474. [CrossRef] [PubMed]
17. Mpiima, D.P.; Wasswa Salongo, G.; Lugobe, H.; Ssemujju, A.; Mumbere Mulisya, O.; Masinda, A.; Twizerimana, H.; Ngonzi, J. Association between prior *Chlamydia trachomatis* infection and ectopic pregnancy at a tertiary care hospital in South Western Uganda. *Obstet. Gynecol. Int.* **2018**, *2018*, 4827353. [CrossRef]
18. Horner, P.J.; Wills, G.S.; Reynolds, R.; Johnson, A.M.; Muir, D.A.; Winston, A.; Broadbent, A.J.; Parker, D.; McClure, M.O. Effect of time since exposure to *Chlamydia trachomatis* on chlamydia antibody detection in women: A cross-sectional study. *Sex Transm. Infect.* **2013**, *89*, 398–403. [CrossRef]
19. Herzog, S.A.; Althaus, C.L.; Heijne, J.C.M.; Oakeshott, P.; Kerry, S.; Hay, P.; Low, N. Timing of progression from *Chlamydia trachomatis* infection to pelvic inflammatory disease: A mathematical modelling study. *BMC Infect. Dis.* **2012**, *12*, 187. [CrossRef]

20. Kuroda, K.; Takeuchi, H.; Kitade, M.; Kikuchi, I.; Shimanuki, H.; Kumakiri, J.; Kobayashi, Y.; Kuroda, M.; Takeda, S. Assessment of tubal disorder as a risk factor for repeat ectopic pregnancy after laparoscopic surgery for tubal pregnancy. *J. Obstet. Gynaecol. Res.* **2009**, *35*, 520–524. [CrossRef]
21. Sindos, M.; Togia, A.; Sergentanis, T.N.; Kabagiannis, A.; Malamas, F.; Farfaras, A.; Sergentanis, I.N.; Bassiotou, V.; Antoniou, S. Ruptured ectopic pregnancy: Risk factors for a life-threatening condition. *Arch. Gynecol. Obstet.* **2008**, *279*, 621. [CrossRef]
22. Gorwitz, R.J.; Wiesenfeld, H.C.; Chen, P.L.; Hammond, K.R.; Sereday, K.A.; Haggerty, C.L.; Johnson, R.E.; Papp, J.R.; Kissin, D.M.; Henning, T.C.; et al. Population-attributable fraction of tubal factor infertility associated with chlamydia. *Am. J. Obstet. Gynecol.* **2017**, *217*, 336.e1–336.e16. [CrossRef] [PubMed]
23. Verweij, S.; Kebbi-Beghdadi, C.; Land, J.; Ouburg, S.; Morre, S.A.; Greub, G. Chondrophila and Chlamydia trachomatis antibodies in screening infertile women for tubal pathology. *Microbes Infect.* **2015**, *17*, 745–748. [CrossRef] [PubMed]
24. Bjartling, C.; Osser, S.; Persson, K. Mycoplasma genitalium in cervicitis and pelvic inflammatory disease among women at a gynecologic outpatient service. *Am. J. Obstet. Gynecol.* **2012**, *206*, 476.e1–476.e8. [CrossRef] [PubMed]
25. Burnett, A.M.; Anderson, C.P.; Zwank, M.D. Laboratory-confirmed gonorrhea and/or chlamydia rates in clinically diagnosed pelvic inflammatory disease and cervicitis. *Am. J. Emerg. Med.* **2012**, *30*, 1114–1117. [CrossRef]
26. Hoenderboom, B.M.; van Benthem, B.H.B.; van Bergen, J.E.A.M.; Dukers-Muijrers, N.H.; Götz, H.M.; Hoebe, C.J.; Hogewoning, A.A.; Land, J.A.; van der Sande, M.A.B.; Morré, S.A.; et al. Relation between Chlamydia trachomatis infection and pelvic inflammatory disease, ectopic pregnancy and tubal factor infertility in a Dutch cohort of women previously tested for chlamydia in a chlamydia screening trial. *Sex Transm. Infect.* **2019**, *95*, 300–306.
27. Roussos, D.; Panidis, D.; Matalliotakis, I.; Mavromatidis, G.; Neonaki, M.; Mamopoulos, M.; Koumantakis, E. Factors that may predispose to rupture of tubal ectopic pregnancy. *Eur. J. Obstet. Gynecol. Reprod. Biol.* **2000**, *89*, 15–17. [CrossRef]

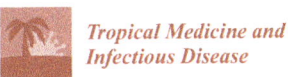 

*Article*

# Combining Immunoassays to Identify Zika Virus Infection in Dengue-Endemic Areas

Pichamon Sittikul, Pimolpachr Sriburin, Jittraporn Rattanamahaphoom, Kriengsak Limkittikul, Chukiat Sirivichayakul and Supawat Chatchen *

Department of Tropical Pediatrics, Faculty of Tropical Medicine, Mahidol University, Bangkok 10400, Thailand
* Correspondence: supawat.cht@mahidol.ac.th; Tel.: +66-2-3549161

**Abstract:** Zika virus (ZIKV) is a mosquito-borne flavivirus that has recently emerged as a global health threat. The rise in ZIKV infections has driven an increased incidence of neonates born with microcephaly or other neurological malformations. Therefore, screening for ZIKV infection can considerably impact pregnant women, especially during the first trimester. The majority of ZIKV infections are mild or asymptomatic, and clinical diagnosis is inaccurate. Moreover, given the high level of cross-reactivity among flaviviruses, serological approaches to distinguish ZIKV from dengue virus (DENV) infections are complicated. We used the combination of DENV and ZIKV nonstructural protein 1 (NS1) IgG enzyme-linked immunosorbent assay (ELISA) and ZIKV NS1 blockade-of-binding (BOB) ELISA to test the convalescent sera of non-flavivirus, primary DENV, secondary DENV, and ZIKV infections. Our findings indicate that primary testing using a ZIKV NS1 IgG ELISA, the test of choice for large-scale ZIKV serosurvey studies, provided relatively high sensitivity. Moreover, the confirmation of positive ELISA results using the ZIKV NS1 BOB ELISA increased average specificity to 94.59% across serum samples. The combined use of two simple ELISAs for ZIKV serosurveys and the monitoring of ZIKV infection during pregnancy can elucidate the epidemiology, pathogenesis, and complications of ZIKV in DENV-endemic areas.

**Keywords:** Zika virus; dengue virus; nonstructural protein 1; serological diagnosis; cross-reactivity

## 1. Introduction

Zika virus (ZIKV) is an enveloped RNA virus in the family *Flaviviridae*, genus *Flavivirus* and is similar to other clinically relevant flaviviruses (e.g., dengue virus (DENV), Japanese encephalitis virus, and yellow fever virus) [1]. ZIKV is transmitted by mosquitoes, primarily the *Aedes aegypti* and the *Aedes albopictus*. ZIKV can be further transmitted through sexual, mother-to-fetus, and blood transfusion routes [2]. With a genome length of approximately 11 kb, the ZIKV is a positive-sense, single-stranded RNA virus that codes for three structural proteins—capsid, pre-membrane, and envelope—and seven nonstructural proteins: nonstructural protein 1 (NS1), NS2a, NS2b, NS3, NS4a, NS4b, and NS5p [3]. NS1 is involved in viral replication, immune evasion, and pathogenesis and is considered an important antigenic marker of ZIKV and other flaviviruses [4]. Antibodies to NS1 have high sensitivity and limited cross-reactivity, suggesting that NS1 may represent an efficient differential assay for DENV and ZIKV infections [5]. ZIKV was originally identified in 1947 in a rhesus monkey in the Zika Forest of Uganda. From there, ZIKV has spread slowly throughout Africa and Asia. The first outbreak of ZIKV infection occurred in 2007 in Yap State, Micronesia, in the western Pacific Ocean [6,7]. The first report on the possible presence of ZIKV in Thailand was published in 1963 [8]. In 2016, small outbreaks of ZIKV infection were reported in Singapore [9], and several hundred cases were detected in Thailand in the same year [10].

ZIKV infections generally cause mild and self-limited illness. However, the infection can cause Guillain–Barré syndrome in adults and microcephaly in infants born to ZIKV-infected women [11]. Therefore, screening for ZIKV infections can considerably impact

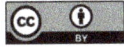

pregnant women, especially during the first trimester [10,12]. The diagnosis of acute ZIKV infection is made through the detection of its viral components (RNA or viral NS1 proteins) within 2 weeks of illness [13]. ZIKV RNA can be detected in a variety of specimens, including blood, serum, plasma, saliva, semen, and cerebrospinal fluid. The detection of viral components is highly sensitive and specific, but the effectiveness of the ZIKV RNA assay is limited by the short period of viremia [14]. Further, serological assays for ZIKV antibodies are widely used for diagnosis, particularly after 2 weeks of the onset of illness, in seroprevalence studies, or in prenatal screening. Unfortunately, ZIKV's cross-reactivity with other antigenically similar flaviviruses—DENV in particular—is a challenging problem in areas such as Thailand, where these viruses co-circulate and where ZIKV infection is considerably less prevalent than DENV infection [15]. Therefore, positive serological test results should be confirmed with tests—such as the plaque reduction neutralization test (PRNT)—that use an alternative platform. However, the PRNT is low-throughput and requires a longer turnaround time (3–7 days) compared with ELISA. Moreover, the need for experienced and highly trained personnel makes the use of the PRNT challenging in a high-volume clinical test setting [1,13,16]. Considerable research has been conducted to develop serological strategies—including the development of the ZIKV NS1 IgG enzyme-linked immunosorbent assay (ELISA) [17,18], the blockade-of-binding (BOB) ELISA [16,19], the microneutralization assay [16], and a cytopathic effect-based virus neutralization test—for more specific ZIKV antibody detection in DENV-endemic areas [15]. In this study, we identified an efficient and practicable strategy that can be used in large-scale ZIKV seroprevalence studies. The strategy relies on primary testing using NS1 IgG ELISA followed by a ZIKV NS1 BOB ELISA for confirmation of positive ELISA results.

## 2. Materials and Methods

*2.1. Serum Samples*

The convalescent sample (1–2 weeks after symptoms onset) in this study was selected from a cohort study of the epidemiology of dengue disease conducted from 2006 to 2009 in school-aged children in Ratchaburi province, Thailand [20]. We used 10 human convalescent sera with primary DENV infections (50% male, age less than 15 years old, DENV serotype 1–4) and 21 human convalescent sera with secondary DENV infections (61.9% male, age less than 15 years old, DENV serotype 1–4) that had a detectable DENV infection by reverse transcription PCR (RT-PCR). Six human convalescent sera with non-flavivirus infection (tested by ELISA and PRNT) were included in the study.

All 30 ZIKV-positive samples (1–2 weeks after symptoms onset) were selected from a study of Zika incidence in dengue epidemiology study in Ratchaburi province, Thailand [20,21]. All samples showed seropositivity using ZIKV NS1 IgG ELISA, and ZIKV infection was confirmed by RT-PCR in acute sera [21]. All procedures were ethically approved before the study (TMEC 21-013).

*2.2. Production of ZIKV and DENV NS1*

Full-length NS1 genes from ZIKV strain SV0127 and DENV serotypes 1, 2, 3, and 4 with NCBI accession numbers KU681081.3, AF180817.1, KU725663.1, KU725665.1, and M14931.2, respectively, were amplified using SuperScrip III One-Step RT-PCR (Invitrogen, Thermo Fisher Scientific, Inc., Waltham, MA, USA) and cloned into pET vectors (Novagen, Sigma-Aldrich, Burlington, MA, USA). The NS1 proteins were over-expressed in *E. coli* BL21 (DE3) in Luria Broth (LB) medium supplemented with 50 μg/mL kanamycin. The optimal conditions for protein expression included keeping cells at 25 °C overnight and inducing them with 1 mM isopropyl β-D-1-thiogalactopyranoside (IPTG) (Bio Basic, Amherst, NY, USA). After expression, cells were harvested by centrifugation at 4000 rpm for 30 min at 4 °C. Cell pellets were resuspended in 1×PBS and were subsequently sonicated by Sonics Vibra Cell VCX750 (Sonics & Material, Inc., Newtown, CT, USA) for 30 min (pulse on 5 s; pulse off 5 s). After sonication, the cell lysate was centrifuged at 10,000 rpm for 30 min at 4 °C. The insoluble protein was solubilized in denatured buffer (50 mM Tris-HCl pH 8, 0.5 M NaCl, 0.03 M imidazole, and 8 M urea). Proteins were purified using the HisTrap column (GE Healthcare, Chicago, IL, USA) under denaturing conditions. The purities of NS1 proteins with a molecular weight of 40 kDa were analyzed using 12% SDS-PAGE. Protein concentrations were measured using a NanoDrop spectrophotometer (Thermo Fisher Scientific, Inc., Waltham, MA, USA), and proteins were kept at −80 °C until used.

### 2.3. Indirect ELISA

Indirect ELISA was performed using a previously described standard protocol [21,22]. In brief, plates were sensitized with ZIKV NS1 (10 µg/mL or 500 ng/well), DENV 1–4 NS1 (5 µg/mL, 250 ng for each serotype or a total of 1000 ng/well), or inactivated ZIKV (MR766) in PBS buffer and incubated at 37 °C overnight. After incubation, plates were washed six times with PBS containing 0.05% Tween20 (200 µL/well) and blocked at 4 °C overnight with 200 µL of PBS containing 5% skim milk. After blocking, plates were washed six times with PBS containing 0.05% Tween20 (200 µL/well), 50 µL of tested serum (dilution 1:1000) was added, and plates were incubated at 37 °C for 1 h. Then, plates were washed six times with PBS containing 0.05% Tween20 (200 µL/well), 50 µL conjugate (goat anti-human IgG-HRP, dilution 1:10,000) was added, and plates were incubated at 37 °C for 1 h. After incubation, plates were washed six times with PBS containing 0.05% Tween20 (200 µL/well), 100 µL substrate (SureBlue TMB microwell peroxidase) was added, and plates were incubated for 30 min at room temperature. The reaction was stopped by adding 0.4 M $H_2SO_4$, and the absorbance was read at 450 nm. P/N ratio is the ratio of the average $OD_{450}$ of the test sample divided by the average $OD_{450}$ of the negative sample. The P/N ratio $\geq 2$ was considered to be positive.

### 2.4. ZIKV NS1 BOB ELISA

ZIKV NS1 BOB ELISA was performed as described in a previous report [19]. The ELISA microplate (Greiner Bio-One, Kremsmünster, Austria) was coated overnight at 4 °C with 1 µg/mL ZIKV NS1 MR766 strain (Aviva Systems Biology, San Diego, CA, USA; 50 µL/well). After incubation, plates were washed twice with PBS containing 0.05% Tween20 (200 µL/well) and blocked at room temperature for 1 h with PBS containing 1% BSA (200 µL/well). After blocking, plates were washed twice with PBS containing 0.05% Tween20 (200 µL/well). Then, 50 µL serum (1:10 dilution) or positive control ZKA35 (Absolute Antibody, UK) was added to ZIKV NS1-coated ELISA plates, and plates were incubated for 1 h at room temperature. Then, 50 µL of ZKA35-HRP conjugate (Absolute Antibody, UK) was added, and the mixture was incubated at room temperature for 1 h. After incubation, plates were washed four times with PBS containing 0.05% Tween20 (200 µL/well). After washing, 50 µL substrate (SureBlue TMB microwell peroxidase substrate) was added, and plates were incubated for 30 min at room temperature. The reaction was stopped by adding 0.4 M $H_2SO_4$, and the absorbance was read at 450 nm. The % inhibition was calculated according to the following equation:

$$\% \text{ inhibition} = ([OD \text{ sample} - OD \text{ neg ctr}]/[OD \text{ pos ctr} - OD \text{ neg ctr}]) \times 100$$

## 3. Results

### 3.1. Analysis of Convalescent Samples of DENV-Infected Patients

In this study, specificity and cross-reactivity were further evaluated using convalescent serum samples derived from DENV-infected patients. The ELISA using the whole ZIKV antigen poorly identified DENV infections, particularly in secondary DENV infection (Figure 1A, Table 1). In the ZIKV NS1 IgG ELISA, one serum sample (10%) from the primary DENV infection group showed cross-reactivity, whereas 10 out of 21 samples (47.6%) from the secondary DENV infection group cross-reacted with ZIKV NS1 (Figure 1B, Table 1). In combined use of the ZIKV and DENV NS1 IgG ELISA, furthermore, the cross-reaction was decreased when the P/N ratio of ZIKV NS1/DENV-NS1 was used. Only two samples (9.52%) of secondary DENV infection showed cross-reactivity with ZIKV (Figure 1C).

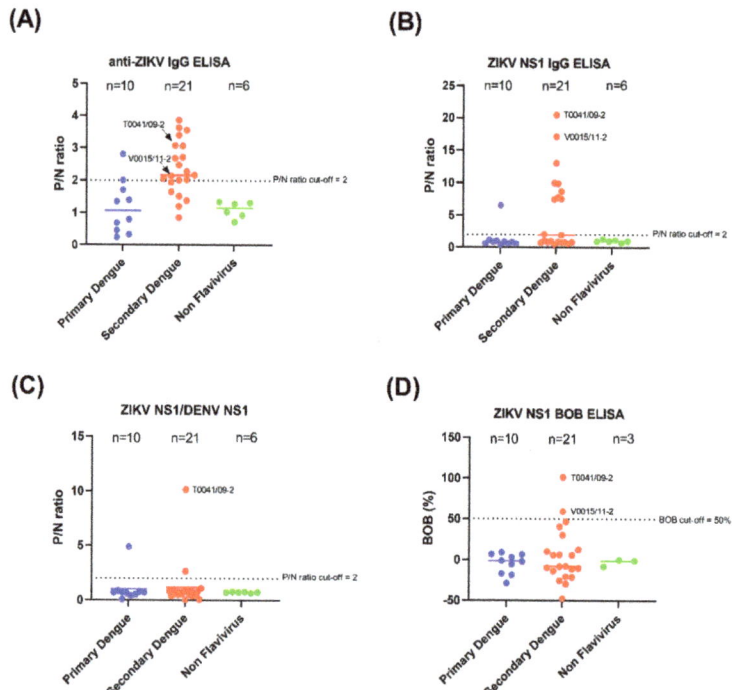

**Figure 1.** The performance of serological assays using DENV infection samples in the convalescent phase. (**A**) anti-ZIKV IgG ELISA. (**B**) ZIKV NS1 IgG ELISA. (**C**) ZIKV NS1/DENV NS1 IgG ELISA. (**D**) ZIKV NS1 BOB ELISA. The dotted line represents the cut-off value of the P/N ratio or %BOB inhibition. ZIKV: Zika virus, DENV: dengue virus, ELISA: enzyme-linked immunosorbent assay, BOB: blockade-of-binding, NS1: nonstructural protein 1, P/N ratio: ratio of average $OD_{450}$ of test sample divided by the average $OD_{450}$ of the negative sample.

**Table 1.** Results of enzyme-linked immunosorbent assays in various serum panels.

| Sample/Test | ZIKV IgG | | | ZIKV NS1-IgG | | | ZIKV NS1-IgG /DENV NS1-IgG | | | BOB | | | ZIKV NS1-IgG followed by BOB | | |
|---|---|---|---|---|---|---|---|---|---|---|---|---|---|---|---|
| | + | − | % | + | − | % | + | − | % | + | − | % | + | − | % |
| Non-flavivirus ($n = 6$) | 0 | 6 | 0% | 0 | 6 | 0% | 0 | 6 | 0% | 0 | 3 | 0% | 0 | 3 | 0% |
| Primary DENV ($n = 10$) | 2 | 8 | 20% | 1 | 9 | 10% | 1 | 9 | 10% | 0 | 10 | 0% | 0 | 10 | 0% |
| Secondary DENV ($n = 21$) | 15 | 6 | 71.4% | 10 | 11 | 47.6% | 2 | 19 | 9.52% | 2 | 19 | 9.52% | 2 | 19 | 9.52% |
| ZIKV ($n = 30$) | 30 | 0 | 100% | 30 | 0 | 100% | 9 | 21 | 30% | 3 | 27 | 10% | 3 | 27 | 10% |

The BOB ELISA relies on the ability of serum antibodies to block the binding of a monoclonal antibody (mAb) to an antigen adsorbed on a microtiter ELISA plate; this assay showed high specificity [19]. Interestingly, the specificity was 90.48% when secondary DENV samples were tested with the ZIKV NS1 BOB ELISA (Figure 1D; Table 2). The combined use of the P/N ratio of ZIKV-NS1/DENV NS1 and the ZIKV NS1 BOB test distinguished ZIKV infections from DENV infections.

**Table 2.** Sensitivity and specificity to ZIKV of enzyme-linked immunosorbent assays.

| ELISA | Sensitivity (95% CI) | Specificity | | |
|---|---|---|---|---|
| | | In Primary DENV Samples (95% CI) | In Secondary DENV Samples (95% CI) | In Overall Serum Samples (95% CI) |
| ZIKV IgG | 100% (88.7–100%) | 80% (49.0–96.5%) | 28.57% (13.8–50%) | 54.05% (38.4–69%) |
| ZIKV NS1-IgG | 100% (88.7–100%) | 90% (59.6–99.5%) | 52.4% (32.4–71.7%) | 70.27% (54.2–82.5%) |
| ZIKV NS1-IgG/DENV NS1-IgG | 30% (16.7–47.9%) | 90% (59.6–99.5%) | 90.48% (71.1–98.3%) | 91.89% (78.7–97.2%) |
| BOB | 10% (3.5–25.6%) | 100% (72.3–100%) | 90.48% (71.1–98.3%) | 94.59% (82.3–99%) |
| ZIKV NS1-IgG followed by BOB | 10% (3.5–25.6%) | 100% (72.3–100%) | 90.48% (71.1–98.3%) | 94.59% (82.3–99%) |

*3.2. Analysis of Zika Infection Samples in the Convalescent Phase*

Recently, our group reported using ZIKV NS1 IgG ELISA screening to identify symptomatic ZIKV infections [21]. However, only the sample with a high P/N ratio (>10) showed a positive score with the ZIKV NS1 BOB ELISA, as shown in Figure 2A,B. We performed a longitudinal study to gain more knowledge of Zika antibody dynamics and the duration of protection after ZIKV infection. We tested three annual blood samples (01-0464, 07-0052, and 01-0493) that were positive for the ZIKV NS1 BOB assay and observed that the antibody can be detected after one year (Figure 2C,D).

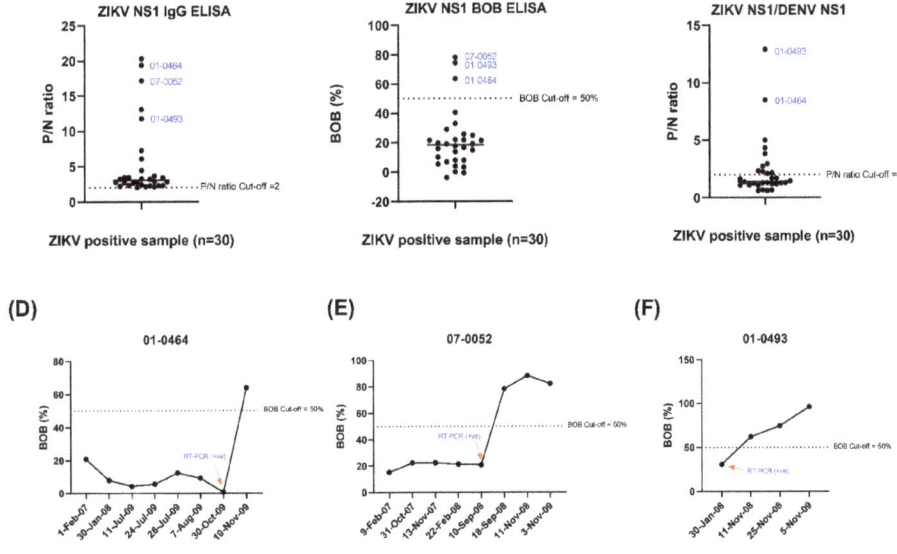

**Figure 2.** Performance of serological assay using ZIKV infection samples in the convalescent phase. (**A**) ZIKV NS1 ELISA. The dotted line represents the cut-off value of the P/N ratio. (**B**) ZIKV NS1 BOB ELISA. The dotted line represents the cut-off value of % BOB inhibition. (**C**) ZIKV NS1/DENV NS1 ELISA. The dotted line represents the cut-off value of the P/N ratio. (**D–F**) ZIKV NS1 BOB ELISA in a sequential annual blood sample of three ZIKV infection patients (01-0464, 07-0052, and 01-0493). The red arrow indicates the date of ZIKV RT-PCR positivity. The dotted lines represent the cut-off value of % BOB inhibition. ZIKV: Zika virus, DENV: dengue virus, ELISA: enzyme-linked immunosorbent assay, BOB: blockade-of-binding, NS1: nonstructural protein 1, P/N ratio: ratio of average $OD_{450}$ of test sample divided by the average $OD_{450}$ of the negative sample.

Our study showed that the ZIKV NS1 BOB test was highly specific in discriminating ZIKV infection from DENV infection and was recommended as the test for confirmation; however, the sensitivity was low compared to that of the ZIKV NS1 IgG ELISA. The combined use of the ZIKV NS1 IgG and the DENV NS1 IgG ELISAs can provide an alternative approach to better determine ZIKV serostatus in DENV-endemic areas.

## 4. Discussion

The serological diagnosis of ZIKV is challenging in dengue-endemic areas. Our study concluded that an effective testing method remains unavailable. The ZIKV IgG and ZIKV NS1 IgG ELISAs provide high sensitivity but low specificity (54% for ZIKV IgG and 70% for ZIKV NS1 IgG), particularly in patients with secondary DENV infection. The low specificity can be explained by the cross-reactivity between DENV and ZIKV antibodies [4]. The lower specificity in patients after secondary DENV infection can be attributed to the characteristically broader antibody response to the antigens of the flavivirus group after secondary DENV infection, while the antibody response after primary DENV infection is predominantly against the type-specific determinant [23]. The sensitivity of the ZIKV NS1 BOB test was lower than that of the ZIKV NS1 IgG ELISA, consistent with a previous study indicating that the sensitivity of a ZIKV NS1 BOB ELISA using F9 mAb was lower than that of the Zika microneutralization assay, especially in samples collected more than 6 months post-infection [16]. The high specificity (90%) of the ZIKV NS1 BOB ELISA is the test's strength. Our results indicated that the ZIKV NS1 BOB ELISA showed no cross-reactivity with primary DENV samples and non-flavivirus infection and that the antibody can be detected after more than one year. However, the ZIKV NS1 BOB ELISA requires monoclonal antibodies and commercial NS1 proteins [19]. In addition, the combined use of ZIKV and DENV NS1 ELISAs was applied to distinguish ZIKV from previous DENV infections [17]. A test using the P/N ratio of ZIKV NS1/DENV NS1 provided specificity comparable to that of the ZIKV BOB ELISA and higher sensitivity (30%); however, this level of sensitivity remains unacceptably low. Primary testing using an NS1 IgG ELISA followed by a ZIKV NS1 BOB ELISA for confirmation of positive ELISA results can decrease the cost of expensive ZIKV NS1 BOB ELISA testing but does not increase sensitivity. Given that the ZIKV NS1 IgG ELISA is cost-effective because it uses an in-house NS1 protein and provides relatively high sensitivity and specificity, we propose this ELISA as the test of choice for Zika seroepidemiological studies. In areas where the incidence of ZIKV is very low, and that of DENV is very high, confirmation of ZIKV infection using the ZIKV NS1 BOB test or the P/N ratio of ZIKV NS1/DENV NS1 can be applied to increase the study accuracy.

The limitations of this study were also considered. The study samples were taken from the previously archived serum from the children in the dengue-endemic area, and the sample numbers for each group were limited.

## 5. Conclusions

This study supports that the combined use of two simple ELISAs (DENV NS1 and ZIKV NS1) for ZIKV serosurveys and the monitoring of ZIKV infection during pregnancy can elucidate the epidemiology, pathogenesis, and complications of ZIKV in DENV-endemic areas.

**Author Contributions:** S.C. conceived and developed the study design. S.C. and P.S. (Pichamon Sittikul) wrote the manuscript. P.S. (Pichamon Sittikul), J.R., and P.S. (Pimolpachr Sriburin) performed ELISA and BOB testing. C.S. and K.L. contributed to the overall research strategy and revised the manuscript. S.C. finalized the manuscript. All authors have read and agreed to the published version of the manuscript.

**Funding:** This study was supported by the Department of Tropical Pediatrics, Faculty of Tropical Medicine, Mahidol University, and the APC was funded by Mahidol University and the Faculty of Tropical Medicine, Mahidol University, Thailand.

**Institutional Review Board Statement:** The study was conducted according to the guidelines of the Declaration of Helsinki, and approved by the ethics committee of the Faculty of Tropical Medicine, Mahidol University (no. TMEC 21-013).

**Informed Consent Statement:** Not applicable.

**Data Availability Statement:** Not applicable.

**Acknowledgments:** The authors would like to thank Arunee Sabchareon for providing the archived samples of a dengue cohort study in children in Ratchaburi, Thailand. We thank Anahid Pinchis for editing a draft of this manuscript.

**Conflicts of Interest:** The authors declare no conflict of interest.

## References

1. Plourde, A.R.; Bloch, E.M. A Literature Review of Zika Virus. *Emerg. Infect. Dis.* **2016**, *22*, 1185–1192. [CrossRef] [PubMed]
2. Shan, C.; Xie, X.; Barrett, A.D.; Garcia-Blanco, M.A.; Tesh, R.B.; Vasconcelos, P.F.; Vasilakis, N.; Weaver, S.C.; Shi, P.Y. Zika Virus: Diagnosis, Therapeutics, and Vaccine. *ACS Infect. Dis.* **2016**, *2*, 170–172. [CrossRef] [PubMed]
3. Ayres, C.F.J.; Guedes, D.R.D.; Paiva, M.H.S.; Morais-Sobral, M.C.; Krokovsky, L.; Machado, L.C.; Melo-Santos, M.A.V.; Crespo, M.; Oliveira, C.M.F.; Ribeiro, R.S.; et al. Zika virus detection, isolation and genome sequencing through Culicidae sampling during the epidemic in Vitória, Espírito Santo, Brazil. *Parasites Vectors* **2019**, *12*, 220. [CrossRef] [PubMed]
4. Silva, I.B.B.; da Silva, A.S.; Cunha, M.S.; Cabral, A.D.; de Oliveira, K.C.A.; Gaspari, E.; Prudencio, C.R. Zika virus serological diagnosis: Commercial tests and monoclonal antibodies as tools. *J. Venom. Anim. Toxins Incl. Trop Dis.* **2020**, *26*, e20200019. [CrossRef] [PubMed]
5. Stettler, K.; Beltramello, M.; Espinosa, D.A.; Graham, V.; Cassotta, A.; Bianchi, S.; Vanzetta, F.; Minola, A.; Jaconi, S.; Mele, F.; et al. Specificity, cross-reactivity, and function of antibodies elicited by Zika virus infection. *Science* **2016**, *353*, 823–826. [CrossRef] [PubMed]
6. Wikan, N.; Smith, D.R. Zika virus: History of a newly emerging arbovirus. *Lancet Infect. Dis.* **2016**, *16*, e119–e126. [CrossRef]
7. Duffy, M.R.; Chen, T.H.; Hancock, W.T.; Powers, A.M.; Kool, J.L.; Lanciotti, R.S.; Pretrick, M.; Marfel, M.; Holzbauer, S.; Dubray, C.; et al. Zika virus outbreak on Yap Island, Federated States of Micronesia. *N. Engl. J. Med.* **2009**, *360*, 2536–2543. [CrossRef] [PubMed]
8. Pond, W.L. Arthropod-Borne virus antibodies in sera from residents of South-East Asia. *Trans. R. Soc. Trop. Med. Hyg.* **1963**, *57*, 364–371. [CrossRef]
9. Ho, Z.J.M.; Hapuarachchi, H.C.; Barkham, T.; Chow, A.; Ng, L.C.; Lee, J.M.V.; Leo, Y.S.; Prem, K.; Lim, Y.H.G.; de Sessions, P.F.; et al. Outbreak of Zika virus infection in Singapore: An epidemiological, entomological, virological, and clinical analysis. *Lancet Infect. Dis.* **2017**, *17*, 813–821. [CrossRef]
10. Khongwichit, S.; Wikan, N.; Auewarakul, P.; Smith, D.R. Zika virus in Thailand. *Microbes. Infect.* **2018**, *20*, 670–675. [CrossRef]
11. Song, B.-H.; Yun, S.-I.; Woolley, M.; Lee, Y.-M. Zika virus: History, epidemiology, transmission, and clinical presentation. *J. Neuroimmunol.* **2017**, *308*, 50–64. [CrossRef] [PubMed]
12. Phatihattakorn, C.; Wongsa, A.; Pongpan, K.; Anuwuthinawin, S.; Mungmanthong, S.; Wongprasert, M.; Tassaneetrithep, B. Seroprevalence of Zika virus in pregnant women from central Thailand. *PLoS ONE* **2021**, *16*, e0257205. [CrossRef]
13. Herrada, C.A.; Kabir, M.A.; Altamirano, R.; Asghar, W. Advances in Diagnostic Methods for Zika Virus Infection. *J. Med. Device.* **2018**, *12*, 0408021–4080211. [CrossRef] [PubMed]
14. Shan, C.; Ortiz, D.A.; Yang, Y.; Wong, S.J.; Kramer, L.D.; Shi, P.Y.; Loeffelholz, M.J.; Ren, P. Evaluation of a Novel Reporter Virus Neutralization Test for Serological Diagnosis of Zika and Dengue Virus Infection. *J. Clin. Microbiol.* **2017**, *55*, 3028–3036. [CrossRef]
15. Nurtop, E.; Villarroel, P.M.S.; Pastorino, B.; Ninove, L.; Drexler, J.F.; Roca, Y.; Gake, B.; Dubot-Peres, A.; Grard, G.; Peyrefitte, C.; et al. Combination of ELISA screening and seroneutralisation tests to expedite Zika virus seroprevalence studies. *Virol. J.* **2018**, *15*, 192. [CrossRef] [PubMed]
16. Nascimento, E.J.M.; Bonaparte, M.I.; Luo, P.; Vincent, T.S.; Hu, B.; George, J.K.; Áñez, G.; Noriega, F.; Zheng, L.; Huleatt, J.W. Use of a Blockade-of-Binding ELISA and Microneutralization Assay to Evaluate Zika Virus Serostatus in Dengue-Endemic Areas. *Am. J. Trop. Med. Hyg.* **2019**, *101*, 708–715. [CrossRef] [PubMed]
17. Tsai, W.Y.; Youn, H.H.; Brites, C.; Tsai, J.J.; Tyson, J.; Pedroso, C.; Drexler, J.F.; Stone, M.; Simmons, G.; Busch, M.P.; et al. Distinguishing Secondary Dengue Virus Infection from Zika Virus Infection with Previous Dengue by a Combination of 3 Simple Serological Tests. *Clin. Infect. Dis.* **2017**, *65*, 1829–1836. [CrossRef]
18. Pereira, S.S.; Andreata-Santos, R.; Pereira, L.R.; Soares, C.P.; Félix, A.C.; de Andrade, P.; Durigon, E.L.; Romano, C.M.; Ferreira, L.C.S. NS1-based ELISA test efficiently detects dengue infections without cross-reactivity with Zika virus. *Int. J. Infect. Dis.* **2021**, *112*, 202–204. [CrossRef] [PubMed]
19. Balmaseda, A.; Stettler, K.; Medialdea-Carrera, R.; Collado, D.; Jin, X.; Zambrana, J.V.; Jaconi, S.; Cameroni, E.; Saborio, S.; Rovida, F.; et al. Antibody-based assay discriminates Zika virus infection from other flaviviruses. *Proc. Natl. Acad. Sci. USA* **2017**, *114*, 8384–8389. [CrossRef]

20. Sabchareon, A.; Sirivichayakul, C.; Limkittikul, K.; Chanthavanich, P.; Suvannadabba, S.; Jiwariyavej, V.; Dulyachai, W.; Pengsaa, K.; Margolis, H.S.; Letson, G.W. Dengue infection in children in Ratchaburi, Thailand: A cohort study. I. Epidemiology of symptomatic acute dengue infection in children, 2006–2009. *PLoS Negl. Trop. Dis.* **2012**, *6*, e1732. [CrossRef]
21. Sriburin, P.; Sittikul, P.; Kosoltanapiwat, N.; Sirinam, S.; Arunsodsai, W.; Sirivichayakul, C.; Limkittikul, K.; Chatchen, S. Incidence of Zika Virus Infection from a Dengue Epidemiological Study of Children in Ratchaburi Province, Thailand. *Viruses* **2021**, *13*, 1802. [CrossRef] [PubMed]
22. Sirinam, S.; Chatchen, S.; Arunsodsai, W.; Guharat, S.; Limkittikul, K. Seroprevalence of Zika Virus in Amphawa District, Thailand, after the 2016 Pandemic. *Viruses* **2022**, *14*, 476. [CrossRef] [PubMed]
23. Russell, P.K.; Udomsakdi, S.; Halstead, S.B. Antibody response in dengue and dengue hemorrhagic fever. *Jpn. J. Med. Sci. Biol.* **1967**, *20*, 103–108. [PubMed]

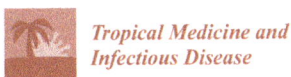 

*Article*

# Importation, Local Transmission, and Model Selection in Estimating the Transmissibility of COVID-19: The Outbreak in Shaanxi Province of China as a Case Study

Xu-Sheng Zhang [1,*], Huan Xiong [2], Zhengji Chen [2] and Wei Liu [2]

1. Statistics, Modelling and Economics, Data, Analytics & Surveillance, UK Health Security Agency, London NW9 5EQ, UK
2. School of Public Health, Kunming Medical University, Kunming 650500, China
* Correspondence: xu-sheng.zhang@ukhsa.gov.uk

**Abstract:** **Background**: Since the emergence of the COVID-19 pandemic, many models have been applied to understand its epidemiological characteristics. However, the ways in which outbreak data were used in some models are problematic, for example, importation was mixed up with local transmission. **Methods**: In this study, five models were proposed for the early Shaanxi outbreak in China. We demonstrated how to select a reasonable model and correctly use the outbreak data. Bayesian inference was used to obtain parameter estimates. **Results**: Model comparison showed that the renewal equation model generates the best model fitting and the Susceptible-Exposed-Diseased-Asymptomatic-Recovered (SEDAR) model is the worst; the performance of the SEEDAR model, which divides the exposure into two stages and includes the pre-symptomatic transmission, and SEEDDAAR model, which further divides infectious classes into two equally, lies in between. The Richards growth model is invalidated by its continuously increasing prediction. By separating continuous importation from local transmission, the basic reproduction number of COVID-19 in Shaanxi province ranges from 0.45 to 0.61, well below the unit, implying that timely interventions greatly limited contact between people and effectively contained the spread of COVID-19 in Shaanxi. **Conclusions**: The renewal equation model provides the best modelling; mixing continuous importation with local transmission significantly increases the estimate of transmissibility.

**Keywords:** basic reproduction number; Bayesian inference; COVID-19; mathematical modelling; model selection; local transmission; importation

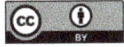

## 1. Introduction

The emerging coronavirus disease, COVID-19, has been circulated worldwide since January 2020 [1–3]. To control its spread, it is crucial to accurately estimate its important epidemiological characteristics such as transmissibility and to predict its further potential spread under different control measures. For this, mathematics and statistics have been used to model the transmission dynamic processes [4–7]. To obtain reliable estimates of the epidemiological characteristics from modelling analyses, correctly distinguishing and using different outbreak data in an appropriate transmission model is essential [8–13].

The transmissibility of an infectious agent describes how easy and fast an infectious disease can spread within a population. It is usually measured by the basic reproduction number (denoted as $R_0$), which is defined as the average number of secondary infections generated by an infectious person introduced into a completely susceptible population [5]. Although many methods of estimating $R_0$ have been developed [14,15], the difficulty in measuring $R_0$ of COVID-19 lies in the fact that it is a novel coronavirus. The knowledge of the well-known coronaviruses such as severe acute respiratory syndrome (SARS) and Middle East respiratory syndrome (MERS) has been borrowed to understand the early transmission dynamics of COVID-19 [11]. Nevertheless, the epidemiological characteristics of COVID-19 appear quite different from those of both SARS and MERS [16]. Further, as $R_0$ is determined by the infectiousness of SARS-CoV-2 and the contact rate between individuals, its value should be different among regions that implemented different control measures. Therefore, the basic knowledge of COVID-19 epidemiological features should be obtained from the epidemic data during outbreaks.

During the initial outbreaks of COVID-19 in China from January to March 2020, the national and provincial governments and public health authorities collected lots of data about the outbreaks and individual cases. These data undoubtedly provide a good chance for us to understand the transmissibility of COVID-19 and the impact of control measures implemented on stopping the spread. The reliable and accurate estimates depend on our understanding of how SARS-CoV-2 is transmitted in the population and the appropriate inference methods to calibrate the transmission models. We noticed that although some modelling studies have been published [17–24], they might have problems in obtaining reliable estimates of epidemiological parameters because of inappropriate use of the outbreak data. For example, when estimating $R_0$, those studies used the daily number of cases, which implicitly summarised local and imported cases. During the early stages of the COVID-19 pandemic, one common feature among the outbreaks, except that in the epicentre, Wuhan city, was the continuous importation due to quick and easy modern transportation. During the outbreaks, the role played by imported cases is different from that of local cases when counting the transmissibility of SARS-CoV-2: local cases as a result of local transmission can increase $R_0$, while imported cases as a potential source of transmission should reduce the estimate of $R_0$. A previous modelling study of the spatial transmission of pandemic flu [25] shows that early importation plays a relatively more important role in estimating transmissibility. Models that mixed up continuous importation with local transmission enlarged the estimate of $R_0$ [18–24,26], and mislead our assessment. To get a reliable estimate of $R_0$, it is crucial to separate imported cases from local cases [13,21,26–29].

Many different models have been proposed to describe the transmission dynamics of COVID-19, such as compartmental transmission dynamics models [8–13,28,30,31], the renewal equation model [32], machine learning [31], the Richards growth model [33,34], and time series models, such as the ARIMA model [35]. In theory, we need to ask: which one is better to approximate the spread of infection among the population given the data collected? In practice, we must search for the one that can provide a simple and accurate tool for us to estimate the essential epidemiological parameters and predict the trend of spread within the population.

In this study, we took the COVID-19 outbreak from January to February 2020 in Shaanxi province, China as an example to show how to avoid the common pitfall in estimating $R_0$ during the early stage of the COVID-19 pandemic in mainland China and other similar situations and show how to select the best transmission model by comparing their fitting to outbreak data. Two models [17,24] have been used for analysing the Shaanxi outbreak. Bai et al. [17] proposed a Susceptible-Exposed-Diseased-Asymptomatic-Recovered (SEDAR) compartmental transmission model, and Yang et al. [24] used the Richards growth model. The same implicit and problematic assumption in their modelling is that the Shaanxi outbreak was caused by one importation event at the very beginning of the outbreak. Based on this assumption, they obtained nearly the same estimate of the basic reproduction number (2.95 and 3.11, respectively). In view of these two models, we will propose five models to analyze the Shaanxi outbreak: the Richards growth model, the renewal equation model, the SEDAR model, the SEEDAR model in which the exposure interval in SEDAR is divided into two with the latter one being infectious, and the SEEDDAAR model in which not only two exposed classes are present as in the SEEDAR model but there are two classes in both diseased and asymptomatic infections, so infectious periods following gamma-distributions. As we show below, the estimate of the basic reproduction number of COVID-19 during the Shaanxi outbreak under the actual continuous importation is below the critical level, 1.0, which is the consequence of the timely and draconian control measures implemented in Shaanxi province.

Although the Shaanxi outbreak was relatively small over a short period of about one month and might be out of date, it was a typical situation of local outbreaks in mainland China except for the epicentre, Wuhan city, and it represented many similar situations in other countries during the early phases of COVID-19 pandemic. It is therefore hoped that this study provides some useful modelling methods in dealing with similar outbreak situations in future.

## 2. Materials and Methods

### 2.1. Data

The outbreak data for COVID-19 were collected from the Shaanxi provincial government website from 23 January to 20 February 2020. Variables used in the line list data for COVID-19 included age, gender, place of origin, exposure date, symptom onset date, hospital admission date, close contacts, cluster number, medical history, symptoms, and travel history. The serial interval and incubation period are estimated by applying the R language function *fitdistr* to the line list data of the Shaanxi outbreak. Among 245 cases reported during the period, 113 were imported from outside of Shaanxi (Figure 1A). The dates of symptom onset were recorded for 210 cases, from which the delay from symptom onset to reporting was estimated to have a mean of 7.54 days and a standard deviation of 4.12 days. The other 35 cases whose dates of symptom onset were missed were imputed from their reporting dates and the distribution of delays from symptom onset to reporting. The timeline of dates of symptom onset of 245 cases is shown in Figure 1B.

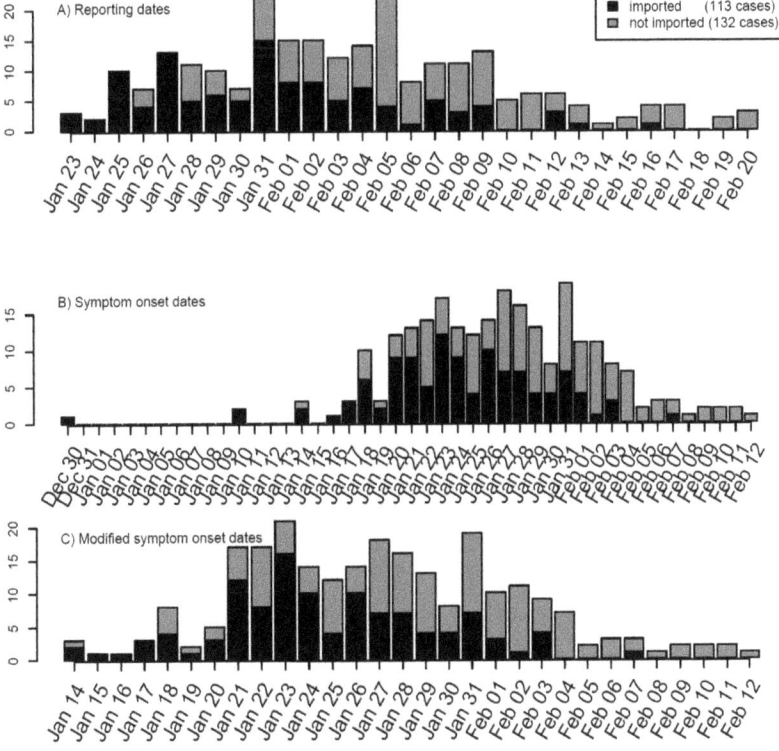

**Figure 1.** Timeline of the COVID-19 outbreak in Shaanxi province, China based on (**A**) reported dates, (**B**) dates of symptom onset, and (**C**) modified dates of symptom onset. For modelling's sake, the daily numbers of imported and local cases have been marked separately.

To provide the direct dates for local transmission modelling, we constructed modified dates of symptom onset for imported cases. If the date of symptom onset of one imported case was earlier than the date of entry into Shaanxi province, then its modified date of symptom onset is its entry date; otherwise, the modified date of symptom onset is its date of symptom onset. There are 19 cases whose dates of the symptom onset were earlier than their entry dates. This modification of symptom onset dates of imported cases will help in modelling the transmission within Shaanxi province. With these arrangements, the timeline of modified dates of symptom onset is shown in Figure 1C.

Once person-to-person transmission of COVID-19 was confirmed and announced on 20 January 2020 in mainland China, the Shaanxi provincial government took rapid actions to launch control measures for COVID-19 containment from 21 January 2020 [36]. The measures implemented in Shaanxi included strict traffic health quarantine, strictly limiting public gathering activities, timely and effective medical treatments, overall coordination of personnel and material allocation, timely release of information according to the law, strengthening publicity and education, professional training, and resolutely safeguarding social stability. These measures effectively controlled the local transmission and quickly reduced the number of importations, as reflected in the epidemic curve shown in Figure 1.

## 2.2. Models

We proposed five models for analysing the SARS-CoV-2 outbreak in Shaanxi: the Richards growth model, the renewal equation model, and three compartmental models: the Susceptible-Exposed-Diseased-Asymptomatic-Recovered (SEDAR), Susceptible-Exposed-Exposed-Diseased-Asymptomatic-Recovered (SEEDAR), and Susceptible-Exposed-Exposed-Diseased-Diseased-Asymptomatic-Asymptomatic-Recovered (SEEDDAAR) models. Bayesian inference via Markov chain Monte-Carlo (MCMC) sampling was used to estimate $R_0$ by calibrating the five models to Shaanxi outbreak data. The details of models and inference methods are given below.

### 2.2.1. Richards Growth Model

The Richards growth model is an extended form of logistic growth model, an ecological population growth model used to describe the growth of a population under competition for resources due to carrying capacity [37,38]. It has been widely used in population biology, including infectious disease dynamics [32,33]. For an outbreak caused by $C_0$ seeds of infection at time $t_0$, the Richards growth model states that the cumulative number of cases at time $t$ is given by the following equation [24,33,39]:

$$C(t) = K\left(1 + \left(\left(\frac{K}{C_0}\right)^\nu - 1\right)\exp(-r\nu(t-t_0))\right)^{-\frac{1}{\nu}}.$$

Here, $r$ is the growth rate, $\nu$ is the scaling exponent, and $K$ is the final epidemic size given $C_0 = C(t_0)$ seeds. If importation is continuing (e.g., there are $C_i$ cases that are imported at $t_i$, $i = 0, \ldots, n-1$) and the outbreaks that importation at different times can cause are of the same final size $K$ and growth rate $r$, then the total cumulative number of cases should be summarized as:

$$C(t) = K\sum_{i=0}^{n-1} H(t-t_i)\left(1 + \left(\left(\frac{K}{C_i}\right)^\nu - 1\right)\exp(-r\nu(t-t_i))\right)^{-\frac{1}{\nu}}. \quad (1)$$

Here, $H(t-t_i)$ is the Heaviside function: which is 1 if $t > t_i$ and 0 otherwise. The daily number of new local cases can be calculated as $\mu(t) = C(t) - C(t-1)$. The basic reproductive number $R_0$ can be calculated from the growth rate and serial interval which is assumed to follow gamma-distribution $g(\tau;\alpha,\beta)$ by [40,41]

$$R_0 = \frac{1}{\int_0^\infty g(\tau;\alpha,\beta)e^{-r\tau}d\tau} = \left(1 + \frac{r}{\beta}\right)^\alpha. \quad (2)$$

### 2.2.2. Renewal Equation Model

It is assumed that, once infected, individuals have an infectivity profile given by a probability distribution $w_s$, dependent on time since infection of the case, $s$, but independent of calendar time, $t$. The distribution $w_s$ typically depends on individual biological factors such as pathogen shedding or symptom severity. For simplicity, the distribution $w_s$ is approximated by the distribution of serial interval (SI), the lag in onset dates of symptoms between an infector and its infectee. In the original renewal equation model, Fraser [42] considers a situation where the only importation is index case(s) at the very beginning of the outbreak and other cases are generated by local transmission (this assumption was also made in its direct application software for estimating the time-varying reproduction number [43]). During the spread of COVID-19 in 2020, the outbreak within a region (except the epicentre, Wuhan) took place with continuous importation. To take this into account, Fraser's model is slightly modified as in the following (c.f., [44]). Let $c_t$ be the number of local cases whose symptoms onset at day $t$, its expected value is approximated by:

$$E(c_t) = R_0 \sum_{j=1}^{\min(t-1, SI\_max)} w_s (c_{t-s} + I_{t-s}). \qquad (3)$$

Here, $I_{t-s}$ is the number of imported cases that have the onset date of symptoms on day $t_{-s}$ and $w_s$ represents the probability mass function of the SI of length $s$ days, which can be obtained by $w_s = G(s) - G(s-1)$, with $G(.)$ representing the cumulative distribution function of the gamma distribution. The gamma distribution is characterized by its mean SI_mean and standard deviation SI_sd, both of which are to be estimated jointly with $R_0$ from the outbreak data [45]. Because only 19 cases among 113 imported cases had symptom onset before entering Shaanxi province, the assumption that all cases started their infectivity duration within Shaanxi province, which is implicitly required in Equation (3), should be approximately satisfied.

In Equation (3) an implicit assumption made is that the transmissibility (i.e., $R_0$) remained constant during the outbreak duration. This should be reasonable in view of the timely control measures implemented in Shaanxi province: control measures started on 21 January 2021 [36] and raised to their first-class emergency responses on 25 January 2020, just 2 days after the reporting of the first three imported cases in Shaanxi province [16,23]. To estimate the daily-varying transmissibility $R_t$, Equation (3) is rearranged as:

$$R_t = c_t / \sum_{j=1}^{\min(t-1, SI\_max)} w_s (c_{t-s} + I_{t-s}).$$

That is, $R_t$ can be estimated by the ratio of the number of new infections produced at time step $t$, $c_t$, to the total infectiousness of infected individuals at time $t$, given by $\sum_{j=1}^{\min(t-1, SI\_max)} w_s (c_{t-s} + I_{t-s})$, the sum of infection incidence, including both imported and locally generated, up to time step $t-1$ or the maximum of SI (whichever is the smallest), weighted by the infectivity function $w_s$. $R_t$ is the average number of secondary cases that each infected individual would infect if the conditions remained as they were at time $t$ [43], and it is used to monitor the change in transmissibility along the course of an outbreak.

### 2.2.3. SEDAR Transmission Model

Figure 2A shows the schematic for the SEDAR compartmental model: susceptible individuals ($S$) contract SARS-CoV-2 virus from infectious people and then it enters the latent class ($E$); a fraction ($\theta$) of those exposed after an average latent period ($L_1$) progress to become diseased ($I$) and the other fraction ($1 - \theta$) remains asymptomatic ($A$) but becomes infectious after an average latent period ($L_2$). The diseased infections will be detected and admitted to hospital and isolated from the community after an average period of $D_1$ and the asymptomatic cases recover after an average infectious period of $D_2$. The model can be described by the following set of differential equations:

$$\frac{d}{dt}S(t) = -\beta S(t)(I(t) + \xi A(t))/N$$

$$\frac{d}{dt}E(t) = \beta S(t)(I(t) + \xi A(t))/N - \theta E(t)/L_1 - (1-\theta)E(t)/L_2$$

$$\frac{d}{dt}I(t) = \theta E(t)/L_1 - I(t)/D_1 + Imported(t) \qquad (4)$$

$$\frac{d}{dt}A(t) = (1-\theta)E(t)/L_2 - A(t)/D_2$$

$$\frac{d}{dt}R(t) = I(t)/D_1 + A(t)/D_2$$

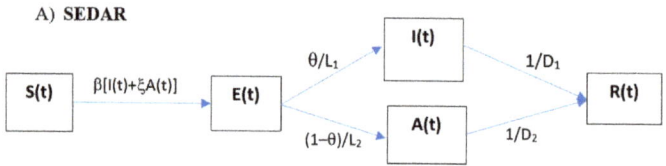

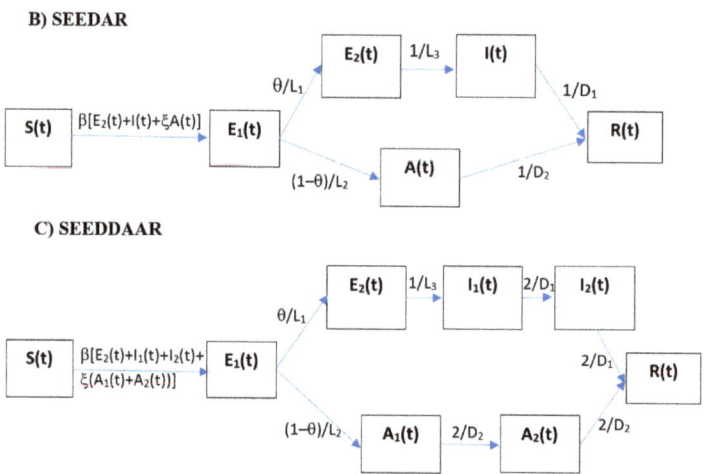

**Figure 2.** Flow chart of (**A**) SEDAR transmission model, (**B**) SEEDAR transmission model, and (**C**) SEEDDAAR transmission model.

Here, $N$ is the size of the population under investigation ($N$ = 37,330,000 for Shaanxi province) and is assumed to be constant during the outbreak. The definitions of model parameters are given in Table 1. Importantly, the model includes an item for imported cases (i.e., *Imported(t)* in equation for $I(t)$) from outside of the population as reported [16]. This is to treat imported cases as the source rather than the results of local transmission from the region under investigation, therefore removing the importation as a result of the local transmissibility.

Table 1. Parameter estimates of five transmission models.

| Parameter | Richards Growth Prior | Richards Growth Posterior | Renewal Equation Prior | Renewal Equation Posterior | SEDAR Prior | SEDAR Posterior | SEEDAR Prior | SEEDAR Posterior | SEEDDAAR Posterior |
|---|---|---|---|---|---|---|---|---|---|
| Growth rate ($r$) | [0,1.0] | 0.02 [0.012,0.032] | - | - | - | - | - | - | - |
| Final epidemic size ($K$) | [1,6600] | 3315 [56,6521] | - | - | - | - | - | - | - |
| Scaling exponent ($v$) | [0.1,50] | 24.51 [0.72,48.81] | - | - | - | - | - | - | - |
| Mean of SI (SI_mean) | - | - | U [3.5,10.0] | 4.66 [3.53,7.18] | - | - | - | - | - |
| Standard deviation of SI (SI_sd) | - | - | U [3.0,15.0] | 11.73 [5.85,14.88] | - | - | - | - | - |
| Transmission coefficient ($\beta$) | - | - | - | - | U [.001,0.5] | 0.155 [0.117,0.186] | U [.001,0.5] | 0.066 [0.029,0.154] | 0.072 [0.032,0.180] |
| Latent period ($L_1$) * | - | - | - | - | U [1.6,14.0] | 1.81 [1.61,2.82] | U [1.0,10.0] | 5.04 [1.25,9.65] | 5.25 [1.28,9.76] |
| Pre-symptomatic infectious period ($L_3$) | - | - | - | - | - | - | U [1.0,10.0] | 1.45 [1.04,4.43] | 1.45 [1.04,4.43] |
| Infectious period ($D_1$) of diseased infections * | - | - | - | - | U [3.5,25.0] | 3.75 [3.51,5.16] | U [1.5,15.0] | 4.78 [1.61,14.06] | 5.40 [1.68,13.97] |
| Dispersion parameter ($\eta$) | - | - | U [1.01,50.0] | 1.58 [1.06,2.86] | U [1.01,50.0] | 2.47 [1.56,4.431] | U [1.01,50.0] | 1.73 [1.08,3.26] | 1.71 [1.09,3.18] |
| $R_0$ ♦ | - | 1.13 [1.08,1.21] | U [0.05,3.0] | 0.61 [0.54,0.68] | - | 0.59 [0.50,0.70] | - | 0.45 [0.30,0.76] | 0.53 [0.35,0.85] |
| DIC ♣ | - | 140.2 | - | 127.9 | - | 175.1 | - | 160.5 | 160.8 |

*: For three compartmental transmission models, the relative infectivity ($\xi$) of asymptomatic infections to symptomatic infection is set at 0.5, and the incubation and infectious period for asymptomatic infections are set to be equal to the counterparts of symptomatic infections (i.e., $L_2 = L_1$ and $D_2 = D_1$). As the proportion of asymptomatic infections is very small (i.e., $1 - \theta = 1.1\%$), the other choices of these three parameters (say $\xi = 1$, $L_2 = 2L_1$ and $D_2 = 2D_1$) do not noticeably change the estimates of the model parameters listed here. The priors for the SEEDAR and SEEDDAAR models are the same. ♦: $R_0$ for the Richards growth model is calculated via equation (2) with the gamma-distributed serial interval of mean = 6.29 days and SD = 4.11 days (shape parameter = 2.343, rate parameter = 0.372). ♣: Deviance information criterion (DIC) is a measure of model fitting.

The steady-state solution of the equation system (4) can be easily obtained. The expression for $S^*$ (the size of the population susceptible to infection at equilibrium) is:

$$S^* = N \frac{\theta/L_1 + (1-\theta)/L_2}{\beta[\theta D_1/L_1 + \xi(1-\theta)D_2/L_2]}.$$

From this, we can obtain the expression of basic reproduction number:

$$R_0 N/S^* = \beta[\theta D_1/L_1 + \xi(1-\theta)D_2/L_2]/[\theta/L_1 + (1-\theta)/L_2] \tag{5}$$

Ref [14,30]. In the special situation where $L_1 = L_2$, expression (5) reduces to:

$$R_0 = \beta[\theta D_1 + \xi(1-\theta)D_2].$$

2.2.4. SEEDAR Transmission Model

Ferretti et al. [46] show that 30% to 50% of all transmissions are pre-symptomatic transmissions. To take the pre-symptomatic transmission into account, we modify the above SEDAR model by including a secondary exposure compartment (see Figure 2B). For simplicity, this new compartment is assumed to be asymptomatic but of the same infectivity as the symptomatic infections. The corresponding equations are modified as:

$$\frac{d}{dt}S(t) = -\beta S(t)(E_2(t) + I(t) + \xi A(t))/N,$$

$$\frac{d}{dt}E_1(t) = \beta S(t)(E_2(t) + I(t) + \xi A(t))/N - \theta E_1(t)/L_1 - (1-\theta)E_1(t)/L_2,$$

$$\frac{d}{dt}E_2(t) = \theta E_1(t)/L_1 - E_2(t)/L_3,$$

$$\frac{d}{dt}I(t) = E_2(t)/L_3 - I(t)/D_1 + Imported(t), \qquad (6)$$

$$\frac{d}{dt}A(t) = (1-\theta)E_1(t)/L_2 - A(t)/D_2,$$

$$\frac{d}{dt}R(t) = I(t)/D_1 + A(t)/D_2.$$

Compared with the SEDAR model, a new parameter $L_3$, the duration of the late incubation period in which the infected person can pass the virus on, is introduced and is to be estimated (See Table 1).

Similarly, the basic reproduction number $R_0$ for the SEEDAR model can be obtained by deriving the expression of the equilibrium number of susceptible people, and it is given by:

$$R_0 = \beta[\theta(L_3 + D_1)/L_1 + \xi(1-\theta)D_2/L_2]/[\theta/L_1 + (1-\theta)/L_2]. \qquad (7)$$

2.2.5. SEEDDAAR Transmission Model

In view of the empirical observations that the infectious period follows the gamma distribution rather than the usual exponential distribution [47–52], we introduce the intermediate compartments by evenly dividing diseased compartment $I(t)$ into $I_1(t)$ and $I_2(t)$, and dividing asymptomatic compartment $A(t)$ into $A_1(t)$ and $A_2(t)$. Adding the two new compartments to Equation (6), the model equations for the SEEDDAAR model are given as:

$$\frac{d}{dt}S(t) = -\beta S(t)(E_2(t) + I_1(t) + I_2(t) + \xi(A_1(t) + A_2(t)))/N,$$

$$\frac{d}{dt}E_1(t) = \beta S(t)(E_2(t) + I_1(t) + I_2(t) + \xi(A_1(t) + A_2(t)))/N - \theta E_1(t)/L_1 - (1-\theta)E_1(t)/L_2,$$

$$\frac{d}{dt}E_2(t) = \theta E_1(t)/L_1 - E_2(t)/L_3,$$

$$\frac{d}{dt}I_1(t) = E_2(t)/L_3 - 2I_1(t)/D_1 + Imported(t), \qquad (8)$$

$$\frac{d}{dt}I_2(t) = 2I_1(t)/D_1 - 2I_2(t)/D_1,$$

$$\frac{d}{dt}A_1(t) = (1-\theta)E_1(t)/L_2 - 2A_1(t)/D_2,$$

$$\frac{d}{dt}A_2(t) = 2A_1(t)/D_2 - 2A_2(t)/D_2,$$

$$\frac{d}{dt}R(t) = 2I_2(t)/D_1 + 2A_2(t)/D_2.$$

The inclusion of additional compartments in diseased and asymptomatic infections does not change the expression of the basic reproduction number, and the SEEDDAAR model has its basic reproduction number as in Equation (7).

2.3. Inference Method by Calibration to Shaanxi Outbreak

Inference is carried out within the Bayesian framework [53,54], obtained through the combination of the prior distributions and the likelihood function. We denote the set of model parameters to be inferred as $\Theta = \{r, \nu, K\}$ for the Richards growth model, $\Theta = \{R_0,$ SI_mean, SI_sd$\}$ for the renewal equation model, $\Theta = \{\beta, L_1, D_1\}$ for the SEDAR model and $\Theta = \{\beta, L_1, L_3, D_1\}$ for the SEDAR and SEEDDAAR models under the special situation where both asymptomatic and symptomatic infections are of the same latent period and infectious period (i.e., $L_2 = L_1$ and $D_2 = D_1$). For simplicity, the proportion of symptomatic infections ($\theta$) is set at 98.9% as reported [16]. Given the values of parameters $\Theta$ for the Richards growth model and the renewal equation model, simulating the time series of local infections, denoted as $\mu(t)$, $t = t_{start}, \ldots, t_{end}$, is straightforward. Here, $t_{start}$ and $t_{end}$ represent the start day and end day of the outbreak data collected, respectively. For each set of parameter values of SEDAR, SEEDAR, and SEEDDAAR models, the Runge–Kutta fourth order method is used to solve the model equations and to obtain predicted time series of infections. In the inference of model parameters, directly observed cases of modified symptom onset dates (see the definition in the data above) are used as illustrated in the following. The likelihood function for the observed time series of local cases $x(t)$, $t = t_{start}, \ldots, t_{end}$, is given as:

$$L(\Theta|\text{Data}) = \prod_{t=t_{start}}^{t_{end}} \frac{\Gamma(x(t)+r(t))}{\Gamma(r(t))\Gamma(x(t)+1)} \left(\frac{1}{\eta}\right)^{r(t)} \left(1-\frac{1}{\eta}\right)^{x(t)}.$$

Here, $r(t) = \frac{\mu(t)}{\eta-1}$ with $\eta$ being the dispersion parameter of the negative binomial distribution. The parameters are estimated using MCMC methods with Gibbs sampling and non-informative flat priors. The boundaries of uniformly distributed priors are set forth as in the literature [16] and the data collected from Shaanxi province (Figure 3). The details of the MCMC sampling method are given below.

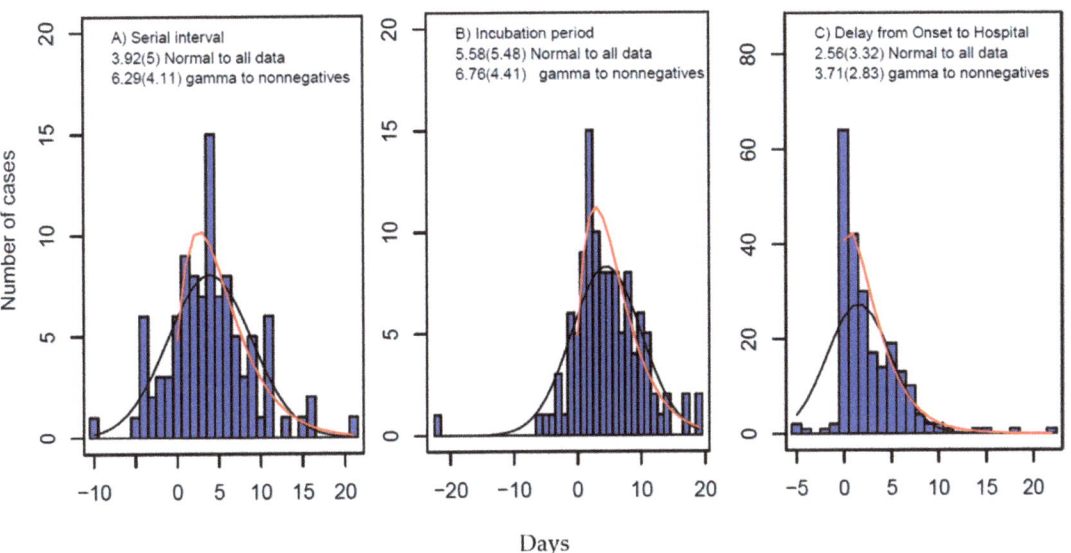

**Figure 3.** Distributions of (**A**) serial interval (SI), (**B**) incubation period, and (**C**) delay from date of symptom onset to hospital visit. The blue pillars represent the data, and the estimate of the mean and its standard deviation in brackets are obtained by fitting gamma distribution to nonnegative data (red curve) and normal distribution to all data (black curves shown in the graphs).

MCMC Sampling

To propose new values for parameters, we use normal random walk. Suppose the current value of the $j$th parameter of $\Theta$ is $\Theta_j^{(t-1)}$, the new proposal is:

$$\Theta_j^* = \Theta_j^{(t-1)} + \sigma_j z.$$

Here, $z$ is a standard normal variable and $\sigma_j$ is the step size of the $j^{th}$ parameter. The normal proposal density is given by:

$$q(\Theta^*|\Theta^{(t-1)}) = \frac{1}{\sigma\sqrt{2\pi}} \exp\left[-\frac{\left(\Theta^* - \Theta^{(t-1)}\right)^2}{2\sigma^2}\right].$$

That is, $\Theta_j^*$ follows $N(\Theta_j^{(t-1)}, \sigma_j^2)$ (normal distribution with mean = $\Theta_j^{(t-1)}$, and standard deviation = $\sigma_j$). The proposal is accepted as the next step of the Markov chain with probability $\alpha = \min(A,1)$, where:

$$A = \frac{\pi(\Theta^*)}{\pi(\Theta^{t-1})} \frac{L(\Theta^*|y)}{L(\Theta^{(t-1)}|y)} \frac{q(\Theta^{(t-1)}|\Theta^*)}{q(\Theta^*|\Theta^{(t-1)})}.$$

Here, $\pi(.)$ denotes the prior density, $L(\Theta_j^*|y)$ the likelihood of parameter $\Theta_j^*$ given data $y$. For a truncated normal walk on the range $(a,b)$, the proposal density is given by:

$$q\left(\Theta^*|\Theta^{(t-1)}\right)|_{(a,b)} = \frac{q\left(\Theta^*|\Theta^{(t-1)}\right)}{\Phi\left(\frac{b-\Theta^{(t-1)}}{\sigma}\right) - \Phi\left(\frac{a-\Theta^{(t-1)}}{\sigma}\right)}.$$

where $\Phi(.)$ is the cumulative distribution function of standard normal. The expression for $A$ is consequently modified as:

$$A = \frac{\pi(\Theta^*)}{\pi(\Theta^{t-1})} \frac{L(\Theta^*|y)}{L(\Theta^{(t-1)}|y)} \frac{\Phi\left(\frac{b-\Theta^{(t-1)}}{\sigma}\right) - \Phi\left(\frac{a-\Theta^{(t-1)}}{\sigma}\right)}{\Phi\left(\frac{b-\Theta^*}{\sigma}\right) - \Phi\left(\frac{a-\Theta^*}{\sigma}\right)}.$$

Sample a uniformly distributed random number ($r$) between 0 and 1,

$\Theta_j^{(t)} = \Theta_j^*$ if $r < \alpha$ (accepted);
$\Theta_j^{(t)} = \Theta_j^{(t-1)}$ otherwise (rejected).

To generate nearly independent samples of model parameters, the samples are to be thinned every 400th observation. To respond to the acceptance rate, the following adaptive procedure is applied: if the acceptance ratio over 400 × 200 iterations is less than 12%, then decrease the jump step to 80% of its current size (i.e., $\sigma_j = 0.8\sigma_j$); if it exceeds 40%, then $\sigma_j = 1.2\sigma_j$. Otherwise, the jump step $\sigma_j$ remains unchanged. To allow the MCMC process to fully converge, a burn-in period of 400,000 iterations is chosen, and the estimates of model parameters are obtained from the further 400,000 iterations.

To compare the performance of the five models [55], the deviance information criterion (DIC), which combines the goodness of fit and model complexity [56], is used. It measures fit via the deviance $Dev(\Theta) = -2\log L(\Theta | Data)$ and complexity by an estimate of the 'effective number of parameters' $p_D = \text{mean}(Dev(\Theta)) - Dev(\text{mean}(\Theta))$ (i.e., posterior mean deviance minus deviance evaluated at the posterior mean of the parameters). The DIC is calculated as:

$$\text{DIC} = Dev(\text{mean}(\Theta)) + 2p_D = \text{mean}(Dev(\Theta)) + p_D.$$

The model that has the smallest DIC is the best.

## 3. Results

*3.1. Estimates of SI and Incubation Period from Line List Data*

The results are shown in Figure 3. Fitting the nonnegative data to gamma distributions, the estimates are: From 85 pairs of infector–infectees observed during the outbreak, the SI is estimated to have a mean of 6.29 days and a SD of 4.11 days (so the fitted gamma distribution has a shape parameter of $\alpha = 2.34$ and a rate parameter of $\beta = 0.37$). From 100 cases that had dates of exposure and symptom onset, the incubation period is estimated to have a mean of 6.76 days and a SD of 4.41 days, and the delay from the onset of symptoms to hospitalization from 222 cases has a mean of 3.71 days and a SD of 2.83 days. If fitting all collected data (including both negative and positive) to normal distributions, the estimates will be shorter (Figure 3). These estimates are consistent with the system review of both the serial interval and the incubation period [57].

### 3.2. Estimate of $R_0$ in Shaanxi Outbreak

#### 3.2.1. Richards Growth Model

Model fitting to the daily number of local cases suggests the growth rate $r = 0.020$ with a 95% confidence interval (95% CI): 0.012, 0.032, and the final epidemic size $K = 3315$ (95% CI: 56, 6521) (Table 1). Based on the estimate of gamma-distributed serial interval (Figure 3), the basic reproduction number is calculated using Formula (2) to be 1.13 (95% CI: 1.08, 1.21). We note that although the prediction of the Richards growth model can be fitted to the daily number of local cases within the outbreak period of 30 days, the continuing increase in the daily number of local cases that the model predicts obviously deviated from the actual observations after the outbreak (Figure 4A). That is, even though the model calibration performs well, the external validation is bad. Our estimate of the growth rate is very near to zero, the nonnegative limit. This is in sharp contrast with Yang et al. 2021 [24] who obtained an estimate of growth rate $r = 0.23$ per day by assuming one importation event and mixing up imported cases thereafter with local cases in their modelling study. This points out the limitation of applying the Richards growth model to infection spread processes. In general, infections can either increase, decrease, or remain the same within a population (i.e., $r$ can be positive, negative, or zero, with $R_0$ being larger, less than, or equal to 1.0). Applying the Richards growth model to an infection spread process, it is implicitly assumed that its growth rate is positive and $R_0 > 1$, which is wrong for the situation of well-controlled infections such as COVID-19 in Shaanxi province during January and February of 2020.

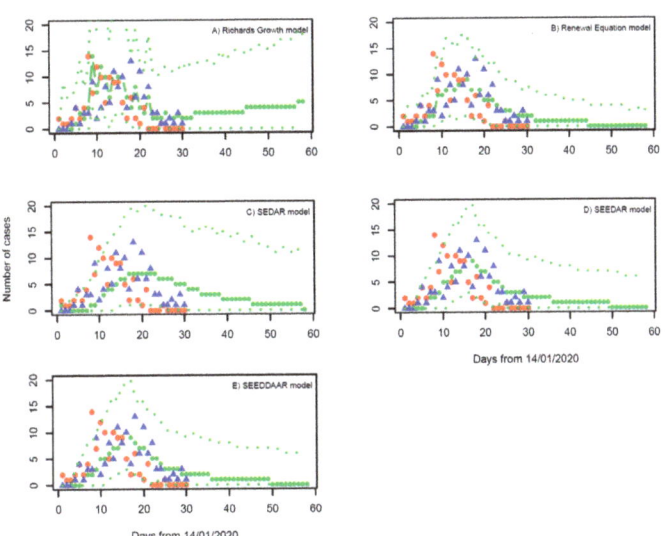

**Figure 4.** Fitting of (**A**) the Richards growth model, (**B**) the renewal equation model, (**C**) the SEDAR model, (**D**) the SEEDAR model, and (**E**) the SEEDDAAR model to outbreak data of symptom onset dates. Red dots represent the imported cases, and the blue triangles are the cases locally transmitted in Shaanxi province. The thick green line represents the median of MCMC samples, and the thin lines represent their upper and lower levels of 95% confidence intervals.

### 3.2.2. Renewal Equation Model

Bayesian inference suggests the basic reproduction number ($R_0$) has a median of 0.61 and 95% CI from 0.54 to 0.68 (Table 1). The SI is estimated to have a mean of 4.66 days and an SD of 11.73 days, which is shorter than but comparable with the direct observation of SI from the outbreak (Figure 3). The model projection into next month (Figure 4B) indicates that the outbreak will die out within two weeks (i.e., the end of February 2020) and is unlikely to generate any further local cases under the current restriction measures.

The time-varying reproduction number $R_t$ shown in Figure 5 demonstrates how the transmissibility changed along the course of the outbreak. $R_t$ increased to about 2.0 within the first week, and then reduced to low values, but occasionally exceeding the critical value of 1.0. Its overall average is 0.61, which is equal to the median of posterior $R_0$ in the above model fitting. The change of $R_t$ reflects the stochasticity of transmission events within the Shaanxi outbreak.

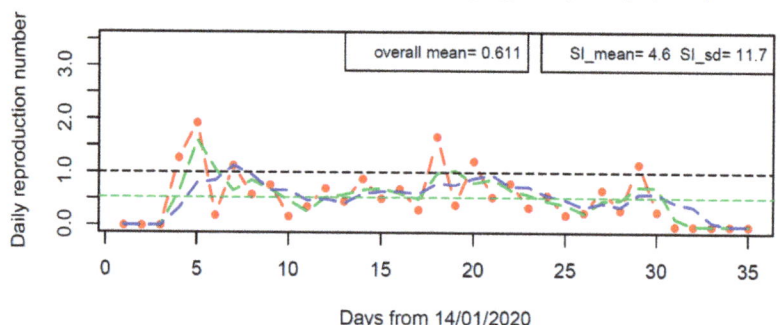

**Figure 5.** The effective reproductive number ($R_t$) along the course of the outbreak in Shaanxi province, China under the SI distributions of SI_mean = 4.6 days, SI_sd = 11.7 days (the Maximum likelihood estimate of SI from model calibration of the renewal equation). $R_t$ is evaluated by averaging over one, two, and four days.

### 3.2.3. SEDAR Model

The calibration of the SEDAR model under the situation with equal incubation and infectious periods for both symptomatic and asymptomatic infection shows that: $R_0$ is estimated at 0.59 with 95% CI from 0.51 to 0.71 (Table 1). The incubation period is 1.8 days (95% CI: 1.6, 2.9), and the infectious period is 3.8 days (95% CI: 3.5, 5.3). The SEDAR model fitting and its prediction over one month ahead are shown in Figure 4C. Sensitivity analyses (data not shown) show that nearly the same estimates of model parameters are obtained when considering different values of latent period ($L_2$) and infectious period ($D_2$) for asymptomatic infections and the relative infectivity ($\xi$) of asymptomatic infections to symptomatic infections. This reflects the fact that, in the Shaanxi outbreak, the asymptomatic infections occupied a very small proportion of all infections (1.1%) [16] and therefore had small effects on model performance.

### 3.2.4. SEEDAR Model

The $R_0$ is estimated at 0.45 with 95% CI from 0.30 to 0.76 (Table 1). The incubation period of symptomatic infection is 5.0 days (95% CI: 1.3, 9.7), which is consistent with the observed values (mean = 6.76 days and sd = 4.41 days), and the infectious period of symptomatic infections is 4.8 days (95% CI: 1.6, 14.1), which is longer than the delay from the onset date of symptoms to hospitalization: mean = 3.71 days and sd=2.83 days (Figure 3). The duration of pre-symptomatic transmission ($L_3$) is estimated at 1.5 days (95% CI: 1.0, 4.4 days); this suggests the fraction of transmission from strictly pre-symptomatic infections was about 1.5/(1.5 + 4.8) =24%, which is in agreement with previous estimates [46]. The

SEEDAR model fits well with the observed data and predicts that the outbreak will die out within about three weeks (Figure 4D).

3.2.5. SEEDDAAR Model

The $R_0$ is estimated at 0.53 with 95% CI from 0.35 to 0.85 (Table 1). The incubation period of symptomatic infection is 5.3 days (95% CI: 1.3, 9.8), and the infectious period of symptomatic infection is 5.4 days (95% CI: 1.7, 14.0). The duration of pre-symptomatic transmission ($L_3$) is estimated at 1.5 days (95% CI: 1.0 to 4.4 days). Those estimates of model parameters are very similar to those of the SEEDAR model. Similar to the SEEDAR model, the SEEDDAAR model equally well fits the observed data and predicts that the outbreak will die out within about three weeks (Figure 4E).

## 4. Discussion

In this study, five transmission models were proposed to model the COVID-19 epidemic within Shaanxi province of China from early January to late February 2020. By distinguishing imported and local cases in their contribution to local transmission dynamics, we show that the basic reproduction number $R_0$ of COVID-19 in the Shaanxi outbreak was well below the critical value of 1.0. This indicates that SARS-CoV-2 cannot self-sustain under the current control measures within Shaanxi province, China, and would stop once the importation of COVID-19 cases was halted. Our model successfully predicted the actual epidemic situation in Shaanxi province from late February 2020.

The estimates of $R_0$ from the renewal equation and the SEDAR models are close to each other, and its estimates from the SEEDAR and SEEDDAAR models are lower; nevertheless, their 95% CIs are closely overlapped. Overall, the estimate of $R_0$ is in the range from 0.45 to 0.61. The model fittings to the local cases, shown in Figure 4, indicate that the renewal equation model provides the best fit to the observations and the SEDAR model is the worst. This is further confirmed by the values of DIC in Table 1 [55]: 127.9, 175.1, 160.5, and 160.8 for the renewal equation, and the SEDAR, SEEDAR, and SEEDDAAR models, respectively. Furthermore, the better performance of the SEEDAR and SEEDDAAR models than the SEDAR model confirms the existence of pre-symptomatic transmission [46]. It is worth mentioning that the SEEDDAAR model that has its infectious periods following gamma distribution does not appear better than SEEDAR that has its infectious period following simple exponential distribution. The Richards growth model, which is borrowed from ecological population dynamics [37,38], can provide a better model fit to the daily number of local cases than three compartmental transmission models (i.e., SEDAR, SEEDAR, and SEEDDAAR). However, the increasing trend of infections after the first month, which the Richards growth model predicts, deviates from the actual observation and hence invalidates the Richards growth model as an appropriate model for the Shaanxi outbreak.

It is worth emphasizing that although the renewal equation model is the simplest in its structure, it gives the best model fit [52]. Given the distribution of SI of COVID-19, it is straightforward to obtain the estimate of the $R_0$ [58]. In this study, we perform a joint estimation of $R_0$ and SI, and the results agree well with three compartmental models in estimation of $R_0$ and the empirical knowledge of SI [16,57]. Nevertheless, it should be kept in mind that the successful performance of the joint estimation of $R_0$ and SI in this study may be conditional on the very low proportion (i.e., 1.1%) of asymptomatic infections [58].

One important issue worth pointing out is the continuous importation along the course of an outbreak within one region, except for the epicenter, Wuhan city, China, during the early stages of the COVID-19 pandemic in mainland China. This spectacular feature, unlike previous infectious disease pandemics (such as the 2003 SARS pandemic and the 2009 influenza pandemic), may reflect the rapid and huge movements of modern human beings. If assuming the earliest importation as the only index case(s), the transmission dynamics cannot be appropriately investigated and might be misled [17,24]. Both Bai et al. [17] and Yang et al. [24] also modelled the Shaanxi outbreak but mixed up imported cases with local cases; they obtained estimates of $R_0$ of about 3.0. Simple reasoning will show that this estimate is problematic. Let us consider a situation where all the 132 cases were generated within Shaanxi province only by the 113 imported cases, a rough estimate is $R_0 = 132/113 \approx 1.2$. Some local cases might have been infected by other early local cases rather than directly from imported cases, which implies that the actual $R_0$ should be less than 1.2. With the similar treatments of continuous importation, the high and problematic estimates of $R_0$ for outbreaks in the major cities of China (except the epicentre, Wuhan city) were also reported [20,21]. Based on estimates of their SEDAR model parameters, Bai et al. [17] predicted that the Shaanxi outbreak would last until April 2020, which is more than one month longer than the actual occurrence. Our analyses show that the occurrence of the Shaanxi outbreak was mainly due to the large and continuous importation rather than the high local transmissibility of COVID-19 within the province. Furthermore, our prediction is consistent with what happened in Shaanxi province.

In modelling the COVID-19 transmission over the whole of mainland China, we found that $R_0$ was estimated at 2.23 before 8th February 2020 and then it dropped to 0.04 [30]. Hao et al. [8] also confirmed the effectiveness of the timely prevention and control measures implemented in China in bringing the $R_0$ well below the critical level of 1.0. To check whether there was any potential breaking point in the transmissibility of COVID-19 within the Shaanxi outbreak, we calculated the instantaneous reproduction number $R_t$ [43]. The result shown in Figure 5 indicates that no clear pattern emerged that supported a potential breaking point in transmissibility although $R_t$ exceeded 1.0 on five days. In contrast, having mixed up imported cases with local cases, Yang et al. [24] used the renewal equation method [43] to obtain a time-varying reproduction number ($R_t$), which persistently decreased over time and stayed beyond the critical level of 1.0 over more than half the course of the outbreak.

Our estimate of $R_0$ for the Shaanxi outbreak sharply differs from other studies which suggest $R_0 = 2–7$ [16,49,59,60] for SARS-CoV-2. In theory, $R_0$ is determined by the infectiousness of SARS-CoV-2 as well as the contact rate between people [5]. In the situation where no vaccine and effective drugs were available to protect people against the virus, the result of $R_0 < 1$ is due to the highly reduced contact rate between people [30]. This resulted from the timely and strong control measures implemented within Shaanxi province soon after it was announced in public on 20 January 2020 that COVID-19 could be transmitted among people. On the other hand, this indicates the success of the interventions executed in Shanxi province, China.

## 5. Conclusions

Modern inference methodology and mathematical theory can help reveal the unobserved transmission dynamic process and hence provide valuable information for us to understand and control the spread of COVID-19. However, it is important to separate continuous importation from local transmission when modelling the local transmission dynamics of COVID-19. The renewal equation model, albeit being simple in model structure, provides better model fitting and therefore is a practical candidate for analyzing transmission dynamics and monitoring the change in transmissibility.

**Author Contributions:** Conceptualization, X.-S.Z. and W.L.; methodology, X.-S.Z.; software, X.-S.Z.; validation, X.-S.Z., H.X. and Z.C.; formal analysis, X.-S.Z., H.X., Z.C. and W.L.; investigation, X.-S.Z. and H.X.; resources, X.-S.Z.; data curation, H.X. and Z.C.; writing—original draft preparation, X.-S.Z.; writing—review and editing, X.-S.Z.; visualization, X.-S.Z.; project administration, W.L.; funding acquisition, W.L. All authors have read and agreed to the published version of the manuscript.

**Funding:** This research was funded by UKHSA, National Nature Science Foundation of China, grant number 81860607; and Innovative Research Team of Yunnan Province (2019(6)), China. The APC was funded by Innovative Research Team of Yunnan Province (2019(6)).

**Institutional Review Board Statement:** Ethical review and approval were waived for this study since this is a theoretical study with the personal identifications being removed from the outbreak data.

**Informed Consent Statement:** Patient consent was waived due to patients' identification being removed from the outbreak data.

**Data Availability Statement:** The data supporting reported results are provided in Figures 1 and 3.

**Conflicts of Interest:** The authors declare no conflict of interest. The funders had no role in the design of the study; in the collection, analyses, or interpretation of data; in the writing of the manuscript; or in the decision to publish the results.

## References

1. Worldometer Coronavirus. Available online: https://www.worldometers.info/coronavirus/ (accessed on 19 September 2021).
2. World Health Organization. Available online: https://www.who.int/publications/m/item/weekly-epidemiological-update-on-COVID-19 (accessed on 31 August 2021).
3. Hale, T.; Angrist, N.; Goldszmidt, R.; Kira, B.; Petherick, A.; Phillips, T.; Webster, S.; Cameron-Blake, E.; Hallas, L.; Majumdar, S.; et al. A global panel database of pandemic policies (Oxford COVID-19 Government Response Tracker). *Nat. Hum. Behav.* **2021**, *5*, 529–538. [CrossRef] [PubMed]
4. Ross, R. *The Prevention of Malaria*; John Murray: London, UK, 1911.
5. Anderson, R.M.; May, R.M. *Infectious Diseases of Humans: Dynamics and Control*; Oxford University Press: Oxford, UK, 1991.
6. Heesterbeek, J.A.P.; Diekmann, O. *Mathematical Epidemiology of Infectious Diseases: Model Building, Analysis and Interpretation*; John Wiley & Sons: Hoboken, NJ, USA, 2000.
7. Keeling, M.J.; Rohani, P. *Modelling Infectious Diseases in Human and Animals*; Princeton University Press: Princeton, NJ, USA, 2007.
8. Hao, X.; Cheng, S.; Wu, D.; Wu, T.; Lin, X.; Wang, C. Reconstruction of the full transmission dynamics of COVID-19 in Wuhan. *Nature* **2020**, *584*, 420–424. [CrossRef] [PubMed]
9. Kucharski, A.J.; Russell, T.W.; Diamond, C.; Liu, Y.; Edmunds, J.; Funk, S.; Eggo, R.M.; Sun, F.; Jit, M.; Munday, J.D.; et al. Early dynamics of transmission and control of COVID-19: A mathematical modelling study. *Lancet Infect. Dis.* **2020**, *20*, 553–558. [CrossRef]
10. Lai, S.; Ruktanonchai, N.W.; Zhou, L.; Proper, O.; Luo, W.; Floyd, J.R.; Wesolowski, A.; Santillana, M.; Zhang, C.; Du, X.; et al. Effect of non-pharmaceutical interventions for containing the COVID-19 outbreak in China. *Nature* **2020**, *585*, 410–413. [CrossRef]
11. Wu, J.T.; Leung, K.; Leung, G.M. Nowcasting and forecasting the potential domestic and international spread of the 2019-nCoV outbreak originating in Wuhan, China: A modelling study. *Lancet* **2020**, *395*, 689–697. [CrossRef]
12. Zhang, J.; Litvinova, M.; Wang, W.; Wang, Y.; Deng, X.; Chen, X.; Li, M.; Zheng, W.; Yi, L.; Chen, X.; et al. Evolving epidemiology and transmission dynamics of coronavirus disease 2019 outside Hubei province, China: A descriptive and modelling study. *Lancet Infect. Dis.* **2020**, *20*, 793–802. [CrossRef]
13. Adekunle, A.I.; Adegboye, O.A.; Gayawan, E.; McBryde, E.S. Is Nigeria really on top of COVID-19? Message from effective reproduction number. *Epidemiol. Infect.* **2020**, *148*, e166. [CrossRef]
14. Heffernan, J.M.; Smith, R.J.; Wahl, L.M. Perspectives on the basic reproductive ratio. *J. R. Soc. Interface* **2005**, *2*, 281–293. [CrossRef]
15. Vynnycky, E.; White, R.G. *An Introduction to Infectious Disease Modelling*; Oxford University Press: Oxford, UK, 2010.
16. Biggerstaff, M.; Cowling, B.J.; Cucunubá, Z.M.; Dinh, L.; Ferguson, N.M.; Gao, H.; Hill, V.; Imai, N.; Johansson, M.A.; Kada, S.; et al. Early Insights from Statistical and Mathematical Modeling of Key Epidemiologic Parameters of COVID-19. *Emerg. Infect. Dis.* **2020**, *26*, e201074. [CrossRef]
17. Bai, Y.; Liu, K.; Chen, Z.; Chen, B.; Shao, Z. Early transmission dynamics of novel coronavirus pneumonia Epidemic in Shaanxi Province. *Chin. J. Nosocomiol.* **2020**, *30*, 834–838.
18. Wu, W.; Bai, R.; Li, D.; Feng, A.; Xu, A.; Lü, J. Preliminary prediction of the epidemic trend of 2019 novel coronavirus (2019-nCoV) pneumonia in Guangdong province. *J. Jinan Univ.* **2020**, *41*, 1–6.
19. D'Arienzo, M.; Coniglio, A. Assessment of the SARS-CoV_2 basic reproduction number, R0, based on the early phase of COVID-19 outbreak in Italy. *Biosaf. Health* **2020**, *2*, 57–59. [CrossRef]
20. Cheng, Q.; Liu, Z.; Cheng, G.; Huang, J. Heterogeneity and effectiveness analysis of COVID-19 prevention and control in major cities in China through time-varying reproduction number estimation. *Sci. Rep.* **2020**, *10*, 21953. [CrossRef]
21. Han, K.; Jia, W.; Cai, W.; Wang, S.; Song, Y.; Yang, S.; Li, J.; Kou, F.; Liu, M.; He, Y.; et al. Estimation of real-time basic reproduction number and epidemic status of 20-19 novel coronavirus disease (COVID-19) in first-tier cities. *Acad. J. Chin. PLA Med. Sch.* **2020**, *4*, 421–426.
22. Song, P.; Chen, C.; Lou, Y.; Jiang, H.; Li, W.; Zhu, L. Assessing effectiveness of integrated strategies for preventing and controlling the outbreak of COVID-19 and predicting impact of opening exit channels to leave Hubei Province. *Chin. J. Appl. Prob. Stat.* **2020**, *36*, 321–330.
23. Yuan, J.; Li, M.; Lv, G.; Lu, Z.K. Monitoring transmissibility and mortality of COVID-19 in Europe. *Int. J. Infect Dis.* **2020**, *95*, 311–315. [CrossRef]
24. Yang, L.; Wang, C.; Shang, H.; Zhang, X.; Zhang, L.; Wang, K. Epidemiological parameter estimation and characteristics of the novel coronavirus (COVID-19) transmission in Shaanxi Province. *J. Pub. Health Prev. Med.* **2021**, *32*, 195–199.
25. Birrell, P.J.; Zhang, X.-S.; Pebody, R.G.; Gay, N.J.; De Angelis, D. Reconstructing a spatially heterogeneous epidemic: Characterising the geographic spread of 2009 A/H1N1pdm infection in England. *Sci. Rep.* **2016**, *6*, 29004. [CrossRef] [PubMed]

26. Chong, K.C.; Cheng, W.; Zhao, S.; Ling, F.; Mohammad, K.N.; Wang, M.; Zee, B.C.; Wei, L.; Xiong, X.; Liu, H.; et al. Transmissibility of coronavirus disease 2019 in Chinese cities with different dynamics of imported cases. *PeerJ* **2020**, *8*, e10350. [CrossRef]
27. Yuan, H.Y.; Blakemore, C. The impact of multiple non-pharmaceutical interventions on controlling COVID-19 outbreak without lockdown in Hong Kong: A modelling study. *Lancet Reg. Health West. Pac.* **2021**, *20*, 100343. [CrossRef]
28. Yuan, H.Y.; Blakemore, C. The impact of contact tracing and testing on controlling COVID-19 outbreak without lockdown in Hong Kong: An observational study. *Lancet Reg. Health West. Pac.* **2022**, *20*, 100374. [CrossRef] [PubMed]
29. Bernal, J.L.; Panagiotopoulos, N.; Byers, C.; Vilaplana, T.G.; Boddington, N.; Zhang, X.-S.; Charlett, A.; Elgohari, S.; Coughlan, L.; Whillock, R.; et al. Transmission dynamics of COVID-19 in household and community settings in the United Kingdom, January to March 2020. *Eurosurveillance* **2022**, *27*, 2001551.
30. Zhang, X.S.; Vynnycky, E.; Charlett, A.; De Angelis, D.; Chen, Z.J.; Liu, W. Transmission dynamics and control measures of COVID-19 outbreak in China: A modelling study. *Sci. Rep.* **2021**, *11*, 2652. [CrossRef] [PubMed]
31. Yang, Z.; Zeng, Z.; Wang, K.; Wong, S.-S.; Liang, W.; Zanin, M.; Liu, P.; Cao, X.; Gao, Z.; Mai, Z.; et al. Modified SEIR and AI prediction of the epidemics trend of COVID-19 in China under public health interventions. *J. Torac. Dis.* **2020**, *12*, 165–174. [CrossRef] [PubMed]
32. Flaxman, S.; Mishra, S.; Gandy, A.; Unwin, H.J.T.; Mellan, T.A.; Coupland, H.; Whittaker, C.; Zhu, H.; Berah, T.; Eaton, J.W.; et al. Estimating the effects of non-pharmaceutical interventions on COVID-19 in Europe. *Nature* **2020**, *584*, 257–261. [CrossRef] [PubMed]
33. Lee, S.Y.; Lei, B.; Mallick, B. Estimation of COVID-19 spread curves integrating global data and borrowing information. *PLoS ONE* **2020**, *15*, e0236860. [CrossRef] [PubMed]
34. Dahal, S.; Luo, R.; Subedi, R.K.; Dhimal, M.; Chowell, G. Transmission Dynamics and Short-Term Forecasts of COVID-19: Nepal 2020/2021. *Epidemiologia* **2021**, *2*, 639–659. [CrossRef]
35. Swaraj, A.; Verma, K.; Kaur, A.; Singh, G.; Kumar, A.; Melo, L.; Sale, D. Implementation of stacking based ARIMA model for prediction of COVID-19 cases in India. *J. Biomed. Inform.* **2021**, *121*, 103887. [CrossRef]
36. Shaanxi Provincial Health Committee. Available online: http://sxwjw.shaanxi.gov.cn/sy/wjyw/index_66.html (accessed on 18 October 2020).
37. Richards, F. A flexible growth function for empirical use. *J. Exp. Bot.* **1959**, *10*, 290–300. [CrossRef]
38. Nelder, J.A. 182. note: An alternative form of a generalized logistic equation. *Biometrics* **1962**, *18*, 614–616. [CrossRef]
39. Hsieh, Y.-H. 2015 Middle East Respiratory Syndrome Coronavirus (MERS-CoV) nosocomial outbreak in South Korea: Insights from modeling. *PeerJ* **2015**, *3*, e1505. [CrossRef]
40. Wallinga, J.; Lipsitch, M. How generation intervals shape the relationship between growth rates and reproductive number. *Proc. Biol. Sci.* **2007**, *27*, 599–604. [CrossRef]
41. Nishiura, H.; Chowell, G.; Safan, M.; Castillo-Chavez, C. Pros and cons of estimating the reproduction number from early epidemic growth rate of influenza A (H1N1) 2009. *Theor. Biol. Med. Model.* **2010**, *7*, 1. [CrossRef]
42. Fraser, C. Estimating Individual and Household Reproduction Numbers in an Emerging Epidemic. *PLoS ONE* **2007**, *2*, e758. [CrossRef]
43. Cori, A.; Ferguson, N.M.; Fraser, C.; Cauchemez, S. A new Framework and software to estimate time varying reproduction numbers during epidemics. *Am. J. Epidemiol.* **2013**, *178*, 1505–1512. [CrossRef] [PubMed]
44. Roberts, M.G.; Nishiura, H. Early Estimation of the Reproduction Number in the Presence of Imported Cases: Pandemic Influenza H1N1-2009 in New Zealand. *PLoS ONE* **2011**, *6*, e17835. [CrossRef]
45. Griffin, J.T.; Garske, T.; Ghani, A.C.; Clarke, P.S. Joint estimation of the basic reproduction number and generation time parameters for infectious disease outbreaks. *Biostatistics* **2011**, *12*, 303–312. [CrossRef]
46. Ferretti, L.; Ledda, A.; Wymant, C.; Zhao, L.; Ledda, V.; Abeler-Dörner, L.; Kendall, M.; Nurtay, A.; Cheng, H.-Y.; Ng, T.-C.; et al. The timing of COVID-19 transmission. *medRxiv* **2020**. [CrossRef]
47. Wearing, H.J.; Rohani, P.; Keeling, M.J. Appropriate models for the management of infectious diseases. *PLoS Med.* **2005**, *2*, e174. [CrossRef]
48. Pasetto, D.; Lemaitre, J.C.; Bertuzzo, E.; Gatto, M.; Rinaldo, A. Range of reproduction number estimates for COVID-19 spread. *Biochem. Biophys. Res. Commun.* **2021**, *538*, 253–258. [CrossRef]
49. Xiang, Y.; Jia, Y.; Chen, L.; Guo, L.; Shu, B.; Long, E. COVID-19 epidemic prediction and the impact of public health interventions: A review of COVID-19 epidemic models. *Infect. Dis. Model.* **2021**, *6*, 324–342. [CrossRef] [PubMed]
50. Röst, G.; Bartha, F.A.; Bogya, N.; Boldog, P.; Dénes, A.; Ferenci, T.; Horváth, K.J.; Juhász, A.; Nagy, C.; Tekeli, T.; et al. Early phase of the COVID-19 outbreak in Hungary and post-lockdown scenarios. *Viruses* **2020**, *12*, 708. [CrossRef] [PubMed]
51. Polver, M.; Previdi, F.; Mazzoleni, M.; Zucchi, A. A SIAT3 HE model of the COVID-19 pandemic in Bergamo, Italy. *IFAC Pap.* **2021**, *54*, 263–268. [CrossRef]
52. Champredon, D.; Dushoff, J.; Earn, D.J.D. Equivalence of the Erlang-distributed SEIR epidemicmodel and the renewal equation. *SIAM J. Appl. Math.* **2018**, *78*, 3258–3278. [CrossRef]
53. Bettencourt, L.M.A.; Ribeiro, R.M. Real time Bayesian estimation of the epidemic potential of emerging infectious diseases. *PLoS ONE* **2008**, *3*, e2185. [CrossRef]
54. Cauchemez, S.; Carrat, F.; Viboud, C.; Valleron, A.J.; Boëlle, P.Y. A Bayesian MCMC approach to study transmission of influenza: Application to household longitudinal data. *Stat. Med.* **2004**, *23*, 3469–3487. [CrossRef]

55. Burnham, K.P.; Anderson, D.R. *Model Selection and Multimodel Inference: A Practical Information—Theoretic Approach*, 2nd ed.; Springer: New York, NY, USA, 2002.
56. Spiegelhalter, D.J.; Best, N.; Carlin, B.P.; van der Linde, A. Bayesian measures of model complexity and fit. *J. Roy. Stat. Soc. B* **2002**, *64*, 583–639. [CrossRef]
57. Alene, M.; Yismaw, L.; Assemie, M.A.; Ketema, D.B.; Gietaneh, W.; Birhan, T.Y. Serial interval and incubation period of COVID-19: A systematic review and meta-analysis. *BMC Infect. Dis.* **2021**, *21*, 257. [CrossRef]
58. Chen, Z.J.; Wei, T.; Li, H.D.; Feng, L.H.; Liu, H.N.; Li, N.; Gu, R.; Zhang, N.; Lu, W.; Zhang, X.-S. Renewal equation model for the COVID-19 in Yunnan. *Chin. Med. Humanit.* **2021**, *7*, 53–55.
59. Liu, Y.; Gayle, A.A.; Wilder-Smith, A.; Rocklov, J. The reproductive number of COVID-19 is higher compared to SARS coronavirus. *J. Travel Med.* **2020**, *27*, taaa021. [CrossRef]
60. Achaiah, N.C.; Subbarajasetty, S.B.; Shetty, R.M. R0 and Re of COVID-19: Can We Predict When the Pandemic Outbreak will be Contained? *Indian J. Crit. Care Med.* **2020**, *24*, 1125. [CrossRef]

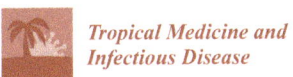 

*Article*

# Prevalence of *Escherichia coli* ST1193 Causing Intracranial Infection in Changsha, China

Yi-Ming Zhong [1,2], Xiao-He Zhang [3], Zheng Ma [3] and Wen-En Liu [1,2,*]

[1] Department of Clinical Laboratory, Xiangya Hospital, Central South University, Changsha 410008, China
[2] National Clinical Research Center for Geriatric Disorders, Xiangya Hospital, Central South University, Changsha 410008, China
[3] Faculty of Laboratory Medicine, Xiangya School of Medicine, Central South University, Changsha 410013, China
* Correspondence: wenenliuxycsu@163.com; Tel.: +86-731-84327437

**Abstract:** ST1193 is an emerging new virulent and resistant clone among *Escherichia coli* with a tendency to spread rapidly across the globe. However, the prevalence of intracranial infection-causing *E. coli* ST1193 is rarely reported. This study aimed at determining the prevalence of *E. coli* ST1193 isolates, causing intracranial infections in Changsha, central China. A total of 28 *E. coli* isolates were collected from the cerebrospinal fluid of patients with intracranial infection over a four-year period. All isolates were differentiated using multilocus sequence typing (MLST), and phylogenetic grouping, and tested for antibiotic resistance. MLST analysis showed 11 sequence types (ST) among the 28 *E. coli* isolates. The most prevalent ST was B2-ST1193 (28.6%, 8/28), followed by B2-ST131 (21.4%, 6/28) and F-ST648 (10.7%, 3/28). Of the eight ST1193 isolates, three carried CTX-M-55, and one carried CTX-M-27. All eight ST1193 isolates were resistant to Ciprofloxacin, showing *gyr*A1AB/*par*C4A mutations. Two ST1193 isolates carried the *aac(6′)-Ib-cr* gene. All ST1193 isolates were recovered from infants with meningitis, with a fatal outcome for one three-month-old infant. ST1193 has emerged as the predominant type of *E. coli* strain causing intracranial infections in Changsha, China. This study highlights the importance of implementing appropriate surveillance measures to prevent the spread of this emerging public health threat.

**Keywords:** *E. coli* ST1193; intracranial infections; antibiotic resistant; meningitis; clinical characteristics

## 1. Introduction

*Escherichia coli* is usually considered to be a part of the normal intestinal flora of humans. However, extraintestinal pathogenic *E. coli* (ExPEC) can cause a range of diseases, including sepsis, meningitis, and urinary tract infections [1–3]. *E. coli* is a major cause of neonatal bacterial meningitis and is responsible for approximately 33% of the cases [4]. Although less common, *E. coli* can also cause meningitis in adults [5]. Neonatal meningitis caused by *E. coli* is associated with fatality rates ranging from 5 to 30% in infants and a high incidence of neurological sequelae [6–8].

ST1193 is emerging as a new virulent clone among fluoroquinolone-resistant *E. coli* in several countries [9–13]. Most studies detected this lineage as a dominant clinical *E. coli* isolate, collected from urine and bloodstream samples [10–12]. Few studies have focused on the prevalence of this ST in cerebrospinal fluid [14]. A recent Chinese study reported that ST1193 was the most frequent sequence type in neonatal invasive *E. coli* infections, but not limited to cerebrospinal fluid [14]. Thus, whether ST1193 was also the predominant clone in cerebrospinal fluid is still uncertain. Recently, Oldendorff et al. reported a case in which ST1193 infection in a preterm newborn with meningitis led to a fatal outcome [15]. Therefore, more studies are warranted to broaden our knowledge on ST1193 causing intracranial infections.

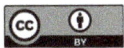

In this study, we aim to determine the prevalence of ST1193 isolates causing intracranial infections collected from the cerebrospinal fluid of patients with intracranial infections over the period of four years in a large university-affiliated hospital in China. The clinical characteristics and outcomes of infections caused by *E. coli* ST1193 were also assessed.

## 2. Materials and Methods

### 2.1. Bacterial Isolates

From January 2013 to December 2016, a total of 28 non-duplicate *E. coli* clinical isolates were consecutively collected from cerebrospinal fluid from patients with intracranial infections at a general teaching hospital affiliated with Central South University (Changsha, Hunan Province, China). The 28 samples were collected as a routine sampling procedure and represent the total number of these types of infections over a four-year period. The diagnosis of intracranial infection and meningitis were defined according to established diagnostic criteria [16,17]. This study was performed in line with the principles of the Declaration of Helsinki. Approval was granted by the Ethics Committee of the Xiangya Hospital of Central South University (reference number 202112178).

### 2.2. Multilocus Sequence Typing and Phylogenetic Group

Multilocus sequence typing (MLST) was performed on all isolates. Primers and PCR conditions for the seven housekeeping genes commonly used in *E. coli* MLST schemes (*adk*, *fumC*, *icd*, *mdh*, *purA*, *recA*, and *gyrB*) were obtained from databases at the University of Warwick (http://mlst.warwick.ac.uk/mlst/dbs/Ecoli) (accessed on 4 August 2022). The sequences of primers and annealing temperature were presented in Supplementary Table S1. Sequence data were analyzed using the *E. coli* MLST database. The phylogenetic groups of *E. coli* were determined by quadruplex PCR [18].

### 2.3. Antimicrobial Susceptibility Testing

Susceptibility testing was performed using the Vitek 2 system (bioMérieux, Marcy-l'Étoile, France). Susceptibilities to the following drugs were determined: ampicillin, cefazolin, ceftriaxone, ampicillin/sulbactam, piperacillin/tazobactam, imipenem, gentamicin, ciprofloxacin, aztreonam, trimethoprim/sulfamethoxazole. The results were interpreted according to Clinical and Laboratory Standards Institute (CLSI) criteria [19]. Extended-spectrum β-lactamase (ESBL) production was confirmed using the double disc synergy test. The *E. coli* ATCC 25922 strain was used as standard quality control. The intermediate susceptibility of isolates towards antibiotics was considered resistant.

### 2.4. Molecular Characterization of ST1193

For ST1193 isolates, detection of $bla_{CTX-M}$ was performed using PCR and amplicon sequencing [20,21]. The quinolone-resistance determining regions (QRDRs) in *gyrA* and *parC* genes were identified and amplicon sequencing was performed as previously described [22]. The screening of plasmid-mediated quinolone resistance (PMQR) determinants [*qnrA*, *qnrB*, *qnrC*, *qnrS*, *aac(6')-Ib-cr*, and *qepA*] was also conducted using PCR [23]. The sequences of primers for PCR amplification and annealing temperature are shown in Supplementary Table S1. The amplified PCR products were sequenced, and the results were analyzed by comparing them to sequences in GenBank (https://blast.ncbi.nlm.nih.gov/Blast.cgi) (accessed on 4 August 2022).

### 2.5. Clinical Data Collection

We reviewed the medical records of the patients with ST1193 infection and collected patient data, including data on demographic characteristics, clinical manifestations, laboratory tests, treatments, and clinical outcomes.

### 2.6. Statistical Analysis

Comparisons of proportions between groups were assessed via Fisher's exact test. A value of $p < 0.05$ was considered to be statistically significant.

## 3. Results

### 3.1. Multilocus Sequence Typing and Phylogenetic Group

MLST analysis revealed a total of 11 STs in the 28 E. coli isolates. Table 1 presents the distribution of ST types among the 28 E. coli isolates. The main STs were ST1193, ST131, and ST648, accounting for 28.6% (8/28), 21.4% (6/28), and 10.7% (3/28), respectively. The other types were ST354, ST38, and ST457, each ST accounting for 7.1% (2/28); ST58, ST69, ST23, ST95, and ST394, each ST accounting for 3.6% (1/28).

**Table 1.** Distribution of ST types and phylogenetic groups among the 28 E. coli isolates.

| MLST | Allelic Profile | | | | | | | Phylogenetic Group | No. (%) of Strains |
|---|---|---|---|---|---|---|---|---|---|
|  | adk | fumC | gyrB | icd | mdh | purA | recA | | |
| ST1193 | 14 | 14 | 10 | 200 | 17 | 7 | 10 | B2 | 8 (28.6) |
| ST131 | 53 | 40 | 47 | 13 | 36 | 28 | 29 | B2 | 6 (21.4) |
| ST648 | 92 | 4 | 87 | 96 | 70 | 58 | 2 | F | 3 (10.7) |
| ST354 | 85 | 88 | 78 | 29 | 59 | 58 | 62 | F | 2 (7.1) |
| ST38 | 4 | 26 | 2 | 25 | 5 | 5 | 19 | D | 2 (7.1) |
| ST457 | 101 | 88 | 97 | 108 | 26 | 79 | 2 | F | 2 (7.1) |
| ST58 | 6 | 4 | 4 | 16 | 24 | 8 | 14 | B1 | 1 (3.6) |
| ST69 | 21 | 35 | 27 | 6 | 5 | 5 | 4 | D | 1 (3.6) |
| ST23 | 6 | 4 | 12 | 1 | 20 | 13 | 7 | C | 1 (3.6) |
| ST95 | 37 | 38 | 19 | 37 | 17 | 11 | 26 | B2 | 1 (3.6) |
| ST394 | 21 | 35 | 61 | 52 | 5 | 5 | 4 | E | 1 (3.6) |

MLST: multi-locus sequence typing; ST: sequence type.

Phylogenetic analysis of the 28 E. coli strains showed that 15 (53.6%) belonged to phylogroup B2, 7 (25.0%) to phylogroup F, 3 (10.7%) to phylogroup D, 1 (3.6%) to phylogroup B1, 1 (3.6%) to phylogroup C, and 1 (3.6%) to phylogroup E.

### 3.2. Antimicrobial Susceptibility

Of the 28 isolates, 26 (92.9%) were found to be resistant to ampicillin, 22 (78.6%) to trimethoprim/sulfamethoxazole and cefazolin, 21 (75%) to ampicillin/sulbactam, and 19 (67.9%) to ceftriaxone and gentamicin (Table 2). Out of the 28 isolates, 60.7% (17/28) were ESBL producers.

**Table 2.** Antimicrobial resistance of the 28 E. coli isolates.

| Antimicrobial Resistance | No. (%) of Strains (n = 28) | No. (%) of Strains | | p-Value * |
|---|---|---|---|---|
|  |  | ST1193 (n = 8) | Non-ST1193 (n = 20) |  |
| Ampicillin | 26 (92.9) | 7 (87.5) | 19 (95.0) | 0.497 |
| Cefazolin | 22 (78.6) | 5 (62.5) | 17 (85.0) | 0.311 |
| Ceftriaxone | 19 (67.9) | 4 (50.0) | 15 (75.0) | 0.371 |
| Ampicillin/sulbactam | 21 (75.0) | 6 (75.0) | 15 (75.0) | 1.000 |
| Piperacillin/tazobactam | 1 (3.6) | 1 (12.5) | 0 (0) | 0.286 |
| Imipenem | 1 (3.6) | 0 (0) | 1 (5.0) | 1.000 |
| Gentamicin | 19 (67.9) | 5 (62.5) | 14 (70.0) | 1.000 |
| Ciprofloxacin | 17 (60.7) | 8 (100) | 9 (45.0) | 0.010 |
| Aztreonam | 12 (42.9) | 3 (37.5) | 9 (45.0) | 1.000 |
| Trimethoprim/sulfamethoxazole | 22 (78.6) | 7 (87.5) | 15 (75.0) | 0.640 |
| ESBLs | 17 (60.7) | 4 (50.0) | 13 (65.0) | 0.671 |

* ST1193 versus non-ST1193.

As shown in Table 2, the ST1193 isolates had a significantly higher prevalence of resistance to ciprofloxacin compared with non-ST1193. Ciprofloxacin resistance was found in 100% of the ST1193 isolates, whereas 45% of the non-ST1193 isolates were resistant.

### 3.3. Molecular Characterization of ST1193

Four of the eight ST1193 strains (50%) were recognized as ESBL producers. Three ESBL-producing isolates carried CTX-M-55, and the remaining carried CTX-M-27. All eight ciprofloxacin-resistant ST1193 isolates possessed a set of three amino acid replacement mutations (*gyr*A1AB Ser-83-Leu, Asp-87-Asn, and *par*C4A Ser-80-Ile) in QRDRs. Two ST1193 isolates carried the $aac(6')$-Ib-cr gene. None of the other types of PMQR determinants was detected in the tested isolates.

### 3.4. Clinical Characteristics of the Patients with ST1193 Infection

The demographical and clinical parameters of the eight patients with intracranial infections carrying ST1193 isolate are summarized in Table 3. All ST1193 isolates were recovered from infants with meningitis. They all exhibited typical manifestations, and their laboratory test results supported their diagnosis. Meropenem treatment was provided to all the selected patients; wherein, all except one patient showed recovery, and one had a fatal outcome. The patient with a fatal outcome was a three-month-old female exhibiting the symptoms of fever, neonatal coma, and convulsion. She was diagnosed with meningitis accompanying subdural effusion, hydrocephalus, and cerebral hernia. The disease progressed rapidly and led to an eventual fatality.

**Table 3.** Clinical characteristics and CTX-M genotype status in the eight patients with intracranial infections carrying ST1193 isolate.

| Clinical Characteristics | Patient 1 | Patient 2 | Patient 3 | Patient 4 | Patient 5 | Patient 6 | Patient 7 | Patient 8 |
|---|---|---|---|---|---|---|---|---|
| Age (days) | 85 | 26 | 12 | 61 | 6 | 92 | 13 | 79 |
| Gender | Male | Female | Male | Female | Female | Female | Female | Female |
| Fever | + | + | + | + | + | + | + | + |
| Convulsion | - | - | + | - | - | + | - | - |
| Meningitis | + | + | + | + | + | + | + | + |
| Subdural effusion | - | + | - | - | - | + | - | + |
| Laboratory test (CSF) | | | | | | | | |
| WBC ($\times 10^6$/L) | 7250 | 1280 | 2220 | 1020 | 2100 | 12820 | 2900 | 1310 |
| Glucose (mmol/L) | 0.20 | 0.43 | 0.24 | 0.25 | 0.71 | 0.06 | 0.02 | 0.14 |
| Protein (mg/L) | 2880 | 2140 | 2660 | 3370 | 2370 | 3520 | 2840 | 3010 |
| Treatment | MEM, TZP | MEM, CRO, AMC | MEM, SAM, CRO | MEM | MEM, CRO, AMC | MEM, CRO | MEM | MEM, CRO |
| Length of stay (days) | 38 | 30 | 56 | 26 | 29 | 8 | 38 | 43 |
| Outcome | Survived | Survived | Survived | Survived | Survived | Death | Survived | Survived |
| CTX-M genotype | CTX-M-27 | - | - | CTX-M-55 | - | CTX-M-55 | CTX-M-55 | - |

CSF: cerebrospinal fluid; MEM: meropenem; TZP: piperacillin/tazobactam; CRO: ceftriaxone; AMC: amoxicillin/clavulanic acid; SAM: ampicillin/sulbactam.

## 4. Discussion

ST1193 is an emerging new virulent and resistant clone among fluoroquinolone-resistant *E. coli* with a tendency to spread rapidly across the globe. Initial studies on ST1193 reported their isolation mostly from adult urine and a few from blood samples [10–12]. Ding et al. initially detected ST1193 isolate in neonatal blood and cerebrospinal fluid specimens of patients with meningitis [14]. Although the study provided the first evidence for the involvement of ST1193 in intracranial infections, it did not provide evidence for its predominance over other isolates in the cerebrospinal fluid of meningitis patients [14]. In the present study, we focused on determining the predominant ST of *E. coli* isolated from CSF of patients with intracranial infections. This is the first study to provide evidence to substantiate the prevalence and predominance of ST1193 (28.6%) over other STs in CSF of patients with intracranial infections. Berman et al. reported that the STs of *E. coli* isolates that were involved in causing meningitis included, ST131, ST69, ST405, and ST62, with no evidence for the detection of ST1193 [24]. These disparities may be due to geographical or host population differences. This finding implies that ST1193 may be poised to emerge as a major type of *E. coli* in patients with intracranial infections in China. A recent review described that ST1193 is following in the footsteps of the most successful MDR *E. coli* clone named ST131 [9]. Our study demonstrated that ST1193 has surpassed ST131 in *E. coli* intracranial infections in Changsha, China, which means this clone has become a public health threat and should be a concern. In order to investigate the emergence of ST1193, basic characteristics, surveillance, and clinical studies must be conducted on an urgent basis [9]. The information will be useful for managing and preventing this infectious disease.

Previous studies have reported that CTX-M-14 is the most prevalent ESBL genotype in China [25–27]. Wu et al. described that the CTX-M-14 genotype accounted for more than 50% of the $bla_{CTX-M}$ positive ST1193 isolates [28]. However, in the present study, CTX-M-55 (a single locus variant (SLV) of CTX-M-15) was a more popular genotype among the ESBL-producing ST1193 isolates. A previous study speculated that dissemination of the $bla_{CTX-M-55}$ in China may be partly because of the widespread prevalence of the *E. coli* ST1193 clone [29]. It has been reported in recent years that the worldwide increase in *E.coli*-producing CTXM-15 enzymes has been linked to epidemic clone ST131 [30]. CTX-M-55 has higher hydrolytic activity than CTX-M-15 and increased catalytic efficiency against ceftazidime and cefotaxime [31,32]. In this study, however, there was not enough data to determine whether CTX-M-55 was related to ST1193 due to the small sample size. Therefore, more studies with larger sample sizes are required to determine a putative association between ST1193 and the presence of CTX-M-55.

Consistent with the findings of Ding et al. [14], we found that all the ST1193 isolates were resistant to ciprofloxacin. The emergence of fluoroquinolone resistance of *E. coli* may be caused as a result of precise, analogous point mutations within the QRDRs of GyrA and ParC, the fluoroquinolone targets [22]. In the present study, all ciprofloxacin-resistance ST1193 isolates harbored the same distinctive mutations of three amino acid substitutions (*gyr*A1AB Ser-83-Leu, Asp-87-Asn, and *par*C4A Ser-80-Ile), complying with the previous reports [12,28,33]. The homogeneity of the ST1193 isolates suggests that this clone probably derived and spread from a common ancestor [12,28]. Johnson et al. reported that distinctive mutations in *gyr*A and *par*C may confer a fitness advantage for ST131 H30 isolates over non-H30 fluoroquinolone-resistant isolates [34]. Similarly, the particular *gyr*A/*par*C mutations of ST1193 may give this clone an advantage and promote its spread. Further research is necessary to verify this speculation and elucidate the role of these *gyr*A/*par*C mutations in ST1193. It seems that ST1193 isolates have some common features such as fluoroquinolone resistance, and QRDR mutations [9]. A high degree of homogeneity between ST1193 strains from different infection sites and geographical locations suggests they are likely descendants of the same ancestor [28]. Further studies are required to elucidate and monitor the evolution of ST1193.

In this study, all ST1193 isolates were collected from infants with meningitis. Although neonatal meningitis is an important cause of neonatal mortality, only a few studies have reported ST1193 infection in this fatal disease [14,15,35]. Ding et al. reported that ST1193 was the most common and invasive neonatal *E. coli* clone recovered from blood and CSF [14]. Only two recent case reports have described the fatal cases of neonatal meningitis caused by *E. coli* ST1193, one each in America and Sweden [15,35]. In our study, one patient who had a fatal outcome also suffered a similar fulminant course as that described in previous studies [15,35]. Therefore, considering the potential of this isolate in rapidly emerging, spreading, and causing severe outcomes, it requires adequate attention and implementation of appropriate measures to prevent its spread, especially in neonatal meningitis.

One limitation of this study was the small number of *E. coli* isolates due to the precious specimen source. Thus, a multicenter study with larger sample sizes is needed to further explore the characterization of ST1193 in CSF.

## 5. Conclusions

In summary, ST1193 has emerged as the predominant type of E. coli strain causing intracranial infections in patients in Changsha, China. It is an important public health issue, especially since this clone became the dominant strain of E. coli that caused this infectious disease. Considering the virulence and multidrug resistance, effective surveillance should be implemented to prevent the spread of ST1193 isolates in patients with intracranial infections.

**Supplementary Materials:** The following supporting information can be downloaded at: https://www.mdpi.com/article/10.3390/tropicalmed7090217/s1, Table S1: Sequences of primers for PCR amplification and annealing temperature.

**Author Contributions:** Conceptualization, W.-E.L. and Y.-M.Z.; methodology, X.-H.Z.; software, Z.M.; validation, W.-E.L. and Y.-M.Z.; formal analysis, Z.M.; investigation, X.-H.Z.; resources, W.-E.L.; data curation, X.-H.Z.; writing—original draft preparation, X.-H.Z. and Y.-M.Z.; writing—review and editing, W.-E.L. and Y.-M.Z.; visualization, W.-E.L.; supervision, W.-E.L.; project administration, W.-E.L. funding acquisition, W.-E.L. and Y.-M.Z. All authors have read and agreed to the published version of the manuscript.

**Funding:** This research was funded by the National Natural Science Foundation of China (81672066) and the Hunan Provincial Natural Science Foundation of China (2022JJ40847).

**Institutional Review Board Statement:** The study was conducted in accordance with the Declaration of Helsinki and approved by the Ethics Committees of the Xiangya Hospital of Central South University (reference number 202112178).

**Informed Consent Statement:** Patient consent was waived because the study was retrospective and used a database that ensured confidentiality.

**Data Availability Statement:** The data that support the findings of this study are available from the corresponding author (W.-E.L.) on reasonable request.

**Acknowledgments:** We thank all staff in the Microbiology Department of Xiangya Hospital for their support and assistance in bacteria collection and storage.

**Conflicts of Interest:** The authors declare no conflict of interest.

## References

1. Lipworth, S.; Vihta, K.-D.; Chau, K.; Barker, L.; George, S.; Kavanagh, J.; Davies, T.; Vaughan, A.; Andersson, M.; Jeffery, K.; et al. Ten-Year Longitudinal Molecular Epidemiology Study of Escherichia Coli and Klebsiella Species Bloodstream Infections in Oxfordshire, UK. Genome Med. **2021**, 13, 144. [CrossRef] [PubMed]
2. Liu, Y.; Zhu, M.; Fu, X.; Cai, J.; Chen, S.; Lin, Y.; Jiang, N.; Chen, S.; Lin, Z. Escherichia Coli Causing Neonatal Meningitis During 2001-2020: A Study in Eastern China. Int. J. Gen. Med. **2021**, 14, 3007–3016. [CrossRef] [PubMed]
3. Zhong, Y.-M.; Liu, W.-E.; Meng, Q.; Li, Y. Escherichia Coli O25b-ST131 and O16-ST131 Causing Urinary Tract Infection in Women in Changsha, China: Molecular Epidemiology and Clinical Characteristics. Infect. Drug Resist. **2019**, 12, 2693–2702. [CrossRef]
4. Ouchenir, L.; Renaud, C.; Khan, S.; Bitnun, A.; Boisvert, A.-A.; McDonald, J.; Bowes, J.; Brophy, J.; Barton, M.; Ting, J.; et al. The Epidemiology, Management, and Outcomes of Bacterial Meningitis in Infants. Pediatrics **2017**, 140, e20170476. [CrossRef]
5. Choi, C. Bacterial Meningitis in Aging Adults. Clin. Infect. Dis. **2001**, 33, 1380–1385. [CrossRef]
6. van de Beek, D.; Drake, J.M.; Tunkel, A.R. Nosocomial Bacterial Meningitis. N. Engl. J. Med. **2010**, 362, 146–154. [CrossRef]
7. Croxen, M.A.; Finlay, B.B. Molecular Mechanisms of Escherichia Coli Pathogenicity. Nat. Rev. Microbiol. **2010**, 8, 26–38. [CrossRef]
8. Kim, K.S. Acute Bacterial Meningitis in Infants and Children. Lancet Infect. Dis. **2010**, 10, 32–42. [CrossRef]
9. Pitout, J.D.D.; Peirano, G.; Chen, L.; DeVinney, R.; Matsumura, Y. Escherichia Coli ST1193: Following in the Footsteps of E. Coli ST131. Antimicrob. Agents Chemother. **2022**, 66, e0051122. [CrossRef]
10. Zhao, L.; Zhang, J.; Zheng, B.; Wei, Z.; Shen, P.; Li, S.; Li, L.; Xiao, Y. Molecular Epidemiology and Genetic Diversity of Fluoroquinolone-Resistant Escherichia Coli Isolates from Patients with Community-Onset Infections in 30 Chinese County Hospitals. J. Clin. Microbiol. **2015**, 53, 766–770. [CrossRef]
11. Kim, Y.; Oh, T.; Nam, Y.S.; Cho, S.Y.; Lee, H.J. Prevalence of ST131 and ST1193 Among Bloodstream Isolates of Escherichia Coli Not Susceptible to Ciprofloxacin in a Tertiary Care University Hospital in Korea, 2013–2014. Clin. Lab. **2017**, 63, 1541–1543. [CrossRef]
12. Platell, J.L.; Trott, D.J.; Johnson, J.R.; Heisig, P.; Heisig, A.; Clabots, C.R.; Johnston, B.; Cobbold, R.N. Prominence of an O75 Clonal Group (Clonal Complex 14) among Non-ST131 Fluoroquinolone-Resistant Escherichia Coli Causing Extraintestinal Infections in Humans and Dogs in Australia. Antimicrob. Agents Chemother. **2012**, 56, 3898–3904. [CrossRef]

13. Tchesnokova, V.L.; Rechkina, E.; Larson, L.; Ferrier, K.; Weaver, J.L.; Schroeder, D.W.; She, R.; Butler-Wu, S.M.; Aguero-Rosenfeld, M.E.; Zerr, D.; et al. Rapid and Extensive Expansion in the United States of a New Multidrug-Resistant *Escherichia Coli* Clonal Group, Sequence Type 1193. *Clin. Infect. Dis. Off. Publ. Infect. Dis. Soc. Am.* **2019**, *68*, 334–337. [CrossRef]
14. Ding, Y.; Zhang, J.; Yao, K.; Gao, W.; Wang, Y. Molecular Characteristics of the New Emerging Global Clone ST1193 among Clinical Isolates of *Escherichia Coli* from Neonatal Invasive Infections in China. *Eur. J. Clin. Microbiol. Infect. Dis.* **2021**, *40*, 833–840. [CrossRef]
15. Oldendorff, F.; Linnér, A.; Finder, M.; Eisenlauer, P.; Kjellberg, M.; Giske, C.G.; Nordberg, V. Case Report: Fatal Outcome for a Preterm Newborn With Meningitis Caused by Extended-Spectrum β-Lactamase-Producing *Escherichia Coli* Sequence Type 1193. *Front. Pediatr.* **2022**, *10*, 866762. [CrossRef]
16. Lin, C.; Zhao, X.; Sun, H. Analysis on the Risk Factors of Intracranial Infection Secondary to Traumatic Brain Injury. *Chin. J. Traumatol.* **2015**, *18*, 81–83. [CrossRef]
17. da Silva, L.P.A.; Cavalheiro, L.G.; Queirós, F.; Nova, C.V.; Lucena, R. Prevalence of Newborn Bacterial Meningitis and Sepsis during the Pregnancy Period for Public Health Care System Participants in Salvador, Bahia, Brazil. *Braz. J. Infect. Dis.* **2007**, *11*, 272–276. [CrossRef]
18. Clermont, O.; Christenson, J.K.; Denamur, E.; Gordon, D.M. The Clermont Escherichia Coli Phylo-Typing Method Revisited: Improvement of Specificity and Detection of New Phylo-Groups. *Environ. Microbiol. Rep.* **2013**, *5*, 58–65. [CrossRef]
19. Clinical and Laboratory Standards Institute. *Performance Standars for Antimicrial Susceptiblity Testing*, 26th ed.; CLSI Supplement M100; Clinical and Laboratory Standards Institute: Wayne, PA, USA, 2016.
20. Woodford, N.; Fagan, E.J.; Ellington, M.J. Multiplex PCR for Rapid Detection of Genes Encoding CTX-M Extended-Spectrum β-Lactamases. *J. Antimicrob. Chemother.* **2006**, *57*, 154–155. [CrossRef]
21. Kim, J.; Lim, Y.-M.; Jeong, Y.-S.; Seol, S.-Y. Occurrence of CTX-M-3, CTX-M-15, CTX-M-14, and CTX-M-9 Extended-Spectrum β-Lactamases in *Enterobacteriaceae* Clinical Isolates in Korea. *Antimicrob. Agents Chemother.* **2005**, *49*, 1572–1575. [CrossRef]
22. Johnson, J.R.; Tchesnokova, V.; Johnston, B.; Clabots, C.; Roberts, P.L.; Billig, M.; Riddell, K.; Rogers, P.; Qin, X.; Butler-Wu, S.; et al. Abrupt Emergence of a Single Dominant Multidrug-Resistant Strain of *Escherichia Coli*. *J. Infect. Dis.* **2013**, *207*, 919–928. [CrossRef] [PubMed]
23. Kim, H.B.; Park, C.H.; Kim, C.J.; Kim, E.-C.; Jacoby, G.A.; Hooper, D.C. Prevalence of Plasmid-Mediated Quinolone Resistance Determinants over a 9-Year Period. *Antimicrob. Agents Chemother.* **2009**, *53*, 639–645. [CrossRef]
24. Berman, H.; Barberino, M.G.; Moreira, E.D.; Riley, L.; Reis, J.N. Distribution of Strain Type and Antimicrobial Susceptibility of *Escherichia Coli* Isolates Causing Meningitis in a Large Urban Setting in Brazil. *J. Clin. Microbiol.* **2014**, *52*, 1418–1422. [CrossRef]
25. Zhong, Y.-M.; Liu, W.-E.; Liang, X.-H.; Li, Y.-M.; Jian, Z.-J.; Hawkey, P.M. Emergence and Spread of O16-ST131 and O25b-ST131 Clones among Faecal CTX-M-Producing *Escherichia Coli* in Healthy Individuals in Hunan Province, China. *J. Antimicrob. Chemother.* **2015**, *70*, 2223–2227. [CrossRef] [PubMed]
26. Yu, Y.; Ji, S.; Chen, Y.; Zhou, W.; Wei, Z.; Li, L.; Ma, Y. Resistance of Strains Producing Extended-Spectrum β-Lactamases and Genotype Distribution in China. *J. Infect.* **2007**, *54*, 53–57. [CrossRef]
27. Zeng, Q.; Xiao, S.; Gu, F.; He, W.; Xie, Q.; Yu, F.; Han, L. Antimicrobial Resistance and Molecular Epidemiology of Uropathogenic Escherichia Coli Isolated From Female Patients in Shanghai, China. *Front. Cell. Infect. Microbiol.* **2021**, *11*, 653983. [CrossRef] [PubMed]
28. Wu, Y.; Lan, F.; Lu, Y.; He, Q.; Li, B. Molecular Characteristics of ST1193 Clone among Phylogenetic Group B2 Non-ST131 Fluoroquinolone-Resistant Escherichia Coli. *Front. Microbiol.* **2017**, *8*, 2294. [CrossRef]
29. Xia, L.; Liu, Y.; Xia, S.; Kudinha, T.; Xiao, S.; Zhong, N.; Ren, G.; Zhuo, C. Prevalence of ST1193 Clone and IncI1/ST16 Plasmid in E-Coli Isolates Carrying BlaCTX-M-55 Gene from Urinary Tract Infections Patients in China. *Sci. Rep.* **2017**, *7*, 44866. [CrossRef]
30. Peirano, G.; Pitout, J.D.D. Molecular Epidemiology of Escherichia Coli Producing CTX-M Beta-Lactamases: The Worldwide Emergence of Clone ST131 O25:H4. *Int. J. Antimicrob. Agents.* **2010**, *35*, 316–321. [CrossRef]
31. Poirel, L. Biochemical Analysis of the Ceftazidime-Hydrolysing Extended-Spectrum Beta-Lactamase CTX-M-15 and of Its Structurally Related Beta-Lactamase CTX-M-3. *J. Antimicrob. Chemother.* **2002**, *50*, 1031–1034. [CrossRef] [PubMed]
32. Po, K.H.L.; Chan, E.W.C.; Chen, S. Functional Characterization of CTX-M-14 and CTX-M-15 β-Lactamases by In Vitro DNA Shuffling. *Antimicrob. Agents Chemother.* **2017**, *61*, e00891-17. [CrossRef]
33. Chang, J.; Yu, J.; Lee, H.; Ryu, H.; Park, K.; Park, Y.-J. Prevalence and Characteristics of Lactose Non-Fermenting Escherichia Coli in Urinary Isolates. *J. Infect. Chemother.* **2014**, *20*, 738–740. [CrossRef] [PubMed]
34. Johnson, J.R.; Johnston, B.; Kuskowski, M.A.; Sokurenko, E.V.; Tchesnokova, V. Intensity and Mechanisms of Fluoroquinolone Resistance within the *H* 30 and *H* 30Rx Subclones of Escherichia Coli Sequence Type 131 Compared with Other Fluoroquinolone-Resistant E. Coli. *Antimicrob. Agents Chemother.* **2015**, *59*, 4471–4480. [CrossRef] [PubMed]
35. Iqbal, J.; Dufendach, K.R.; Wellons, J.C.; Kuba, M.G.; Nickols, H.H.; Gómez-Duarte, O.G.; Wynn, J.L. Lethal Neonatal Meningoencephalitis Caused by Multi-Drug Resistant, Highly Virulent *Escherichia Coli*. *Infect. Dis.* **2016**, *48*, 461–466. [CrossRef] [PubMed]

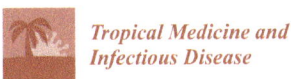 *Tropical Medicine and Infectious Disease*

*Communication*

# Can Biomarkers of Oxidative Stress in Serum Predict Disease Severity in West Nile Virus Infection? A Pilot Study

Maxim Van Herreweghe [1,*], Annelies Breynaert [1], Tess De Bruyne [1], Corneliu Petru Popescu [2], Simin-Aysel Florescu [2], Yaniv Lustig [3], Eli Schwartz [4], Federico Giovanni Gobbi [5], Nina Hermans [1] and Ralph Huits [1,5,6,*]

1. NatuRA Research Group, Department of Pharmaceutical Sciences, University of Antwerp, 2610 Wilrijk, Belgium
2. Department of Adult Infectious and Tropical Diseases, Carola Davila University of Medicine and Pharmacy and Dr Victor Babeș Clinical Hospital of Infectious and Tropical Diseases, 030303 Bucharest, Romania
3. The Central Virology Laboratory, Public Health Services, Ministry of Health, Sheba Medical Center, Tel Hashomer, Israel & Sackler Faculty of Medicine, Tel Aviv University, Tel Aviv 52621, Israel
4. Center for Geographic Medicine and Tropical Diseases, Sheba Medical Center, Tel Hashomer & Sackler Faculty of Medicine, Tel Aviv University, Tel Aviv 52621, Israel
5. IRCCS Ospedale Sacro Cuore Don Calabria, Department of Infectious Tropical Diseases and Microbiology, 37024 Verona, Italy
6. Institute of Tropical Medicine Antwerp, Department of Clinical Sciences, 2000 Antwerpen, Belgium
* Correspondence: maxim.vanherreweghe@uantwerpen.be (M.V.H.); ralph.huits@sacrocuore.it (R.H.); Tel.: +31-6-1884-6086 (R.H.)

**Abstract:** West Nile virus (WNV) can cause asymptomatic infection in humans, result in self-limiting febrile illness, or lead to severe West Nile Neuroinvasive disease (WNND). We conducted a pilot study to compare selected biomarkers of oxidative stress in sera of viremic West Nile virus patients and asymptomatic infected blood donors to investigate their potential as predictors of disease severity. We found that total oxidant status was elevated in WNND and in uncomplicated WNV infections (median 9.05 (IQR 8.37 to 9.74) and 7.14 (7.03 to 7.25) µmol $H_2O_2$ equiv./L, respectively) compared to asymptomatic infections (0.11 (0.07 to 0.19) µmol $H_2O_2$ equiv./L) ($p = 0.048$). MDA levels showed a similar trend to TOS, but differences were not significant at $\alpha = 0.05$. Total antioxidant status did not differ significantly between different disease severity groups. Oxidative stress appears to be associated with more severe disease in WNV-infected patients. Our preliminary findings warrant prospective studies to investigate the correlation of oxidative stress with clinical outcomes and severity of WNV infection.

**Keywords:** oxidative stress; West Nile virus; West Nile Fever; West Nile Neuroinvasive disease; *Flaviviridae*; biomarkers

## 1. Introduction

West Nile virus (WNV) is a single-stranded, positive sense RNA virus part of the genus *Flaviviridae*. It is one of multiple arboviruses of growing public health importance [1]. It is transmitted in bird populations by *Culex* mosquitoes, and several larger mammals, including humans, are considered dead-end hosts. WNV is endemic in the United States and an increasing public health threat across Europe and other continents, mainly due to climate change and global travel [1,2].

Human infections are frequently asymptomatic but lead to West Nile Fever (WNF) in 20% of infected patients, and in approximately 1% of infections to more serious pathologies such as meningitis, encephalitis, or flaccid paralysis [1,3]. Neurological presentations, commonly referred to as West Nile Neuroinvasive Disease (WNND), have fatality rates of approximately 10% [1,4]. Many WNND survivors report significant neurological sequelae that may persist for years after acute infection, including abnormal reflexes, muscle weakness, chronic fatigue, and hearing and sensory loss [1,4]. Age is the main risk factor for severe WNV infection, and WNND incidence increases 1.5-fold with each decade [3].

Our understanding of the pathogenesis, predictors of disease severity and neurological sequelae of neuronal injury in WNV infection remains incomplete. Previous studies implicated oxidative stress (OS), an imbalance between antioxidative defense mechanisms and production of cell-damaging reactive oxygen species (ROS), in *Flavivirus* pathogenesis [5–7]. Several studies have observed an increase in ROS in dengue-infected patients by comparing patients' OS markers to healthy controls [6,7]. However, data about OS in WNV infected patients are scarce. We hypothesized that OS plays an important role in the pathogenesis and severity of WNV disease [8,9]. In this pilot study, we evaluated selected OS biomarkers on a panel of stored human sera from patients with West Nile virus infection of varying severity.

## 2. Materials and Methods

The study protocol was approved by the relevant ethics committees (see ethics statement) and informed consent was provided by all participants. We obtained WNV-RNA qRT-PCR-positive serum samples from blood donors and patients with varying disease severity, i.e., asymptomatic (AS), WNF or WNND, at Sheba Medical Center, Tel Hashomer, Israel, during the 2020 transmission season. The qRT-PCR used primers and probes that targeted the envelope and capsid protein coding regions and the 5′ untranslated region, as described elsewhere [10,11]. Disease severity was assessed by the attending physicians. Patients were classified as WNF when febrile (temperature $\geq$ 38 °C), presenting with headache, rash or myalgia, and no signs of WNND. Patients were classified as WNND when they presented with encephalitis (altered mental status lasting $\geq$ 24 h with no alternative cause identified, generalized or partial seizures, new onset of focal neurologic findings, MRI abnormalities suggestive of encephalitis), meningitis (fever and headache AND/OR signs of meningeal irritation), or flaccid paralysis (as acute onset of progressive limb weakness over 48 h AND without sensory abnormalities). AS viremic individuals were identified among blood donors via Magen David Alom, during routine safety evaluation by the central virology lab at Sheba Medical Centre. All blood donors in Israel are screened for WNV RNA during the WNV transmission season using the Procleix WNV assay, a nucleic acid test (NAT) performed on the Procleix Panther system (Grifols, Spain) [12]. Positive NAT results are then confirmed using qRT-PCR (as mentioned above). Samples were collected at one time point only, handled, frozen and stored on-site until shipment to and analysis in the NatuRA lab in Antwerp in 2021. All OS markers were analyzed using commercially available kits, per manufacturer's instructions: Total Oxidant Status (TOS) and Total Antioxidant Status (TAS) using colorimetric kits (RelAssay Diagnostics, Şehitkamil, Turkey), malondialdehyde (MDA) was quantified using ELISA (My Biosource, San Diego, CA, USA).

SPSS Statistics (IBM; Armonk, NY, USA) was used for statistical analyses. The association of disease severity and markers of OS was analyzed using Kruskal–Wallis tests. All hypotheses were tested at significance level $\alpha$ = 0.05.

## 3. Results

Eight patients were recruited, six of which (75%) were female. Cycle-threshold values (Ct-values) for WNV RNA by qRT-PCR ranged from 32.63 to 41.25. Patients were categorized based on disease severity: four were asymptomatic (age range 18 to 59 years old), two had WNF (aged 23 and 43 years old), and two developed WNND (11 and 84 years old). Patient characteristics, WNV viral loads and serum concentrations of OS markers are shown in Table 1.

TOS in the WNND and WNF patients was significantly higher than in AS; 9.05 (8.37 to 9.74) (median, IQR) and 7.14 (7.03 to 7.25) and 0.11 (0.07 to 0.19) μmol $H_2O_2$ equiv./L, respectively ($p$ = 0.048) (Figure 1a). Median TAS was 1.12 (1.05 to 1.19), 1.64 (1.45 to 1.84) and 1.34 (0.95 to 1.80) mmol Trolox equiv./L, respectively (Figure 1b). TAS was slightly lower in the two WNND patients, but differences were less pronounced than with TOS or MDA. MDA concentrations were 749.04 (696.74 to 801.33) ng/mL in WNND, 772.65 (751.47 to 793.82) ng/mL in WNF and 420.26 (312.23 to 425.01) ng/mL in the AS group. While MDA levels showed a similar trend to TOS, differences were not statistically significant ($p = 0.105$) (Figure 1c).

**Table 1.** Serum concentrations of markers of oxidative stress in 8 WNV-infected patients from Israel.

| Patient | Age | Sex | WNV (Ct-Value) | Disease Severity | TOS (µmol $H_2O_2$ Equiv./L) | TAS (mmol Trolox Equiv./L) | MDA (ng/mL) |
|---|---|---|---|---|---|---|---|
| 1 | 84 | female | 32.63 | WNND | 10.42 | 1.26 | 644.44 |
| 2 | 11 | female | 41.25 | WNND | 7.69 | 0.99 | 853.63 |
| 3 | 23 | female | 38.38 | WNF | 7.36 | 2.04 | 730.30 |
| 4 | 43 | female | 33.13 | WNF | 6.92 | 1.25 | 814.99 |
| 5 | 59 | female | 36.64 | AS | 0.07 | 1.71 | 204.19 |
| 6 | 21 | female | 35.29 | AS | 0.07 | 0.97 | [a] |
| 7 | 18 | male | 35.58 | AS | 0.20 | 1.83 | 420.26 |
| 8 | 20 | male | 37.50 | AS | 0.15 | 0.94 | 429.76 |

Legend. WNV = West Nile virus, Ct-value = cycle threshold value, WNND = West Nile Neuroinvasive Disease, WNF = West Nile Fever, AS = asymptomatic, TOS = Total Oxidant Status, $H_2O_2$ = hydrogen peroxide, TAS = Total Antioxidant Status, MDA = malondialdehyde, [a] = measurement omitted due to spurious results. Each value for TOS, TAS and MDA is the mean of 2 measurements.

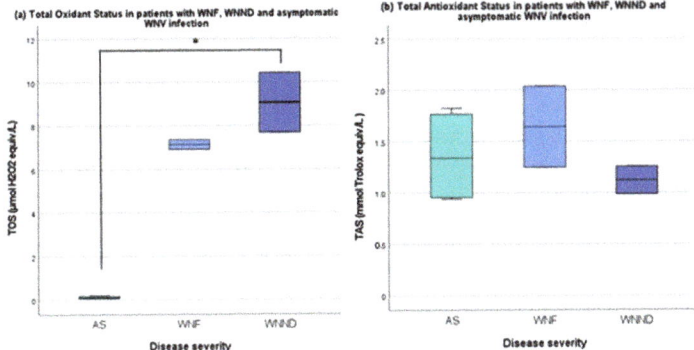

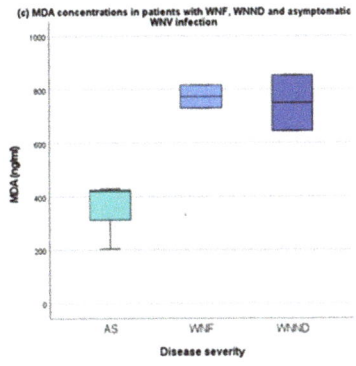

**Figure 1.** Boxplots of TOS (**a**), TAS (**b**) and MDA levels (**c**) in WNV-infected patients from Israel,

per disease severity subgroup. Legend. (**a**) TOS (median) 9.1, IQR [8.4–9.7], 7.1 [7.0–7.3] and 0.1 [0.1–0.12] µmol $H_2O_2$ equiv./L in WNND, WNF and AS groups, respectively. TOS was significantly higher in the WNND and WNF groups ($p$ = 0.048) compared to AS. (**b**) TAS (median) 1.1 [1.1–1.2], 1.6 [1.5–1.8] and 1.3 [1.0–1.8] mmol Trolox equiv./L, respectively. TAS was lower in the WNND patients (not significant). (**c**) MDA concentrations were higher in WNND (median) 749.0 ng/mL [696.7–801.3] and in WNF 772.7 [751.5–793.8] ng/mL than in AS (420.3 [312.2–425.0] ng/mL. (not significant, $p$ = 0.105). AS = asymptomatic, WNF = West Nile Fever, WNND = West Nile Neuroinvasive Disease, TOS = Total Oxidant Status, $H_2O_2$ = hydrogen peroxide, MDA = malondialdehde, TAS = Total Antioxidant Status. * = $p$ < 0.05 (Kruskal–Wallis test).

## 4. Discussion

We observed a significant increase in TOS in WNF and WNND compared to AS. The increased TOS, a summary parameter of the total oxidative capacity in a sample, suggests that oxidation is more prominent in WNF and WNND than in AS [13]. Because of the very small sample size, we were not able to discriminate between WNF and WNND using TOS in this pilot study. However, using a larger study population and parametric tests, a significant difference in TOS between WNF and WNND might still be observable. Still, the marked difference in TOS between symptomatic WNV disease and AS individuals calls for a detailed assessment of the redox status in WNV infections and an investigation of more specific biomarkers than TOS as a potential predictor of severe WNV disease.

Whereas TOS does not necessarily reflect oxidative damage (OD) to the host, MDA, the most widely studied end-product of lipid peroxidation, is a highly relevant marker of OD in neuronal toxicity studies [7,14]. The observed histopathology of the brain in WNND resembles that of neurodegenerative diseases, where brain cell damage results from lipid peroxidation [9,15]. This similarity may indicate that WNV-induced OS is an important contributor to the observed brain injury in WNND. We observed higher MDA levels in symptomatic patients, suggesting that lipid peroxidation was increased, although not significant, at $\alpha$ = 0.05. Therefore, our pilot study does not allow us to conclude that disease severity is positively correlated with the extent of OD to the host.

Studies of more specific biomarkers of OS than TOS in dengue virus (another member of the *Flavivirus* genus) infections detected significant differences in subgroups with varying disease severities. Protein carbonylation (PCO) was higher in dengue hemorrhagic fever (DHF) than in dengue fever in two studies by Soundravally et al. [16,17]. Patra et al. found higher intracellular ROS levels in erythrocytes of severely ill dengue patients than in patients with mild disease [18].

TAS levels did not follow the same distinctive trends as TOS and MDA, as shown in Figure 1. In other studies, TAS was significantly lower in patients with DHF and dengue shock syndrome than in those with uncomplicated dengue, but only later in the course of infection (day 5 and 7 after symptom onset) [16]. While TAS summarizes the total capacity of the antioxidant defense against ROS, TAS levels are more difficult to interpret because of a variety of confounders, such as dietary antioxidant intake and lifestyle [13]. Our results may indicate that the antioxidant capacity across different groups is comparable, but the investigation into the relationship between TAS and disease severity requires further study. Prospective, controlled studies are needed to establish if there is a correlation between the age-related declining efficiency of endogenous antioxidant systems and increased susceptibility to WNV-induced oxidative stress [19,20].

Because we studied single samples only, no changes in OS biomarkers over time could be established within the different severity subgroups. Longitudinal follow-up of WNV-infected patients is needed to study the intra-host kinetics of these biomarkers. Only markers that differentiate between patients at risk for WNND and patients with mild disease in the early stages of infection are likely to have diagnostic utility for clinical management. We do know that all patients here were in the acute stage of infection during sampling, as shown by their Ct values. These values are indicative of acute WNV infection in serum: in a paper from Lustig et al., WNV viral load in serum was shown to be less than 100 copies/mL on average [12]. A low viral load in the sample leads to high Ct values. Ct values in serum, plasma or cerebrospinal fluid of WNV-infected patients are almost always higher than 30, due to the low levels or even absence of viraemia at the time of symptom onset [12].

Important limitations apply to our study. First and foremost, the small sample size seriously limited statistical analysis. The limited number of subjects required the use of non-parametric tests, with less power compared to parametric testing. This makes it difficult to detect significant differences between the different disease severity groups. Second, while all samples were stored at $-80\ °C$ immediately after being received in the lab, OS marker measurements are susceptible to pre-analytical variations, and we cannot exclude this to have occurred in our pilot study. Third, variations in the duration of infection at the time of sampling could account for the observed differences in biomarker assays between individual patients. Nonetheless, all patients were in the acute, viremic stage of WNV infection, with viral loads in a similar range (Ct values 32.6–41.3). This duration could affect biomarker measurements. Still, we think these pilot results warrant further research into using more selective biomarkers for OS as potential predictors, reflecting its role in the neurological symptoms seen in WNF/WNND, and to see whether this OS could lie at the base of the observed pathology.

## 5. Conclusions

In our pilot study, we observed higher TOS levels in WNF and WNND patients than in asymptomatic WNV-infected controls. Prospective studies are warranted to investigate the association of increased lipid peroxidation and declining total antioxidant capacity with disease severity in WNV infections. We are planning an adequately powered prospective controlled cohort study to evaluate the clinical relevance of an extensive panel of peripheral OS biomarkers as predictors of disease severity in patients with WNV and related *Flavivirus* infections. In the projected study, we will also look at intra-host kinetics of the selected OS biomarkers at pre-specified timepoints since symptom onset. The identification of OS biomarkers as predictors of disease severity and long-term outcomes of WNND may assist physicians in the clinical management of patients with WNV infection.

**Author Contributions:** Writing—Original Draft: M.V.H.; Writing—Review and Editing: M.V.H., A.B., T.D.B., C.P.P., Y.L., E.S., F.G.G., N.H. and R.H.; Conceptualization: A.B., T.D.B., C.P.P., S.-A.F., N.H. and R.H.; Investigation: A.B., T.D.B., Y.L., E.S. and R.H.; Methodology: A.B., T.D.B., N.H. and R.H.; Formal Analysis: M.V.H., A.B., T.D.B., Y.L. and R.H.; Project Administration: A.B., N.H. and R.H.; Funding Acquisition: N.H. and R.H. All authors have read and agreed to the published version of the manuscript.

**Funding:** This work was supported by the Institute of Tropical Medicine and the University of Antwerp's Joint Pump Priming Proposal program (Antigoon ID 43642), funded by the Department of Economics, Science & Innovation of the Flemish Government, Belgium.

**Institutional Review Board Statement:** The study protocol was approved by the Institutional Review Board of the Institute of Tropical Medicine and the Ethics Committees of the University Hospital in Antwerp, Belgium and Sheba Medical Centre, Tel Hashomer, Israel (EC number: 20/19/253, 29 June 2020).

**Informed Consent Statement:** Informed consent was waived because of the retrospective nature of the study and the analysis used anonymous clinical data.

**Data Availability Statement:** All data generated or analyzed during this study are included in this published article.

**Conflicts of Interest:** The authors declare no conflict of interest.

## References

1. Petersen, L.R.; Brault, A.C.; Nasci, R.S. West Nile Virus: Review of the Literature. *JAMA* **2013**, *310*, 308–315. [CrossRef] [PubMed]
2. Rizzoli, A.; Jiménez-Clavero, M.A.; Barzon, L.; Cordioli, P.; Figuerola, J.; Koraka, P.; Martina, B.; Moreno, A.; Nowotny, N.; Pardigon, N.; et al. The challenge of West Nile virus in Europe: Knowledge gaps and research priorities. *Eurosurveillance* **2015**, *20*, 21135. [CrossRef]
3. Habarugira, G.; Suen, W.W.; Hobson-Peters, J.; Hall, R.A.; Bielefeldt-Ohmann, H. West Nile Virus: An Update on Pathobiology, Epidemiology, Diagnostics, Control and "One Health" Implications. *Pathogens* **2020**, *9*, 589. [CrossRef] [PubMed]
4. Weatherhead, J.E.; Miller, V.E.; Garcia, M.N.; Hasbun, R.; Salazar, L.; Dimachkie, M.M.; Murray, K.O. Long-term neurological outcomes in West Nile virus-infected patients: An observational study. *Am. J. Trop. Med. Hyg.* **2015**, *92*, 1006–1012. [CrossRef] [PubMed]
5. Zhang, Z.; Rong, L.; Li, Y.-P. Flaviviridae Viruses and Oxidative Stress: Implications for Viral Pathogenesis. *Oxid. Med. Cell. Longev.* **2019**, *2019*, 1409582. [CrossRef] [PubMed]
6. Gil, L.; Martínez, G.; Tápanes, R.; Castro, O.; González, D.; Bernardo, L.; Vázquez, S.; Kourí, G.; Guzmán, M.a.G. Oxidative stress in adult dengue patients. *Am. J. Trop. Med. Hyg.* **2004**, *71*, 652–657. [CrossRef] [PubMed]
7. Soundravally, R.; Hoti, S.L.; Patil, S.A.; Cleetus, C.C.; Zachariah, B.; Kadhiravan, T.; Narayanan, P.; Kumar, B.A. Association between proinflammatory cytokines and lipid peroxidation in patients with severe dengue disease around defervescence. *Int. J. Infect. Dis.* **2014**, *18*, 68–72. [CrossRef] [PubMed]
8. Koh, W.-L.; Ng, M.-L. Molecular mechanisms of West Nile virus pathogenesis in brain cell. *Emerg. Infect. Dis.* **2005**, *11*, 629–632. [CrossRef] [PubMed]
9. Liu, Z.; Zhou, T.; Ziegler, A.C.; Dimitrion, P.; Zuo, L. Oxidative Stress in Neurodegenerative Diseases: From Molecular Mechanisms to Clinical Applications. *Oxid. Med. Cell. Longev.* **2017**, *2017*, 2525967. [CrossRef] [PubMed]
10. Lanciotti Robert, S.; Kerst Amy, J.; Nasci Roger, S.; Godsey Marvin, S.; Mitchell Carl, J.; Savage Harry, M.; Komar, N.; Panella Nicholas, A.; Allen Becky, C.; Volpe Kate, E.; et al. Rapid Detection of West Nile Virus from Human Clinical Specimens, Field-Collected Mosquitoes, and Avian Samples by a TaqMan Reverse Transcriptase-PCR Assay. *J. Clin. Microbiol.* **2000**, *38*, 4066–4071. [CrossRef] [PubMed]
11. Linke, S.; Ellerbrok, H.; Niedrig, M.; Nitsche, A.; Pauli, G. Detection of West Nile virus lineages 1 and 2 by real-time PCR. *J. Virol. Methods* **2007**, *146*, 355–358. [CrossRef] [PubMed]
12. Lustig, Y.; Mannasse, B.; Koren, R.; Katz-Likvornik, S.; Hindiyeh, M.; Mandelboim, M.; Dovrat, S.; Sofer, D.; Mendelson, E. Superiority of West Nile Virus RNA Detection in Whole Blood for Diagnosis of Acute Infection. *J. Clin. Microbiol.* **2016**, *54*, 2294–2297. [CrossRef] [PubMed]
13. Wu, R.; Feng, J.; Yang, Y.; Dai, C.; Lu, A.; Li, J.; Liao, Y.; Xiang, M.; Huang, Q.; Wang, D.; et al. Significance of Serum Total Oxidant/Antioxidant Status in Patients with Colorectal Cancer. *PLoS ONE* **2017**, *12*, e0170003. [CrossRef] [PubMed]
14. Katerji, M.; Filippova, M.; Duerksen-Hughes, P. Approaches and Methods to Measure Oxidative Stress in Clinical Samples: Research Applications in the Cancer Field. *Oxid. Med. Cell. Longev.* **2019**, *2019*, 1279250. [CrossRef] [PubMed]
15. Grubaugh, N.D.; Massey, A.; Shives, K.D.; Stenglein, M.D.; Ebel, G.D.; Beckham, J.D. West Nile Virus Population Structure, Injury, and Interferon-Stimulated Gene Expression in the Brain From a Fatal Case of Encephalitis. In *Open Forum Infectious Diseases*; Oxford University Press: Oxford, UK, 2015; Volume 3. [CrossRef]
16. Soundravally, R.; Sankar, P.; Bobby, Z.; Hoti, S.L. Oxidative stress in severe dengue viral infection: Association of thrombocytopenia with lipid peroxidation. *Platelets* **2008**, *19*, 447–454. [CrossRef] [PubMed]
17. Rajendiran, S.; Lakshamanappa, H.S.; Zachariah, B.; Nambiar, S. Desialylation of plasma proteins in severe dengue infection: Possible role of oxidative stress. *Am. J. Trop. Med. Hyg.* **2008**, *79*, 372–377. [CrossRef] [PubMed]
18. Patra, G.; Saha, B.; Mukhopadhyay, S. High titres of IgM-bound circulating immune complexes and erythrocytic oxidative damage are indicators of dengue severity. *Clin. Exp. Immunol.* **2019**, *198*, 251–260. [CrossRef] [PubMed]
19. Montgomery, R.R. Age-related alterations in immune responses to West Nile virus infection. *Clin. Exp. Immunol.* **2017**, *187*, 26–34. [CrossRef] [PubMed]
20. Tan, B.L.; Norhaizan, M.E.; Liew, W.-P.-P.; Sulaiman Rahman, H. Antioxidant and Oxidative Stress: A Mutual Interplay in Age-Related Diseases. *Front. Pharmacol.* **2018**, *9*, 1162. [CrossRef] [PubMed]

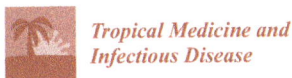

*Tropical Medicine and Infectious Disease*

Article

# Gender and Cutaneous Leishmaniasis in Israel

Michal Solomon [1,*], Inbal Fuchs [2], Yael Glazer [3] and Eli Schwartz [4]

1. Department of Dermatology, Chaim Sheba Medical Center, Tel Hashomer, The Sackler School of Medicine, Tel Aviv University, Tel Aviv 8436322, Israel
2. Clalit Health Services-Southern District Department of Family Medicine, Faculty of Health Sciences, Ben Gurion University, Beer Sheva 84105, Israel
3. Division of Epidemiology, Ministry of Health, Jerusalem 9462401, Israel
4. Center for Geographic Medicine and Tropical Diseases, Chaim Sheba Medical Center, Tel Hashomer, The Sackler School of Medicine, Tel Aviv University, Tel Aviv 6997801, Israel
* Correspondence: michal.solomon2@sheba.health.gov.il; Tel.: +972-52-8629799

**Abstract:** Leishmaniasis is estimated to be more common in males than in females. Our purpose was to evaluate differences in preponderance in relation to sex and gender across cutaneous and mucocutaneous leishmaniasis in Israel. An observational study was performed, including cases of endemic CL (cutaneous leishmaniasis) in Israel, and imported MCL (mucocutaneous leishmaniasis). CL is a notifiable disease and is supposed to be reported to the Ministry of Health (MOH). The MOH database shows that males as more likely to be infected by leishmania, with an incidence of 5/100,000 in males vs. 3.5/100,000 in females. However, while conducting a demographic house-to-house survey in several locations in Israel where CL is highly endemic, among 608 people who were screened only 49% were males in *Leishmania major* (*L. major*) endemic regions and 41% were males in *Leishmania tropica* (*L. tropica*) endemic regions, while among 165 cases of imported New-World cutaneous leishmaniasis in Israeli travelers freturning from abroad, 142 (86%) were males. It may be postulated that there is no real gender difference in leishmanial infection, but, perhaps, infections are more commonly seen in men because of referral/reported bias, due to more risk-taking behaviors by men or, perhaps, men are less likely to strictly adhere to recommended preventive measures and thus increase their risk of contracting the disease.

**Keywords:** cutaneous leishmaniasis; mucocutaneous leishmaniasis; *Leishmania major*; *Leishmania tropica*; *Leishmania braziliensis*; gender

**Citation:** Solomon, M.; Fuchs, I.; Glazer, Y.; Schwartz, E. Gender and Cutaneous Leishmaniasis in Israel. *Trop. Med. Infect. Dis.* **2022**, *7*, 179. https://doi.org/10.3390/tropicalmed7080179

Academic Editor: Yannick Simonin

Received: 6 July 2022
Accepted: 6 August 2022
Published: 12 August 2022

**Publisher's Note:** MDPI stays neutral with regard to jurisdictional claims in published maps and institutional affiliations.

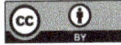

**Copyright:** © 2022 by the authors. Licensee MDPI, Basel, Switzerland. This article is an open access article distributed under the terms and conditions of the Creative Commons Attribution (CC BY) license (https://creativecommons.org/licenses/by/4.0/).

## 1. Introduction

Cutaneous leishmaniasis (CL) is endemic to Israel and is caused mainly by Old-World cutaneous leishmaniasis (OWCL). In the past, CL in Israel was almost exclusively attributed to *Leishmania major* (*L. major*) [1,2]. The disease is typically more common in the Arava, along the Jordan River Valley and in the rural areas of the Negev Desert. However, over the last two decades or so there have been increasing reports of CL due to *Leishmania tropica* (*L. tropica*) in several other regions of Israel, including the hilly and mountainous regions, Samaria in the center of the country and in northern Israel [3,4].

Additionally, travel to Central and South America has increased over the past two decades, mainly among young Israeli adults, increasing potential exposure to various tropical diseases, including leishmaniasis [5]. New-World cutaneous leishmaniasis (NWCL), which is endemic to some parts of the Americas, is caused by *Leishmania viannia* and *Leishmania mexicana* species complexes. Infection with *L. viannia* species, particularly *Leishmania viannia braziliensis* (*L. (V) braziliensis*), results in cutaneous leishmaniasis (CL) which tends to be persistent and may be further complicated by mucocutaneous leishmaniasis (MCL) [6]. Among Israeli travelers *L. (V) braziliensis* was found to be the dominant species, acquired mostly in the Amazon region of Bolivia, causing CL and MCL [7].

Most studies of CL and MCL provide minimal data on sex and gender. Differences between the sexes in the incidence and severity of infection might be related to physiological or genetic constitutions [8], but could also result from differences in exposure, use of preventive strategies [9], participation in high-risk activities, attractiveness to vectors, routes of pathogen entry, or processing of pathogens and cellular responses. A recent study of sex-related differences in leishmaniasis, showed that environmental exposure and healthcare access [10] alone do not explain the variance. Moreover, transcriptomic evidence reveals that biological sex is a variable which impacts physiology, drug metabolism, immune response, and, consequently, the progression of disease [10].

In this paper, we sought to evaluate gender and sex differences among CL patients in Israel as well as returning Israeli travelers with CL/MCL.

## 2. Materials and Methods

Leishmaniasis is a notifiable disease in Israel. All cases reported to the Ministry of Health (MOH) were analyzed based on Leishmania species and gender. Because many cases are not reported, in certain areas where CL is highly endemic, we chose to carry out a demographic survey. One such region was in Southern Israel (Negev) where *L. major* is the common species, and where, starting in 2010, a dramatic increase in CL cases was observed by the primary clinic staff of three kibbutzim.

Clinical and demographic data of patients who presented to the three kibbutzim clinics were recorded. In the context of outbreak investigation, a questionnaire was sent to all kibbutz members including those who had not presented to the clinic, inquiring if any household members had cutaneous leishmanial lesions and did not present to the clinic. Demographic and clinical data concerning those additional patients were completed by phone interviews conducted by the kibbutz nurses.

The other region was in Samaria, in the central part of Israel, where *L. tropica* is the common species and where similar house-to-house enquiries were made.

In addition, we analyzed data from returning travelers with CL and MCL due to *L. (V) braziliensis* who presented at Sheba Medical Center, a tertiary medical center in Israel.

OWCL was diagnosed when patients from endemic areas developed cutaneous lesions (ulcers, nodules, or papules) that were clinically similar to leishmaniasis, when biopsy or smear specimens revealed Leishmania amastigotes within a dermal infiltrate, or when a polymerase chain reaction (PCR) assay revealed positive results for *L. major* or *L. tropica*.

NWCL was diagnosed when (i) cutaneous lesions (ulcers, nodules, or papules) that were clinically compatible with leishmaniasis were observed, and one or both of the following tests came back positive, (ii) a smear or biopsy specimen showed Leishmania amastigotes within a dermal or mucosal infiltrate, and (iii) a polymerase chain reaction (PCR) assay tested positive for *Leishmania vianna braziliensis*. [5]

MCL: All cases of MCL were symptomatic with either nasal or oral symptoms and proven by PCR, culture, or biopsy for leishmaniasis [11].

*Statistical Analysis*

Data entry and analysis was performed using the statistical package for the social sciences (SPSS) version 23.0 for Windows software. Interquartile range (IQR) and the median were used to express continuous variables, whereas percentages were used to indicate categorical variables. Fisher's exact test (two-tailed) was used to compute the $p$-value in the prevalence assessment. A $p$-value < 0.05 was considered significant.

## 3. Results

The nationally reported cases of CL in the MOH registry showed 382 cases of *L. major* during the years 2012–2016, among them 203 (53%) males and 179 (47%) females. There were 348 cases of *L. tropica*, among them 191 (55%) males and 157 (45%) females

The MOH database shows that males are also more likely to be infected with leishmania, with a male incidence of 5/100,000 vs. a female incidence of 3.5/100,000 in 2015.

In our house-to-house survey, among the total population of three Kibbutzim in the Negev in southern Israel—which is known to be an endemic area for *L. major*—1146 people were screened, and 330 patients with *L. major* CL were identified between the years 2010 and 2013; 164/330 (49.6%) were males. Demographic data are presented in Table 1. The median age at diagnosis was 48 years (range 0.6–87 years).

**Table 1.** CL in three kibbutzim and one village endemic for Leishmania in Israel.

| | *L. major* | | | | *L. tropica* | Total Old-World Leishmaniasis (*L. major* and *L. tropica*) |
|---|---|---|---|---|---|---|
| | Kibbutz 1 | Kibbutz 2 | Kibbutz 3 | Total | Village (Sample) | |
| Cases/total population (%) | 160/346 (46.2) | 148/380 (39) | 22/420 (5.2) | 330/1146 (28.7) | 278/1096 (25.3) | 608 |
| Gender | | | | | | |
| Male * | 78 (48.8) | 75 (50.7) | 11 (50) | 164 (49.6) | 114 (41) | 278 (45.7) |
| Female | 82 (51.2) | 73 (49.3) | 11 (50) | 166 (50.3) | 164 (59) | 330 (54.2) |
| Age | | | | | | |
| 0–15 | 10 (6.2) | 19 (12.8) | 3 (13.6) | 32 (9.6) | 143 (51.4) | 176 |
| 15–64 | 98 (61.2) | 101 (68.2) | 16 (72.7) | 215 (65.1) | 134 (48.2) | 351 |
| 65+ | 52 (32.5) | 28 (18.9) | 3 (13.6) | 83 (25.1) | 1 (0.4) | 85 |

\* $p$-value between males and females is non-significant. *L. major* = Leishmania major and *L. tropica* = Leishmania tropica.

In Peduel, a village in Samaria, in central Israel, an endemic area for *L. tropica*, between the years 2008 and 2012; 1096 people (25% of the total village population) were screened. Among them, 278 (25.3%) were diagnosed with CL. Gender distribution was 114 (41%) males and 164 (59%) females in comparison to 49% males in the *L. major* group ($p$ value = 0.03).

Altogether, in these population-based screenings of four villages, 278 males (45.7%) and 330 females (54.2%) were diagnosed. Most of the patients in the *L. major* group were between the ages of 15 and 64 years (65%), however in the *L. tropica* group most of the patients were children between the ages of 0 and 15 years (51.4%) (Table 1).

Among travelers, the total number of patients diagnosed with NWCL from South America at Sheba Medical Center during the years 1993–2021 was 165. All the cases were acquired in Bolivia's Amazon region, where *Leishmania (V.) braziliensis* is known to be endemic. In this cohort, the majority were males 140 (85%).

MCL: Nineteen patients (11.5%) were diagnosed with MCL among the cohort of travelers returning from Latin America with leishmaniasis. Among them the majority (18 patients (95%)) were also males. The high rate of males in the MCL group was non-significantly higher than that of the other NWCL cases (95% vs. 84%) (Table 2).

**Table 2.** Comparison between New-World CL patients and MCL patients with cutaneous leishmaniasis and mucocutaneous leishmaniasis.

| | Total New-World Leishmania Cases | Cutaneous LeishmaniAsis | Mucocutaneous LeishManiasis | Percentage of Mucocutaneous Leishmaniasis * |
|---|---|---|---|---|
| No. of patients | 165 | 146 | 19 | 11.5% |
| Males | 142 | 124 (84%) | 18 (95%) | 12.6% |
| Females | 23 | 22 (15%) | 1 (5%) | 4.3% |
| Mean age (years) | | 24.2 | 27.6 | |

\* $p$ value is insignificance. CL, cutaneous leishmaniasis and MCL, mucocutaneous leishmaniasis.

## 4. Discussion

Gender relates to a person's self-representation as male or female and to the way that social institutions influence that person, and it is shaped by environment and experience [9], while sex is biologically determined (the sexual genotype is XX in the female and XY in the male). Most studies of NWCL and MCL provide scant information regarding gender and sex in relation to leishmania infection. Disparities between the sexes in the incidence and severity of infection might be attributed to 'sex' differences such as genetic and physiological constitutions [8], or to 'gender'/cultural differences such as participation in high-risk activities [9].

In this study we examined three cohorts of leishmanial patients regarding their gender distribution. Each cohort gave a different result. The most striking difference between males and females was found among travelers returning from South America where NWCL was acquired.

There is epidemiological evidence of a sex bias in NWCL [12]. Data from the New World documented a higher incidence of CL in males than in females in Mexico and Colombia, and similar studies from all around Brazil reveal males developing cutaneous manifestations of leishmaniasis more frequently than females [12–18]. A nationwide study found that in infants under the age of one year, males had a higher rate of CL in comparison to females. Minipuberty, a transient postnatal rise in sex steroid levels that exhibits clear hormonal variations between boys and girls has been linked to other sex-biased infectious diseases [19,20] and may be the cause of the predominance in male infants. Overall, the prevalence of CL among males increased at puberty, peaked during adulthood, and then decreased in the elderly. This occurred even though it is unlikely that males experience increased parasite exposure, suggesting that the observed sex dichotomy has a biological basis [19,21]. Together, these data lend credence to the hypothesis that innate biological characteristics place males at higher risk of New-World CL.

Reported leishmaniasis cases in travelers show that most cases are in males [22]. The rate of infected males among returning Israeli travelers was 84% of all those diagnosed with NWCL. This high proportion of males is far greater than the known distribution of Israelis visiting the tropics, which is about 50% of each gender [23]. However, all these infections were contracted while on adventure trips in the Amazon region in Bolivia, an area known to be endemic for *Leishmania (V.) braziliensis* [22,24]. We therefore cannot rule out the possibility that female travelers are less likely to visit this region specifically or that they take stricter precautions. Indeed, the Geosentinel report about NWCL also reported a high rate of male travelers (72%) [22]. The additional observation we made among these patients was assessing the rate of mucosal leishmania among those who contracted NWCL. Among the cohort mentioned above, 11% (19/165) of travelers developed MCL. Although the rate of MCL was higher in males (12%) vs. 4% in females, this was a non-significant difference (Table 2). A higher rate of MCL in males was also documented in the local population [24]. Whether the lack of a clear gender difference regarding this severe complication in our cohort is due to the small sample size or due to a real lack of difference should be further investigated.

Among OWCL we presented two cohorts; one was the reported cases to the MOH while the other was the house-to-house survey.

Israel is endemic for CL and all cases must be reported to the Ministry of Health (MOH), whose database also shows males as more prone to leishmania infection, with an incidence of 5/100,000 in males vs. 3.5/100,000 in females. We chose to carry out a demographic survey in several areas where CL is highly endemic because it is an established fact that there is significant under-reporting of the condition. One of these regions was in Southern Israel (Negev) where *L. major* is the common species, while the other was in Central Israel where the common species is *L. tropica*. A total of 608 people was screened, and results showed that altogether there were 278 males (45.7%) and 330 females (54.2%) infected. However, in the *L. major* endemic region, 49% were males and 51% were females, while in the *L. tropica* endemic region 41% were males and 59% were females (Table 1).

Multiple endemic regions of the Old World have documented CL incidence varying between the sexes. It is argued that whether there is a sex bias, and its direction if there is, is determined by a complex interaction between environmental, host gender, and biological factors, and the infective Leishmania species [25–29]. Our data clearly demonstrate that the rate of infection is relatively comparable across males and females when population-based screening is carried out, avoiding referral and reporting biases, and or/risky travel to endemic regions.

Patient and animal models of infection of Old-World species have both shown sex-based differences [30]. It was estimated that CL due to *L. major* is more common in males [28,31], while in some endemic areas *L. tropica* infection seems to be more prevalent among females, and that males are more likely to develop viscerotropic leishmaniasis [10,27,32]. However, the mechanisms responsible for this variability are elusive [30].

Although in animal models sex was found to be a risk factor, we did not find it in our results. It was estimated that leishmaniasis is more common in males. However, in our cohort when house-to-house screening was done, the rate of infection in males and females was comparable. The reason for this difference is the avoidance of referral and reporting biases, or/risky travel to endemic regions.

## 5. Conclusions

In order to check the rate of CL and MCL infections, house-to-house screening is the preferred method. Our research in Israel demonstrates that there are no real differences between the sexes in cutaneous leishmaniasis infection rate, but infections are more frequently seen in men, possibly due to reporting and referral bias, riskier behavior, and travel to more remote destinations where the risk of contracting tropical diseases is higher. Men may also be less likely to adhere to preventive measures, which increases their risk of contracting the disease.

**Author Contributions:** Conceptualization M.S. and E.S. Methodology M.S. and E.S. Software I.F. Validation M.S. and E.S. Formal analysis I.F. and E.S. Investigation, E.S.; resources, Y.G. and I.F.; data curation, M.S., E.S. and I.F. Y.G.; writing—original draft preparation, M.S.; writing—review and editing, M.S.; visualization, M.S.; supervision, E.S.; project administration, E.S.; funding acquisition, NO. All authors have read and agreed to the published version of the manuscript.

**Funding:** This research received no external funding.

**Institutional Review Board Statement:** The study was conducted in accordance with the Declaration of Helsinki, and approved by the Institutional Review Board Sheba Medical Center (protocol code 7274-09, 2009l).

**Informed Consent Statement:** Not applicable.

**Data Availability Statement:** No new data were created or analyzed in this study. Data sharing is not applicable to this article.

**Conflicts of Interest:** The authors have no conflict of interest to declare.

## Abbreviations

| | |
|---|---|
| NWCL | New-World cutaneous leishmaniasis |
| OWCL | Old-World cutaneous leishmaniasis |
| *L. (V.) braziliensis* | *Leishmania viannia braziliensis* |
| *L. Major* | *Leishmania major* |
| *L. Tropica* | *Leishmania tropica* |
| CL | Cutaneous leishmaniasis |
| MCL | Mucocutaneous leishmaniasis |
| PCR | Polymerase chain reaction |

## References

1. Jaffe, C.L.; Baneth, G.; Abdeen, Z.A.; Schlein, Y.; Warburg, A. Leishmaniasis in Israel and the Palestinian Authority. *Trends. Parasitol.* **2004**, *20*, 328–332. [CrossRef] [PubMed]
2. Schlein, Y.; Warburg, A.; Schnur, L.F.; Le Blancq, S.M.; Gunders, A.E. Leishmaniasis in Israel: Reservoir hosts, sandfly vectors and leishmanial strains in the Negev, Central Arava and along the Dead Sea. *Trans. R Soc. Trop. Med. Hyg.* **1984**, *78*, 480–484. [CrossRef]
3. Shani-Adir, A.; Kamil, S.; Rozenman, D.; Schwartz, E.; Ramon, M.; Zalman, L.; Nasereddin, A.; Jaffe, C.L.; Ephros, M. Leishmania tropica in northern Israel: A clinical overview of an emerging focus. *J. Am. Acad. Dermato.l* **2005**, *53*, 810–815. [CrossRef]
4. Azmi, K.; Schönian, G.; Nasereddin, A.; Schnur, L.F.; Sawalha, S.; Hamarsheh, O.; Ereqat, S.; Amro, A.; Qaddomi, S.E.; Abdeen, Z. Epidemiological and clinical features of cutaneous leishmaniases in Jenin District, Palestine, including characterisation of the causative agents in clinical samples. *Trans. R Soc. Trop. Med. Hyg.* **2012**, *106*, 554–562. [CrossRef]
5. Schonian, G.; Nasereddin, A.; Dinse, N.; Schweynoch, C.; Schallig, H.D.; Presber, W.; Jaffe, C.L. PCR diagnosis and characterization of Leishmania in local and imported clinical samples. *Diagn. Microbiol. Infect. Dis.* **2003**, *47*, 349–358. [CrossRef]
6. Herwaldt, B.L. Leishmaniasis. *Lancet* **1999**, *354*, 1191–1199. [CrossRef]
7. Scope, A.; Trau, H.; Anders, G.; Barzilai, A.; Confino, Y.; Schwartz, E. Experience with New World cutaneous leishmaniasis in travelers. *J. Am. Acad. Dermatol.* **2003**, *49*, 672–678. [CrossRef]
8. Jansen, A.; Stark, K.; Schneider, T.; Schoneberg, I. Sex differences in clinical leptospirosis in Germany: 1997–2005. *Clin. Infect. Dis.* **2007**, *44*, e69–e72. [CrossRef] [PubMed]
9. Schlagenhauf, P.; Chen, L.H.; Wilson, M.E.; Freedman, D.O.; Tcheng, D.; Schwartz, E.; Pandey, P.; Weber, R.; Nadal, D.; Berger, C.; et al. Sex and gender differences in travel-associated disease. *Clin. Infect. Dis.* **2010**, *50*, 826–832. [CrossRef] [PubMed]
10. Lockard, R.D.; Wilson, M.E.; Rodríguez, N.E. Sex-Related Differences in Immune Response and Symptomatic Manifestations to Infection with *Leishmania* Species. *J. Immunol. Res.* **2019**, *2019*, 4103819. [CrossRef]
11. Solomon, M.; Sahar, N.; Pavlotzky, F.; Barzilai, A.; Jaffe, C.L.; Nasereddin, A.; Schwartz, E. Mucosal Leishmaniasis in Travelers with Leishmania braziliensis Complex Returning to Israel. *Emerg. Infect. Dis.* **2019**, *25*, 642–648. [CrossRef] [PubMed]
12. Lezama-Davila, C.M.; Oghumu, S.; Satoskar, A.R.; Isaac-Marquez, A.P. Sex-associated susceptibility in humans with chiclero's ulcer: Resistance in females is associated with increased serum-levels of GM-CSF. *Scand. J. Immunol.* **2007**, *65*, 210–211. [CrossRef] [PubMed]
13. Medina-Morales, D.A.; Machado-Duque, M.E.; Machado-Alba, J.E. Epidemiology of Cutaneous Leishmaniasis in a Colombian Municipality. *Am. J. Trop. Med. Hyg.* **2017**, *97*, 1503–1507. [CrossRef] [PubMed]
14. Munoz, G.; Davies, C.R. Leishmania panamensis transmission in the domestic environment: The results of a prospective epidemiological survey in Santander, Colombia. *Biomedica* **2006**, *26* (Suppl. S1), 131–144. [CrossRef] [PubMed]
15. Brilhante, A.F.; Melchior, L.A.K.; Nunes, V.L.B.; Cardoso, C.O.; Galati, E.A.B. Epidemiological aspects of American cutaneous leishmaniasis (ACL) in an endemic area of forest extractivist culture in western Brazilian Amazonia. *Rev. Inst. Med. Trop. Sao. Paulo.* **2017**, *59*, e12. [CrossRef] [PubMed]
16. Gosch, C.S.; Marques, C.P.; Resende, B.S.; Souza, J.D.S.; Rocha, R.; Lopes, D.S.S.; Gosch, M.S.; Dias, F.R.; Dorta, M.L. American tegumentary leishmaniasis: Epidemiological and molecular characterization of prevalent Leishmania species in the State of Tocantins, Brazil, 2011–2015. *Rev. Inst. Med. Trop. Sao Paulo* **2017**, *59*, e91. [CrossRef] [PubMed]
17. Guimaraes, L.H.; Queiroz, A.; Silva, J.A.; Silva, S.C.; Magalhaes, V.; Lago, E.L.; Machado, P.R.; Bacellar, O.; Wilson, M.E.; Beverley, S.M.; et al. Atypical Manifestations of Cutaneous Leishmaniasis in a Region Endemic for Leishmania braziliensis: Clinical, Immunological and Parasitological Aspects. *PLoS Negl. Trop. Dis.* **2016**, *10*, e0005100. [CrossRef]
18. Turetz, M.L.; Machado, P.R.; Ko, A.I.; Alves, F.; Bittencourt, A.; Almeida, R.P.; Mobashery, N.; Johnson, W.D., Jr.; Carvalho, E.M. Disseminated leishmaniasis: A new and emerging form of leishmaniasis observed in northeastern Brazil. *J. Infect. Dis.* **2002**, *186*, 1829–1834. [CrossRef]
19. Guerra-Silveira, F.; Abad-Franch, F. Sex bias in infectious disease epidemiology: Patterns and processes. *PLoS ONE* **2013**, *8*, e62390. [CrossRef]
20. Johannsen, T.H.; Main, K.M.; Ljubicic, M.L.; Jensen, T.K.; Andersen, H.R.; Andersen, M.S.; Petersen, J.H.; Andersson, A.M.; Juul, A. Sex Differences in Reproductive Hormones During Mini-Puberty in Infants With Normal and Disordered Sex Development. *J. Clin. Endocrinol. Metab.* **2018**, *103*, 3028–3037. [CrossRef]
21. Soares, L.; Abad-Franch, F.; Ferraz, G. Epidemiology of cutaneous leishmaniasis in central Amazonia: A comparison of sex-biased incidence among rural settlers and field biologists. *Trop. Med. Int. Health* **2014**, *19*, 988–995. [CrossRef] [PubMed]
22. Boggild, A.K.; Caumes, E.; Grobusch, M.P.; Schwartz, E.; Hynes, N.A.; Libman, M.; Connor, B.A.; Chakrabarti, S.; Parola, P.; Keystone, J.S.; et al. Cutaneous and mucocutaneous leishmaniasis in travellers and migrants: A 20-year GeoSentinel Surveillance Network analysis. *J. Travel Med.* **2019**, *26*, taz055. [CrossRef] [PubMed]
23. Solomon, M.; Benenson, S.; Baum, S.; Schwartz, E. Tropical skin infections among Israeli travelers. *Am. J. Trop. Med. Hyg.* **2011**, *85*, 868–872. [CrossRef] [PubMed]
24. Jones, T.C.; Johnson, W.D., Jr.; Barretto, A.C.; Lago, E.; Badaro, R.; Cerf, B.; Reed, S.G.; Netto, E.M.; Tada, M.S.; Franca, F.; et al. Epidemiology of American Cutaneous Leishmaniasis Due to Leishmania braziliensis braziliensis. *J. Infect. Dis.* **1987**, *156*, 73–83. [CrossRef] [PubMed]

25. Aara, N.; Khandelwal, K.; Bumb, R.A.; Mehta, R.D.; Ghiya, B.C.; Jakhar, R.; Dodd, C.; Salotra, P.; Satoskar, A.R. Clinco-epidemiologic study of cutaneous leishmaniasis in Bikaner, Rajasthan, India. *Am. J. Trop. Med. Hyg.* **2013**, *89*, 111–115. [CrossRef]
26. Bamba, S.; Gouba, A.; Drabo, M.K.; Nezien, D.; Bougoum, M.; Guiguemdé, T.R. Epidemiological profile of cutaneous leishmaniasis: Retrospective analysis of 7444 cases reported from 1999 to 2005 at Ouagadougou, Burkina Faso. *Pan. Afr. Med. J.* **2013**, *14*, 108. [CrossRef] [PubMed]
27. Hakkour, M.; Hmamouch, A.; El Alem, M.M.; Rhalem, A.; Amarir, F.; Touzani, M.; Sadak, A.; Fellah, H.; Sebti, F. New epidemiological aspects of visceral and cutaneous leishmaniasis in Taza, Morocco. *Parasit Vectors* **2016**, *9*, 612. [CrossRef]
28. Moein, D.; Masoud, D.; Saeed, M.; Abbas, D. Epidemiological Aspects of Cutaneous Leishmaniasis during 2009-2016 in Kashan City, Central Iran. *Korean J. Parasitol.* **2018**, *56*, 21–24. [CrossRef]
29. Turan, E.; Yeşilova, Y.; Sürücü, H.A.; Ardic, N.; Doni, N.; Aksoy, M.; Yesilova, A.; Oghumu, S.; Varikuti, S.; Satoskar, A.R. A Comparison of Demographic and Clinical Characteristics of Syrian and Turkish Patients with Cutaneous Leishmaniasis. *Am. J. Trop. Med. Hyg.* **2015**, *93*, 559–563. [CrossRef]
30. Kobets, T.; Havelkova, H.; Grekov, I.; Volkova, V.; Vojtiskova, J.; Slapnickova, M.; Kurey, I.; Sohrabi, Y.; Svobodova, M.; Demant, P.; et al. Genetics of host response to Leishmania tropica in mice–different control of skin pathology, chemokine reaction, and invasion into spleen and liver. *PLoS Negl. Trop. Dis.* **2012**, *6*, e1667. [CrossRef]
31. Solomon, M.; Greenberger, S.; Baum, S.; Pavlotsky, F.; Barzilai, A.; Schwartz, E. Unusual forms of cutaneous leishmaniasis due to Leishmania major. *J. Eur. Acad. Dermatol. Venereol.* **2016**, *30*, 1171–1175. [CrossRef] [PubMed]
32. Reithinger, R.; Mohsen, M.; Aadil, K.; Sidiqi, M.; Erasmus, P.; Coleman, P.G. Anthroponotic cutaneous leishmaniasis, Kabul, Afghanistan. *Emerg. Infect. Dis.* **2003**, *9*, 727–729. [CrossRef] [PubMed]

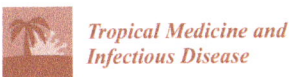 

*Article*

# Expression Profile Analysis of Circular RNAs in Leishmaniasis

Zhongqiu Li [1], Wenbo Zeng [1], Yufeng Yang [2], Peijun Zhang [3], Zhengbing Zhou [1], Yuanyuan Li [1], Yunhai Guo [1] and Yi Zhang [1,4,*]

[1] National Institute of Parasitic Diseases, Chinese Center for Disease Control and Prevention (Chinese Center for Tropical Diseases Research), NHC Key Laboratory of Parasite and Vector Biology, WHO Collaborating Center for Tropical Diseases, National Center for International Research on Tropical Diseases, Shanghai 200025, China
[2] Rizhang Center for Disease Control and Prevention, Rizhao 276803, China
[3] Yangquan Center for Disease Control and Prevention, Yangquan 045000, China
[4] School of Global Health, Chinese Center for Tropical Diseases Research, Shanghai Jiao Tong University School of Medicine, Shanghai 200025, China
* Correspondence: zhangyi@nipd.chinacdc.cn

**Abstract:** Leishmaniasis is a neglected tropical disease that seriously influences global public health. Among all the parasitic diseases, leishmaniasis is the third most common cause of morbidity after malaria and schistosomiasis. Circular RNAs (circRNAs) are a new type of noncoding RNAs that are involved in the regulation of biological and developmental processes. However, there is no published research on the function of circRNAs in leishmaniasis. This is the first study to explore the expression profiles of circRNAs in leishmaniasis. GO and KEGG analyses were performed to determine the potential function of the host genes of differentially expressed circRNAs. CircRNA–miRNA–mRNA (ceRNA) regulatory network analysis and protein–protein interaction (PPI) networks were analyzed by R software and the STRING database, respectively. A total of 4664 significant differentially expressed circRNAs were identified and compared to those in control groups; a total of 1931 were up-regulated and 2733 were down-regulated. The host genes of differentially expressed circRNAs were enriched in ubiquitin-mediated proteolysis, endocytosis, the MAPK signaling pathway, renal cell carcinoma, autophagy and the ErbB signaling pathway. Then, five hub genes (*BRCA1*, *CREBBP*, *EP300*, *PIK3R1*, and *CRK*) were identified. This study provides new evidence of the change of differentially expressed circRNAs and its potential function in leishmaniasis. These results may provide novel insights and evidence for the diagnosis and treatment of leishmaniasis.

**Keywords:** leishmaniasis; circular RNA; neglected tropical diseases; zoonotic diseases

**Citation:** Li, Z.; Zeng, W.; Yang, Y.; Zhang, P.; Zhou, Z.; Li, Y.; Guo, Y.; Zhang, Y. Expression Profile Analysis of Circular RNAs in Leishmaniasis. *Trop. Med. Infect. Dis.* **2022**, *7*, 176. https://doi.org/10.3390/tropicalmed7080176

Academic Editor: Yannick Simonin

Received: 12 July 2022
Accepted: 7 August 2022
Published: 10 August 2022

**Publisher's Note:** MDPI stays neutral with regard to jurisdictional claims in published maps and institutional affiliations.

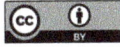

**Copyright:** © 2022 by the authors. Licensee MDPI, Basel, Switzerland. This article is an open access article distributed under the terms and conditions of the Creative Commons Attribution (CC BY) license (https:// creativecommons.org/licenses/by/ 4.0/).

## 1. Introduction

Leishmaniasis, a zoonotic disease, is one of the neglected tropical diseases that can seriously influence global public health [1]. There are three main types of leishmaniasis: visceral leishmaniasis, cutaneous leishmaniasis and mucocutaneous leishmaniasis. It is widely distributed around the world, present in 101 countries, and is transmitted through the bite of infected female sandflies, whose hosts are animals such as canids, rodents, marsupials, hyraxes, and human beings [2]. Leishmaniasis is an obligate intracellular pathogen that is mainly parasitic on host cells, and it is one of the parasitic diseases that can be dangerous to human health [3]. Among all the parasitic diseases, leishmaniasis is the third highest cause of morbidity after malaria and schistosomiasis in terms of disability adjusted life years (DALYs) [4]. However, it is the second most common cause of mortality after malaria. According to publication reports, there are 101 countries and approximately 350 million people living in leishmaniasis-endemic areas [5]. Most leishmaniasis patients live in impoverished areas, which makes prevention, diagnosis, and treatment very difficult [6]. Therefore, more than 2 million people are afflicted by leishmaniasis worldwide each year, resulting in an estimated 40,000 deaths [7]. This parasite also has a high recurrence rate;

patients may relapse after 6–12 months despite receiving the appropriate treatment [8]. Moreover, if untreated, patients can develop multisystem disease or a secondary infection, potentially leading to death [9]. Detecting pathogens is the traditional way to diagnose leishmaniasis through the smear or culture tests of bone marrow aspirate [10]. However, bone marrow aspiration is not only painful, but its protozoa density is also extremely low, and it is easy to miss the diagnosis. In addition to this, visceral leishmaniasis has no specific clinical symptoms; it is easy to confuse it with other diseases, especially in endemic areas [11,12]. Therefore, it is also necessary to conduct epidemiological investigations. Furthermore, the occurrence of minimally symptomatic and completely asymptomatic and subclinical disease is considered an important aspect of the epidemiology of visceral leishmaniasis, which requires clinicians to determine more epidemiological characteristics of leishmaniasis [13]. Hence, it is important to research the mechanism of visceral leishmaniasis in order to find effective diagnostic biomarkers.

Circular RNAs (circRNAs) were first discovered in RNA viruses in 1976 [14]. With the development of high-throughput sequencing technology, thousands of circRNAs species have been detected, and this number is still increasing. Although circRNAs are a new type of the non-coding RNAs with covalent closed-loop structures, some circRNAs have protein-coding potential [15,16]. He et al. first discovered that circRNAs have protein-coding capacity in his research on the hepatitis D virus [17]. Published research shows that the post-translation products of circRNA can participate in multiple physiological processes in the human body, for example, preventing the linear translation product from being degraded by ubiquitin proteases [18]. Moreover, circRNAs can competitively bind with microRNA (miRNA) and act as a miRNA sponge, thereby affecting the regulation of miRNA on target genes [19]. Previous research has found that when circACVR2A is overexpressed, it can act as a sponge for miRNA-626 to regulate EYA4 gene expression through the enhancement of cell proliferation, migration, and invasion in bladder cancer cells [20]. Rong et al. found that has_circ_0002577 can act as an miR-197 sponge to regulate the proliferation and invasion of endometrial cancer cells [21]. CircRNAs are more resistant to exonuclease degradation than linear RNA. Therefore, circRNAs have greater stability [22]. Many studies have shown that they are related to various diseases, including cancer [23], cerebrovascular diseases [24], systemic lupus erythematosus [25] and so on. However, there is no published study on the function and molecular mechanisms of circRNAs in leishmaniasis.

Zoonotic diseases seriously influence human health through spillover effects from their impact on animals and the environment [26]. In order to reduce the harm of zoonotic diseases, this study, according to the different expressions of circRNAs in patients, finds biomarkers of leishmaniasis. Therefore, the differentially expressed circRNAs and miRNAs were screened by high-throughput sequencing. Furthermore, the functionals and pathways of host genes were analyzed by gene ontology (GO) and the Kyoto Encyclopedia of Genes and Genomes (KEGG). In addition, the correlation of all genes was performed though protein–protein interaction (PPI) and the competing endogenous RNAs (ceRNA) network. This study may provide assistance for leishmaniasis diagnosis and expand the horizons of targeted gene therapy.

## 2. Materials and Methods

### 2.1. Clinical Samples

According to data from the Infectious Disease Reporting Information Management System of the Chinese Center for Disease Control and Prevention, leishmaniasis is most prevalent in Yangquan, China. The sera of 3 leishmaniasis patients and 3 healthy persons (controls) were obtained from the Yangquan Center for Disease Control and Prevention.

### 2.2. RNA Extraction

Total RNA was extracted using TRIzol reagent (Thermo Fisher Scientific, Waltham, MA, USA). Additionally, the concentrations of RNA samples were measured, and purity was determined with an ultraviolet spectrophoto-meter (NanoDrop ND-1000, NanoDrop, Wilmington, DE, USA). RNA integrity and gDNA contamination were assessed by agarose gel electrophoresis.

*2.3. Library Construction and RNA Sequence Analysis*

The RNA libraries were constructed using RNA samples with the RNA Integrity Number (RIN) $\geq 8$. Subsequently, the RNA libraries were controlled for quality by the Bio-Analyzer 2100 system. The RNA-Seq libraries were performed in NovaSeq6000 (San Diego, CA, USA). RNA-seq data were analyzed using the Tuxedo protocol. The reads were aligned to GRCh38.p13 (http://asia.ensembl.org/Homo_sapiens/Info/Index (accessed on 12 March 2022)) by TopHat (version 2.1.1, Daehwan Kim and Steven Salzberg, MD, USA). Additionally, the transcript assembly and abundance were determined using Cufflinks (version 2.1.1, the lab of Cole Trapnell, Washington, DC, USA). circRNAs/miRNAs were analyzed as significantly different expressions with an absolute fold change $\geq 2$ and with $p < 0.05$.

*2.4. Screening od Differentially Expressed circRNAs and miRNAs*

Differentially expressed circRNAs-/-miRNAs were determined and data were normalization using R software (v4.0.3, Hadley Wickham, IA, USA). A $t$-test was used to identify differentially expressed circRNAs and miRNAs with a significance level $\leq 0.05$. The differentially expressed circRNAs and miRNAs thresholds were analyzed with a fold change $\geq 2$. Moreover, the fold change and $p$-value were used to identify the top 10 up-and down-regulated differentially expressed circRNAs and miRNAs in leishmaniasis patients and local normal health persons. Volcano plots were visualized by ggplot2 in R software (v4.0.3).

*2.5. Functional and Pathway Enrichment Analyses*

Gene ontology (GO) analysis was used to highlight the biological processes (BP), molecular functions (MF), and cellular components (CC) of genes. Hence, the host genes of differentially expressed circRNAs were analyzed for their potential function. Kyoto Encyclopedia of Genes and Genomes (KEGG) pathway analyses were performed to find the functional attributes of the host genes using clusterProfiler (v4.0.2, Vince Carey, Boston, MA, USA); $p < 0.05$ was set as the statistically significant difference.

*2.6. PPI Network Construction and Regulation ceRNA Network*

The STRING database (https://string-db.org/ (accessed on 23 March 2022)), an online biological database, can display interactions of proteins and genes. Then, the potential relationship of hosts genes and proteins for differentially expressed circRNAs was determined. The PPI network (PPI score > 0.8) was used to accomplish this Cytoscape (version 3.6.1, NIGMS, Bethesda, USA). The interactions between circRNAs and miRNA were identified by TargetScan and miRanda databases. Subsequently, mRNAs were predicted through response elements-MiRNAs by miRTarBase (version 2, Hsien-Da Huang, HongKong, China), miRWalk (version 3, University of Heidelberg, Heidelberg, Germany), miRDB (Xiaowei Wang, Washington University School of Medicine in St. Louis, Washington, DC, USA) and TargetScan (version 7.1, Bartel laboratory, MA, USA) software. Finally, an endogenous competitive ceRNA (circRNAs–miRNA–mRNA) network was constructed using Cytoscape software, with a $p$ value $< 0.05$.

**3. Results**

*3.1. The Differential Expression of Serum circRNAs and miRNAs*

According to the statistical criteria of fold change $\geq 2$ and $p < 0.05$, a total of 4664 significant differentially expressed circRNAs were identified compared with those in the control groups, of which 1931 were up-regulated and 2733 were down-regulated. Stratified cluster analysis showed that the circRNA expression patterns were distinguishable between leishmaniasis patients and healthy control group (Figure 1A), and volcano plots were used to show the significant differentially expressed circRNAs in the leishmaniasis patients' group (Figure 1B). The top 10 up- (Table 1) and down-regulated (Table 2) circRNAs are listed in the tables in this paper. Under the same statistical screening conditions, there were 57 significant differentially expressed miRNAs, including 28 that were up-regulated and 29 that were down-regulated (Figure 2A,B). Similarly, the details of the top 10 up- (Table 3) and down-regulated (Table 4) differentially expressed miRNAs are listed.

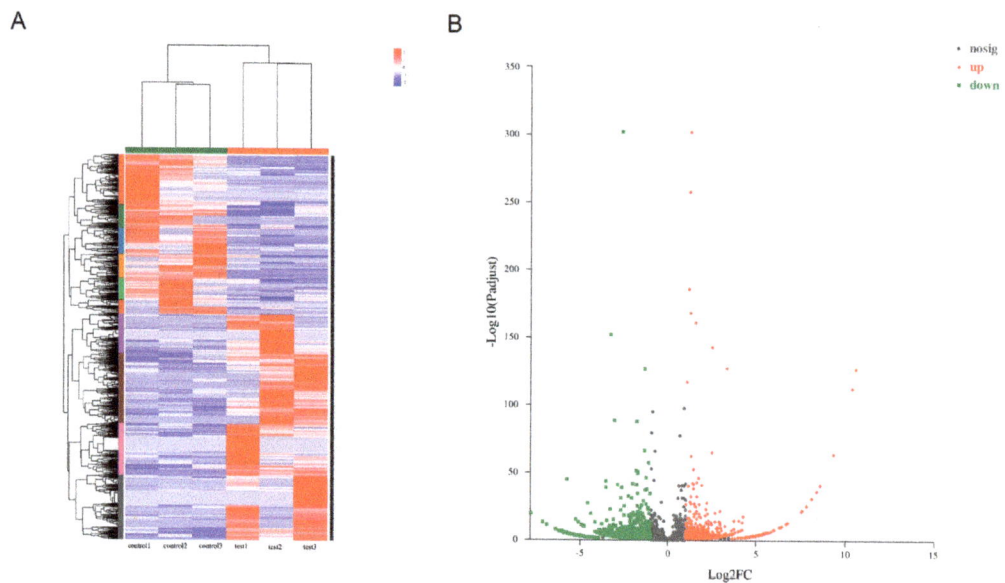

**Figure 1.** Differentially expressed circRNAs profiles. The heatmap (cluster analysis) was used to detect the significant differentially expressed circRNAs (**A**). Red represents high expression and blue represents low expression of circRNAs. Volcano plots were used to assess the circRNAs (**B**) expression variation. The values of X- and Y-axes in the scatter plot are averaged normalized values of each sample. Fold change $\geq 2$, $p < 0.05$.

**Table 1.** The top 10 up-regulated circRNAs in Leishmaniasis patients compared to healthy control group.

| circRNA ID | logFC | p Value | Regulate | Significant |
|---|---|---|---|---|
| chr13: 30251931_30257867 | 10.54691 | $1.03 \times 10^{-130}$ | up | yes |
| chr 6: 31271073_31355592 | 10.32427 | $3.57 \times 10^{-116}$ | up | yes |
| chr 13: 30280063_30283791 | 9.30495 | $4.25 \times 10^{-67}$ | up | yes |
| chr 6: 29887955_29942626 | 8.557338 | $2.02 \times 10^{-44}$ | up | yes |
| chr 6: 29829418_29888742 | 8.551388 | $2.84 \times 10^{-44}$ | up | yes |
| chr13: 30621764_30647057 | 8.339884 | $2.45 \times 10^{-39}$ | up | yes |
| chr 1: 35850157_35851053 | 8.100131 | $2.25 \times 10^{-34}$ | up | yes |
| chr1: 244408712_244430099 | 7.772076 | $1.52 \times 10^{-28}$ | up | yes |
| chr 7: 77083887_77098951 | 7.563262 | $2.43 \times 10^{-25}$ | up | yes |
| chr 6: 3410188_3438555 | 7.515168 | $1.18 \times 10^{-24}$ | up | yes |

**Table 2.** The top 10 down-regulated circRNAs in leishmaniasis patients compared to healthy control group.

| circRNA ID | logFC | $p$ Value | Regulate | Significant |
|---|---|---|---|---|
| chr 6: 32521905_32581838 | −7.77687 | $1.49 \times 10^{-22}$ | down | yes |
| chr 12: 2866393_2872244 | −7.14883 | $7.86 \times 10^{-16}$ | down | yes |
| chr17: 16034765_16040494 | −7.14883 | $7.86 \times 10^{-16}$ | down | yes |
| chr 1: 11016844_11020599 | −6.89104 | $1.11 \times 10^{-13}$ | down | yes |
| chr11: 20407911_20426865 | −6.36747 | $3.68 \times 10^{-10}$ | down | yes |
| chr17: 63666940_63685578 | −6.36747 | $3.68 \times 10^{-10}$ | down | yes |
| chr 1: 23971573_23972012 | −6.17483 | $4.15 \times 10^{-9}$ | down | yes |
| chr2: 171435083_171458075 | −6.12236 | $7.68 \times 10^{-9}$ | down | yes |
| chr1: 235812971_235833667 | −6.06791 | $1.43 \times 10^{-8}$ | down | yes |
| chr12: 102269600_102315490 | −6.06791 | $1.43 \times 10^{-8}$ | down | yes |

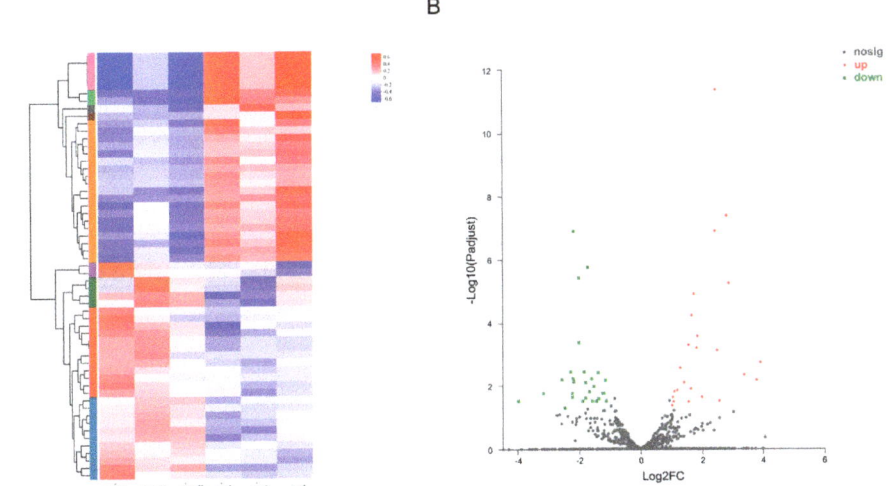

**Figure 2.** Differentially expressed miRNAs profiles. The heatmap (cluster analysis) was used to detect the significant differentially expressed miRNAs (**A**). Red represents high expression and blue represents low expression of miRNAs. Volcano plots were used to assess the miRNAs (**B**) expression variation. The values of $X$- and $Y$-axes in the scatter plot are averaged normalized values of each sample. Fold change ≥ 2, $p < 0.05$.

**Table 3.** The top 10 up-regulated miRNAs in leishmaniasis patients compared to healthy control group.

| miRNA ID | logFC | $p$ Value | Regulate | Significant |
|---|---|---|---|---|
| hsa-miR-483-3p | 3.906015 | $6.71 \times 10^{-5}$ | up | yes |
| hsa-let-7b-3p | 3.784429 | 0.000352 | up | yes |
| hsa-miR-486-3p | 3.369297 | 0.000199 | up | yes |
| hsa-miR-16-2-3p | 2.870342 | $1.19 \times 10^{-7}$ | up | yes |
| hsa-miR-25-5p | 2.467263 | $2.58 \times 10^{-5}$ | up | yes |
| hsa-let-7d-3p | 2.430329 | $7.36 \times 10^{-15}$ | up | yes |
| hsa-miR-5100 | 2.400199 | $1.86 \times 10^{-9}$ | up | yes |
| hsa-miR-6877-5p | 1.977799 | 0.001816 | up | yes |
| hsa-miR-1260b | 1.82933 | $6.81 \times 10^{-6}$ | up | yes |
| hsa-miR-877-5p | 1.79051 | $2.06 \times 10^{-5}$ | up | yes |

**Table 4.** The top 10 down-regulated miRNAs in leishmaniasis patients compared to healthy control group.

| miRNA ID | logFC | p Value | Regulate | Significant |
|---|---|---|---|---|
| hsa-miR-4482-5p | −4.00131 | 0.002571 | down | yes |
| hsa-miR-411-5p | −3.16776 | 0.001176 | down | yes |
| hsa-miR-487b-3p | −2.57252 | 0.000307 | down | yes |
| hsa-miR-381-3p | −2.47089 | 0.005327 | down | yes |
| hsa-miR-654-3p | −2.29163 | 0.000147 | down | yes |
| hsa-miR-2355-3p | −2.24553 | 0.00178 | down | yes |
| hsa-miR-382-5p | −2.24167 | 0.001283 | down | yes |
| hsa-miR-494-3p | −2.21251 | 0.000269 | down | yes |
| hsa-miR-1-3p | −2.18407 | 0.000411 | down | yes |
| hsa-miR-146a-5p | −2.1812 | $1.68 \times 10^{-9}$ | down | yes |

*3.2. Functional and Pathway Enrichment Analyses*

Briefly, GO analysis describes the host genes' function and relationships between these. The enrichment results with regard to biological processes (BP) showed that nuclear envelope reassembly, $G_2/M$ transition of the mitotic cell cycle and microtubule cytoskeleton organization are involved in mitosis and other processes (Figure 3A). As for cellular components (CC), the host genes were enriched in chromosomes, the centromeric region, the chromosomal region and the transferase complex, as well as others (Figure 3B). Additionally, MF analysis showed that the host genes were enriched in histone binding, nucleoside-triphosphatase regulator activity and protein serine/threonine kinase activity, and others (Figure 3C). Furthermore, KEGG pathway enrichment analysis was enriched in some biological pathways, including ubiquitin-mediated proteolysis, endocytosis, MAPK signaling pathway, renal cell carcinoma, autophagy and the ErbB signaling pathway, and others (Figure 3D).

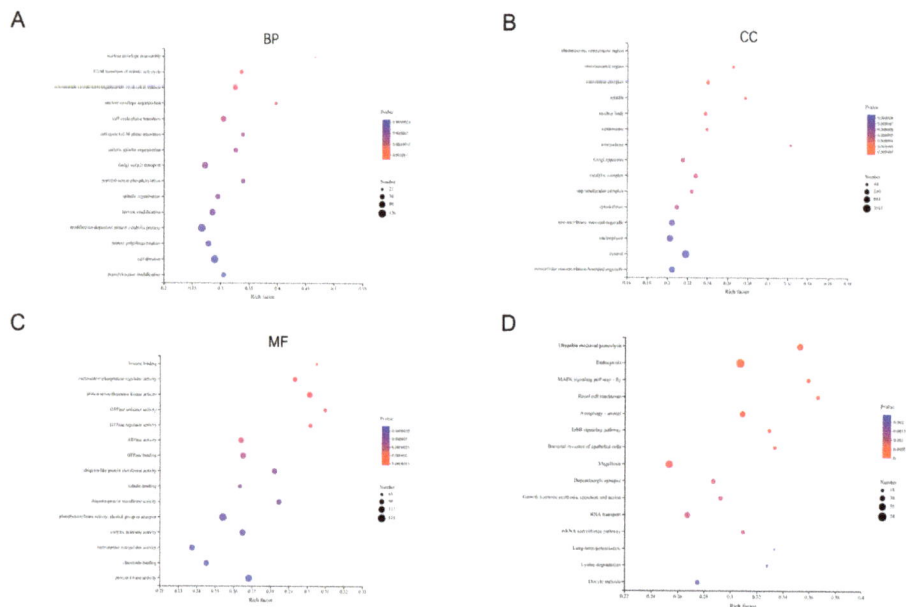

**Figure 3.** GO analysis and KEGG Pathway analysis. The target genes significantly enrich molecular function (MF), biological process (BP) and cellular component (CC) as shown in (**A–C**). The target genes significantly enrich signal pathways (**D**).

## 3.3. PPI Network Module Analysis of Host Genes

A total of 142 nodes and 185 edges were found in down-regulated host genes with a PPI score ≥ 0.9 and experiments ≥ 0.6 (Figure 4A). In addition, 197 nodes and 254 edges were found in down-regulated host genes with a PPI score ≥ 0.9 and experiments ≥ 0.6 (Figure 4B). In total, the top five hub genes were calculated as hub genes using the plugin CytoHubba: *BRCA1*, *CREBBP*, *EP300*, *PIK3R1*, and *CRK*.

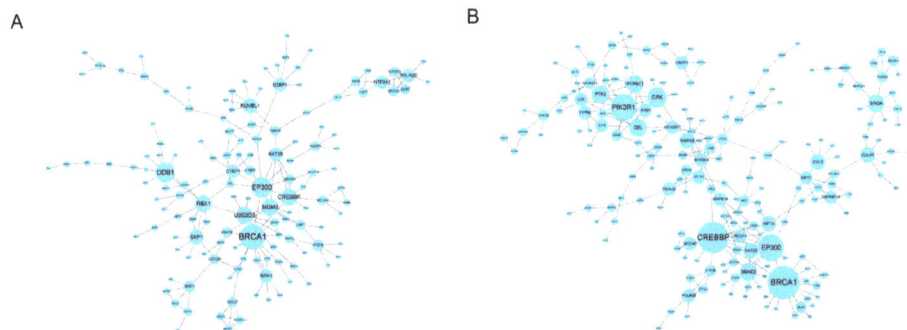

**Figure 4.** PPI network analysis of host genes. (**A**) The host genes of up-regulated circRNAs from the protein–protein interaction network. (**B**) The host genes of down-regulated circRNAs from the protein–protein interaction network.

## 3.4. circRNA–miRNA–mRNA Network

The ceRNA network was built to research the relationship among circRNAs, miRNAs and mRNAs. In total, 208 circRNAs, 52 miRNAs, 713 mRNAs, and 2034 edges had differentially expressed profiles, as shown in Figure 5.

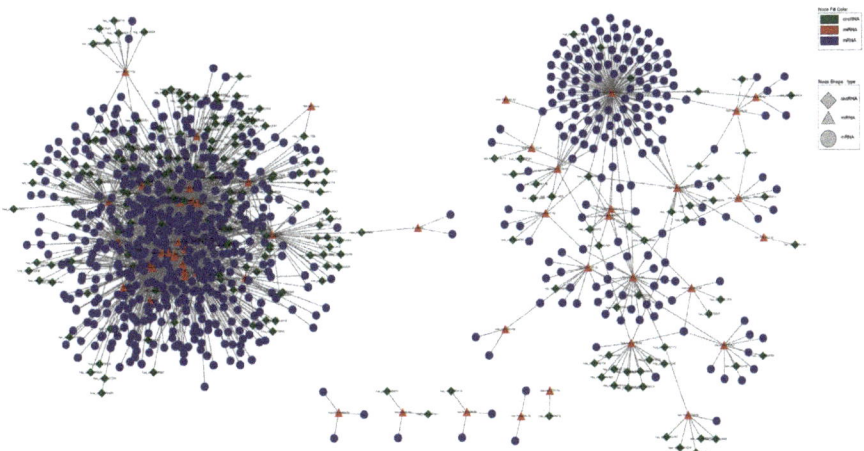

**Figure 5.** The circRNAs–miRNA–mRNA competing endogenous RNA network. Overall regulatory networks of circRNAs, miRNAs and mRNAs containing high-score interactions. Red triangles indicate up-regulated circRNAs, pink triangles indicate the down-regulated circRNAs, green circles represent miRNAs, blue rectangles indicate the mRNAs and a link between the nodes indicates the target relationship.

## 4. Discussion

There is no published study on the function and molecular mechanisms of circRNAs in leishmaniasis. This is the first study to explore the different expressions of the circRNAs profile of leishmaniasis. In this study, a total of 4664 significant differentially expressed circRNAs were identified, which were compared with those in healthy persons through high-throughput sequencing, of which 1931 were up-regulated and 2733 were down-regulated. In recent years, many studies found that circRNAs have several special characteristics, including variety, structural stability, sequence conservation and specific expression that may play an important role in a variety of diseases [27], and participate in important biological processes, such as: neurogenesis [28], neuronal differentiation [29], and immune response [30,31]. Moreover, as a proto-oncogene or tumor-suppressor gene, circRNA is closely related to the occurrence of various tumors [32]. CircNUP210L (has_circ_0014359) influences on the miR-153/PI3K pathway to facilitate glioma cell proliferation [33]. As for lung cancer, Zhu et al. discovered specifically expressed circRNAs, 39 of which were up-regulated, and 20 were down-regulated [34]. They also found that has_circ_0013958 was up-regulated in the adenocarcinoma tissue and plasma of patients through further research; when knock down has_circ_0013958 is present, the proliferation and invasion ability of lung adenocarcinoma cells is promoted, and apoptosis is inhibited. However, circZFR plays the role of an oncogene by promoting the expression of CUL4B (cullin-4B) by sponging miR-101-3p [35]. In addition, Lai et al. found that has_circ_0047905, has_circ_0138960 and has_circRNA7690-15 are up-regulated in stomach cancer. The proliferation and invasion of gastric cancer cells are inhibited when knocking down the three circRNAs [36]. Furthermore, overexpressed circPSMC3 can inhibit the growth and proliferation of gastric cancer cells by targeting miR-654-3p and miR-296-5p, which affect the p21and PTEN signaling pathways [37]. Previous research found that the down-regulation of circTFF1 can inhibit the occurrence of breast cancer by sponging miR-326 and increasing the expression level of TFF1 [38]. Another study found that highly expressed circGFRA1 has a very important relationship with the prognosis of triple-negative breast cancer [39]. Qin et al. found that the expression of has_circ_0001649 is associated with tumor size and tumor emboli occurrence in hepatocellular carcinoma, which also suggests that has_circ_0001649 may serve as a potential new biomarker for hepatocellular carcinoma and play an important role in the occurrence and metastasis of hepatocellular carcinoma [40]. Furthermore, circUSP25 (hsa_circ_0001178) can induce hepatocellular carcinoma progression by regulating the miR-382/VEGFA axis [41]. However, circMALAT1 (hsa_circ_0002082) acts as a proto-oncogene or tumor-suppressor gene, and circMALAT1 can inhibit the translation of the tumor-suppressor gene PAX5 and also act as a sponge of miR-6887-3p, activate the JAK/STAT3 signaling pathway and promote the self-renewal of cancer stem cells [42]. The above research revealed that due to their characteristics, circRNAs can act as biomarkers in a variety of tumors. However, there is currently no research on the functions and mechanisms of circRNAs in leishmaniasis.

Therefore, this study discovered the functions of the host genes of significant differentially expressed circRNAs through GO and KEGG analyses. According to the results of the GO enrichment analysis, the host genes may play an important role in the occurrence of leishmaniasis. The results of KEGG pathway analysis showed that the top five significant signal pathways are enrich in ubiquitin-mediated proteolysis, endocytosis, the MAPK signaling pathway, renal cell carcinoma, autophagy and the ErbB signaling pathway. Among these five significant signaling pathways, three pathways have been shown to be associated with leishmaniasis. Previous research found that the endocytic pathway of *Leishmania* is achieved by clathrin, followed by the internalization of host hemoglobin (Hb) via a high-affinity receptor (HbR) [43]. Kumar et al. discovered that the endocytic pathway of *Leishmania* into host macrophages is through clathrin- and caveolin-mediated endocytosis [44]. In addition, *Leishmania* generally affects the CD40/MAPK pathway, and increases ERK1/2 and decreases IL-10 and IL-12 production [45]. Moreover, multiple studies demonstrate that enhanced LC3 labeling in vitro and in vivo is evidence that all

*Leishmania* can induce autophagy [46–48]. Taken together, KEGG pathway analysis reveals the possible biological functions of these host genes of leishmaniasis.

In the present study, we also identify the five hub genes of those host genes of the PPI network, including: BRCA1, CREBBP, EP300, PIK3R1, and CRK. According to published literature reports, these 10 hub genes all play important roles in tumors or other diseases. However, only EP300 has been studied in leishmaniasis. Pragya et al. found that when *Leishmania* infected BMMFs, time-dependence is increased in EP300 binding to the Bcl2L12 promoter [49]. This suggests that the other four hub genes may also play important roles in leishmaniasis infection, which needs to be further studied.

## 5. Conclusions

This study is the first report of circRNA in leishmaniasis, and may provide novel insights and evidence for the diagnosis and treatment of leishmaniasis. However, these findings are preliminary, we will conduct further research on the corresponding circRNAs.

There are also several limitations in our study, the number of high-throughput sequencing samples in this study was relatively small and only met the requirements for publication. Moreover, the differentially expressed outer circular RNAs we screened require further validation in vivo and in vitro.

**Author Contributions:** Z.L. and Y.Z. designed the study. W.Z., Y.Y., P.Z. and Y.L. collected the serum sample. Z.L. analyzed the data and prepared draft figures. Z.L. and Z.Z. prepared the manuscript draft with important intellectual input from Y.Z., Y.G., Z.L., W.Z., Y.Y., P.Z., Z.Z., Y.L., Y.G. and Y.Z. had complete access to the study data. All authors have read and agreed to the published version of the manuscript.

**Funding:** This study was financially sponsored by Shanghai Sailing Program (21YF1452200) and National Key Research and Development Program of China (No. 2021YFC2300800, 2021YFC2300804) and Ministry of Science and Technology of China basic platform (No. 2019-194-30).

**Institutional Review Board Statement:** The medical ethics committee of the National Institute of Parasitic Diseases (NIPD), Chinese Center for Disease Control and Prevention (Chinese Center for Tropical Dis-eases Research) approved this study (2021019). Six subjects gave written informed consent.

**Informed Consent Statement:** Informed consent was obtained from all subjects involved in the study and written informed consent has been obtained from the patient(s) to publish this paper.

**Data Availability Statement:** The RNA sequencing data has been uploaded to the SRA database (https://www.ncbi.nlm.nih.gov/sra/?term= (accessed on 26 April 2022)). With accession number: PRJNA824834 and PRJNA827265.

**Acknowledgments:** We are very grateful to the staff from Yangquan Center for Disease Control and Prevention, as well as Jing Lu, Jingjing Shi and Yongchao Shang for serum sample collection. We greatly thank volunteers for their participation and cooperation. All individuals included in this section have consented to the acknowledgement.

**Conflicts of Interest:** The authors have no conflict of interest to declare.

## References

1. Mersha, T.T.; Mekonnen Wolde, B.; Shumuye, N.A.; Hailu, A.B.; Mohammed, A.H.; Redda, Y.T.; Abera, B.H.; Menghistu, H.T. Prioritization of neglected tropical zoonotic diseases: A one health perspective from Tigray region, Northern Ethiopia. *PLoS ONE* **2021**, *16*, e0254071. [CrossRef] [PubMed]
2. Singh, O.P.; Tiwary, P.; Kushwaha, A.K.; Singh, S.K.; Singh, D.K.; Lawyer, P.; Rowton, E.; Chaubey, R.; Singh, A.K.; Rai, T.K.; et al. Xenodiagnosis to evaluate the infectiousness of humans to sandflies in an area endemic for visceral leishmaniasis in Bihar, India: A transmission-dynamics study. *Lancet Microbe* **2021**, *2*, e23–e31. [CrossRef]
3. Mohammed, A.S.A.; Tian, W.; Zhang, Y.; Peng, P.; Wang, F.; Li, T. Leishmania lipophosphoglycan components: A potent target for synthetic neoglycoproteins as a vaccine candidate for leishmaniasis. *Carbohydr. Polym.* **2020**, *237*, 116120. [CrossRef] [PubMed]
4. de Vlas, S.J.; Stolk, W.A.; le Rutte, E.A.; Hontelez, J.A.; Bakker, R.; Blok, D.J.; Cai, R.; Houweling, T.A.; Kulik, M.C.; Lenk, E.J.; et al. Concerted Efforts to Control or Eliminate Neglected Tropical Diseases: How Much Health Will Be Gained? *PLoS Negl. Trop. Dis.* **2016**, *10*, e0004386. [CrossRef]

5. Babat, S.O.; Cavus, I.; Ozbilgin, A.; Kayalar, H.; Gunduz, C.; Ceylan, S.S.; Girginkardesler, N. Investigation of the Anti-Leishmanial Effects of Prangos ferulacea and Ferula orientalis Extracts Collected from Sirnak Province Against Leishmania tropica Isolated in Turkey. *Mikrobiyol. Bul.* **2022**, *56*, 339–348. [CrossRef]
6. Yasmeen, N.; Jabbar, A.; Shah, T.; Fang, L.X.; Aslam, B.; Naseeb, I.; Shakeel, F.; Ahmad, H.I.; Baloch, Z.; Liu, Y. One Health Paradigm to Confront Zoonotic Health Threats: A Pakistan Prospective. *Front. Microbiol.* **2021**, *12*, 719334. [CrossRef]
7. Rodrigues, V.; Cordeiro-da-Silva, A.; Laforge, M.; Silvestre, R.; Estaquier, J. Regulation of immunity during visceral Leishmania infection. *Parasit. Vectors* **2016**, *9*, 118. [CrossRef]
8. Goyal, V.; Das, V.N.R.; Singh, S.N.; Singh, R.S.; Pandey, K.; Verma, N.; Hightower, A.; Rijal, S.; Das, P.; Alvar, J.; et al. Long-term incidence of relapse and post-kala-azar dermal leishmaniasis after three different visceral leishmaniasis treatment regimens in Bihar, India. *PLoS Negl. Trop. Dis.* **2020**, *14*, e0008429. [CrossRef]
9. Soyal, A.; Gokmen, T.G.; Kayar, B.; Koksal, F. Comparison of convensional and molecular methods used to determine Leishmania species. *Trop. Biomed.* **2016**, *33*, 260–267.
10. Machado de Assis, T.S.; Azeredo-da-Silva, A.L.; Werneck, G.L.; Rabello, A. Cost-effectiveness analysis of diagnostic tests for human visceral leishmaniasis in Brazil. *Trans. R. Soc. Trop. Med. Hyg.* **2016**, *110*, 464–471. [CrossRef]
11. Abass, E.; Kang, C.; Martinkovic, F.; Semiao-Santos, S.J.; Sundar, S.; Walden, P.; Piarroux, R.; El Harith, A.; Lohoff, M.; Steinhoff, U. Heterogeneity of Leishmania donovani parasites complicates diagnosis of visceral leishmaniasis: Comparison of different serological tests in three endemic regions. *PLoS ONE* **2015**, *10*, e0116408. [CrossRef] [PubMed]
12. Srividya, G.; Kulshrestha, A.; Singh, R.; Salotra, P. Diagnosis of visceral leishmaniasis: Developments over the last decade. *Parasitol. Res.* **2012**, *110*, 1065–1078. [CrossRef] [PubMed]
13. Faleiro, R.J.; Kumar, R.; Hafner, L.M.; Engwerda, C.R. Immune regulation during chronic visceral leishmaniasis. *PLoS Negl. Trop. Dis.* **2014**, *8*, e2914. [CrossRef]
14. Eger, N.; Schoppe, L.; Schuster, S.; Laufs, U.; Boeckel, J.N. Circular RNA Splicing. *Adv. Exp. Med. Biol.* **2018**, *1087*, 41–52. [CrossRef]
15. Ebbesen, K.K.; Hansen, T.B.; Kjems, J. Insights into circular RNA biology. *RNA Biol.* **2017**, *14*, 1035–1045. [CrossRef] [PubMed]
16. Bagchi, A. Different roles of circular RNAs with protein coding potentials. *Biochem. Biophys. Res. Commun.* **2018**, *500*, 907–909. [CrossRef] [PubMed]
17. Li, J.; Sun, D.; Pu, W.; Wang, J.; Peng, Y. Circular RNAs in Cancer: Biogenesis, Function, and Clinical Significance. *Trends Cancer* **2020**, *6*, 319–336. [CrossRef]
18. Yang, Y.; Gao, X.; Zhang, M.; Yan, S.; Sun, C.; Xiao, F.; Huang, N.; Yang, X.; Zhao, K.; Zhou, H.; et al. Novel Role of FBXW7 Circular RNA in Repressing Glioma Tumorigenesis. *J. Natl. Cancer Inst.* **2018**, *110*, 304–315. [CrossRef]
19. Liu, Y.C.; Hong, H.C.; Yang, C.D.; Lee, W.H.; Huang, H.T.; Huang, H.D. Ouroboros resembling competitive endogenous loop (ORCEL) in circular RNAs revealed through transcriptome sequencing dataset analysis. *BMC Genom.* **2018**, *19*, 171. [CrossRef] [PubMed]
20. Dong, W.; Bi, J.; Liu, H.; Yan, D.; He, Q.; Zhou, Q.; Wang, Q.; Xie, R.; Su, Y.; Yang, M.; et al. Circular RNA ACVR2A suppresses bladder cancer cells proliferation and metastasis through miR-626/EYA4 axis. *Mol. Cancer* **2019**, *18*, 95. [CrossRef]
21. Rong, D.; Sun, H.; Li, Z.; Liu, S.; Dong, C.; Fu, K.; Tang, W.; Cao, H. An emerging function of circRNA-miRNAs-mRNA axis in human diseases. *Oncotarget* **2017**, *8*, 73271–73281. [CrossRef]
22. Xiao, M.S.; Wilusz, J.E. An improved method for circular RNA purification using RNase R that efficiently removes linear RNAs containing G-quadruplexes or structured 3' ends. *Nucleic Acids Res.* **2019**, *47*, 8755–8769. [CrossRef] [PubMed]
23. Zhang, Z.; Xie, Q.; He, D.; Ling, Y.; Li, Y.; Li, J.; Zhang, H. Circular RNA: New star, new hope in cancer. *BMC Cancer* **2018**, *18*, 834. [CrossRef]
24. Min, X.; Liu, D.L.; Xiong, X.D. Circular RNAs as Competing Endogenous RNAs in Cardiovascular and Cerebrovascular Diseases: Molecular Mechanisms and Clinical Implications. *Front. Cardiovasc. Med.* **2021**, *8*, 682357. [CrossRef] [PubMed]
25. Liu, H.; Zou, Y.; Chen, C.; Tang, Y.; Guo, J. Current Understanding of Circular RNAs in Systemic Lupus Erythematosus. *Front. Immunol.* **2021**, *12*, 628872. [CrossRef] [PubMed]
26. Sanchez, C.A.; Venkatachalam-Vaz, J.; Drake, J.M. Spillover of zoonotic pathogens: A review of reviews. *Zoonoses Public Health* **2021**, *68*, 563–577. [CrossRef]
27. Li, T.R.; Jia, Y.J.; Wang, Q.; Shao, X.Q.; Lv, R.J. Circular RNA: A new star in neurological diseases. *Int. J. Neurosci.* **2017**, *127*, 726–734. [CrossRef]
28. Rybak-Wolf, A.; Stottmeister, C.; Glazar, P.; Jens, M.; Pino, N.; Giusti, S.; Hanan, M.; Behm, M.; Bartok, O.; Ashwal-Fluss, R.; et al. Circular RNAs in the Mammalian Brain are Highly Abundant, Conserved, and Dynamically Expressed. *Mol. Cell* **2015**, *58*, 870–885. [CrossRef]
29. Suenkel, C.; Cavalli, D.; Massalini, S.; Calegari, F.; Rajewsky, N. A Highly Conserved Circular RNA is Required to Keep Neural Cells in a Progenitor State in the Mammalian Brain. *Cell Rep.* **2020**, *30*, 2170–2179. [CrossRef]
30. Lu, S.; Zhu, N.; Guo, W.; Wang, X.; Li, K.; Yan, J.; Jiang, C.; Han, S.; Xiang, H.; Wu, X.; et al. RNA-Seq Revealed a Circular RNA-microRNA-mRNA Regulatory Network in Hantaan Virus Infection. *Front. Cell. Infect. Microbiol.* **2020**, *10*, 97. [CrossRef]
31. Wesselhoeft, R.A.; Kowalski, P.S.; Parker-Hale, F.C.; Huang, Y.; Bisaria, N.; Anderson, D.G. RNA Circularization Diminishes Immunogenicity and Can Extend Translation Duration In Vivo. *Mol. Cell* **2019**, *74*, 508–520. [CrossRef]

32. Anastasiadou, E.; Faggioni, A.; Trivedi, P.; Slack, F.J. The Nefarious Nexus of Noncoding RNAs in Cancer. *Int. J. Mol. Sci.* **2018**, *19*, 72. [CrossRef] [PubMed]
33. Shi, F.; Shi, Z.; Zhao, Y.; Tian, J. CircRNA hsa-circ-0014359 promotes glioma progression by regulating miR-153/PI3K signaling. *Biochem. Biophys. Res. Commun.* **2019**, *510*, 614–620. [CrossRef] [PubMed]
34. Zhu, X.; Wang, X.; Wei, S.; Chen, Y.; Chen, Y.; Fan, X.; Han, S.; Wu, G. hsa_circ_0013958: A circular RNA and potential novel biomarker for lung adenocarcinoma. *FEBS J.* **2017**, *284*, 2170–2182. [CrossRef] [PubMed]
35. Chen, D.; Ma, W.; Ke, Z.; Xie, F. CircRNA hsa_circ_100395 regulates miR-1228/TCF21 pathway to inhibit lung cancer progression. *Cell Cycle* **2018**, *17*, 2080–2090. [CrossRef] [PubMed]
36. Lai, Z.; Yang, Y.; Yan, Y.; Li, T.; Li, Y.; Wang, Z.; Shen, Z.; Ye, Y.; Jiang, K.; Wang, S. Analysis of co-expression networks for circular RNAs and mRNAs reveals that circular RNAs hsa_circ_0047905, hsa_circ_0138960 and has-circRNA7690-15 are candidate oncogenes in gastric cancer. *Cell Cycle* **2017**, *16*, 2301–2311. [CrossRef]
37. Rong, D.; Lu, C.; Zhang, B.; Fu, K.; Zhao, S.; Tang, W.; Cao, H. CircPSMC3 suppresses the proliferation and metastasis of gastric cancer by acting as a competitive endogenous RNA through sponging miR-296-5p. *Mol. Cancer* **2019**, *18*, 25. [CrossRef]
38. Pan, G.; Mao, A.; Liu, J.; Lu, J.; Ding, J.; Liu, W. Circular RNA hsa_circ_0061825 (circ-TFF1) contributes to breast cancer progression through targeting miR-326/TFF1 signalling. *Cell Prolif.* **2020**, *53*, e12720. [CrossRef]
39. He, R.; Liu, P.; Xie, X.; Zhou, Y.; Liao, Q.; Xiong, W.; Li, X.; Li, G.; Zeng, Z.; Tang, H. circGFRA1 and GFRA1 act as ceRNAs in triple negative breast cancer by regulating miR-34a. *J. Exp. Clin. Cancer Res.* **2017**, *36*, 145. [CrossRef]
40. Qin, M.; Liu, G.; Huo, X.; Tao, X.; Sun, X.; Ge, Z.; Yang, J.; Fan, J.; Liu, L.; Qin, W. Hsa_circ_0001649: A circular RNA and potential novel biomarker for hepatocellular carcinoma. *Cancer Biomark.* **2016**, *16*, 161–169. [CrossRef]
41. Gao, S.; Hu, W.; Huang, X.; Huang, X.; Chen, W.; Hao, L.; Chen, Z.; Wang, J.; Wei, H. Circ_0001178 regulates miR-382/VEGFA axis to facilitate hepatocellular carcinoma progression. *Cell Signal.* **2020**, *72*, 109621. [CrossRef] [PubMed]
42. Chen, L.; Kong, R.; Wu, C.; Wang, S.; Liu, Z.; Liu, S.; Li, S.; Chen, T.; Mao, C.; Liu, S. Circ-MALAT1 Functions as Both an mRNA Translation Brake and a microRNA Sponge to Promote Self-Renewal of Hepatocellular Cancer Stem Cells. *Adv. Sci.* **2020**, *7*, 1900949. [CrossRef] [PubMed]
43. Ansari, I.; Basak, R.; Mukhopadhyay, A. Hemoglobin Endocytosis and Intracellular Trafficking: A Novel Way of Heme Acquisition by Leishmania. *Pathogens* **2022**, *11*, 585. [CrossRef] [PubMed]
44. Kumar, G.A.; Karmakar, J.; Mandal, C.; Chattopadhyay, A. Leishmania donovani Internalizes into Host Cells via Caveolin-mediated Endocytosis. *Sci. Rep.* **2019**, *9*, 12636. [CrossRef] [PubMed]
45. Soares-Silva, M.; Diniz, F.F.; Gomes, G.N.; Bahia, D. The Mitogen-Activated Protein Kinase (MAPK) Pathway: Role in Immune Evasion by Trypanosomatids. *Front. Microbiol.* **2016**, *7*, 183. [CrossRef]
46. Cyrino, L.T.; Araujo, A.P.; Joazeiro, P.P.; Vicente, C.P.; Giorgio, S. In vivo and in vitro Leishmania amazonensis infection induces autophagy in macrophages. *Tissue Cell* **2012**, *44*, 401–408. [CrossRef] [PubMed]
47. Franco, L.H.; Fleuri, A.K.A.; Pellison, N.C.; Quirino, G.F.S.; Horta, C.V.; de Carvalho, R.V.H.; Oliveira, S.C.; Zamboni, D.S. Autophagy downstream of endosomal Toll-like receptor signaling in macrophages is a key mechanism for resistance to Leishmania major infection. *J. Biol. Chem.* **2017**, *292*, 13087–13096. [CrossRef]
48. Dias, B.R.S.; de Souza, C.S.; Almeida, N.J.; Lima, J.G.B.; Fukutani, K.F.; Dos Santos, T.B.S.; Franca-Cost, J.; Brodskyn, C.I.; de Menezes, J.P.B.; Colombo, M.I.; et al. Autophagic Induction Greatly Enhances Leishmania major Intracellular Survival Compared to Leishmania amazonensis in CBA/j-Infected Macrophages. *Front. Microbiol.* **2018**, *9*, 1890. [CrossRef] [PubMed]
49. Chandrakar, P.; Seth, A.; Rani, A.; Dutta, M.; Parmar, N.; Descoteaux, A.; Kar, S. Jagged-Notch-mediated divergence of immune cell crosstalk maintains the anti-inflammatory response in visceral leishmaniasis. *J. Cell Sci.* **2021**, *134*, jcs252494. [CrossRef] [PubMed]

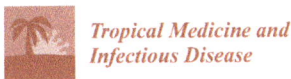
*Tropical Medicine and Infectious Disease*

*Article*

# West Nile Virus Lineage 2 Overwintering in Italy

Giulia Mencattelli [1,2,3,*], Federica Iapaolo [1], Andrea Polci [1], Maurilia Marcacci [1], Annapia Di Gennaro [1], Liana Teodori [1], Valentina Curini [1], Valeria Di Lollo [1], Barbara Secondini [1], Silvia Scialabba [1], Marco Gobbi [4], Elisabetta Manuali [4], Cesare Cammà [1], Roberto Rosà [2], Annapaola Rizzoli [3], Federica Monaco [1] and Giovanni Savini [1]

1 Istituto Zooprofilattico Sperimentale dell'Abruzzo e del Molise, 64100 Teramo, Italy; f.iapaolo@izs.it (F.I.); a.polci@izs.it (A.P.); m.marcacci@izs.it (M.M.); a.digennaro@izs.it (A.D.G.); l.teodori@izs.it (L.T.); v.curini@izs.it (V.C.); v.dilollo@izs.it (V.D.L.); b.secondini@izs.it (B.S.); s.scialabba@izs.it (S.S.); c.camma@izs.it (C.C.); f.monaco@izs.it (F.M.); g.savini@izs.it (G.S.)
2 Center Agriculture Food Environment, University of Trento, 38098 Trento, Italy; roberto.rosa@unitn.it
3 Fondazione Edmund Mach, Research and Innovation Centre, San Michele all'Adige, 38098 Trento, Italy; annapaola.rizzoli@fmach.it
4 Istituto Zooprofilattico Sperimentale dell'Umbria e delle Marche "Togo Rosati", 06126 Perugia, Italy; m.gobbi@izsum.it (M.G.); e.manuali@izsum.it (E.M.)
* Correspondence: giulia.mencattelli@unitn.it

**Abstract:** In January 2022, West Nile virus (WNV) lineage 2 (L2) was detected in an adult female goshawk rescued near Perugia in the region of Umbria (Italy). The animal showed neurological symptoms and died 15 days after its recovery in a wildlife rescue center. This was the second case of WNV infection recorded in birds in the Umbria region during the cold season, when mosquitoes, the main WNV vectors, are usually not active. According to the National Surveillance Plan, the Umbria region is included amongst the WNV low-risk areas. The necropsy evidenced generalized pallor of the mucous membranes, mild splenomegaly, and cerebral edema. WNV L2 was detected in the brain, heart, kidney, and spleen homogenate using specific RT-PCR. Subsequently, the extracted viral RNA was sequenced. A Bayesian phylogenetic analysis performed through a maximum-likelihood tree showed that the genome sequence clustered with the Italian strains within the European WNV strains among the central-southern European WNV L2 clade. These results, on the one hand, confirmed that the WNV L2 strains circulating in Italy are genetically stable and, on the other hand, evidenced a continuous WNV circulation in Italy throughout the year. In this report case, a bird-to-bird WNV transmission was suggested to support the virus overwintering. The potential transmission through the oral route in a predatory bird may explain the relatively rapid spread of WNV, as well as other flaviviruses characterized by similar transmission patterns. However, rodent-to-bird transmission or mosquito-to-bird transmission cannot be excluded, and further research is needed to better understand WNV transmission routes during the winter season in Italy.

**Keywords:** West Nile virus; flavivirus; birds of prey; overwintering; bird-to-bird transmission; rodent-to-bird transmission; hybrid mosquitoes; surveillance

**Citation:** Mencattelli, G.; Iapaolo, F.; Polci, A.; Marcacci, M.; Di Gennaro, A.; Teodori, L.; Curini, V.; Di Lollo, V.; Secondini, B.; Scialabba, S.; et al. West Nile Virus Lineage 2 Overwintering in Italy. *Trop. Med. Infect. Dis.* **2022**, 7, 160. https://doi.org/10.3390/tropicalmed7080160

Academic Editor: Yannick Simonin

Received: 27 June 2022
Accepted: 29 July 2022
Published: 31 July 2022

**Publisher's Note:** MDPI stays neutral with regard to jurisdictional claims in published maps and institutional affiliations.

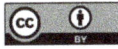

**Copyright:** © 2022 by the authors. Licensee MDPI, Basel, Switzerland. This article is an open access article distributed under the terms and conditions of the Creative Commons Attribution (CC BY) license (https://creativecommons.org/licenses/by/4.0/).

## 1. Introduction

West Nile virus (WNV) is a mosquito-borne flavivirus, belonging to the family *Flaviviridae*, genus *Flavivirus* [1]. It is part of the Japanese encephalitis serocomplex, which includes other related viruses such as Usutu, Murray Valley encephalitis, Stratford, Alfui, Kunjin, and Saint Louis encephalitis [2]. WNV is transmitted in nature by vector-competent mosquitoes mainly belonging to the *Culex* genus [3]. Its transmission cycle involves several bird species and orders as main-amplifier hosts and humans, equids, and other animals as incidental, dead-end hosts [3,4]. In humans, 80% of cases are generally asymptomatic, while in about 20% of cases, infection causes mild, flu-like symptoms known as West Nile fever (WNF). West Nile neuro-invasive disease (WNND) occurs in less than 1% of cases, reporting WNV meningitis, encephalitis, or poliomyelitis [2,5]. Among birds, several avian species can be infected by WNV, but corvids and raptors appear to be the most susceptible ones, showing neurological symptoms and deaths [5]. Once infected, horses usually do not have symptoms. In 20% of cases, they can develop clinical and neurological forms [6], which can lead to 30–50% deaths in unvaccinated animals [5]. The severity of symptoms has been often correlated to WNV genetic diversity [7]. Up to now, 8 lineages have been recognized. Among them, WNV lineage 1 (WNV L1) and lineage 2 (WNV L2) are by far the most widely spread and the most virulent, capable of causing numerous cases worldwide [2,8,9].

Nowadays, WNV represents a serious public health concern in Europe. In the last decades, WNV has expanded its geographical range. The number of West Nile disease (WND) cases have been increasing in animals and humans, especially in southern, central, and eastern Europe, where many countries have become endemic [10,11].

Italy is one of the European countries most affected by WNV circulation [12]. Since 2002, four years after the first incursion in the Tuscany region [13,14], the Italian Ministry of Health has implemented a veterinary surveillance plan to monitor the viral introduction and circulation of WNV in the whole country. In Italy, the WNV circulation is currently monitored through an annually updated preparedness and response plan, aiming at limiting the risk of WNV transmission to humans either by mosquitoes or by substances of human origin. The current program, modulated on the basis of seasonality and local epidemiology, includes national integrated human, animal (equids and birds), and entomological surveillance (One Health Surveillance). Viral circulation is monitored from April to November by testing vector-competent mosquitoes, resident birds belonging to target species (*Pica pica*, *Corvus corone cornix*, and *Garrulus glandarius*) or sentinel chickens, wild birds found dead, horses showing nervous symptoms, and humans presenting neuro-invasive disease signs. On the basis of WNV occurrence and the eco-climatic characteristics of the territory, Italy is divided in three areas: (1) high-risk areas, where WNV is circulating or has circulated in at least one of the previous five years and where, therefore, episodes of infection have been repeatedly observed; (2) low-risk areas, where WNV has circulated sporadically in the past or has never circulated but whose eco-climatic characteristics are favorable for viral circulation; and (3) minimum-risk areas, where WNV has never circulated and where, given the eco-climatic characteristics of the territory, the probability of its circulation is considered as minimal (National Plan for Prevention, Surveillance, and Response to Arbovirus 2020–2025).

The Umbria region is classified as a low-risk area. WNV circulation has never been reported, at least up to 2019, when the death of a little grebe (*Tachybaptus ruficollis* subsp. *ruficollis*) was associated with WNV L2 infection [15].

In this report, a second clinical case associated with WNV L2 infection observed in a northern goshawk (*Accipiter gentilis*) in Umbria during the winter season is described.

## 2. Materials and Methods
### 2.1. Case Report

On 4 January 2022, a female adult northern goshawk was rescued in Torgiano, a municipality in the province of Perugia, Italy (Figure 1).

The bird was found on the roof of a private house while trying to defend itself from a mobbing attack by crows. The noise caused by the crows attacking the stunned goshawk attracted the homeowner, who recovered the bird and brought it to a wildlife rescue center (WRC). The northern goshawk showed classical neurological symptoms, including stupor, blepharospasm, and an inability to maintain a normal posture. After an initial improvement of symptoms in which the bird restarted feeding on its own, the clinical signs suddenly worsened, and the bird died on 19 January 2022. The necropsy evidenced a good state of nutrition, generalized pallor of the mucous membranes, and mild splenomegaly. Cerebral edema was also observed. The picture and video of the WNV-infected northern goshawk are reported in Figure S1 and Video S1 (Supplementary Materials).

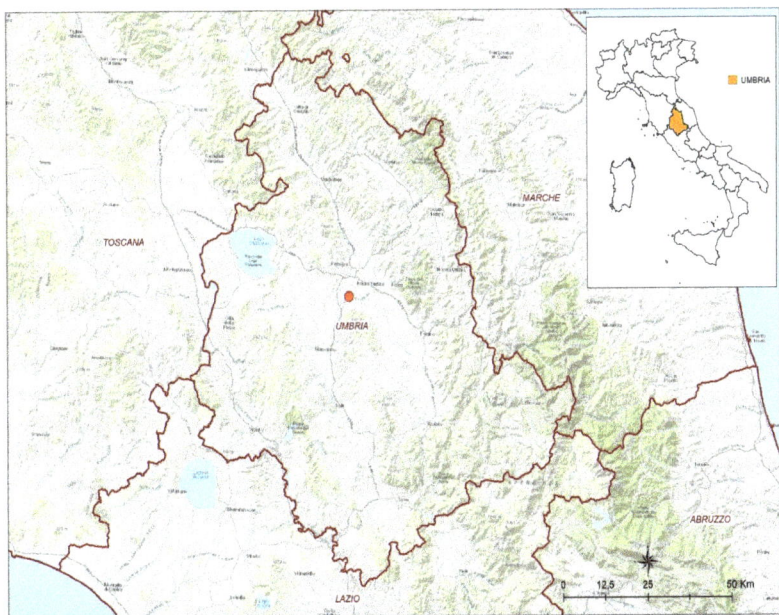

**Figure 1.** Map of geo-localization site. The northern goshawk was found in the Torgiano municipality (43.0893° N, 12.4410° E) in the Umbria region.

*2.2. Laboratory Analyses*

2.2.1. Real-Time PCR for WNV and USUV

The brain, heart, kidney, and spleen were collected, pooled, and homogenized in sterile phosphate-buffered saline (PBS). The viral RNA was extracted from 200 µL supernatant using Qiasymphony® DSP automatic instrumentation (Germantown, MD, USA) according to the manufacturer instructions. The extracted RNA was then tested using one-step quantitative reverse transcription polymerase chain reactions (qRT-PCRs) specific for USUV, all known lineages of West Nile virus, and West Nile virus L1 and L2 [16–18].

2.2.2. Illumina and Sanger Sequencing

A WNV-positive sample was selected for Illumina and Sanger sequencing. The total RNA was subjected to Turbo DNase treatment (Thermo Fisher Scientific, Waltham, MA, USA) at 37 °C for 20 min and then purified with an RNA Clean and Concentrator-5 Kit (Zymo Research, Irvine, CA, USA). The purified RNA was used for the assessment of the sequence independent single primer amplification (SISPA) protocol [19,20]. In detail, a single-strand cDNA was obtained using reverse transcription (RT) in 20 µL reaction mixture with 5X SSIV buffer, 50 µM random hexamer FR26RV-N 50-GCCGGAGCTCTGCAGATATCNNN NNN-30, 10 mM dNTPs mix, 100 mM DTT, 200 units SuperScript® IV Reverse Transcriptase (Thermo Fisher Scientific, Waltham, MA, USA), and 40 U RNAse OUT RNase inhibitor (Thermo Fisher Scientific, Waltham, MA, USA) following the manufacturer instructions. The reaction was incubated at 23 °C for 10 min, 50 °C for 50 min, and 80 °C for 10 min. To convert the single-stranded cDNA into double-stranded (ds) cDNA, 1 µL (2.5 U) 3′-5′ Klenow Polymerase (New England Biolabs, Ipswich, MA, USA) was directly added to the reaction. The incubation was carried out at 37 °C for 1 h and 75 °C for 10 min. Next, 5 µL of ds cDNA was amplified with a PCR master mix containing 5X Q5 reaction buffer, 10 mM dNTPs, 40 µM random primer FR20 Rv 50 -GCCGGAGCTCTGCAGATATC-30, 0.01 U/µL Q5® High Fidelity DNA polymerase (NEB, New England Biolabs, Ipswich, MA, USA), and 5X Q5 High Enhancer. The reaction was incubated at 98 °C for 10 s, 65 °C for 30 s, 72 °C for 3 min, and 72 °C for 2 min. The PCR product was purified using Expin ™ PCR SV (GeneAll Biotechnology CO., Seoul, Korea) and then quantified using a Qubit® DNA HS Assay Kit (Thermo Fisher Scientific, Waltham, MA, USA). The sample was diluted to obtain a concentration of 100–500 ng, then used for library preparation with an Illumina DNA prep kit, and sequenced with a NextSeq 500 (Illumina Inc., San Diego, CA, USA) using a NextSeq 500/550 Mid Output Reagent Cartridge v2, 300 cycles, and standard 150 bp paired-end reads. After quality control and trimming with Trimmomatic v0.36 (Usadellab, Düsseldorf, Germany) [21] and FastQC tool v0.11.5 (Bioinformatics Group, Babraham Institute, Cambridge, UK) [22,23], reads were *de novo* assembled using SPADES v3.11.1 (Algorithmic Biology Lab, St Petersburg, Russia) [24]. The contigs obtained were analyzed with BLASTn to identify the best match reference. Mapping of the trimmed reads was then performed using the iVar computational tool [25] to obtain a consensus sequence. In order to close some large gaps, the WNV-positive sample was further sequenced using the Sanger method [26]. Briefly, the total RNA was extracted from the collected sample using a High Pure Viral Nucleic Acid Kit (Roche Diagnostics GmbH, Roche Applied Science, 68298 Mannheim, Germany) according to the manufacturer instructions and collected in 45 µL elution buffer prewarmed at 72 °C. The complete WNV-coding DNA sequences (cds) of the polyprotein precursor gene was amplified using 13 WNV primer pairs able to amplify 13 overlapping regions of the genome (the primer sequences are available upon request). Gel-based RT-PCR was performed using a Transcriptor One-Step RT-PCR kit (Roche Diagnostics Deutschland GmbH, Mannheim, Germany) as described by the manufacturer instructions. The RT-PCR cycling conditions for the amplification were 50 °C for 15 min and 94 °C for 7 min, followed by 35 cycles of denaturation at 94 °C for 10 s, annealing at 57.5 °C for 30 s, and extension at 68 °C for 4 min and 30 s, followed by 1 extension cycle performed at 68 °C for 7 min. The gel-based RT-PCR amplicons were purified with a Qiaquick PCR Purification kit (Qiagen, Leipzig, Germany). The purified amplicons and the 13 WNV sequencing primers were sent to an external service, Eurofins Genomics (Eurofins Genomics, Germany GmbH, Anzinger Str. 7a, 85560 Ebersberg, Germany), to perform sequencing in both directions. The obtained sequences were analyzed with SeqScape v3.0 (Thermo Fisher Scientific, Waltham, MA, USA).

2.2.3. Phylogenetic Analysis

A phylogenetic analysis was conducted including 62 WNV L2 genome sequences publicly available. Specifically, 57 complete and 5 partial genome sequences representative of different geographic regions and identified in different hosts were downloaded from Genbank. In addition, three sequences were added as outgroups: WNV L1 Italy 2020 (MW627239), WNV L1 France 2015 (MT863559), and Koutango virus (KOUTV) Senegal 2013 (EU082200). All 66 sequences were aligned using the MAFFT online alignment program (https://mafft.cbrc.jp/alignment/server/, accessed on: 15 April 2022) and curated using BioEdit v. 7.2.5.0 software (https://bioedit.software.informer.com/7.2/, Bioedit Company, Manchester, UK, accessed on: 15 April 2022). The WNV sequence alignment and the metadata of the WNV strains used for the present study are reported in File S1 and Table S1, respectively (Supplementary Materials). Bayesian phylogenetic inference (BI) was performed using a Bayesian Evolutionary Analysis by Sampling Tree (BEAST) software package version 2.6.3 (http://www.beast2.org/, University of Auckland, Auckland 1142, New Zealand) [27,28]. In detail, using the interface program called Bayesian Evolutionary Analysis Utility (BEAUti) included in the BEAST package, the amino acid sequence alignment was uploaded by choosing a gamma-site model with a gamma category count of 4, as well as invariant sites model (GTR + Γ + I) [28]. A family of Bayesian Markov chain Monte Carlo (MCMC) algorithms with 10 independent MCMC runs with up to 100,000,000 generations was used to perform the inference. Using TreeAnnotator v.2.6.3 (https://www.beast2.org/treeannotator/), trees were summarized in a maximum-clade-credibility tree with common ancestor heights after a 10% burnin percentage [28]. Tracer v 1.7.1 (available at http://beast.bio.ed.ac.uk/Tracer, accessed on: 16 April 2022) was used to ensure convergence during the MCMC runs. Finally, the FigTree v2.6.3 program (http://tree.bio.ed.ac.uk/software/) allowed the estimation of a maximum-likelihood tree [29].

## 3. Results

The northern goshawk rescued in the Umbria region in January 2022 was positive for WNV L2 (Ct 25) and turned out negative for WNV L1 and USUV.

The Illumina sequencing run produced a total of 15,763,124 reads. BLASTn analysis was performed to identify the closest publicly available sequence in the GenBank database. The best match (99.49%) was with the West Nile virus isolate of Nea Santa-Greece-2010 (accession no. HQ537483), and this sequence was used to perform mapping with the iVar tool [25]. This analysis produced a consensus sequence with a horizontal coverage (HCov) of 57% and a mean vertical coverage of 575,535, probably due to the low quality of the RNA sample.

The large gaps were partially filled with Sanger sequencing data, and a consensus sequence of 11.056 nt in length was obtained (HCov 91%) and published in the NCBI database under acc. no ON032498 and the NCBI sequence name of 15935/22.

Phylogenetic analysis placed 15935/22 NCBI in the same cluster as the other central-southern European WNV L2 sequences [30] (highlighted in pink in Figure 2) with a posterior probability of 100%.

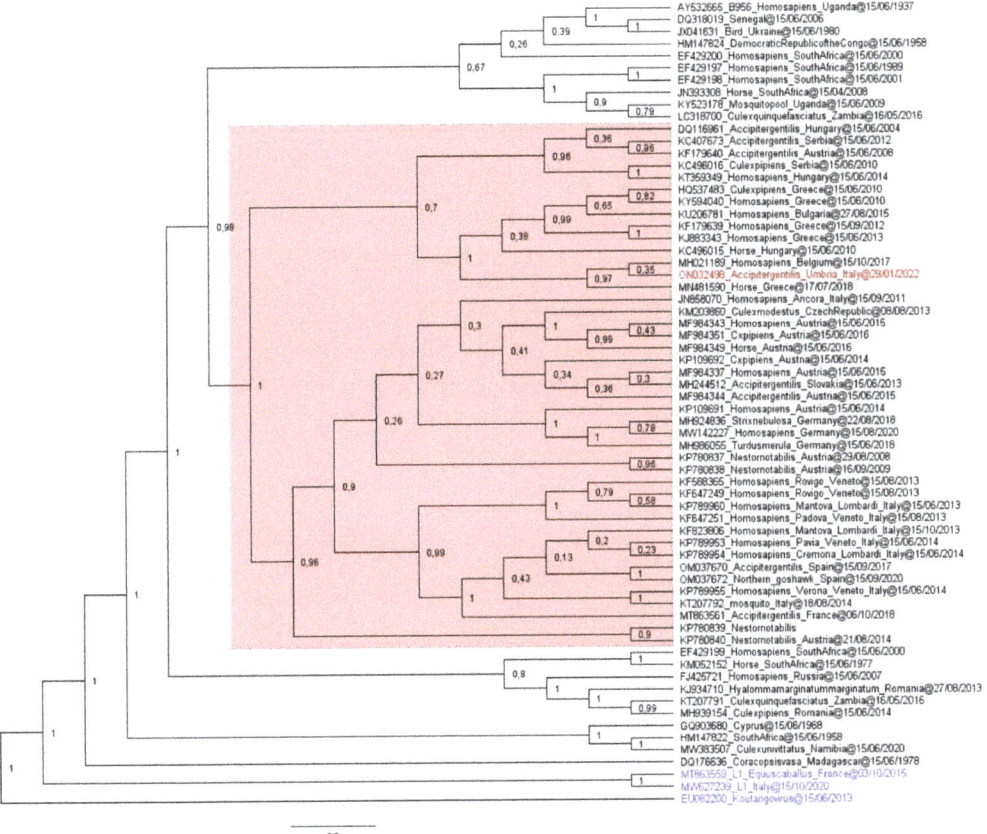

**Figure 2.** The evolutionary analysis inferred by using the maximum-likelihood method and the general time reversible model is illustrated. The tree with the highest log-likelihood is shown. The

percentage of trees in which the associated taxa clustered together is displayed next to the branches. Initial trees for the heuristic search were obtained by applying the neighbor-joining method to a matrix of pairwise distances estimated using the maximum composite likelihood (MCL) approach. A discrete Gamma distribution was used to model evolutionary rate differences among the sites (4 categories). The evolutionary distances were computed using the optimal GTR + Γ + I model, with 2000 Γ-rate categories and 5000 bootstrap replications using the Shimodaira–Hasegawa (SH) test. Ten independent MCMC runs with up to 100 million generations were performed to ensure the convergence of the estimates. GenBank accession numbers are indicated for each strain, with country, lineage, and year of isolation. The genome sequence ON032498 WNV L2 (HCov 91%), obtained from the goshawk organ homogenate, is highlighted in red. The WNV L1 MW627239 (Italy 2020) and MT863559 (France 2015), and Koutango virus (KOUTV) EU082200 (Senegal 2013), chosen as outgroups, are highlighted in blue. The new strain (ON032498) showed high genetic similarity with the central-southern European WNV L2 clade, highlighted in pink, with a posterior probability of 100%.

## 4. Discussion

This study reported the second evidence of WNV L2 circulation in the Umbria region. The current National Surveillance Plan includes Umbria amongst those areas whose eco-climatic characteristics are favorable for viral circulation but where WNV has never or sporadically circulated in the past (National Plan for Prevention, Surveillance, and Response to Arbovirus 2020–2025). In fact, no WNV circulation has ever been reported in the territory, neither in humans [31] nor in animals, before 2019, when the virus was detected for the first time in a little grebe [15]. Interestingly, in both reported Umbrian cases, WNV was detected in the winter months (December and January), a period when, normally, the most common vector, *Culex pipiens*, is less active.

The northern goshawk (*Accipiter gentilis*) is a medium-sized bird of prey belonging to the family of *Accipitridae*. The family also includes other diurnal raptors, such as eagles, buzzards, and harriers [32]. With regard to WNV infection, northern goshawks have been demonstrated to be highly susceptible. In fact, following WNV infection, severe clinical symptoms have often been described in this species and, in general, in raptors [19,30,33,34]. The clinical signs described in this report were compatible with WNV infection. Moreover, the absence of fractures in the bird skull excluded a possible traumatic origin of the observed neurological disorders.

The first aspect that needs to be clarified is the time of infection: did it really occur in winter? In this regard, the occurrence of clinical signs and the direct detection of WNV in the goshawk organs indicates that this case was related to a recent infection. WNV infections in periods of mosquito inactivity have been described, particularly in raptors [33,35,36]. This group of birds is, in fact, characterized by predatory habits [32] and the transmission of WNV by the predation of infected birds has been frequently observed [33,37]. In this reported case, it is then highly probable that the Umbrian goshawk became infected by eating an infected bird. If, on the one hand this explanation indeed clarifies the way the goshawk obtained the infection, on the other hand, it does not explain how the supposed goshawk prey was still infectious in a period of mosquito inactivity. The persistence of infectious WNV for prolonged periods in the organs of birds and, in particular, of *Passeriformes* has been evidenced by many authors [35,38–42]. Persistent infection has been defined as the detection of a virus in host tissues after viremia has subsided [43]. The persistent, high viral loads in organs of birds and, in particular, in those belonging to prey species might sustain WNV transmission to predators also months after mosquito season. The recent finding of WNV L2 in a little grebe collected in the winter months in Umbria [15] indicates that finding birds with WNV-infected organs in the winter months is not uncommon [33,34,38,41,43]. Thus, the symptomatic goshawk found in Umbria last January can be regarded as a case of bird-to-bird WNV oral transmission.

This transmission route has been considered as one of the possible ways of overwintering for WNV [33,34,38,41,43]. Bearing in mind that common prey of goshawks also include rodents and that, also, in these animals infectious WNV has been detected months after infection [44,45], a possible rodent-to-bird transmission cannot be excluded.

Further attention should be given to the *Culex pipiens* complex because of its vector role in WNV transmission [46,47]. Among this complex, the *Culex pipiens* (rural, mainly ornithophilic) and *Culex molestus* (urban, mainly mammophilic) biotypes can interbreed, giving birth to a hybrid form with intermediate ecological features found in a wide set of environments and acting as a WNV bridge-vector from birds to humans [46,47]. Interestingly, while *Cx. pipiens* are well-known to enter diapause during winter, *Cx. molestus* and *Cx. Pipiens–Cx. molestus* hybrids actively feed all year round [46] and might, for this reason, have been responsible for the goshawk WNV infection.

Irrespective of whether the goshawk was infected by hybrid mosquitoes or by the predation of infected animals, WNV has indeed been circulating in the winter months. Therefore, the second important issue to be clarified in this report is where the goshawk was infected. According to the National Surveillance Plan, Umbria is classified as a WNV low-risk area, while the neighboring regions (parts of Tuscany, Marche, and Lazio) are high-risk areas (National Plan for Prevention, Surveillance, and Response to Arbovirus 2020–2025). In most parts of Europe, the northern goshawk is a sedentary species [32,48]. In Italy, it is a rather scarce, localized breeder, mainly present in mature forests of the Apennines and the Alps that are especially rich in large trees and are particularly suitable for nest-building, where its common prey are abundant (e.g., squirrels, wood pigeons, woodpeckers, corvids, and rabbits) [32]. In January, even if it further reduces its movements, it can still keep moving for hundreds of kilometers [32]. Because of that and in view of the fact that Umbria has a very small surface (8.456 Km$^2$), it is very difficult to determine whether the goshawk became infected in Umbria or in the neighboring regions. Interestingly, during the WNV season 2021, there was no evidence for the circulation of WNV, not only in Umbria but also in the nearby area of central Italy [49]. The lack of WNV infection cases in high-risk areas (Latium and Tuscany) also in wintertime [15,50], when mosquitoes are less active, might suggest that birds have an important role in WNV overwintering. The potential transmission through the oral route in a predatory bird might explain the relatively rapid spread of WNV and of other similar flaviviruses, such as Tick-borne encephalitis virus and Usutu virus (USUV) [50–52]. It has to be said that Umbria is endemic for USUV [53] (National Plan for Prevention, Surveillance, and Response to Arbovirus 2020–2025), which is a mosquito-borne virus that shares the same life cycle and patterns of transmissibility with WNV [4]. If the eco-climatic conditions of Umbria are suitable for maintaining the USUV life cycle, they should also be favorable for WNV.

Based on these features and due to recent WNV positivities detected in the territory, the Umbria region was included among the high-risk areas in 2022 by the WNV National Surveillance Plan (National Plan for Prevention, Surveillance, and Response to Arbovirus 2020–2025).

## 5. Conclusions

In conclusion, our study highlighted the circulation of WNV L2 during the winter in Italy. Even though the reported cases remain rare during the cold season, this report is of fundamental importance because it evidences the potential for human transmission when veterinary active surveillance is suspended. It means that we cannot rely on the early warning system for WNV circulation mainly provided by mosquito and bird surveillance to prevent human infection. Further research is needed to better understand the transmission routes and the role of overwintering birds, rodents, and mosquitoes, as well as WNV infection per *os.* in WNV transmission and epidemiology in Italy. Considering the strong WNV circulation in the Italian territory and the observed changes in the seasonal and regional patterns of WNV, with the virus observed lately in winter times, as well as in WNV low-risk areas, this work also highlighted the strong importance of the passive surveillance of wildlife. This should be coupled with the implementation of a harmonized protocol for necroscopies and biological sample collection, including gastro-intestinal contents, in order to obtain additional data needed to clarify the potential cause of death, especially in winter, when the National Surveillance Plan does not include an active search for the virus.

**Supplementary Materials:** The following supporting information can be downloaded at: https://www.mdpi.com/article/10.3390/tropicalmed7080160/s1, Figure S1: Picture of WNV-infected Northern goshawk; Video S1: Video of WNV-infected Northern goshawk; File S1: WNV List of Sequence dataset; Table S1: Metadata of WNV strains used for the present study.

**Author Contributions:** Conceptualization, G.M., F.I., F.M. and G.S.; methodology, G.M., F.M., A.P., M.M. and G.S.; validation, F.M., A.P., M.M., V.C. and G.S.; formal analysis, G.M., A.P., F.M. and M.M.; investigation, A.D.G., L.T., A.P., M.M., M.G., E.M., S.S., B.S., V.D.L. and G.M.; resources, F.M. and G.S.; data curation, M.G., E.M., A.P. and G.M.; writing—original draft, G.M., F.I., F.M. and G.S.; writing—review and editing, G.M., F.M., M.M., R.R., A.R. and G.S.; visualization, G.M., F.I., F.M., A.D.G., L.T., V.C., M.M., A.P., M.G., E.M., V.D.L., S.S., B.S., C.C., R.R., A.R. and G.S.; supervision, F.M. and G.S.; project administration, G.S.; funding acquisition, G.S. All authors have read and agreed to the published version of the manuscript.

**Funding:** This research was funded by the Italian Ministry of Health (law 19 January 2001). This research was financially supported by an international PhD initiative including the Fondazione Edmund Mach, the University of Trento, and the Istituto Zooprofilattico Sperimentale dell'Abruzzo e Molise.

**Institutional Review Board Statement:** Not applicable.

**Informed Consent Statement:** Not applicable.

**Data Availability Statement:** Sequence data are available via NCBI. The accession numbers for the sequences used can be found in Table S1, Supplementary Materials.

**Acknowledgments:** The authors acknowledge all personnel in the lab and in the field for their skill and technical support. The authors also wish to thank Sandro Pelini for the creation of the map included in the text, as well as Massimo Balducci and CRAS Lipu Umbria for providing the iconographic material.

**Conflicts of Interest:** All the authors declare no conflict of interest.

## References

1. Habarugira, G.; Suen, W.W.; Hobson-Peters, J.; Hall, R.A.; Bielefeldt-Ohmann, H. West Nile Virus: An Update on Pathobiology, Epidemiology, Diagnostics, Control and "One Health" Implications. *Pathogens* **2020**, *9*, 589. [CrossRef] [PubMed]
2. Mencattelli, G.; Ndione, M.H.D.; Rosà, R.; Marini, G.; Diagne, C.T.; Diagne, M.M.; Fall, G.; Faye, O.; Diallo, M.; Faye, O.; et al. Epidemiology of West Nile Virus in Africa: An Underestimated Threat. *PLoS Negl. Trop. Dis.* **2022**, *16*, e0010075. [CrossRef]
3. Popescu, C.P.; Florescu, S.A.; Ruta, S.M. West Nile Virus in Central Europe—Pandora's Box Is Wide Open! *Travel Med. Infect. Dis.* **2020**, *37*, 101864. [CrossRef]
4. Mancuso, E.; Cecere, J.G.; Iapaolo, F.; Di Gennaro, A.; Sacchi, M.; Savini, G.; Spina, F.; Monaco, F. West Nile and Usutu Virus Introduction via Migratory Birds: A Retrospective Analysis in Italy. *Viruses* **2022**, *14*, 416. [CrossRef] [PubMed]
5. Byas, A.D.; Ebel, G.D. Comparative Pathology of West Nile Virus in Humans and Non-Human Animals. *Pathogens* **2020**, *9*, 48. [CrossRef] [PubMed]
6. Reisen, W.K.; Hahn, D.C. Comparison of Immune Responses of Brown-Headed Cowbird and Related Blackbirds to West Nile and Other Mosquito-Borne Encephalitis Viruses. *J. Wildl. Dis.* **2007**, *43*, 439–449. [CrossRef] [PubMed]
7. Fall, G.; Di Paola, N.; Faye, M.; Dia, M.; Freire, C.C.d.M.; Loucoubar, C.; Zanotto, P.M.d.A.; Faye, O.; Sall, A.A. Biological and Phylogenetic Characteristics of West African Lineages of West Nile Virus. *PLoS Negl. Trop Dis.* **2017**, *11*, e0006078. [CrossRef]
8. Bakonyi, T.; Ivanics, É.; Erdélyi, K.; Ursu, K.; Ferenczi, E.; Weissenböck, H.; Nowotny, N. Lineage 1 and 2 Strains of Encephalitic West Nile Virus, Central Europe. *Emerg. Infect. Dis.* **2006**, *12*, 618–623. [CrossRef]
9. Beck, C.; Leparc Goffart, I.; Franke, F.; Gonzalez, G.; Dumarest, M.; Lowenski, S.; Blanchard, Y.; Lucas, P.; de Lamballerie, X.; Grard, G.; et al. Contrasted Epidemiological Patterns of West Nile Virus Lineages 1 and 2 Infections in France from 2015 to 2019. *Pathogens* **2020**, *9*, 908. [CrossRef]
10. West Nile Virus Infection. Available online: https://www.ecdc.europa.eu/en/west-nile-virus-infection (accessed on 3 May 2022).
11. Bakonyi, T.; Haussig, J.M. West Nile Virus Keeps on Moving up in Europe. *Euro Surveill* **2020**, *25*, 2001938. [CrossRef]
12. Rizzo, C.; Napoli, C.; Venturi, G.; Pupella, S.; Lombardini, L.; Calistri, P.; Monaco, F.; Cagarelli, R.; Angelini, P.; Bellini, R.; et al. West Nile Virus Transmission: Results from the Integrated Surveillance System in Italy, 2008 to 2015. *Eurosurveillance* **2016**, *21*, 30340. [CrossRef]
13. Cantile, C.; Di Guardo, G.; Eleni, C.; Arispici, M. Clinical and Neuropathological Features of West Nile Virus Equine Encephalomyelitis in Italy. *Equine Vet. J.* **2000**, *32*, 31–35. [CrossRef]

14. Monaco, F.; Lelli, R.; Teodori, L.; Pinoni, C.; Di Gennaro, A.; Polci, A.; Calistri, P.; Savini, G. Re-Emergence of West Nile Virus in Italy. *Zoonoses Public Health* **2010**, *57*, 476–486. [CrossRef] [PubMed]
15. Giglia, G.; Mencattelli, G.; Lepri, E.; Agliani, G.; Gobbi, M.; Gröne, A.; van den Brand, J.M.A.; Savini, G.; Mandara, M.T. West Nile Virus and Usutu Virus in Wild Birds from Rescue Centers, a Post-Mortem Monitoring Study from Central Italy. *bioRxiv* **2022**. [CrossRef]
16. Del Amo, J.; Sotelo, E.; Fernández-Pinero, J.; Gallardo, C.; Llorente, F.; Agüero, M.; Jiménez-Clavero, M.A. A Novel Quantitative Multiplex Real-Time RT-PCR for the Simultaneous Detection and Differentiation of West Nile Virus Lineages 1 and 2, and of Usutu Virus. *J. Virol. Methods* **2013**, *189*, 321–327. [CrossRef]
17. Vázquez, A.; Herrero, L.; Negredo, A.; Hernández, L.; Sánchez-Seco, M.P.; Tenorio, A. Real Time PCR Assay for Detection of All Known Lineages of West Nile Virus. *J. Virol. Methods* **2016**, *236*, 266–270. [CrossRef]
18. Cavrini, F.; Della Pepa, M.E.; Gaibani, P.; Pierro, A.M.; Rossini, G.; Landini, M.P.; Sambri, V. A Rapid and Specific Real-Time RT-PCR Assay to Identify Usutu Virus in Human Plasma, Serum, and Cerebrospinal Fluid. *J. Clin. Virol.* **2011**, *50*, 221–223. [CrossRef]
19. Mencattelli, G.; Iapaolo, F.; Monaco, F.; Fusco, G.; de Martinis, C.; Portanti, O.; Di Gennaro, A.; Curini, V.; Polci, A.; Berjaoui, S.; et al. West Nile Virus Lineage 1 in Italy: Newly Introduced or a Re-Occurrence of a Previously Circulating Strain? *Viruses* **2022**, *14*, 64. [CrossRef]
20. Marcacci, M.; De Luca, E.; Zaccaria, G.; Di Tommaso, M.; Mangone, I.; Aste, G.; Savini, G.; Boari, A.; Lorusso, A. Genome Characterization of Feline Morbillivirus from Italy. *J. Virol. Methods* **2016**, *234*, 160–163. [CrossRef] [PubMed]
21. Bolger, A.M.; Lohse, M.; Usadel, B. Trimmomatic: A Flexible Trimmer for Illumina Sequence Data. *Bioinformatics* **2014**, *30*, 2114–2120. [CrossRef]
22. Cito, F.; Pasquale, A.D.; Cammà, C.; Cito, P. The Italian Information System for the Collection and Analysis of Complete Genome Sequence of Pathogens Isolated from Animal, Food and Environment. *Int. J. Infect. Dis.* **2018**, *73*, 296–297. [CrossRef]
23. Aprea, G.; Scattolini, S.; D'Angelantonio, D.; Chiaverini, A.; Di Lollo, V.; Olivieri, S.; Marcacci, M.; Mangone, I.; Salucci, S.; Antoci, S.; et al. Whole Genome Sequencing Characterization of HEV3-e and HEV3-f Subtypes among the Wild Boar Population in the Abruzzo Region, Italy: First Report. *Microorganisms* **2020**, *8*, 1393. [CrossRef] [PubMed]
24. Bankevich, A.; Nurk, S.; Antipov, D.; Gurevich, A.A.; Dvorkin, M.; Kulikov, A.S.; Lesin, V.M.; Nikolenko, S.I.; Pham, S.; Prjibelski, A.D.; et al. SPAdes: A New Genome Assembly Algorithm and Its Applications to Single-Cell Sequencing. *J. Comput. Biol.* **2012**, *19*, 455–477. [CrossRef]
25. Grubaugh, N.D.; Gangavarapu, K.; Quick, J.; Matteson, N.L.; De Jesus, J.G.; Main, B.J.; Tan, A.L.; Paul, L.M.; Brackney, D.E.; Grewal, S.; et al. An Amplicon-Based Sequencing Framework for Accurately Measuring Intrahost Virus Diversity Using PrimalSeq and IVar. *Genome Biol.* **2019**, *20*, 8. [CrossRef] [PubMed]
26. Verma, M.; Kulshrestha, S.; Puri, A. Genome Sequencing. *Methods Mol. Biol.* **2017**, *1525*, 3–33. [CrossRef]
27. Nei, M.; Kumar, S. *Molecular Evolution and Phylogenetics*; Oxford University Press: New York, NY, USA, 2000.
28. Drummond, A.J.; Suchard, M.A.; Xie, D.; Rambaut, A. Bayesian Phylogenetics with BEAUti and the BEAST 1.7. *Mol. Biol. Evol.* **2012**, *29*, 1969–1973. [CrossRef]
29. Price, M.N.; Dehal, P.S.; Arkin, A.P. FastTree 2—Approximately Maximum-Likelihood Trees for Large Alignments. *PLoS ONE* **2010**, *5*, e9490. [CrossRef]
30. Aguilera-Sepúlveda, P.; Napp, S.; Llorente, F.; Solano-Manrique, C.; Molina-López, R.; Obón, E.; Solé, A.; Jiménez-Clavero, M.Á.; Fernández-Pinero, J.; Busquets, N. West Nile Virus Lineage 2 Spreads Westwards in Europe and Overwinters in North-Eastern Spain (2017–2020). *Viruses* **2022**, *14*, 569. [CrossRef]
31. Riccò, M.; Peruzzi, S.; Balzarini, F. Epidemiology of West Nile Virus Infections in Humans, Italy, 2012-2020: A Summary of Available Evidences. *Trop Med. Infect. Dis.* **2021**, *6*, 61. [CrossRef]
32. Peterson, R.; Mountfort, G.; Hollom, P.A.; Pandolfi, M.; Frugis, S. Guida Degli Uccelli d'Europa. Atlante Illustrato a Colori. Libri—Amazon.It. Available online: https://www.amazon.it/uccelli-dEuropa-Atlante-illustrato-colori/dp/8874130473 (accessed on 28 April 2022).
33. Vidaña, B.; Busquets, N.; Napp, S.; Pérez-Ramírez, E.; Jiménez-Clavero, M.Á.; Johnson, N. The Role of Birds of Prey in West Nile Virus Epidemiology. *Vaccines* **2020**, *8*, 550. [CrossRef]
34. Nemeth, N.M.; Kratz, G.E.; Bates, R.; Scherpelz, J.A.; Bowen, R.A.; Komar, N. Clinical Evaluation and Outcomes of Naturally Acquired West Nile Virus Infection in Raptors. *J. Zoo Wildl. Med.* **2009**, *40*, 51–63. [CrossRef] [PubMed]
35. Garmendia, A.E.; Van Kruiningen, H.J.; French, R.A.; Anderson, J.F.; Andreadis, T.G.; Kumar, A.; West, A.B. Recovery and Identification of West Nile Virus from a Hawk in Winter. *J. Clin. Microbiol.* **2000**, *38*, 3110–3111. [CrossRef] [PubMed]
36. Ip, H.S.; Van Wettere, A.J.; McFarlane, L.; Shearn-Bochsler, V.; Dickson, S.L.; Baker, J.; Hatch, G.; Cavender, K.; Long, R.; Bodenstein, B. West Nile Virus Transmission in Winter: The 2013 Great Salt Lake Bald Eagle and Eared Grebes Mortality Event. *PLoS Curr.* **2014**, *6*, 3110. [CrossRef] [PubMed]
37. Nemeth, N.; Gould, D.; Bowen, R.; Komar, N. Natural and Experimental West Nile Virus Infection in Five Raptor Species. *J. Wildl. Dis.* **2006**, *42*, 1–13. [CrossRef]
38. Komar, N.; Langevin, S.; Hinten, S.; Nemeth, N.; Edwards, E.; Hettler, D.; Davis, B.; Bowen, R.; Bunning, M. Experimental Infection of North American Birds with the New York 1999 Strain of West Nile Virus. *Emerg. Infect. Dis.* **2003**, *9*, 311–322. [CrossRef]

39. Montecino-Latorre, D.; Barker, C.M. Overwintering of West Nile Virus in a Bird Community with a Communal Crow Roost. *Sci. Rep.* **2018**, *8*, 6088. [CrossRef]
40. Wheeler, S.S.; Vineyard, M.P.; Woods, L.W.; Reisen, W.K. Dynamics of West Nile Virus Persistence in House Sparrows (Passer Domesticus). *PLoS Negl. Trop. Dis.* **2012**, *6*, e1860. [CrossRef]
41. Reisen, W.K.; Fang, Y.; Lothrop, H.D.; Martinez, V.M.; Wilson, J.; Oconnor, P.; Carney, R.; Cahoon-Young, B.; Shafii, M.; Brault, A.C. Overwintering of West Nile Virus in Southern California. *J. Med. Entomol.* **2006**, *43*, 344–355. [CrossRef]
42. Conte, A.; Candeloro, L.; Ippoliti, C.; Monaco, F.; Massis, F.D.; Bruno, R.; Sabatino, D.D.; Danzetta, M.L.; Benjelloun, A.; Belkadi, B.; et al. Spatio-Temporal Identification of Areas Suitable for West Nile Disease in the Mediterranean Basin and Central Europe. *PLoS ONE* **2015**, *10*, e0146024. [CrossRef]
43. Wheeler, S.S.; Langevin, S.A.; Brault, A.C.; Woods, L.; Carroll, B.D.; Reisen, W.K. Detection of Persistent West Nile Virus RNA in Experimentally and Naturally Infected Avian Hosts. *Am. J. Trop Med. Hyg.* **2012**, *87*, 559–564. [CrossRef]
44. Tesh, R.B.; Siirin, M.; Guzman, H.; Travassos da Rosa, A.P.A.; Wu, X.; Duan, T.; Lei, H.; Nunes, M.R.; Xiao, S.-Y. Persistent West Nile Virus Infection in the Golden Hamster: Studies on Its Mechanism and Possible Implications for Other Flavivirus Infections. *J. Infect. Dis.* **2005**, *192*, 287–295. [CrossRef]
45. Appler, K.K.; Brown, A.N.; Stewart, B.S.; Behr, M.J.; Demarest, V.L.; Wong, S.J.; Bernard, K.A. Persistence of West Nile Virus in the Central Nervous System and Periphery of Mice. *PLoS ONE* **2010**, *5*, e10649. [CrossRef]
46. Vogels, C.B.F.; van de Peppel, L.J.J.; van Vliet, A.J.H.; Westenberg, M.; Ibañez-Justicia, A.; Stroo, A.; Buijs, J.A.; Visser, T.M.; Koenraadt, C.J.M. Winter Activity and Aboveground Hybridization Between the Two Biotypes of the West Nile Virus Vector Culex Pipiens. *Vector Borne Zoonotic Dis.* **2015**, *15*, 619–626. [CrossRef]
47. Di Luca, M.; Toma, L.; Boccolini, D.; Severini, F.; La Rosa, G.; Minelli, G.; Bongiorno, G.; Montarsi, F.; Arnoldi, D.; Capelli, G.; et al. Ecological Distribution and CQ11 Genetic Structure of Culex Pipiens Complex (Diptera: Culicidae) in Italy. *PLoS ONE* **2016**, *11*, e0146476. [CrossRef] [PubMed]
48. Brown, L.; Amadon, D. *Eagles, Hawks and Falcons of the World*; Wellfleet: Secaucus, NJ, USA, 1989; ISBN 978-1-55521-472-2.
49. Bollettino_WND_2021_19 (1).Pdf—Adobe Cloud Storage. Available online: https://acrobat.adobe.com/link/file/?x_api_client_id=chrome_extension_viewer&uri=urn%3Aaaid%3Asc%3AUS%3A9868069d-ee54-4d0a-9351-4da5a42ffa6b&filetype=application%2Fpdf&size=1302218 (accessed on 25 July 2022).
50. Bollettino_WND_2022_3.Pdf—Adobe Cloud Storage. Available online: https://acrobat.adobe.com/link/file/?x_api_client_id=chrome_extension_viewer&uri=urn%3Aaaid%3Asc%3AUS%3A359a79f6-a813-4fdd-90b8-b52904f3ca1b&filetype=application%2Fpdf&size=1468985 (accessed on 25 July 2022).
51. Riccò, M. Epidemiology of Tick-Borne Encephalitis in North-Eastern Italy (2017–2020): International Insights from National Notification Reports. *Acta Biomed.* **2021**, *92*, e2021229. [CrossRef]
52. Toscana_2020.Pdf—Adobe Cloud Storage. Available online: https://acrobat.adobe.com/link/file/?x_api_client_id=chrome_extension_viewer&uri=urn%3Aaaid%3Asc%3AUS%3A35ca9c99-25e9-406b-b502-28c485af700&filetype=application%2Fpdf&size=344881 (accessed on 25 July 2022).
53. Mancini Mosquito Species Involved in the Circulation of West Nile and Usutu Viruses in Italy. *Vet. Ital.* **2017**, *53*, 97–110. [CrossRef]

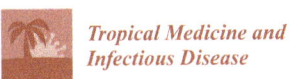 

*Review*

# Dengue in Pregnancy: A Southeast Asian Perspective

Vanessa Chong [1,†], Jennifer Zi Ling Tan [1,†] and Valliammai Jayanthi Thirunavuk Arasoo [2,*]

1. Monash School of Medicine, Faculty of Medicine, Nursing & Health Sciences, Monash University Australia, Clayton 3168, Australia
2. Clinical School Johor Bahru, Jeffrey Cheah School of Medicine and Health Sciences, Monash University Malaysia, Johor Bahru 80100, Malaysia
* Correspondence: t.jayanthi@monash.edu
† These authors contributed equally to this work.

**Abstract:** Dengue cases have been rising in recent years. In 2019 alone, over 658,301 of the 5.6 million reported cases originated from Southeast Asia (SEA). Research has also shown detrimental outcomes for pregnant infected women. Despite this, existing literature describing dengue's effects on pregnancy in SEA is insufficient. Through this narrative review, we sought to describe dengue's effects on pregnancy systemically and emphasize the existing gaps in the literature. We extensively searched various journals cited in PubMed and Ovid Medline, national clinical practice guidelines, and governmental reports. Dengue in pregnancy increases the risk of pre-eclampsia, Dengue Hemorrhagic Fever (DHF), fetal distress, preterm delivery, Caesarean delivery, and maternal mortality. Vertical transmission, intrauterine growth restriction, and stillbirth are possible sequelae of dengue in fetuses. We found that trimester-specific physiological impacts of dengue in pregnancy (to both mother and child) and investigations and management methods demanded further research, especially in the SEA region.

**Keywords:** dengue; pregnancy; Southeast Asia; trimester; physiology; investigations; management

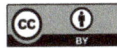

## 1. Introduction

Dengue is endemic to the Southeastern geographical area of Asia (SEA), spreading through the mosquito vector *Aedes aegypti* [1]. The countries included in the geographical region of SEA include Brunei, Myanmar, Cambodia, Timor-Leste, Indonesia, Laos, Malaysia, Philippines, Singapore, Thailand, and Vietnam [2]. Globally, the incidence of dengue increased from 30,668,000 in 1990 to 56,879,000 in 2019 [3]. In SEA alone, there were 7,700,000 cases of dengue in 2019 [4].

Dengue cases were seen more often in females than males, with the age-standardized incidence rate (ASIR) female-to-male ratio of 1.10 in 1990 and 1.08 in 2019 [3]. In 2019, the ASIR per 100,000 in SEA was 1153.57, the 3rd highest after Oceania and South Asia [4].

The 15–49-year-old age group had the most significant incidence of cases, with deaths and disability-adjusted life years (DALY) shifting from children to this age group as well. Pregnancies occur in this age group, and with the incidence being higher in women, it is crucial to have a clear understanding of the physiological changes in pregnancy and the natural progression of dengue to appreciate the potential complications of dengue in pregnancy.

There is also evidence to suggest a higher percentage of severe dengue infections happening to pregnant women than non-pregnant women. Many pregnant women with dengue infection may progress to have Dengue Shock Syndrome (DSS), and the mortality rate triples in this scenario [5].

Dengue has undergone a change in classification by the World Health Organization (WHO). In 1997, symptomatic dengue was divided into undifferentiated fever, dengue fever (DF), and Dengue Hemorrhagic Fever (DHF). DHF was subclassified by severity into four grades. Grades III and IV were known as DSS. The diagnosis of DHF requires a person to have a fever, hemorrhagic manifestation, thrombocytopenia, and evidence of plasma leakage [6].

In addition to the signs seen in DHF, patients who develop DSS additionally have signs of shock, hypotension, a further narrowing of pulse pressure, and an increase in hematocrit (HCT) levels [7,8]. The difficulty in fulfilling the strict criteria of DHF led to the introduction of new criteria in 2009.

In the new criteria, symptomatic dengue was classified as dengue without warning signs, dengue with warning signs (DWS), and severe dengue (SD). Warning signs include abdominal pain and tenderness, persistent vomiting, clinical fluid accumulation, mucosal bleeding, lethargy, restlessness, liver enlargement of more than 2 cm, or laboratory findings of increased HCT value concurrent with a rapid decrease in platelet count. SD is diagnosed when severe plasma leakage leading to shock or respiratory distress, severe bleeding, or severe organ involvement is present [9].

The 2009 WHO classification has less emphasis on pathophysiology and is more like a case management tool. This posed difficulties for dengue research, and the DHF classification continued to be used by researchers [10]. Due to limited research papers following the new classification, this paper includes references to the older classification system.

Despite the high prevalence of dengue in SEA and potentially severe clinical implications in pregnancy, no SEA-specific review is available. Due to varying population genetics, we endeavored to determine the effects of dengue on pregnancy, specifically in SEA, the management options, and the differences in approaches between SEA countries, and further highlight crucial areas for research.

In this review, we discuss the incidence of dengue in SEA, systems-based physiological changes of dengue in pregnancy by trimester, maternal–fetal complications, and relevant investigations and treatments. We aim to provide a concise, up-to-date resource on dengue in pregnancy for healthcare professionals. Simultaneously, we highlight significant gaps in the literature for future research focus.

At the time of writing, we found limited research available to extract data from almost all review sections. Namely, those on the incidence of dengue in pregnancy in SEA, trimester-specific and general pathophysiological changes in dengue, the use of aspirin, preconception vaccination, and impact on the fetus demand a significant proportion of future research.

## 2. Materials and Methods

Our search strategy involved using Google Scholar, PubMed, and Ovid Medline. The latter two were utilized through searching with the following combinations of MESH keywords: "(dengue OR dengue virus) AND (pregnant OR pregnant women) AND (Southeast Asia)." We searched by each country in the geographical SEA (Brunei, Cambodia, Indonesia, Laos, Malaysia, Myanmar, Philippines, Singapore, Thailand, Timor-Leste, and Vietnam). This was used with other relevant keywords using the "OR" conjunction: dengue hemorrhagic fever, dengue shock syndrome, trimester, incidence, investigations, management, monitoring, complications, vaccination, post-partum, fetal/fetal impacts, pre-eclampsia, gestational thrombocytopenia, and gestational diabetes. For two sections, pathophysiology (Section 4) and effect on fetus (Section 5), the data reviewed were not specific to SEA due to the lack of availability. For these sections, the location of origin is disclosed at the start of each section. For the rest of the areas (Management and Preconception Vaccination), data from SEA were primarily targeted for utilization in this review. Due to limited studies based in SEA, we also included combinations of keywords without the "(Southeast Asia)" component. Despite broadening our search through this method, the search yield was limited. As such, the major component of our search strategy included hand-searching based on articles we had previously sourced.

Our inclusion criteria for journal articles included peer-reviewed papers in English, systematic reviews, case–control trials, retrospective studies, cohort studies, and case reports. However, due to a lack of literature from the SEA region, information was sourced from countries outside the SEA. Other references include textbook chapters, national clinical practice guidelines, governmental reports, organization reports, United Nations public health reports, and news reports pertaining to epidemiology and physiology. The data presented in the review will state where they are extracted from for relevant areas. The exclusion criteria were non-English articles and articles without full-text access.

We utilized EndNote x9.3.3 (Clarivate, London, UK) to organize our references.

## 3. Incidence of Dengue in Southeast Asia

There were 5.6 million cases of dengue reported in 2019 globally [3]. This was an 8-fold increase from 2000, when only 505,430 cases were reported. Deaths also increased from 960 in 2000 to 4032 in 2015 [1]. Although 70% of dengue cases are from Asia, human factors such as travel have increased the spread risk in other regions [11].

In SEA, 7,700,000 cases of dengue were reported in 2019. This is a 36.5% increase from 1990, with 4,890,000 cases [4]. Trends and incidences of each country are summarized in Figure 1. Nonetheless, there are no available data looking at the incidence of pregnant women with dengue in SEA.

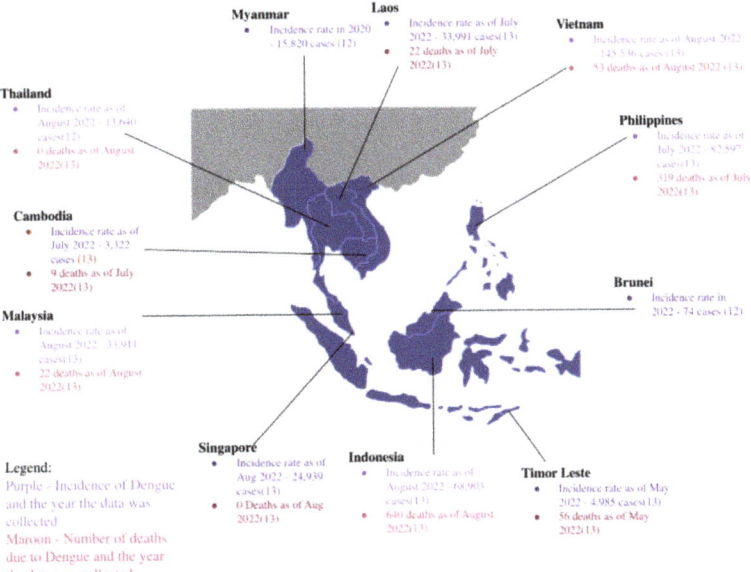

**Figure 1.** Map of geographical Southeast Asia. The incidence of dengue in each country, the year the data were collected, and the number of mortalities due to dengue [12–14].

## 4. Pathophysiology of Uninfected versus Infected Pregnant Women

The first trimester is defined as the period from preconception to 12 weeks, the second trimester of pregnancy from the 13th to the 26th week of pregnancy, and the third trimester from the 27th to the 40th week of pregnancy [15]. Post-partum is defined as the period after the delivery of the fetus. The time frame is not well-specified, but it is generally considered to end around 6 to 8 weeks post-birth [16].

The following tables summarize systemic pathophysiological changes by trimester in pregnancy. Namely, the cardiovascular, endocrinological, hematological, respiratory, and hepatobiliary systems will be discussed. Following each table, further explanation will be given in prose. Physiological changes in thermoregulation will also be addressed.

Careful consideration should be given that the health outcomes measured in the studies referenced may have been complicated by age differences, pre-existing morbidity, different Body Mass Indexes (BMI), healthcare technological advancement variation, or environmental/external factors. Due to varying epigenetics, we attempted to target our search by looking for the pathophysiological changes specific to women in the geographical SEA region. However, due to the lack of research available, we have widened our search to include other demographic data. Such data will be acknowledged in the discussion following every table.

### 4.1. Cardiovascular Physiology

The cardiovascular changes in infected and uninfected mothers are described in Table 1.

**Table 1.** Uninfected versus dengue-infected cardiovascular changes in pregnant women.

| Gestational Stage | Uninfected | Infected |
|---|---|---|
| Trimester 1 | Widened pulse pressure [7]. | Higher risk of pre-eclampsia and eclampsia in severe dengue. Unclear if related to first or second-trimester infection [5,17]. Narrowing of pulse pressure to 25 mm Hg or less with shock [7]. Sepsis or DHF increases capillary permeability, putting infected mothers at an even higher risk of Acute Pulmonary Edema (APO) [7]. Decrease in plasma volume can happen secondary to bleeding in dengue [18]. |
| Trimester 2 | Development of pre-eclampsia in susceptible women. Diastolic BP drops more than systolic BP, causing widened pulse pressure [7]. Mean heart rate = 75 beats per minute (bpm) [19]. Blood pressure (BP) generally reduces [20]. Progressive increase in plasma volume [21]. | Effects on pre-eclampsia and pulse pressures are as above. Refer to above for general altered physiology for dengue in pregnant women. |
| Trimester 3 | The mean heart rate peaks late in the third trimester. However, it should not be >95 bpm [7]. Plasma volume increases until the 30th–34th week and then plateaus or decreases slightly through the term [21]. BP generally increases [22] | No specific altered physiology for dengue in pregnant women in the third trimester can be found. Refer to above for general altered physiology for dengue in pregnant women. |
| Post-partum | Two weeks post-delivery, the mother returns to a hemodynamically same state as pre-pregnancy [23]. Maternal heart rate is fastest on the day of delivery, with a median of 83 bpm. This decreases until Day 14 post-labor [24]. Maternal BP increases until day 5 or 6 post-delivery, reaching a median of 121/79 mm Hg. It then decreases to normal by day 14 post-partum, reaching a median of 116/75 mm Hg [24]. Plasma volume decreases [25]. | No specific altered physiology for dengue in post-partum women can be found. |

The literature for this section was taken from various countries. We heavily referenced the Sri Lankan guidelines for dengue in pregnancy [7]. The guideline was created using data sourced locally, from SEA, and international guidelines (WHO and Up-to-Date). Of note, it lacked in-text citations to distinguish from where each data point was taken.

Additionally, an older classification system was used to classify dengue according to DHF and DSS rather than newer classifications written by WHO. A SEA guideline on dengue from Malaysia [5] is also referenced in this section. As it is not specific to pregnancy, there is limited information on cardiovascular changes in pregnant women with dengue. For the other articles, one from SEA includes a case report from Singapore [26]. Research based in Asia consists of that from China [20] only. Research based on populations outside of Asia was from Mexico [17], Spain [22], and the United Kingdom [24]. Articles [19,21,23,25,27,28] did not consider or stratify by country of origin.

Decreasing systemic vascular resistance during pregnancy results in a disproportionate fall in diastolic compared to systolic pressures, thus widening the pulse pressure to around 30 mm Hg. During shock, compensatory mechanisms reduce pulse pressures (7). With a fall in oncotic pressures and pulmonary resistance, mothers are also vulnerable to developing APO with any fluid overload or increased capillary permeability [7,27].

Plasma volume decreases during hemorrhage. Due to cardiovascular changes during pregnancy [18], signs of hypovolemia may not display until the later stages, endangering both the mother and fetus [7]. Attending doctors should be aware of this possibility.

Severe dengue increases the risk of pre-eclampsia. Placental ischemia in trimester one can occur secondary to capillary leak syndrome. As inadequate spiral artery development leads to pre-eclampsia, concerns about pre-eclampsia development in the second trimester may arise. With dengue, plasma leakage results from inflammatory cytokines, dengue protein non-structural protein-1 (NS1), and inflammatory lipid mediators, increasing capillary permeability [28]. Maternal compensatory mechanisms following pathological plasma leakage and vasodilation may increase the risk of developing pre-eclampsia [26], especially if dengue was severe (15.4%). In non-severe dengue, pre-eclampsia rates were comparable to that of a normal pregnancy (2.9%). This could be due to the disruption of spiral artery development, although the study does not mention whether the illness onset was in the first trimester, so other mechanisms are possible. In addition, the sample size of this study was small, so further research on a larger scale should be considered. If the positive association between dengue and pre-eclampsia is further confirmed, there may be a need for monitoring infected mothers and prescribing aspirin [17].

Overall, there is limited evidence of cardiovascular physiological changes in infected mothers. Available evidence notes that in infected mothers, there could be a narrowing of pulse pressure [7], increased capillary permeability [7], increased risk of pre-eclampsia [17], and decreased plasma volume [18] in some instances. However, the specific mechanisms of why some of these changes happen are not further explained. Furthermore, the data is not trimester-specific or particular to the SEA population. More research can be done focusing on trimester-specific cardiovascular physiological changes in pregnant women infected with dengue from the SEA region, especially regarding changes to maternal heart rate, maternal BP, and the mechanism behind the changes.

### 4.2. Endocrinological Physiology

The endocrinological changes in infected and uninfected mothers are described in Table 2.

**Table 2.** Uninfected versus dengue-infected endocrinological changes in pregnant women.

| Gestational Stage | Uninfected | Infected |
|---|---|---|
| Trimester 1 | Progesterone level increases [29].<br>Human chorionic gonadotropin (hCG) peaks from the 8th to the 10th week before plateauing [30].<br>Relaxin increases [30].<br>Parathyroid hormone levels rise [31].<br>Prolactin levels rise [32]. | There is insufficient research on pathological hormonal changes in infected pregnant mothers. |
| Trimester 2 | GDM can develop in susceptible women.<br>Increase in human Placental Lactogen (hPL) levels [33] stimulates liver production of insulin-like growth factor (IGF-1) [34] for glucose control [35].<br>• High levels of IGF-1 have an insulin-like effect [36]. However, extremely high levels are linked to insulin resistance and could increase the risk of developing Type 2 Diabetes Mellitus [37].<br>Human leukocyte antigen-G (HLA-G) increases to regulate the immunological system [38].<br>• Reduced serum HLA-G increases the risk of pre-eclampsia [39–41].<br>Increase in estrogen levels [42].<br>• Causes vasodilation of blood vessels, thus increasing blood flow to the uterus and placenta [30]. | Lack of evidence to suggest dengue increases the risk of developing GDM [43].<br>No evidence was found on how dengue can affect the hormones discussed. |

**Table 2.** *Cont.*

| Gestational Stage | Uninfected | Infected |
|---|---|---|
| Trimester 3 | hPL levels do not change much from the 2nd trimester [33]. Serum HLA-G levels decrease in concentration (63.31 Units/mL), but remain higher than in non-pregnant women [38]. Estrogen continues to increase [44]. | No specific altered physiology for dengue in pregnant women in the third trimester can be found. Refer to above for general altered physiology for dengue in pregnant women. |
| Post-partum | hPL levels decrease post-birth, becoming undetectable by 18–24 h post-birth [33]. Estrogen levels decrease after placenta removal and return to pre-pregnancy levels by day 5 post-partum [45]. | No specific altered physiology for dengue in post-partum women can be found. |

The literature for this section was sourced from various countries. From Asia, one article took data from Asian countries broadly [46], while others used data from India [43], Sri Lanka [47], and Taiwan [36,48]. The literature on populations outside Asia was based on people from Poland [38], the USA [33,42], Denmark [37], and Brazil [49–51]. Articles [29–32,34,35,39–41,44,45,52,53] did not consider or stratify by country of origin. No study was based on SEA populations alone.

Placental ischemia in the first trimester can occur secondary to capillary leak syndrome. The resulting placental function dysregulation can alter hPL production. Concerns about developing GDM in the second trimester may arise subsequently as hPL levels are interlinked with GDM. GDM occurs in about 11.5% of pregnancies in Asia [46]. Currently, there is inadequate research into changes in placental hPL production levels. Nevertheless, extraplacental effects of dengue have been shown to cause pancreatomegaly, hyperlipemia, and rarely pancreatitis [43] with an unclear pathophysiology. Postulations include direct virulence on the pancreas, ischemia from DSS, secondary autoimmune reactions, or extraluminal edematous obstruction of the ampulla of Vater [43]. However, there is very little evidence for dengue-induced pancreatitis leading to diabetes mellitus [52] or altering hPL levels during pregnancy.

Progression to the critical phase is more likely to occur in females, diabetics, hypertensives, kidney disease, and those with cardiovascular disease [53]. Studies have shown that pregnancy is also a risk factor for progression to DHF/DSS [49]. A case series from Sri Lanka showed that having GDM was associated with more severe infections such as DHF [47]. This is consistent with studies demonstrating increased severity of illness in Type 2 Diabetes Mellitus patients [48], especially those with poor glycemic control [50]. Dengue also aggravates damage in the diabetic pancreas, with evidence of macrophage infiltrates [51,53]. As such, closer monitoring of at-risk individuals can significantly benefit treatment efficacy, although further studies should confirm this.

To summarize, little evidence can be found on endocrinological changes in infected mothers, especially regarding specific endocrine hormones. More research can be done surrounding trimester-specific endocrinology physiological changes in dengue-infected mothers from the SEA region, specifically looking at the possible changes to hormone levels and the impact of dengue on GDM.

### 4.3. Hematological Physiology

Hematological changes in infected and uninfected mothers are described in Table 3.

**Table 3.** Uninfected versus dengue-infected hematological changes in pregnant women.

| Gestational Stage | Uninfected | Infected |
|---|---|---|
| Trimester 1 | Lymphocyte count decreases, although leukocytosis is present [54].<br>Blood volume expansion at 6–12 weeks [54].<br>• Fall in hemoglobin (rise in hemoglobin is outweighed by the increase in plasma volume) [54]. | Leukopenia may not be seen in infected mothers [7].<br>Due to physiological hemodilution during pregnancy, hemoconcentration with plasma leakage in dengue may be masked [55]. Therefore, a rising HCT can mean maternal shock [7]. |
| Trimester 2 | Increased hypercoagulability, particularly in the second trimester [20].<br>• Driven by an elevation of factors VII, VIII, X, von Willebrand factor, and fibrinogen.<br>• Reduced sensitivity to activated protein C and protein S [56] and increased inhibition of fibrinolytic factors [57].<br>• Mechanical factors like increased abdominal pressure on pelvic veins favor hemostasis as the pregnancy progresses [57].<br>• Estrogen is also prothrombotic and increases the risk of venous thrombosis [58].<br>Increased platelet count [20].<br>Gestational thrombocytopenia (GT) may develop in 4.4% to 11.6% of pregnant women [59].<br>• GT happens as platelet counts fall below 130–150.000/µL [60].<br>• It rarely drops <80 × $10^9$/L in GT [7].<br>• Hemodilution from higher plasma volume, placental consumption of platelets [61], and possible inefficacious thrombopoietin action [62] result in GT.<br>• Usually asymptomatic, with no significant consequences from gestational thrombocytopenia [61].<br>Mean white blood cell (WBC) is around 8 × $10^9$/L [19], increased [20].<br>Decreased erythrocyte count [20]. | Thrombocytopenia can occur in dengue [63], and a fall in platelet counts below <80 × $10^9$/L may suggest plasma leakage [7]. |
| Trimester 3 | Mean WBC count approximates 9 × $10^9$/L [19].<br>Leukocyte count remains like the second trimester [20].<br>Platelet count decreases [20].<br>Erythrocyte count increases from the 28th week to the end of pregnancy [20].<br>Remains in a hypercoagulable state [64,65]. | No specific altered physiology for dengue in pregnant women in the third trimester can be found.<br>Refer to above for general altered physiology for dengue in pregnant women. |
| Post-partum | Leukocyte count peaks a week post-partum and subsequently decreases drastically at week 7 post-partum [20].<br>Platelet count increases after birth and peaks a week post-partum [20].<br>Erythrocyte count decreases a week post-partum before increasing again [20].<br>Hypercoagulable state takes approximately 4 weeks to resolve [66]. | No specific altered physiology for dengue in post-partum women can be found. |

The literature for this section was sourced from various countries. From SEA, an Indonesian article [55] and the Malaysia guideline on dengue [5] were used. From Asia, articles used include the Sri Lankan clinical guidelines [7] and research from China if the population discussed was of Chinese ancestry [20,62,64]. Populations outside Asia that were used include England [66]. Articles [7,19,54,56–61,63,65] did not consider or stratify by country of origin. There were no studies found based on SEA exclusively.

Research on pregnant Han Chinese women reported them to be in a hypercoagulable state. Han Chinese is the largest Chinese ethnic group in SEA [64,65]. Therefore, physiological changes in Han Chinese and SEA women may have similarities. This data is also consistent with other sources that state that women are in a hypercoagulable state in the second trimester [20].

Thrombocytopenia occurs due to hematopoietic stem cell inhibition and disruption of plasma kinin systems (non-trimester specific). Consumptive coagulopathy can result due to Disseminated Intravascular Coagulopathy (DIC) in severe dengue [63], and prothrombotic states worsen this in pregnancy. Although uncommon, should bleeding occur, early intervention (while taking caution about fluid overload) is crucial for maternal wellbeing [5].

In essence, there is limited evidence of hematological changes in infected mothers. Current evidence suggests that in dengue-infected mothers, thrombocytopenia can occur [63], and a rising HCT can indicate maternal shock [7]. However, leukopenia might not be present in mothers with dengue [7]. The data found are also not trimester-specific and do not look specifically at the physiological changes in infected SEA mothers [7]. Additional research can be done on trimester-specific hematological changes in pregnant women with dengue from the SEA region, looking particularly at how dengue can affect specific blood components, dengue's impact on coagulability state, and how dengue could further impact mothers with GT.

### 4.4. Respiratory Physiology

Respiratory changes in infected and uninfected mothers are described in Table 4.

**Table 4.** Uninfected versus dengue-infected respiratory changes in pregnant women.

| Gestational Stage | Uninfected | Infected |
|---|---|---|
| Trimester 1 | Minute ventilation increases by up to 48% with higher tidal volume and unchanged respiratory rate [67]. | No specific altered physiology for dengue in pregnant women in the first trimester can be found. Refer below for general altered physiology for dengue in pregnant women. |
| Trimester 2 | Pregnancy leads to compensated respiratory alkalosis. Increased oxygen consumption causes hypoxia susceptibility [7]. Mean respiratory rate is around 15 breaths per minute [19]. Mean partial pressure of carbon dioxide is around 32 mm Hg [19]. | No trimester-specific evidence on the altered respiratory physiology in pregnant women with dengue was found. The fall in oncotic pressure and pulmonary resistance causes vulnerability to developing APO [7]. Additionally, the respiratory rate might increase [7]. |
| Trimester 3 | Continued compensated respiratory alkalosis and oxygen consumption [7]. Respiratory rate ranges between 8–24 breathes per minute [68]. | No specific altered physiology for dengue in pregnant women in the third trimester can be found. Refer to above for general altered physiology for dengue in pregnant women. |
| Post-partum | Respiratory parameters return to normal 6–12 weeks after labor [69]. Respiratory rate returns to pre-pregnancy levels by 2–3 days post-birth [70]. | No specific altered physiology for dengue in post-partum women can be found. |

The literature for this section was sourced from various countries. From Asia, the Sri Lankan guideline was the only Asian guideline found to be useful [7]. Articles [19,67,69,70] did not consider or stratify by country of origin. No studies were found based exclusively on SEA.

Overall, evidence for respiratory changes in infected mothers is lacking. Available evidence states that infected mothers are more vulnerable to developing APO [7], and respiratory rates might increase [7]. However, there is no evidence on how dengue affects other respiratory parameters, such as the mean partial pressure of carbon dioxide. Data found are also neither trimester-specific nor specific to the SEA population. Further research is needed to examine the trimester-specific respiratory changes in pregnant dengue-infected mothers from the SEA region.

### 4.5. Hepatobiliary Physiology

Hepatobiliary changes in infected and uninfected mothers are described in Table 5.

**Table 5.** Uninfected versus dengue-infected hepatobiliary changes in pregnant women.

| Gestational Stage | Uninfected | Infected |
|---|---|---|
| Trimester 1 | Albumin level decreases [71]. Serum total and free bilirubin concentrations are lower in all trimesters [71]. | |
| Trimester 2 | Serum alkaline phosphatase (ALP) activity increases [71]. Serum gamma-glutamyl transferase (GGT) activity levels decrease slightly [71]. | Maternal liver enzyme derangement [17]. |
| Trimester 3 | | |
| Post-partum | Bilirubin concentration increases post-partum, returning to pre-pregnancy levels by day 5 post-partum [72]. GGT levels should return to normal by day 13 post-partum [72]. GGT levels initially decrease, then increase, peaking at either day 5 or 10 post-partum [72]. | |

The literature for this section was sourced from various countries. Articles from populations outside Asia were taken from Mexico [17] and England [72]. Articles [71] and [73] did not consider or stratify by country of origin. There were no studies found based on SEA exclusively.

Dengue can cause maternal liver enzyme derangement. Alanine aminotransferase (ALT) and aspartate transaminase (AST) become elevated [17]. When dengue targets hepatocytes and Kupffer cells, the resultant cell death causes ALT and AST to rise. T-cell-mediated cytotoxicity is precipitated and a brewing cytokine storm of IL-2, IL-6, TNF-α, and IFN-γ (amongst other cytokines), further exacerbates hepatic damage [73].

In summary, some evidence suggests that dengue affects hepatobiliary physiology. Dengue can cause derangement of ALT and AST liver enzymes [17]. However, evidence is lacking on whether ALP, albumin, bilirubin and GGT levels are affected. Furthermore, the data is neither trimester-specific nor SEA population specific. More research is needed on trimester-specific hepatobiliary physiological changes in dengue-infected pregnant women from the SEA region, including looking specifically at changes to the ALP, albumin, bilirubin, and GGT.

### 4.6. Thermoregulatory Physiology

Thermoregulatory changes in infected and uninfected mothers are described in Table 6.

**Table 6.** Uninfected versus dengue-infected thermoregulatory changes in pregnant women.

| Gestational Stage | Uninfected | Infected |
|---|---|---|
| Trimester 1 | Core body temperature increases a few tenths of a degree [74]. | |
| Trimester 2 | Mean body temperature decreases from the first trimester [74] to around 36.9 degrees Celsius [19]. | Dengue causes an increase in body temperature [1]. No trimester-specific data was found. |
| Trimester 3 | Body temperature decreases from the second trimester [74] and ranges between 35.37 to 37.35 degrees Celsius [68]. | |
| Post-partum | Core body temperature remains below pre-pregnancy levels until 3 months post-partum [74]. | |

The literature was sourced from various countries. Articles using populations outside Asia include data from the United Kingdom [68] and Norway [74]. Articles [1,19] did not consider or stratify by country of origin. There were no studies found based on SEA exclusively.

The relatively significant increase in estradiol and progesterone in the first trimester, followed by higher estradiol and low progesterone, explains the temperature change. Estradiol causes peripheral vasodilation, which in turn dissipates heat [74].

In essence, the evidence on thermoregulatory physiological changes in infected mothers is neither trimester-specific nor specific to SEA.

### 4.7. Others

The Malaysia guidelines for pregnancy also note an increased risk of dengue encephalopathy in severe dengue. It is not specific to any trimester of pregnancy [5]. The pathogenesis behind this complication includes hepatic encephalopathy, cerebral hypoperfusion in DSS, increased vascular permeability causing cerebral edema, electrolyte imbalance, and intracranial bleeding, which leads to thrombocytopenia or coagulopathy. However, the exact reason why pregnant women have an increased risk of dengue encephalopathy is still unanswered, with researchers questioning whether it is due to the immune-tolerant state of pregnancy [75].

## 5. Impact on Fetus

### 5.1. Vertical Transmission

Although vertical transmission of dengue can happen [5,76], it is rare [77], especially if mothers are asymptomatic [5]. However, a study involving 54 participants in French Guiana reported vertical transmission in about 18.5–22.7%. Dengue is detected by IgM or viruses in the placental, cord or peripheral blood of the newborn. The rate of transmission is higher in the third trimester [78]. Perinatally, dengue is transmitted through the placenta [79]. New evidence suggest that the virus may also be transmitted by breast milk [80]. Clinical presentations of the vertical transmission of dengue in neonates can range from mild (fever) to severe (DHF, DSS, death), where symptoms of fever and rash are most common, followed by hepatomegaly, thrombocytopenia, and DHF.

In a Malaysian study, 63 pregnant women were dengue-specific IgM positive with a vertical transmission rate of 1.6%. Preterm birth rates, low birth weight, and adverse neonatal outcomes were no different from IgM-negative women [81].

The literature for this section was sourced from various countries. From Asia, data from Sri Lanka [77] and Malaysia [5,81] was used. Articles using populations outside Asia used data from French Guiana [82], West Africa [78], Brazil [79], and Polynesia [80]. Article [76] did not consider or stratify by country of origin.

### 5.2. Fetal Malformation

There is no link between dengue with fetal malformations [5,17]. During the first trimester, vertical transmission may raise concerns about defects in organogenesis. Early studies on dengue have concluded that dengue does not cause birth defects [83] or abortions [84]. In addition, no long-term complications are implicated, with the normal development of infants [83]. Another research article also notes that fever during pregnancy adversely affects offspring health, with a 1.5- to nearly three-fold increased risk of developing neural tube defects, congenital heart defects, and oral clefts with maternal fever in the first trimester. Although not dose-dependent, there was some evidence that using antipyretic medications during febrile episodes may have protective effects. Nonetheless, congenital abnormalities in the offspring of women who had dengue in the first trimester may be caused by pyrexia and not be virus-related [85].

The research here was sourced from SEA regions such as Thailand [83], Asian countries such as China [84], and countries outside Asia such as Mexico [17].

### 5.3. Neurodevelopmental Disorder

The risk of neurodevelopmental disorder (NDD) in offspring exposed to maternal fever during pregnancy is increased with an Odds Ratio (OR) of 1.24 [95% CI: 1.12–1.38]. Further, if fever occurred during the first trimester, the risk for NDD increased with an OR of 1.13 [95% CI:1.02–1.26] [86].

*5.4. Fetal Growth Restriction*

Placental ischemia can affect fetal growth. A descriptive Brazilian study proposes that due to capillary leak syndrome and capillary permeability, inadequate vascular supply to the fetus leads to hypoxic injury (loss of trophoblastic epithelia, edema in villous stroma, chorangiosis, infarction), in addition to inflammatory damage (villitis, deciduitis, choriodeciduitis) [87].

Low birth weight is the most common negative impact on the fetus with dengue during pregnancy, according to a French Guiana study [88]. Brazilian data showed DHF doubles the risk of low birth weight, while mild disease increases the risk by 20%. A Thailand study and the Malaysian guidelines on dengue corroborated the higher chances of low birth weight [5,83]. However, other studies showed that dengue does not increase the risk of intrauterine growth restriction (IUGR) [84]. It can be inferred that hypoxia is sufficient to reduce growth rates, but insufficient to lead to IUGR.

*5.5. Stillbirth*

There are a few reported cases of dengue causing fetal death after vertical virus transmission [89]. The study done in French Guiana suggested that the risk of stillbirth increases when the mother has symptomatic dengue infection [88], while another in Thailand showed a higher risk of stillbirth [83]. The Malaysian Guidelines also note the relationship between dengue and fetal death [5].

After 20 weeks of gestation, monitoring for fetal distress can be helpful. In addition to determining fetal status, it may be the first indication of maternal plasma leakage [7]. Fetal tachycardia is observed with fetal hypoxia. Overall, it also stands out that there is a lack of trimester-specific fetal impact, as most research focused on fetal outcomes cumulatively for all trimesters.

*5.6. Fetal Distress, Delivery, and Maternal Mortality*

In an Indonesian study of 41 participants with confirmed dengue during pregnancy, women with secondary infections had more adverse maternal and neonatal outcomes. This included five maternal deaths [90].

Another study done in Mexico suggested that severe dengue increases the risk of fetal distress, cesarean delivery, and maternal mortality in the third trimester of pregnancy [17]. The Thailand guideline that looks at the effect of dengue infection in pregnancy also concurs with the above findings [91].

However, a Thailand study compared 48 pregnant women with dengue to 500 pregnant women without dengue. It concluded that there was no increased risk of adverse neonatal outcomes or maternal mortality [92].

According to the Malaysian guidelines, pregnant women who have spontaneous vaginal delivery while having dengue do not have an increased risk of adverse outcomes. However, infection during labor increases the chances of needing surgical intervention. If that was the case, surgical interventions such as cesarean section and assisted vaginal delivery would increase the risk of bleeding. An infection during labor would also increase the risk of fetal distress [5].

This discrepancy in outcomes shows that more research is needed before a more definitive conclusion can be made on whether dengue affects neonatal and maternal outcomes.

*5.7. Miscarriage and Preterm Delivery*

In Laos, 76 women with confirmed dengue were studied. Six had miscarriages, and nine had preterm births. One participant with severe dengue died [93]. In the Indonesian study of 41 participants mentioned above, one progressed to term, while the other had a miscarriage. Seven women delivered prematurely [90].

In another descriptive study in Brazil, alarmingly, all patients with dengue in the first trimester had miscarriages, possibly due to inflammatory placental changes, as mentioned earlier [87]. This is concurred by the Malaysian guidelines, which state that first-trimester infections are associated with miscarriages [5].

In the Thailand study described above, there was a two-fold increased risk of preterm labor. This indicates a possible link between dengue and miscarriage/preterm delivery [92]. The Malaysian guidelines also note the association between infections in the third trimester and preterm birth [5]. At the same time, the Thailand guidelines state a possible link between dengue and premature uterine contractions [91].

DHF increases the risk of preterm delivery by 10%, according to Thai and Mexican studies [83,94]. This is especially so if the patient is in the critical phase of DHF. If possible, the delivery should be delayed using tocolytic drugs until the plasma leakage is resolved [7]. Steroids usually used to speed up fetal lung development in preterm delivery [95] can still be used. However, there is insufficient evidence to prove the use of steroids in the treatment of dengue [96].

Sources [95] and [96] did not consider or stratify by country of origin.

### 5.8. Placental Abruption and Hemorrhage

Placental abruptions can happen any time after 20 weeks of pregnancy [97]. Indonesia reported the only placental abruption occurring at 35 weeks of gestation due to DHF [98].

According to the Thailand guidelines, dengue can increase the risk of intrapartum and post-partum hemorrhage [91]. Medical teams should consider how this could impact the management of pregnancy and delivery of infected pregnant women.

## 6. Management

Despite the severe implications of dengue in pregnancy and its increasing prevalence in SEA, data on its management in SEA are scarce, restricting any discourse. There are five guidelines discussing the management of dengue from SEA. They are from Malaysia [5], Singapore [99], the Philippines [100], Myanmar [101], and Thailand [91].

### 6.1. Investigations

In SEA, guidelines on dengue are available from Myanmar [101], the Philippines [100], Thailand [91], Malaysia [5], and Singapore [99]. Investigations recommended by the five countries vary slightly. All guidelines described the general investigations done for adults with dengue. Only the Myanmar [101] and the Philippines [100] guidelines outlined the investigations essential to pregnant individuals. The guidelines from the Philippines [100] and Singapore [99] lacked information on recommended investigations for follow-up. Thailand's [91] guidelines were brief and failed to mention the initial and follow-up tests that should be done. The dengue guidelines from Brunei, Indonesia, Laos, Timor-Leste, and Vietnam were unavailable, while the Cambodian guidelines were inaccessible. Therefore, in this section, we consolidated the available guidelines in Table 7. Information in the table is applicable for dengue in adults unless specified.

The collated information in Table 7 shows that the investigations recommended are relatively similar. Where an initial assessment was mentioned in the guidelines, an FBC including HCT is recommended, and dengue IgM/IgG tests are also generally listed as a diagnostic tool.

Nonetheless, several guidelines still have gaps in the investigation section. This is especially so in the required follow-up investigations. It is essential to highlight that the guidelines were mostly investigations for adults suspected of having dengue and not pregnancy specific. Myanmar [101] and the Philippines [100] are the only two countries that mentioned investigations that should be done on pregnant women. Myanmar's guidelines stated that FBC needs to be repeated daily once the pregnant woman is admitted [101], while the Philippines guidelines said that FBC is essential in a pregnant woman [100]. These guidelines, however, do not adequately address the need for additional pregnancy specific investigations, like a biophysical profile or cardiotocography, to assess fetal wellbeing.

**Table 7.** Comparison of investigations recommended by dengue guidelines from Myanmar [101], the Philippines [100], Malaysia [5], Thailand [91], and Singapore [99].

| Country | Initial Assessment | Diagnostics | Follow-Up |
|---|---|---|---|
| Myanmar | Baseline Full Blood Count (FBC), including HCT<br>• In the presence of leukopenia and/or thrombocytopenia and with signs of dengue should be sent for a medical consultation.<br>• Changes to baseline parameters should be noted as early as possible<br>• If HCT is unavailable, multiply hemoglobin by 3 for an estimate of HCT.<br>Other tests to consider: Blood glucose, serum electrolytes, calcium, urea, creatine, bicarbonate, coagulation profile, liver function tests | Dengue NS1 test<br>Dengue IgM test<br>• Recommended from day 5<br>• Highly suggestive of dengue: Positive in a single serum sample:<br>• Confirmed dengue: IgM seroconversion in paired sera<br>Dengue IgG test<br>• Recommended from day 5<br>• Highly suggestive of dengue: Positive in a single serum sample with hemagglutination inhibition of more than or equal to 1280:<br>• Confirmed dengue: IgG seroconversion in paired sera or fourfold IgG titre increase in paired sera<br>Duo test (NS1 Ag + IgM/IgG)<br>• Recommended from day 4<br>• As a duo test, the sensitivity may increase to >90%<br>Dengue Polymerase Chain Reaction (PCR)<br>• Confirmed: Positive<br>Dengue Virus culture<br>• Confirmed: Positive | FBC<br>• Monitor for signs of DHF—leukopenia, thrombocytopenia, and a rising HCT<br>• FBC Checked daily in pregnant women admitted to the hospital |
| Philippines | History<br>Physical examination<br>• Signs of ascites, tourniquet test, signs of rash and bleedings, hemodynamic status, signs of respiratory distress<br>Investigations: FBC, including HCT (essential in pregnant women) | Viral culture isolation<br>Dengue PCR<br>Diagnostic tests are not necessary for acute management. | Not Applicable (N/A) |
| Malaysia | Baseline FBC (including HCT) for all patients suspected of having dengue. (As per point 1 of Myanmar guideline)<br><br>Other tests to consider performing include liver function test, renal profile, coagulation profile, lactate, blood gases, troponin, and creatine kinase. | Rapid Combo Test (RCT)<br>• Analyzes the presence or absence of dengue NS1 Antigen, dengue IgM and IgG antibodies<br>NS1<br>• Antigen detection test for NS1 antigen is necessary for virus viability.<br>Dengue IgM test<br>• IgM enzyme-linked immunosorbent assay (ELISA)<br>• More helpful in picking up primary infections compared to secondary infections<br>Dengue IgG test<br>• IgG ELISA<br>• Detected 7 days after onset of Fever<br>• Repeat is recommended if dengue IgM is still negative after day 7 and the initial IgG test showed a negative result.<br>• Useful in differentiating primary and secondary dengue infections<br>Dengue Viral RNA Detection (RT-PCR)<br>• Only useful during the viremic stage<br>• Detects viral RNA up to 5 days after symptom onset<br>• Detects dengue serotype<br>Dengue Virus Isolation/Culture<br>• Only carried out for research, surveillance, and genotyping purposes | Serial FBC to monitor disease progression |
| Thailand | N/A | Dengue PCR<br>Dengue NS1<br>Dengue IgM/IgG test | N/A |
| Singapore | FBC (including HCT). (As per point 1 of Myanmar guideline)<br>Liver Function Tests<br>Monitor for elevated transaminases (AST is normally more elevated than ALT) | Dengue IgM<br>• As per the Myanmar guidelines<br>Dengue IgG<br>• As per the Myanmar guidelines<br>Dengue PCR<br>• To be done within 5 days of onset of symptoms | N/A |

Regarding the initial assessment, all guidelines apart from Thailand [91] stated FBC, including HCT, as their investigation of choice. Myanmar [101], Malaysia [5], and Singapore [99] guidelines also mentioned other baseline investigations. The Philippines was the only country that specified history and examinations that should be done to help rule in/out the diagnosis of dengue [100]. Thailand's guidelines failed to mention the initial investigations that should be carried out [91]. While FBC, including HCT, may be adequate in a general adult, medical teams should consider the need for a further initial assessment in pregnant individuals.

All five guidelines mentioned the investigations used for diagnosing dengue. However, as previously mentioned, they are not pregnancy specific and vary slightly between countries. Dengue PCR is the only investigation recommended by all five countries. There are also differences in opinions on when the dengue IgG test should be done, with Myanmar recommending it from day 5 [101], while Malaysia recommends it from day 7 [5]. Although test sensitivity in the different labs might be a reason for the difference, further exploration to determine the day might be helpful. Diagnostic tools for dengue are available, but one specific for dengue in pregnant women is unavailable.

Follow-up investigations that are required for pregnant women with dengue are lacking. Only the Malaysian and Myanmar guidelines mentioned the necessary follow-up investigations, and only FBC was listed [5,101]. All the guidelines require a more in-depth list of follow-up investigations to assist medical teams in managing pregnant women with dengue.

The dengue guidelines available from SEA were not pregnancy specific. Important differential diagnoses such as HELLP (hemolysis, elevated liver enzymes, and thrombocytopenia) syndrome in patients with pre-eclampsia were not discussed.

### 6.2. Treatment

Approaches to dengue in pregnancy vary in the clinical practice guidelines of SEA countries. The guidelines found (Myanmar, Philippines, Malaysia, and Thailand) described general adult management of dengue based on various phases of the disease. Special considerations for pregnant individuals were subsequently described. The guideline from Singapore was brief and did not consider pregnancy status. Similarly, Thailand guidelines had limited information about dengue management and even less about dengue during pregnancy. Some SEA countries had no guidelines available online (Brunei, Indonesia, Laos, Timor-Leste, and Vietnam) or required permission to view (Cambodia). For this section, we will consolidate the guidelines specific to dengue in pregnancy, and a summary table is shown below (Table 8).

**Table 8.** Data from SEA countries with pregnancy-specific information.

| | Malaysia [5] | Thailand [91] | Myanmar [101] | Singapore [99] | Philippines [100] |
|---|---|---|---|---|---|
| Pathophysiology | | | | N/A | N/A |
| Investigations | | | | | |
| Management | | | | | |
| Complications | | | | N/A | N/A |
| Links | https://www.moh.gov.my/moh/resources/penerbitan/GUIDELINE/GUIDELINE%20Dengue%20Infection%20PDF%20Final.pdf | https://www.tm.mahidol.ac.th/seameo/2015-46-1-suppl/c7Annexp169-181.pdf | https://www.mmacentral.org/wp-content/uploads/2022/06/National-Guideline-for-Clinical-Management-of-Dengue-2021.pdf | https://www.ncid.sg/Health-Professionals/Diseases-and-Conditions/Pages/Dengue.aspx | https://pcp.org.ph/images/PSBIM/PSBIM_Local_Guidelines_2019/RevisedDengueClinicalCaseManagementGuidelines2011-DOH.pdf |
| Access Date | 2 December 2021 | 9 December 2022 | 9 December 2022 | 9 December 2022 | 9 December 2022 |

Legend: ■ Pregnancy specific data. ■ Absence of pregnancy specific data. ■ Mixed data (standard dengue management with some evaluation for pregnancy). "N/A" refers to "Not Applicable." Guidelines from Brunei, Indonesia, Laos, Timor-Leste, Vietnam, and Cambodia were not assessed.

Myanmar's and the Philippines' guidelines bear similarities. They designated pregnancy as one of the many indications for in-hospital management, then detailed how the latter should be done. As such, although these guidelines contain the highest quantity of relevant data amongst SEA countries, the management was not specific to dengue in pregnancy. Table 8 summarizes which SEA countries considered pregnancy-specific information in their guidelines and provides links to each guideline.

A comparison of guidelines from SEA is described in Table 9.

From Table 9, it can be inferred that the guidelines bear some similarities. Some examples include higher precaution levels, monitoring parameters, transfusion guidelines, and reduction of traumatic procedures peripartum.

However, many of the guidelines require more management information. This is especially so for dengue and its various phases, and dengue in the pregnant state. While some guidelines appear to fill the gaps of other guidelines, most of the data are not pregnancy-specific. As mentioned earlier, the guidelines from Myanmar and the Philippines [100,101] merely stated pregnancy as one of the indications in an overall management flow without differentiating management for DHF, DSS, or progression of complications in pregnancy. For instance, the Philippines guidelines provide extensive detail about fluid management, but do not consider the hypervolemic state in pregnancy [100]. Fluid management not tailored to pregnancy could overcorrect and cause fluid overload, resulting in acute pulmonary edema [7,27]. Pregnancy-specific comorbidities such as pre-eclampsia and gestational diabetes were not considered. Although the Myanmar guidelines did mention lower platelet levels in pregnancy, gestational thrombocytopenia was not addressed. The Myanmar guidelines were also the only ones to describe physiological changes to vital signs in pregnancy.

Additionally, all the guidelines had neither trimester-specific information nor fetal surveillance advice.

Lastly, only the Myanmar and the Philippines guidelines considered the 2009 WHO classification of dengue (DWS, SD) and stratified management based on this. The Myanmar guidelines included DHF and DSS management, while the Philippines guidelines were entirely based on the 2009 classification. As opposed to the Malaysia guidelines, the Myanmar and Philippines guidelines do not mention the management of organ impairment that can occur in SD. The Malaysia, Thailand, and Singapore guidelines outlined management based on old classifications (DHF, DSS).

No guidelines specific to dengue in pregnancy were available in the SEA region. However, Sri Lankan guidelines (South Asia) have extensive details on dengue in pregnancy and can be helpful as a reference [7].

Ongoing Use of Aspirin

For the use of aspirin, the literature was taken from various populations. From Asia, the Sri Lankan [7] and Indian guidelines [102] were used. Articles [103–105] did not consider or stratify by country of origin.

Patients with a history of pre-eclampsia or antiphospholipid syndrome may already be on prophylactic low-dose aspirin therapy, which without dengue has low risks of bleeding [103]. Low-dose aspirin is an irreversible Cyclooxygenase-1 inhibitor with an antiplatelet effect via thromboxane-A2 [104]. This may potentiate the increased risk of bleeding from dengue.

For those at risk of pre-eclampsia and its complications (such as pulmonary embolism or IUGR), 75–150 mg aspirin is given orally once daily from 12–16 weeks of gestation until delivery [105]. Ongoing use of aspirin can precipitate bleeding [7] and should be withheld if infected with dengue, as it can worsen thrombocytopenia [102]. However, further research is needed to investigate the benefits and costs of using antiplatelet therapy.

Table 9. Comparison of guidelines from Myanmar [100], the Philippines [99], Malaysia [5], Thailand [90] and Singapore [98].

| Country | Initial Assessment | Febrile Phase | DHF | DSS | Complications | Peripartum |
|---|---|---|---|---|---|---|
| Myanmar | • Admit if Day 2 of fever, with multidisciplinary team involvement.<br>• Hemodynamic stability should consider<br>  ○ Lower baseline BP<br>  ○ Higher pulse pressure<br>  ○ Higher heart rates<br>• FBC interpretation should consider<br>  ○ Lower HCT<br>  ○ Lower platelet counts<br>• Fluid management<br>  ○ Calculated based on preconception weights | N/A | DHF with warning signs:<br>• Reference HCT taken<br>• Isotonic intravenous (IV) fluids given<br>• Vital signs, perfusion status, urine output, and blood glucose or organ function tests are monitored for improvement or deterioration into shock.<br>• Same monitoring is done as for DHF with warning signs<br>In DHF without warning signs:<br>• Oral fluids preferred over IV | • Transfer to high dependency or intensive care.<br>• Immediate crystalloid fluid resuscitation. | • If profound thrombocytopenia<br>  ○ Strict bed rest<br>  ○ Avoidance of trauma<br>  ○ Prophylactic platelet transfusion is not evidence-based<br>• Severe hemorrhage<br>  ○ 5–10 mL/kg of fresh packed red blood cells (PRBC) administered as needed, and patient monitoring for improvement | • Avoidance of cesarean sections, induction of labor, and obstetric procedures (due to hemorrhagic risk).<br>• If necessary, interventional delivery<br>  ○ Maintain platelet counts of about 50,000/mm³, with potential platelet single donor transfusion<br>  ○ Episiotomy to prevent perineal tears<br>• Post-partum fever<br>  ○ Early suspicion of dengue and physician referral |
| Philippines | N/A | N/A | As per the Myanmar guidelines.<br>Contains detailed guidelines on fluid management in DHF without warning signs. | Hypotensive shock<br>• Extensive guidelines on IV fluid management<br>• If HCT uncorrected with fluids, suspect hemorrhage. | As per the Myanmar guidelines. | N/A |
| Malaysia | • Close monitoring of vital signs for shock.<br>• Appropriate fluid or blood product administration.<br>• Early referral to intensivist and obstetrician. | • Measure hemodynamic, respiratory, neurological status, and urine output every 4 h.<br>• FBC daily.<br>• Organ function tests, Arterial Blood Gas (ABG), lactate, and coagulation profile, only if indicated. | • Measure hemodynamic, respiratory, neurological status, and urine output every 2 h.<br>• FBC 4–12 hourly.<br>• Renal and liver function tests, creatine kinase daily at least.<br>• Cardiac function tests, ABG, lactate, and coagulation profile, only if indicated. | • Measure hemodynamic, respiratory, and neurological status every 15 min until stable, then hourly.<br>• Measure hourly urine output.<br>• FBC between fluid resuscitation.<br>• ABG, lactate close monitoring.<br>• Organ function tests, and coagulation profile, only as indicated. | • Contains detailed management of hepatic, cardiac, neurological, and immunological complications of dengue, and intensive care management. | • Avoidance of caesarean section, operative vaginal delivery, intramuscular injections.<br>• Blood products, including platelets, on standby if interventional delivery needed.<br>• Spontaneous delivery preferred.<br>• Preterm labor<br>  ○ Tocolysis (nifedipine or atosiban)<br>  ○ Close fetal monitoring.<br>  ○ Group and cross match.<br>• Third stage of labor<br>  ○ IV uterotonic agent.<br>• Breastfeeding recommended only after the viremic phase. |

Table 9. Cont.

| Country | Initial Assessment | Febrile Phase | DHF | DSS | Complications | Peripartum |
|---|---|---|---|---|---|---|
| Thailand | N/A | Monitoring similar to the Malaysian guidelines but does not distinguish between different phases of dengue. | | | N/A | As per the Myanmar guidelines on intrapartum platelet transfusion. |
| | | Antipyretics, hydration, and supportive care (no clear indication of specific phase involved). | N/A | Persistent shock despite fluids - Determine if other causes are present (including extreme hemorrhage) - IV vasopressors like norepinephrine | | |
| Singapore | N/A | As per the Thailand guidelines on supportive care Daily platelet and HCT for platelets less than 100,000/mm$^3$ Complete bed rest for platelets less than 50,000/mm$^3$ | | | N/A | N/A |

Legend: ▇ Pregnancy-specific data. ☐ Lack of pregnancy-specific data. ▨ Mixed data (standard dengue management with some evaluation for pregnancy). "N/A" refers to "Not Applicable".

Overall, investigations and management depend on the resources the hospital has access to and may differ across geographical locations. However, the principles of management (early suspicion of dengue, early monitoring for complications, managing fluid and aspirin use) remain unchanged. Aside from the Sri Lankan guidelines, there is a lack of available management guidelines and evidence about maternal aspirin use in dengue, suggesting a need for an increased focus on managing dengue in pregnancy, especially in endemic SEA countries.

## 7. Preconception Vaccination

For preconception vaccination, the literature was taken from various populations. From SEA, a Malaysian study [106], a Singaporean study [107], and a Vietnamese study [108] were used. Articles [109–111] did not consider or stratify by country of origin.

With pregnant women having poorer outcomes in dengue, is there a role for preconception vaccination?

Dengvaxia® (CYD-TDV), the only licensed dengue vaccine globally, is a live attenuated tetravalent vaccine that can improve immunity against all dengue virus serotypes only for seropositive (70% or higher seroprevalence) individuals in endemic areas.

It is contraindicated in seronegative individuals as it can precipitate poorer outcomes than in the unvaccinated [109]. WHO cautions against Dengvaxia in pregnant or lactating women as there is inadequate research. A small sample size study showed no increase in adverse pregnancy outcomes following the Dengvaxia administration [110]. This finding is consistent with a Malaysian study where seropositive mothers (secondary to infections) tend to transfer IgG cross-placenta without adverse effects on fetuses [106].

A study on mice based in Singapore found that vaccinated pregnant mice are likely to vertically transfer maternal strain-specific antibodies to their offspring for the first few months post-partum. More significantly, the offspring also developed a strong cross-reactive immunoprotective CD8 T cell response that suppressed viral replication. However, they were still susceptible to Antibody Dependent Enhancement (ADE) of infection with heterologous strain infections, causing severe disease [107]. This occurs in secondary infections when antibody–antigen complexes do not neutralize viruses, but facilitate further adsorption into host leukocytes, precipitating higher viral loads [111]. Further research on Vietnamese infants showed that declining maternal IgG to critical levels can lead to ADE and that DHF was likely only to be present in infants if the mothers are seropositive [108]. Further preconception studies are needed to confirm the fetal impact.

Overall, preconception vaccination is not recommended due to a lack of data. For seronegative individuals, maternal antibodies confer immunity to infants through antibody transfer. However, this is short-term and could cause infant predisposition to ADE. Even though there has been no reported adverse neonatal impact from seropositive individuals, there is still insufficient information on vaccination safety. The idea of seropositive preconception vaccination has yet to be explored by research. As there is limited Asian population-based research on preconception vaccination, further studies must be done to investigate the precise cost–benefit ratios.

## 8. Areas for Improvement

This review highlights specific areas for further research.

For epidemiology, the incidence of dengue in pregnant women in SEA is unknown. Regarding physiology, research on infected pregnant women is lacking for all the systems discussed, especially trimester-specific and SEA-specific information. For the cardiovascular system, the mechanisms of physiological changes in infection and trimester-specific pathological effects on vital signs in infection require further research. Future research should focus on gestational BP due to the higher pre-eclampsia risk in severe dengue, especially in SEA women. For the endocrinological system, no data was available detailing dengue's impact on various hormone levels. More importantly, there was inadequate evidence on the effect of dengue on GDM risk. For hematology, there is insufficient trimester-specific data about how dengue affects various blood components, the coagulability state, and the effects on GT. This is important, as they provide parameters for measuring the baseline and scoring severity. Specifically, the effects on GT are crucial due to implications on hemorrhagic risks. Pertaining to hepatobiliary physiology, there is a lack of evidence on changes to ALP, albumin, bilirubin, and GGT levels. In terms of respiratory physiology, more research is needed to determine how dengue affects respiratory parameters, such as the mean partial pressure of carbon dioxide, for baseline and severity scoring.

In terms of management, some SEA guidelines did not consider pregnancy status extensively, if at all. None of the SEA guidelines were wholly pregnancy-specific. Although the various guidelines fill each other's gaps, cross referencing may not be applicable due to variability in consideration of pregnancy status. The management of pregnancy complications in dengue-infected mothers, such as pre-eclampsia, gestational thrombocytopenia, or gestational diabetes, was not explicitly covered. SEA guidelines that were utilized either did not stratify management by the 2009 WHO guidelines' classification of dengue (DWS, SD) or had incomplete information (failure to explain appropriate care in SD with organ failure). Additionally, insufficient research into the outcomes and indications for aspirin cessation in pregnant mothers with pre-eclampsia risks restricts management guidelines.

Moreover, preconception vaccination's maternal and fetal outcomes, especially for pregnant seropositive women in SEA, require further research as no data are available. Regarding fetal complications, there is a lack of trimester-specific effects of DHF and DSS (most articles displayed fetal outcomes cumulatively for all trimesters). Additionally, trimester-specific effects on fetal platelet counts need further research.

Further, insufficient information is available to guide the management of aspirin use for pre-eclampsia in the setting of the hemorrhagic risk of dengue. While the current treatment method is aspirin cessation, perhaps titration to lower doses can achieve optimal therapeutic benefits for the patient. There is also inadequate research on preconception vaccination available to conclude the vaccination benefits versus costs for seropositive and seronegative pregnant women, much less SEA-based conclusions. There is a need to investigate the protective effects versus the ADE risk for vaccination of mothers.

Lastly, larger sample size studies are needed to reduce sampling errors.

## 9. Conclusions

The physiological cardiovascular, respiratory, hematological, and endocrine changes in an infected pregnant woman that are necessary for an uncomplicated pregnancy and birth can be altered, leading to complications such as placental abruption, preterm delivery, low birth weight, and stillbirth. Investigation and management of dengue fever in pregnant women are mostly like those of non-pregnant individuals. Management requires early suspicion of dengue, serology tests, managing fluid status and hemodynamic status, and preparing for progression to critical phases. Without adequate management, DHF or DSS can lead to bleeding, multi-organ failure, fetal distress, and predisposal to miscarriages, especially in the first trimester.

The fetus can be adversely affected through direct vertical transmission or secondary to complications of maternal infection. Although dengue in the fetus does not cause long-term complications, monitoring vertical transmission via infant serum serology is recommended. Therefore, the monitoring of fetal wellbeing in pregnant women with dengue should be considered.

In general, there is a lack of research on dengue in pregnancy, especially in SEA. Thus, reviewing investigation and management guidelines for dengue-infected women in different stages of pregnancy has significant restrictions. We recommend a substantial increase in research on the areas listed above. More data on various aspects of dengue in pregnancy, such as pathophysiological changes, response to the disease processes, and management in SEA women, needs to be explored.

Our review had some limitations. The most relevant limitation is the unavailability of literature based on SEA, necessitating the utility of data from other populations. The literature available also did not utilize WHO guidelines classification of dengue into DWS and SD. Hence, this review was based on the older classification of dengue. Additionally, the Sri Lankan study referenced in this review did not have in-text citations to support their data points, and their bibliography included data from non-native populations.

**Author Contributions:** Conceptualization, V.J.T.A.; methodology, V.J.T.A. software V.C. and J.Z.L.T.; resources, V.C. and J.Z.L.T.; writing—original draft preparation, V.C. and J.Z.L.T.; writing—review and editing, V.C., J.Z.L.T. and V.J.T.A.; visualization, V.C., J.Z.L.T. and V.J.T.A.; supervision, V.J.T.A.; project administration, V.J.T.A. All authors have read and agreed to the published version of the manuscript.

**Funding:** This research received no external funding.

**Institutional Review Board Statement:** Not applicable.

**Informed Consent Statement:** Not applicable.

**Data Availability Statement:** Not applicable.

**Conflicts of Interest:** The authors declare no conflict of interest.

## Abbreviations

| | |
|---|---|
| ABG | Arterial Blood Gas |
| ADE | Antibody Dependent Enhancement |
| ALP | Alkaline Phosphatase |
| ALT | Alanine Transaminase |
| APO | Acute Pulmonary Edema |
| ASIR | Age-Standardized Incidence Rate |
| AST | Aspartate Aminotransferase |
| BMI | Body Mass Index |
| BP | Blood Pressure |
| Bpm | Beats per minute |
| CYD TDV | Dengvaxia |
| DALY | Disability-Adjusted Life Years |
| DHF | Dengue Hemorrhagic Fever |
| DIC | to Disseminated Intravascular Coagulopathy |
| DSS | Dengue Shock Syndrome |
| DWS | Dengue with Warning Signs |
| ELISA | Enzyme-Linked Immunosorbent Assay |
| FBC | Full Blood Count |
| GDM | Gestational Diabetes Mellitus |
| GGT | Gamma-glutamyl Transferase |
| GT | Gestational Thrombocytopenia |
| hCG | Human Chorionic Gonadotropin |
| HCT | Hematocrit |
| HELLP | Hemolysis, Elevated Liver enzymes, Low Platelets |
| HLA-G | Human Leukocyte Antigen G |
| hPL | Human Placental Lactogen |
| IUGR | Intrauterine Growth Restriction |
| IV | Intravenous |
| N/A | Not Applicable |
| NDD | Neurodevelopmental Disorder |
| NS1 | Non-Structural Protein 1 |

| | |
|---|---|
| OR | Odds Ratio |
| PCR | Polymerase Chain Reaction |
| PRBC | Packed Red Blood Cells |
| RCT | Rapid Combo Test |
| SD | Severe Dengue |
| SEA | Southeast Asia |
| WBC | White Blood Cell count |
| WHO | World Health Organisation |

## References

1. World Health Organization. Dengue and Severe Dengue. 2021. Available online: https://www.who.int/news-room/fact-sheets/detail/dengue-and-severe-dengue (accessed on 22 November 2021).
2. University, NI. Southeast Asian Countries College of LIberal Arts and Science. Available online: https://www.niu.edu/clas/cseas/resources/countries.shtml#:~{}:text=Southeast%20Asia%20is%20composed%20of,%2C%20Singapore%2C%20Thailand%20and%20Vietnam (accessed on 6 June 2022).
3. Yang, X.; Quam, M.B.M.; Zhang, T.; Sang, S. Global burden for dengue and the evolving pattern in the past 30 years. *J. Travel Med.* **2021**, *28*, 183. [CrossRef]
4. Tian, N.; Zheng, J.X.; Guo, Z.Y.; Li, L.H.; Xia, S.; Lv, S.; Zhou, X.N. Dengue Incidence Trends and Its Burden in Major Endemic Regions from 1990 to 2019. *Trop. Med. Infect. Dis.* **2022**, *7*, 180. [CrossRef]
5. Sinnadurai, J.T.S. *Management of Dengue Infections In Adults*, 3rd ed.; Malaysia Ministry of Health, Ed.; Malaysia Health Technology Assessment Section (MaHTAS): Putrajaya, Malaysia, 2015; p. 36.
6. World Health Organization. *Dengue Haemorrhagic Fever: Diagnosis, Treatment, Presevent and Control*; World Health Organization: Geneva, Switzerland, 1997.
7. Wijesundere, A.; Wijewickrama, A.; Kaluarachchi, A.; Senanayake, H.; Fernando, L.; Dissanayake, U.; Pallemulla, R.; Jayawardena, P.; Ratnasiri, U.D.; Wijesundere, A.; et al. Guidelines for Clinical Management of Dengue Infection in Pregnancy. Epidemiology Unit, Ministry of Health: Colombo, Sri Lanka, 2019.
8. Gunawardane, N.; Wijewickrama, A.; Dissanayake, U.; Wanigasuriya, K.; Karunanayaka, P.; Gooneratne, L.; Jayawardana, P.; Ragunathan, M.K.; Pinto, V.; Kaluarachchi, A.; et al. *Guidelines on Management of Dengue Fever & Dengue Haemorrhagic Fever In Adults*; Epidemiology Unit, Ministry of Health: Colombo, Sri Lanka, 2012.
9. World Health Organization. *Dengue Guidelines for Diagnosis, Treatment, Prevention and Control: New Edition*; World Health Organization: Geneva, Switzerland, 2009.
10. Srikiatkhachorn, A.; Rothman, A.L.; Gibbons, R.V.; Sittisombut, N.; Malasit, P.; Ennis, F.A.; Nimmannitya, S.; Kalayanarooj, S. Dengue—How Best to Classify It. *Clin. Infect. Dis.* **2011**, *53*, 563–567. [CrossRef] [PubMed]
11. Torres, J.R.; Castro, J. The health and economic impact of dengue in Latin America. *Cad. Saude Publica* **2007**, *23* (Suppl. 1), S23–S31. [CrossRef]
12. Wiyono, L.; Rocha, I.C.N.; Cedeño, T.D.D.; Miranda, A.V.; Lucero-Prisno Iii, D.E. Dengue and COVID-19 infections in the ASEAN region: A concurrent outbreak of viral diseases. *Epidemiol. Health* **2021**, *43*, e2021070. [CrossRef]
13. European Centre for Disease Prevention and Control. Dengue Worldwide Overview. Available online: https://www.ecdc.europa.eu/en/dengue-monthly (accessed on 3 October 2022).
14. Vecteezy. Free State Map of Southeast Asia. Available online: https://static.vecteezy.com/system/resources/previews/000/105/867/original/vector-free-state-map-of-southeast-asia.jpg (accessed on 5 June 2022).
15. UCSF Health. Pregnancy the Three Trimesters. Available online: https://www.ucsfhealth.org/conditions/pregnancy/trimesters#:~{}:text=Pregnancy%20The%20Three%20Trimesters%20%7C%20UCSF,Trimester%20(27%20to%2040%20Weeks (accessed on 2 December 2021).
16. ACOG Committee Opinion No. 736: Optimizing Postpartum Care. *Obstet. Gynecol.* **2018**, *131*, e140–e150. [CrossRef]
17. Machain-Williams, C.; Raga, E.; Baak-Baak, C.M.; Kiem, S.; Blitvich, B.J.; Ramos, C. Maternal, Fetal, and Neonatal Outcomes in Pregnant Dengue Patients in Mexico. *BioMed Res. Int.* **2018**, *2018*, 9643083. [CrossRef]
18. HMP Global Learning Network. Beyond The Basics: Trauma During Pregnancy. Available online: https://www.hmpgloballearningnetwork.com/site/emsworld/article/10320626/beyond-basics-trauma-during-pregnancy (accessed on 3 December 2021).
19. Bauer, M.E.; Bauer, S.T.; Rajala, B.; MacEachern, M.P.; Polley, L.S.; Childers, D.; Aronoff, D.M. Maternal physiologic parameters in relationship to systemic inflammatory response syndrome criteria: A systematic review and meta-analysis. *Obstet. Gynecol.* **2014**, *124*, 535–541. [CrossRef]
20. Zhang, Y.; Zhang, Y.; Zhao, L.; Shang, Y.; He, D.; Chen, J. Distribution of complete blood count constituents in gestational diabetes mellitus. *Medicine* **2021**, *100*, e26301. [CrossRef] [PubMed]
21. Chesley, L.C. Plasma and red cell volumes during pregnancy. *Am. J. Obstet. Gynecol.* **1972**, *112*, 440–450. [CrossRef]
22. Ayala, D.E.; Hermida, R.C.; Mojón, A.; Fernández, J.R.; Silva, I.; Ucieda, R.; Iglesias, M. Blood pressure variability during gestation in healthy and complicated pregnancies. *Hypertension* **1997**, *30*, 611–618. [CrossRef]
23. Robson, S.C.; Hunter, S.; Moore, M.; Dunlop, W. Haemodynamic changes during the puerperium: A Doppler and M-mode echocardiographic study. *Br. J. Obstet. Gynaecol.* **1987**, *94*, 1028–1039. [CrossRef]

24. Green, L.J.; Pullon, R.; Mackillop, L.H.; Gerry, S.; Birks, J.; Salvi, D.; Davidson, S.; Loerup, L.; Tarassenko, L.; Mossop, J.; et al. Postpartum-Specific Vital Sign Reference Ranges. *Obstet. Gynecol.* **2021**, *137*, 295.
25. Barclay, M.L. *Physiology of Pregnancy*; The Global Library of Women's Medicine: London, UK, 2004; Volume 1.
26. Tagore, S.; Yim, C.F.; Kwek, K. Dengue haemorrhagic fever complicated by eclampsia in pregnancy. *Singap. Med. J.* **2007**, *48*, e281–e283. [PubMed]
27. Sanghavi, M.; Rutherford, J.D. Cardiovascular Physiology of Pregnancy. *Circulation* **2014**, *130*, 1003–1008. [CrossRef]
28. Malavige, G.N.; Ogg, G.S. Pathogenesis of vascular leak in dengue virus infection. *Immunology* **2017**, *151*, 261–269. [CrossRef] [PubMed]
29. Csapo, A.I.; Pulkkinen, M.O.; Wiest, W.G. Effects of luteectomy and progesterone replacement therapy in early pregnant patients. *Am. J. Obstet. Gynecol.* **1973**, *115*, 759–765. [CrossRef] [PubMed]
30. Reshef Tal, H.S.T. *Endocrinology of Pregnancy*; Endotext: South Dartmouth, MA, USA, 2021.
31. Kumar, P.; Magon, N. Hormones in pregnancy. *Niger. Med. J.* **2012**, *53*, 179–183. [CrossRef] [PubMed]
32. Mustafa Al-Chalabi, A.N.B.; Alsalman, I. *Physiology, Prolactin*; Statpearls: Treasure Island, FL, USA, 2021.
33. Samaan, N.; Yen, S.C.C.; Friesen, H.; Pearson, O.H. Serum Placental Lactogen Levels During Pregnancy and in Trophoblastic Disease. *J. Clin. Endocrinol. Metab.* **1966**, *26*, 1303–1308. [CrossRef]
34. Handwerger, S.; Freemark, M. The roles of placental growth hormone and placental lactogen in the regulation of human fetal growth and development. *J. Pediatr. Endocrinol. Metab.* **2000**, *13*, 343–356. [CrossRef] [PubMed]
35. Simpson, H.L.; Umpleby, A.M.; Russell-Jones, D.L. Insulin-like growth factor-I and diabetes. A review. *Growth Horm. IGF Res.* **1998**, *8*, 83–95. [CrossRef]
36. Yang, M.-J.; Tseng, J.-Y.; Chen, C.-Y.; Yeh, C.-C. Changes in maternal serum insulin-like growth factor-I during pregnancy and its relationship to maternal anthropometry. *J. Chin. Med. Assoc.* **2013**, *76*, 635–639. [CrossRef]
37. Friedrich, N.; Thuesen, B.; Jørgensen, T.; Juul, A.; Spielhagen, C.; Wallaschofksi, H.; Linneberg, A. The Association Between IGF-I and Insulin Resistance. *Diabetes Care* **2012**, *35*, 768. [CrossRef] [PubMed]
38. Darmochwal-Kolarz, D.; Kolarz, B.; Rolinski, J.; Leszczynska-Gorzelak, B.; Oleszczuk, J. The concentrations of soluble HLA-G protein are elevated during mid-gestation and decreased in pre-eclampsia. *Folia Histochem. Et Cytobiol.* **2012**, *50*, 286–291. [CrossRef]
39. Carosella, E.D.; Moreau, P.; Lemaoult, J.; Rouas-Freiss, N. HLA-G: From biology to clinical benefits. *Trends Immunol.* **2008**, *29*, 125–132. [CrossRef]
40. O'Brien, M.; Dausset, J.; Carosella, E.D.; Moreau, P. Analysis of the role of HLA-G in preeclampsia. *Hum. Immunol.* **2000**, *61*, 1126–1131. [CrossRef]
41. Hackmon, R.; Hallak, M.; Krup, M.; Weitzman, D.; Sheiner, E.; Kaplan, B.; Weinstein, Y. HLA-G Antigen and Parturition: Maternal Serum, Fetal Serum and Amniotic Fluid Levels during Pregnancy. *Fetal Diagn. Ther.* **2004**, *19*, 404–409. [CrossRef]
42. Pritchard, J.A. Changes in the blood volume during pregnancy and delivery. *Anesthesiology* **1965**, *26*, 393–399. [CrossRef] [PubMed]
43. Jain, V.; Gupta, O.; Rao, T.; Rao, S. Acute pancreatitis complicating severe dengue. *J. Glob. Infect. Dis.* **2014**, *6*, 76–78. [CrossRef]
44. Lu, J.; Wang, Z.; Cao, J.; Chen, Y.; Dong, Y. A novel and compact review on the role of oxidative stress in female reproduction. *Reprod. Biol. Endocrinol.* **2018**, *16*, 80. [CrossRef] [PubMed]
45. Hendrick, V.; Altshuler, L.L.; Suri, R. Hormonal Changes in the Postpartum and Implications for Postpartum Depression. *Psychosomatics* **1998**, *39*, 93–101. [CrossRef] [PubMed]
46. Lee, K.W.; Ching, S.M.; Ramachandran, V.; Yee, A.; Hoo, F.K.; Chia, Y.C.; Wan Sulaiman, W.A.; Suppiah, S.; Mohamed, M.H.; Veettil, S.K. Prevalence and risk factors of gestational diabetes mellitus in Asia: A systematic review and meta-analysis. *BMC Pregnancy Childbirth* **2018**, *18*, 494. [CrossRef] [PubMed]
47. Waduge, R.; Malavige, G.N.; Pradeepan, M.; Wijeyaratne, C.N.; Fernando, S.; Seneviratne, S.L. Dengue infections during pregnancy: A case series from Sri Lanka and review of the literature. *J. Clin. Virol.* **2006**, *37*, 27–33. [CrossRef]
48. Lee, I.K.; Hsieh, C.J.; Lee, C.T.; Liu, J.W. Diabetic patients suffering dengue are at risk for development of dengue shock syndrome/severe dengue: Emphasizing the impacts of co-existing comorbidity(ies) and glycemic control on dengue severity. *J. Microbiol. Immunol. Infect.* **2020**, *53*, 69–78. [CrossRef]
49. Machado, C.R.; Machado, E.S.; Rohloff, R.D.; Azevedo, M.; Campos, D.P.; de Oliveira, R.B.; Brasil, P. Is pregnancy associated with severe dengue? A review of data from the Rio de Janeiro surveillance information system. *PLoS Negl. Trop. Dis.* **2013**, *7*, e2217. [CrossRef]
50. Bueno Colman, E.D.; Pozzo, Y.A.; Umpierrez, G.E.; Medina, U.B.; Benitez, A.; Marin, S.N. The Impact of Diabetes and Hyperglycemia in Patients Hospitalized for Dengue. *Diabetes* **2018**, *67*, 1645-P. [CrossRef]
51. Póvoa, T.F.; Alves, A.M.B.; Oliveira, C.A.B.; Nuovo, G.J.; Chagas, V.L.A.; Paes, M.V. The pathology of severe dengue in multiple organs of human fatal cases: Histopathology, ultrastructure and virus replication. *PLoS ONE* **2014**, *9*, e83486. [CrossRef]
52. Sudulagunta, S.R.; Sodalagunta, M.B.; Sepehrar, M.; Bangalore Raja, S.K.; Nataraju, A.S.; Kumbhat, M.; Sathyanarayana, D.; Gummadi, S.; Burra, H.K. Dengue shock syndrome. *Oxf. Med. Case Rep.* **2016**, *2016*, omw074. [CrossRef]
53. Sangkaew, S.; Ming, D.; Boonyasiri, A.; Honeyford, K.; Kalayanarooj, S.; Yacoub, S.; Dorigatti, I.; Holmes, A. Risk predictors of progression to severe disease during the febrile phase of dengue: A systematic review and meta-analysis. *Lancet Infect. Dis.* **2021**, *21*, 1014–1026. [CrossRef] [PubMed]

54. Chandra, S.; Tripathi, A.K.; Mishra, S.; Amzarul, M.; Vaish, A.K. Physiological changes in hematological parameters during pregnancy. *Indian J. Hematol. Blood Transfus.* **2012**, *28*, 144–146. [CrossRef]
55. Hariyanto, H.; Yahya, C.Q.; Wibowo, P.; Tampubolon, O.E. Management of severe dengue hemorrhagic fever and bleeding complications in a primigravida patient: A case report. *J. Med. Case Rep.* **2016**, *10*, 357. [CrossRef] [PubMed]
56. Bremme, K.A. Haemostatic changes in pregnancy. *Best Pract. Res. Clin. Haematol.* **2003**, *16*, 153–168. [CrossRef]
57. Antovic, A.; Blombäck, M.; Bremme, K.; He, S. The assay of overall haemostasis potential used to monitor the low molecular mass (weight) heparin, dalteparin, treatment in pregnant women with previous thromboembolism. *Blood Coagul. Fibrinolysis* **2002**, *13*, 181–186. [CrossRef]
58. Tchaikovski, S.N.; Rosing, J. Mechanisms of Estrogen-Induced Venous Thromboembolism. *Thromb. Res.* **2010**, *126*, 5–11. [CrossRef] [PubMed]
59. Cines, D.B.; Levine, L.D. Thrombocytopenia in pregnancy. *Blood* **2017**, *130*, 2271–2277. [CrossRef] [PubMed]
60. Ankit Mangla, H.H. *Thrombocytopenia in Pregnancy*; StatPearls Publishing: Treasure Island, FL, USA, 2021.
61. Ciobanu, A.M.; Colibaba, S.; Cimpoca, B.; Peltecu, G.; Panaitescu, A.M. Thrombocytopenia in Pregnancy. *Maedica* **2016**, *11*, 55–60.
62. Zhang, X.; Zhao, Y.; Li, X.; Han, P.; Jing, F.; Kong, Z.; Zhou, H.; Qiu, J.; Li, L.; Peng, J.; et al. Thrombopoietin: A potential diagnostic indicator of immune thrombocytopenia in pregnancy. *Oncotarget* **2016**, *7*, 7489–7496. [CrossRef]
63. Azeredo, E.L.d.; Monteiro, R.Q.; de-Oliveira Pinto, L.M. Thrombocytopenia in Dengue: Interrelationship between Virus and the Imbalance between Coagulation and Fibrinolysis and Inflammatory Mediators. *Mediat. Inflamm.* **2015**, *2015*, 313842. [CrossRef]
64. Liu, J.; Yuan, E.; Lee, L. Gestational age-specific reference intervals for routine haemostatic assays during normal pregnancy. *Clin. Chim. Acta* **2012**, *413*, 258–261. [CrossRef]
65. Brenner, B. Haemostatic changes in pregnancy. *Thromb. Res.* **2004**, *114*, 409–414. [CrossRef]
66. Maybury, H.J.; Waugh, J.J.S.; Gornall, A.; Pavord, S. There is a return to non-pregnant coagulation parameters after four not six weeks postpartum following spontaneous vaginal delivery. *Obstet. Med.* **2008**, *1*, 92–94. [CrossRef] [PubMed]
67. LoMauro, A.; Aliverti, A. Respiratory physiology of pregnancy: Physiology masterclass. *Breathe* **2015**, *11*, 297–301. [CrossRef] [PubMed]
68. Green, L.J.; Mackillop, L.H.; Salvi, D.; Pullon, R.; Loerup, L.; Tarassenko, L.; Mossop, J.; Edwards, C.; Gerry, S.; Birks, J.; et al. Gestation-Specific Vital Sign Reference Ranges in Pregnancy. *Obstet. Gynecol.* **2020**, *135*, 653–664. [CrossRef] [PubMed]
69. Datta, S.; Kodali, B.S.; Segal, S. *Obstetric Anesthesia Handbook*; Spring Science+Business Media: New York, NY, USA, 2010. [CrossRef]
70. Chauhan, G.; Tadi, P. *Physiology, Postpartum Changes*; StatPearls Publishing: Treasure Island, FL, USA, 2020.
71. Bacq, Y. The Liver in Normal Pregnancy. In *Madame Curie Bioscience Database*; Landes Bioscience: Austin, TX, USA, 2013.
72. David, A.L.; Kotecha, M.; Girling, J.C. Factors influencing postnatal liver function tests. *BJOG Int. J. Obstet. Gynaecol.* **2005**, *107*, 1421–1426. [CrossRef]
73. Samanta, J.; Sharma, V. Dengue and its effects on liver. *World J. Clin. Cases* **2015**, *3*, 125–131. [CrossRef] [PubMed]
74. Hartgill, T.W.; Bergersen, T.K.; Pirhonen, J. Core body temperature and the thermoneutral zone: A longitudinal study of normal human pregnancy. *Acta Physiol.* **2011**, *201*, 467–474. [CrossRef]
75. Rajagopala, L.; Satharasinghe, R.L.; Karunarathna, M. A rare case of dengue encephalopathy complicating a term pregnancy. *BMC Res. Notes* **2017**, *10*, 79. [CrossRef]
76. Ferreira-de-Lima, V.H.; Lima-Camara, T.N. Natural vertical transmission of dengue virus in Aedes aegypti and Aedes albopictus: A systematic review. *Parasites Vectors* **2018**, *11*, 77. [CrossRef]
77. Sinhabahu, V.P.; Sathananthan, R.; Malavige, G.N. Perinatal transmission of dengue: A case report. *BMC Res. Notes* **2014**, *7*, 795. [CrossRef]
78. Sondo, K.A.; Ouattara, A.; Diendéré, E.A.; Diallo, I.; Zoungrana, J.; Zémané, G.; Da, L.; Gnamou, A.; Meda, B.; Poda, A. Dengue infection during pregnancy in Burkina Faso: A cross-sectional study. *BMC Infect. Dis.* **2019**, *19*, 997. [CrossRef] [PubMed]
79. Ribeiro, C.F.; Lopes, V.G.; Brasil, P.; Coelho, J.; Muniz, A.G.; Nogueira, R.M. Perinatal transmission of dengue: A report of 7 cases. *J. Pediatr.* **2013**, *163*, 1514–1516. [CrossRef] [PubMed]
80. Barthel, A.; Gourinat, A.C.; Cazorla, C.; Joubert, C.; Dupont-Rouzeyrol, M.; Descloux, E. Breast milk as a possible route of vertical transmission of dengue virus? *Clin. Infect. Dis.* **2013**, *57*, 415–417. [CrossRef] [PubMed]
81. Tan, P.C.; Rajasingam, G.; Devi, S.; Omar, S.Z. Dengue infection in pregnancy: Prevalence, vertical transmission, and pregnancy outcome. *Obstet. Gynecol.* **2008**, *111*, 1111–1117. [CrossRef]
82. Basurko, C.; Matheus, S.; Hildéral, H.; Everhard, S.; Restrepo, M.; Cuadro-Alvarez, E.; Lambert, V.; Boukhari, R.; Duvernois, J.-P.; Favre, A.; et al. Estimating the Risk of Vertical Transmission of Dengue: A Prospective Study. *Am. J. Trop. Med. Hyg.* **2018**, *98*, 1826–1832. [CrossRef]
83. Phongsamart, W.; Yoksan, S.; Vanaprapa, N.; Chokephaibulkit, K. Dengue Virus Infection in Late Pregnancy and Transmission to the Infants. *Pediatr. Infect. Dis. J.* **2008**, *27*, 500–504. [CrossRef]
84. Chong, K.Y.; Lin, K.C. A preliminary report of the fetal effects of dengue infection in pregnancy. *Gaoxiong Yi Xue Ke Xue Za Zhi* **1989**, *5*, 31–34.
85. Dreier, J.W.; Andersen, A.M.; Berg-Beckhoff, G. Systematic review and meta-analyses: Fever in pregnancy and health impacts in the offspring. *Pediatrics* **2014**, *133*, e674–e688. [CrossRef]

86. Antoun, S.; Ellul, P.; Peyre, H.; Rosenzwajg, M.; Gressens, P.; Klatzmann, D.; Delorme, R. Fever during pregnancy as a risk factor for neurodevelopmental disorders: Results from a systematic review and meta-analysis. *Mol. Autism* **2021**, *12*, 60. [CrossRef]
87. Ribeiro, C.F.; Lopes, V.G.S.; Brasil, P.; Pires, A.R.C.; Rohloff, R.; Nogueira, R.M.R. Dengue infection in pregnancy and its impact on the placenta. *Int. J. Infect. Dis.* **2017**, *55*, 109–112. [CrossRef]
88. Friedman, E.E.; Dallah, F.; Harville, E.W.; Myers, L.; Buekens, P.; Breart, G.; Carles, G. Symptomatic Dengue infection during pregnancy and infant outcomes: A retrospective cohort study. *PLoS Negl. Trop. Dis.* **2014**, *8*, e3226. [CrossRef]
89. Goldenberg, R.L.; McClure, E.M. Dengue and stillbirth. *Lancet Infect. Dis.* **2017**, *17*, 886–888. [CrossRef] [PubMed]
90. Mulyana, R.S.; Pangkahila, E.S.; Pemayun, T.G.A. Maternal and Neonatal Outcomes during Dengue Infection Outbreak at a Tertiary National Hospital in Endemic Area of Indonesia. *Korean J. Fam. Med.* **2020**, *41*, 161–166. [CrossRef] [PubMed]
91. Royal College Physician of Thailand. *Practical Guideline For Management of Dengue in Adults*; SEAMEO Regional Tropical Medicine and Public Health Network: Bangkok, Thailand, 2014; Volume 46.
92. Singkibutr, T.; Wuttikonsammakit, P.; Chamnan, P. Effects of Dengue Infection on Maternal and Neonatal Outcomes in Thai Pregnant Women: A Retrospective Cohort Study. *J. Med. Assoc. Thai.* **2020**, *103*, 155–162.
93. Chansamouth, V.; Thammasack, S.; Phetsouvanh, R.; Keoluangkot, V.; Moore, C.E.; Blacksell, S.D.; Castonguay-Vanier, J.; Dubot-Pérès, A.; Tangkhabuanbutra, J.; Tongyoo, N.; et al. The Aetiologies and Impact of Fever in Pregnant Inpatients in Vientiane, Laos. *PLoS Negl. Trop. Dis.* **2016**, *10*, e0004577. [CrossRef]
94. Paixão, E.S.; Campbell, O.M.; Teixeira, M.G.; Costa, M.C.; Harron, K.; Barreto, M.L.; Leal, M.B.; Almeida, M.F.; Rodrigues, L.C. Dengue during pregnancy and live birth outcomes: A cohort of linked data from Brazil. *BMJ Open* **2019**, *9*, e023529. [CrossRef]
95. Informed Health.Org. *Pregnancy and Birth: Before Preterm Birth: What do Steroids do?* Institute for Quality and Efficacy in Health Care: Cologne, Germany, 2006.
96. Zhang, F.; Kramer, C.V. Corticosteroids for dengue infection. *Cochrane Database Syst. Rev.* **2014**, *2014*, CD003488. [CrossRef]
97. MarchOfDimes. Placental Abruption. Available online: https://www.marchofdimes.org/complications/placental-abruption.aspx (accessed on 23 January 2022).
98. Kusuma, N.; Kusuma, A. Dengue hemorrhagic fever in pregnancy complicated with placenta abruption and vertical transmission: A case report. *Bali Med. J.* **2017**, *6*, 100. [CrossRef]
99. National Centre for Infectious Diseases. Dengue. Singapore. Available online: https://www.ncid.sg/Health-Professionals/Diseases-and-Conditions/Pages/Dengue.aspx (accessed on 23 January 2022).
100. *Revised Dengue Clinical Case Management Guidelines*, 15th ed.; Republic of the Philippines, Department of Health: Manila, Philippines, 2011; p. 18.
101. *National Guideline for Clinical Management of Dengue*, 1st ed.; Department of Public Health, Ministry of Health and Sports: Naypyidaw, Myanmar, 2021; p. 46.
102. Gupte, S.; Singh, S.; Sheriar, N.; Kurian, R.; Thanawala, U.; Wagh, G.; Tank, P.; Chauhan, A., Kinjawdekar, S.; Vij, A.; et al. Dengue In Pregnancy: Management Protocols. Federation of Obstetric and Gynecological Societies of India: Mumbai, India, 2014.
103. Choi, Y.J.; Shin, S. Aspirin Prophylaxis During Pregnancy: A Systematic Review and Meta-Analysis. *Am. J. Prev. Med.* **2021**, *61*, e31–e45. [CrossRef]
104. Cadavid, A.P. Aspirin: The Mechanism of Action Revisited in the Context of Pregnancy Complications. *Frontiers in Immunology* **2017**, *8*, 261. [CrossRef]
105. Australian Medical Handbook. *Aspirin (Antiplatelet)*; Commonwealth Department of Health and Human Services: Adelaide, Australia, 2021.
106. Mohamed Ismail, N.A.; Wan Abd Rahim, W.E.R.; Salleh, S.A.; Neoh, H.-M.; Jamal, R.; Jamil, M.A. Seropositivity of Dengue Antibodies during Pregnancy. *Sci. World J.* **2014**, *2014*, 436975. [CrossRef]
107. Lam, J.H.; Chua, Y.L.; Lee, P.X.; Martínez Gómez, J.M.; Ooi, E.E.; Alonso, S. Dengue vaccine-induced CD8+ T cell immunity confers protection in the context of enhancing, interfering maternal antibodies. *JCI Insight* **2017**, *2*, e94500. [CrossRef] [PubMed]
108. Simmons, C.P.; Chau, T.N.B.; Thuy, T.T.; Tuan, N.M.; Hoang, D.M.; Thien, N.T.; Lien, L.B.; Quy, N.T.; Hieu, N.T.; Hien, T.T.; et al. Maternal antibody and viral factors in the pathogenesis of dengue virus in infants. *J. Infect. Dis.* **2007**, *196*, 416–424. [CrossRef] [PubMed]
109. Dengue vaccine: WHO position paper, September 2018—Recommendations. *Vaccine* **2019**, *37*, 4848–4849. [CrossRef] [PubMed]
110. Skipetrova, A.; Wartel, T.A.; Gailhardou, S. Dengue vaccination during pregnancy—An overview of clinical trials data. *Vaccine* **2018**, *36*, 3345–3350. [CrossRef] [PubMed]
111. Shukla, R.; Ramasamy, V.; Shanmugam, R.K.; Ahuja, R.; Khanna, N. Antibody-Dependent Enhancement: A Challenge for Developing a Safe Dengue Vaccine. *Front. Cell. Infect. Microbiol.* **2020**, *10*, 572681. [CrossRef]

**Disclaimer/Publisher's Note:** The statements, opinions and data contained in all publications are solely those of the individual author(s) and contributor(s) and not of MDPI and/or the editor(s). MDPI and/or the editor(s) disclaim responsibility for any injury to people or property resulting from any ideas, methods, instructions or products referred to in the content.

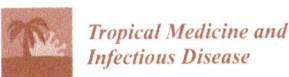 

*Review*

# Climatic and Environmental Factors Influencing COVID-19 Transmission—An African Perspective

Allan Mayaba Mwiinde [1,2,*], Enock Siankwilimba [3], Masauso Sakala [4], Faustin Banda [4,5] and Charles Michelo [2,6]

1. Graduate School of Public Health, Department of Epidemiology Ridgeway Campus, University of Zambia, Lusaka P.O. Box 50516, Zambia
2. Department of Public Health, Mazabuka Municipal Council, Mazabuka P.O. Box 670022, Zambia
3. Graduate School of Business, University of Zambia, Lusaka P.O. Box 50516, Zambia
4. School of Engineering, Department of Geomatic Engineering, University of Zambia, Lusaka P.O. Box 50516, Zambia
5. The National Remote Sensing Centre, Plot Number 15302 Airport Road, Lusaka P.O. Box 310303, Zambia
6. Harvest Research Institute, Lusaka P.O. Box 51176, Zambia
* Correspondence: mayabamwiinde@gmail.com

**Citation:** Mwiinde, A.M.; Siankwilimba, E.; Sakala, M.; Banda, F.; Michelo, C. Climatic and Environmental Factors Influencing COVID-19 Transmission—An African Perspective. *Trop. Med. Infect. Dis.* **2022**, 7, 433. https://doi.org/10.3390/tropicalmed7120433

Academic Editor: Yannick Simonin

Received: 4 October 2022
Accepted: 3 December 2022
Published: 12 December 2022

**Publisher's Note:** MDPI stays neutral with regard to jurisdictional claims in published maps and institutional affiliations.

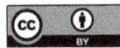

**Copyright:** © 2022 by the authors. Licensee MDPI, Basel, Switzerland. This article is an open access article distributed under the terms and conditions of the Creative Commons Attribution (CC BY) license (https://creativecommons.org/licenses/by/4.0/).

**Abstract:** Since the outbreak of COVID-19 was decreed by the World Health Organization as a public health emergency of worldwide concern, the epidemic has drawn attention from all around the world. The disease has since spread globally in developed and developing countries. The African continent has not been spared from the pandemic; however, the low number of cases in Africa compared to developed countries has brought about more questions than answers. Africa is known to have a poor healthcare system that cannot sustain the emerging infectious disease pandemic. This study explored climatic and environmental elements influencing COVID-19 transmission in Africa. This study involved manuscripts and data that evaluated and investigated the climatic and environmental elements of COVID-19 in African countries. Only articles written in English were considered in the systematic review. Seventeen articles and one database were selected for manuscript write-ups after the review process. The findings indicated that there is evidence that suggests the influence of climatic and environmental elements on the spread of COVID-19 in the continent of Africa; however, the evidence needs more investigation in all six regions of Africa and at the country level to understand the role of weather patterns and environmental aspects in the transmission of COVID-19.

**Keywords:** Africa; COVID-19; climatic factors; environmental factors; transmission

## 1. Introduction

By December 2019, there were a number of pneumonia cases in Wuhan, Hubei Province, China [1]. These illnesses had spread to 19 countries by 31 January 2020 when there were 11,791 confirmed cases, including 213 fatalities [2]. Three months after the initial report, the World Health Organization (WHO) proclaimed a Public Health Emergency of International Concern because it had spread globally [3]. The WHO first referred to the new virus as 2019-nCoV [4] while the International Committee for the Taxonomy of Viruses referred to it as SARS-CoV-2. The WHO declared that the 2019 novel coronavirus was officially known as coronavirus illness (COVID-19) on 11 February 2020 [4,5]. Over 630,601,291 people have been affected globally by the infectious disease COVID-19 as of 10 November 2022 [6].

Since the first confirmed case of COVID-19 was reported in Egypt on 14 February 2020, Africa, home to more than 1 billion people, has been tracking COVID-19 cases [7,8]. From sub-Saharan Africa, the first case was reported in Nigeria on 27 February 2020 in an Italian patient who had travelled to Nigeria by plane from Italy on 25 February 2020. Since then, the continent recorded an increase in the number of cases. As of 23 March 2020, there were 4,116,102 confirmed cases of COVID-19 from 55 African countries [9]. A total of 110,163 deaths were reported in Africa, although 5,599,955 immunizations were given out and 3,690,639 persons made a full recovery [10].

Although the number of COVID-19 cases and fatalities might appear to be lower in Africa than in Europe, the USA, and the Middle East, the impact of the epidemic has caused constraints in the health sector, causing limited diagnostic and manpower due to scarce resources with a higher need for social and economic recovery than in developed countries [11]. The possible strive towards the implementation of public health interventions does not always lower infection rates, but to some extent, it causes a huge social and economic impact that ultimately causes a violation of possible lockdowns in most African countries so individuals can access basic social needs [12].

To stop the spread of COVID-19, many global and local public health measures have been put in place, such as vaccinations, social distancing, masks, and lockdowns that allow for some ventilation in indoor spaces. However, in some places, these actions were seen as punishments because people were reluctant to get vaccinated during vaccination campaigns in Africa, to some extent the majority did not wear masks in public and did not follow lockdowns [10]. The massive movement of people from and between regions and other parts of the world was reported to have increased the geographical distribution of COVID-19 [7].

Environmental and climatic factors like evaporation, humidity, gravity, wind speed, wind direction, and particulate matter have been shown to have a big effect on how respiratory droplets and aerosols spread [13].

COVID-19 has the potential to cause various lung complications, such as pneumonia and, in the most severe cases, acute respiratory distress syndrome, or ARDS, sepsis [14]. People who are exposed to air pollution for a long time are more likely to get sick and die from chronic diseases, which could make them more likely to get COVID-19 [15]. Some studies have established that climatic factors such as temperature, humidity, wind speed, and rainfall are some of the transmission influences of the novel COVID-19 disease whereas other infectious diseases, such as Middle East respiratory syndrome coronavirus (SARS), have differences in seasonal infection rates and deaths [16,17]. Most of the highest peaks of respiratory virus infections have been seen in the winter months [18]. High temperatures and high relative humidity can stop SARS-CoV from infecting people, but low temperatures and low humidity can keep the virus alive on contaminated surfaces for about two weeks [19]. Since COVID-19 spreads through close personal contact between individuals [20], it is important to comprehend the common climatic and environmental factors [21] that influence COVID-19 transmission throughout African nations [22]. Further studies are being carried out to establish the relationship between the climate and environmental factors in association with COVID-19 virus mutation [13]. The parallels, trends, and patterns of the pandemic in the 55 members of the African Union (AU) have not yet been thoroughly examined [23]. There is a lack of understanding of the environmental, climatic, social, and cultural factors that can lessen the transmission of COVID-19 in the majority of modeling estimates, response suggestions, and pandemic transmission in Africa [23].

To improve the effectiveness of the current public health measures, this review intends to examine the literature on climatic and environmental factors that affect the transmission of COVID-19 in African nations.

## 2. Materials and Methods

### 2.1. Eligibility Criteria

Manuscripts published research papers and data that evaluated and investigated the environmental factors that influence the transmission of COVID-19 in Africa were included in the study. Due to the difference in the use of the official language, only articles written in English were considered.

## 2.2. Literature Identification and Data Extraction

Two different authors were responsible for independently identifying relevant literature and extracting relevant data. Where there was disagreement, a third party was consulted to determine the article's eligibility. A literature search was undertaken using the terms 'COVID-19', 'coronavirus', and 'COVID-19' as well as other conjugations of the terms 'environmental variables' and 'Africa' [24]. The titles of each manuscript were used to identify and extract information. After determining the title and determining that the content appeared to discuss environmental indicators influencing the spread of COVID-19 in any of the African countries or at the global level where Africa is included, information was obtained, and its full reference included the author, year, title, and abstract for further evaluation.

## 3. Results

### 3.1. Electronic/Manual Search

The systematic review of the Elsevier and Google Scholar Advanced Search databases generated a total of 17,268 articles. A total of 16,138 records were removed by automation tools, and 55 records were removed for other reasons. Elsevier returned 202 results whereas Google Scholar returned 875. Further evaluation was done where a total of 1077 records were evaluated, and 950 were eliminated because they did not meet the eligibility requirements; they did not study environmental issues. A total of 127 articles were requested for retrieval, of which, 61 were not recovered because they lacked environmental elements.

The articles that passed the title and abstract screening (n = 66) were subjected to a full screening by investigators, which resulted in the exclusion of a total of 39 reports: (n = 6) reviews, (n = 24) does not analyze environmental reasons and Africa, (n = 2) letters to the editor, and (n = 7) duplicates. After the full-text screening, twenty-seven articles (n = 27 articles and 1 database) were included (n = 27 articles and 1 database) (Appendix A). Figure A1 shows a summary of the search procedure.

### 3.2. COVID-19 Epidemic in Africa from 2020 to 2022

From the electronic database of John Hopkins University, Figure 1 below indicates the prevalence of COVID-19 in Africa from February 2020 to November 2022. Figure 2 indicates the mortality recorded in the same period from February 2020 to 11 November 2022 [25].

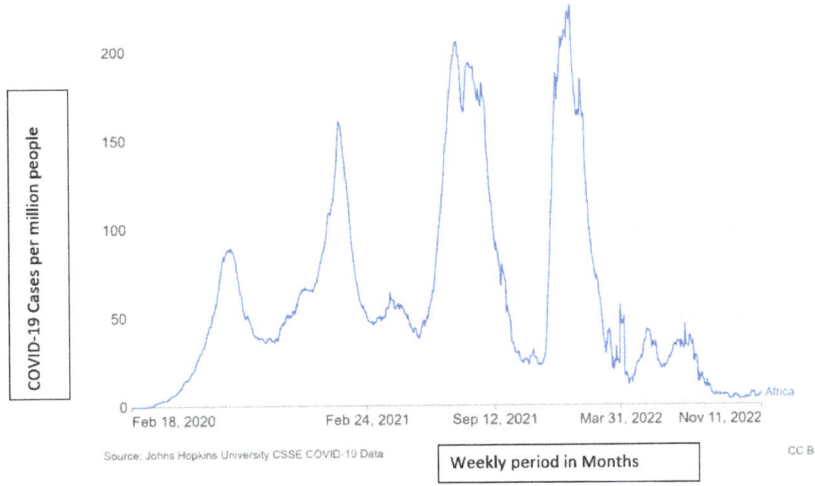

**Figure 1.** This figure is the daily COVID-19 documented cases per million persons in Africa between February 2020 and 11 November 2022.

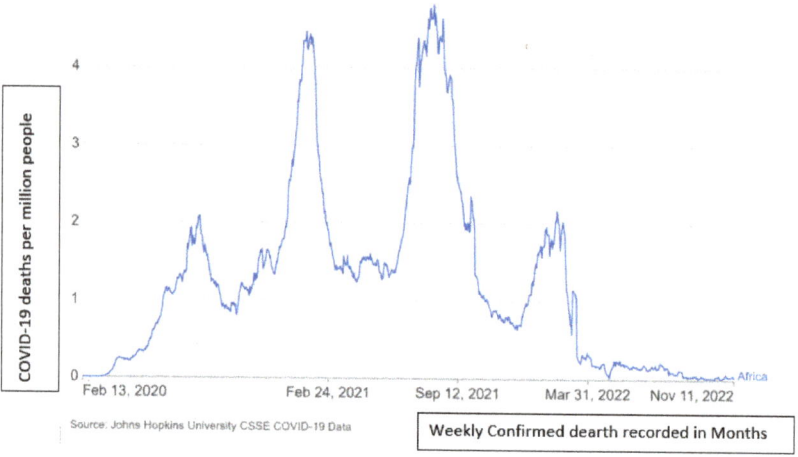

**Figure 2.** This figure indicates the daily confirmed deaths due to COVID-19 per million people in Africa from February 2020 to November 2022.

During the initial wave of the pandemic in Africa, the transmission of the COVID-19 virus was rather slow between February and May 2020. (Figure 1). The ensuing spike was first observed at the end of March and beginning of April when 2.6 million cases were rerecorded with the largest peak occurring on 24 July 2020 when 92.57 million cases were reported in African communities (Figure 1). There was an increase in November with a peak of 68.40 million instances recorded on November 30. A large increase was noticed on 1 December 2020 with the highest peak of the second wave of the epidemic curve reaching 166.89 million cases on 11 January 2021. The second curve reached its lowest point on 5 March 2021 with 47.74 million cases. In April 2021 the number of cases increased to 66.59 before declining to 39.48 on 16 May 2021, signaling the beginning of the third wave, which peaked on 15 July 2021 with 213.56 instances. Towards the end of the month, however, there was an increase to 171.56 million cases and 201.49 cases on 3 August, prior to a sharp decline. On 27 September 2021, there were 57.55 reported cases. November's lowest number in the third wave was 3.41 million, and November's greatest number was 4.70 million before recording 3.46 million, marking the beginning of the fourth wave, which reached 31.4 million by 31 December 2021. The infection rate on January 10 2022, was the highest among the first, second, third, and fourth waves at approximately 33.51 [24]: the highest record since the COVID-19 pandemic. By the end of January, the number of COVID-19 cases had reached 20.73; by the end of February, it had reached 6.09 million [25].

### 3.3. COVID-19 Mortalities in Africa from 2020 to 2022

During the first wave of COVID-19, the death rate between 19 February and 20 March was below 0.01 (Figure 2). There was a spike on 28 July of 2.08 million deaths, and the highest spike was on 9 August 2021. The lowest before the second wave was 0.86, recorded on 5 October 2021. The highest spike in the second wave was 4.64 on 9 January 2021; there was a second spike of 4.60 on 24 January 2021. There was a slight increase from April to 7 June 2021 with a value of 1.42. The highest spike in the third wave of the first spike on 11 June 2021 was 4.55, and the second spike on 26 July 2021 was 4.82 deaths. The third spike during the third wave was on 29 July 2021 at 4.96, and the fourth recorded spike was on 4 August 2021 with 5.02 deaths. The first spike on 17 August 2021 was at 4.83 before dropping to 1.99 on 26 September 2021. October recorded 2.45 as the highest in 2021, which continued to decrease in November and had the highest of 0.93 and the lowest of 0.76 on

22 November 2021. On 13 December 2021, the lowest number of deaths recorded in the month was 0.67, which began to increase to 1.12 by 31 December. On 24 January 2022, the recorded number of deaths was 2.01, and February recorded 2.24 as the highest in the fourth wave before decreasing to 1.07 by 28 February 2022 [25].

*3.4. Temperature, Humidity, and Wind Speed*

Based on the analysis of the publications included in this review (Appendix B), it has been concluded that temperature is one of the major elements and the strongest environmental predictor of whether a region will have a smaller prevalence of COVID-19 cases [26,27]. A study was done in 16 Africa Union member states, including South Africa, Ghana, Nigeria, Egypt, Algeria, Morocco, Kenya, Congo, Côte d'Ivoire, Cameroon, Niger, Somalia, Tanzania, Zambia, Mozambique, and Madagascar [28]. The results showed that the temperature and the number of COVID-19 cases ($r = -0.25$, $p = 0.001$) and deaths ($r = -0.18$, $p = 0.001$) were linked in a statistically significant way. Moreover, a regression analysis showed that the number of cases and deaths dropped by 15.1% and 10.5%, respectively, for every 1 °C increase in temperature [28].

According to studies, regions in Zambia with temperatures above 22 degrees Celsius had a very low number of COVID-19 cases whereas those with temperatures below 22 degrees Celsius had a high number of cases [29]. When the daily mean temperature was below the global mean temperature, which is approximately 21.07 °C, the chance of COVID-19 transmission increased, according to global studies that included Africa [30]. In Mozambique, too, the number of confirmed cases of COVID-19 seems to be related to the temperature and pressure of the air [31].

Diouf et al. [32] found statistically significant inverse correlations between COVID-19 cases and temperature in the Maghreb and Gulf of Guinea. Niger and Mali, however, exhibited positive relationships [32]. Correlations with humidity and water vapor characteristics exhibited significant and positive values over the Sahelian and Gulf of Guinea countries and negative values over the Maghreb countries. The results also demonstrated that COVID-19 pandemic transmission is affected differently by the three climatic regions: (i) cold and dry environmental conditions; (ii) warm and humid environmental conditions; and (iii) cold and humid environmental conditions [32].

Other investigations indicated that the average temperature was statistically correlated negatively with the increase in confirmed cases of COVID-19 in Africa, but the average wind speed was statistically correlated favorably with the growth of COVID-19 [33].

According to [34], a 1 °C increase in average temperature was related to a 25.44% (95 CI: 1.12–3.65) decrease in COVID-19 growth in Africa. Similarly, a one percent increase in average wind speed was associated with a 22.13% (95 CI: 0.22–1.43) rise in confirmed COVID-19 cases in Africa [35].

When many cases were discovered in South Africa's Western Cape (from 12 March 2020 to 30 June 2020), the average daily temperature was 15 °C, the relative humidity was 70%, the UV index was 7, and the wind speed was 17 km/h [36,37].

There was an average daily count of 343 confirmed cases in 127 African nations when the mean temperature was 20.5 °C, the relative humidity was 66.54%, and the wind speed was 1.94 m per second [38]. In some studies, issues related to temperature were still significantly negatively correlated with daily new cases when the temperature was below 20 °C [21] and positively correlated with daily new cases when the temperature was above 20 °C [29].

A global study revealed that the coefficients divulge a strong (positive and negative) association between weather conditions and COVID-19 infections in approximately 67.2% of the selected states [36]. In two African nations, Egypt and Ethiopia, a strong positive association was established between the number of new cases and temperature [35].

The number of daily new cases of COVID-19 was negatively correlated with temperature (r = 0.25), wind speed (r = 0.06), absolute humidity (r = 0.19), and relative humidity (r = 0.10) at the global level whereas the diurnal temperature range was positively correlated (r = 0.1) [38].

Other studies indicated that population size, average temperature, and median age do not have a significant impact on the number of cases when evaluated individually; nevertheless, their interactions with other determinants had a substantial effect on the transmission of COVID-19 [39].

It has been determined that countries located 1000 km closer to the equator can anticipate 33% fewer instances of COVID-19 per million population, all else being equal (given that a degree of latitude translates on average to 111 km). Changes occur in the number of COVID-19 cases per million for every degree of latitude shift [40]. Since temperature was substantially correlated with other climatic variables, such as solar irradiance and precipitation, this indicated that humidity would also have similar impacts even though it was not included as one of the explanatory factors in the datasets [29].

Note that we are not arguing that temperature is the only or main factor: in fact, there must be other conditions such as humidity, wind speed, air pressure and pollution which could also possibly play a role in the transmission of COVID-19, as temperature explains just 18% of the variability in disease spread [40].

It must be noted that the degree of influence differs in different situations and environments [41]. In Cape Town, South Africa, it was found that the influence of meteorological variables such as temperature and humidity is not always homogeneous, providing room for other intervening variables to have an influence [42]. Similarly, in Ghanaian studies, results show that wind speed and pressure have a positive linear relationship with the risk of COVID-19 spread whereas temperature and humidity have a nonlinear relationship [43].

The 16 African Union member states revealed a significant inverse correlation between humidity and the number of cases (r = −0.192, $p$ 0.001) and deaths (r = −0.213, $p$ 0.001). Furthermore, the regression results showed that with a 1% increase in humidity, the number of cases and deaths significantly reduced by 3.6% and 3.7%, respectively [28].

The influence of COVID-19 on relative humidity established that the cases of COVID-19 are oscillating between negative and positive from one country to another in four countries, namely South Africa, Morocco, Tunisia, and Ethiopia. The rise in relative humidity was associated with high COVID-19 infections in Morocco and Tunisia; however, the rise in relative humidity was associated with low cases in South Africa and Ethiopia. The relative humidity rises by 1 (%) in Morocco and 0.111 in Tunisia. The opposite was recorded in South Africa and Ethiopia when the relative humidity increased by 1% [44].

African countries have recorded that a 1% increase in average wind speed (m/s) is associated with an 11.21% (95 CI: 0.51–1.19) increase in confirmed cases of COVID-19 in Africa [34].

Wind speed has been recognized to play a critical role in the dispersal of bacterial and viral pathogens through the troposphere. The long-range transmission of viruses and bacteria contributes to increasing their distribution ranges in dormant or inactive states; this happens when more viruses are attached to the smallest airborne organic particles at heights of 3 km (Reche et al. [45]). Using the spatiotemporal credence for the exposure-response curve of meteorological factors and COVID-19 growth in Africa using the generalized additive model (GAM), the findings suggested that mean temperature and average wind speed are inversely related to the growth curve of COVID-19 in Africa [34].

### 3.5. COVID-19 and UV Radiation

Studies have also revealed that the substantial correlation between latitude and COVID-19 deaths may be explained by the involvement of sunshine in the production of vitamin D5 by the skin and the studies associating vitamin D insufficiency and COVID-19 fatalities. This demonstrated that the known increase in UV radiation intensity closer to the equator increases the likelihood that populations closer to the equator have more adequate endogenous vitamin D than populations farther away, thereby decreasing the likelihood of fatal immune dysfunction in the presence of COVID-19 [41].

A study by [36] shows that UV rays have direct lethal effects on microorganisms, and as such, the COVID-19 pandemic is seen to be more severe in places with lower UV indices and had a limited lifetime in the open-air dependent on sunlight and humidity. A global analysis study illustrated a smaller effect on seasonal changes in UV rays and their influence on regional patterns of COVID-19 growth rates from January to June [46]. However, there is a need for a comprehensive analysis to understand how COVID-19 cases are influenced by UV rays in all seasons [46].

### 3.6. COVID-19 and Air Quality

In Africa, it had been estimated that air pollution would be responsible for 1 to 1 million deaths by 2019. Over 697,000 people died because of air pollution in their homes while 394,000 died because of air pollution in the environment. Deaths caused by air pollution in the environment have been going up, and new records have been set in the continent of Africa [47]. However, most of the deaths linked to ambient air pollution are caused by non-infectious diseases, such as high blood pressure, diabetes, and lung cancer [47]. Air pollution is believed to be a further factor contributing to the high mortality rate associated with COVID-19 transmission. A study in Mozambique determined that the air quality is moderately hazardous, especially in Maputo, where the annual mean concentration of 2.5 micrometer (PM2.5) is 21 g/m$^3$, exceeding the WHO-recommended maximum of 10 g/m$^3$ [39]. In general, the reviewed research indicates that nations with more air pollution (PM2.5) and larger obese populations have a higher probability of severe COVID-19 infection and death [48].

Environmental health problems are getting worse because both outdoor and indoor air pollution is getting worse [49]. However, it has been seen that the level of air pollution inside households is a bigger cause of early death and illness in most parts of Africa. The challenge of inadequate clean energy for households, such as electricity and solar systems, causes high exposure to air pollution, a mixture of fine particulate matter and gases that result from burning fuels inside homes in rural and urban areas with limited ventilation. The environmental health problems existing at the household level due to the burning of solid fuels are the same as being exposed to about PM2.5 pollution outside [15].

As of 2019, the proportion of households using solid fuels for cooking was high in Eastern Africa (95%, UI: 94–95%), Western Africa (83%, UI: 81–86%), and Central Africa (77%, UI: 74–79%) respectively. The lowest proportions were recorded in Southern Africa (32%, UI: 29–35%) [15].

Most people across Africa live in areas with PM2.5 levels that exceed the World Health Organization (WHO) Air Quality Guidelines of 5 g/m$^3$, often by a large margin. Particulate matter pollution, such as ambient PM2.5 and air pollution from homes, is suspected to be the leading cause of death in sub-Saharan African countries [49]. Moreover, it is known that about 7 million people die every year from air pollution, making it the fourth leading cause of death in the world [50]. High levels of ground-level ozone accelerated the global spread of COVID-19 [51]. Other studies have established that PM10 was positively linked with daily COVID-19 instances over the study period (PM10: 0.02, 95% CI: (0.06, 0.26); $p$ = 0.002) even after the underlying models adjusted for the previously indicated collection of covariables [52].

PM2.5 demonstrated the same trend as the temperature in other parts of Africa with a significant relationship between particulate matter and COVID-19 cases [26,42]. Higher PM2.5 concentrations were related to rapid growth rates when only early outbreaks were considered [26].

Some studies [33] show that four bioclimatic factors (BIO) primarily influence the transmission of COVID-19: isothermality, i.e., day and night temperature (BIO3), precipitation in the wettest month (BIO14), the maximum temperature in the warmest month (BIO5), and mean temperature in the driest month (BIO10), with respective AUCs of 0.618, 0.615, 0.610, and 0.610.

*3.7. COVID-19 and Land Cover*

Land cover is also related to COVID-19 in a variety of ways, including elevation, slope, and aspect, all of which influence the habitability of an area. Therefore, population and socioeconomic activity (such as migration) are determined according to the study by [29]. In addition, the data indicate that an increase of 1 percentage point in the urbanization rate is associated with a 3.1% to 3.7% rise in the number of active COVID-19 cases [52]. The first lesson is recognizing urban planning as a public health activity that requires urgent attention in African cities. The COVID-19 crisis has highlighted the limitations of urban planning for most of Africa's urban poor in informal settlements and sectors where there is poor sanitation and other essential public health incentives which are important for COVID-19 control [53].

## 4. Discussion

This study investigated the impact of environmental conditions on COVID-19 transmission in Africa. The impact of environmental determinants on the transmission of COVID-19 in Africa was demonstrated by a systematic literature review in this study. Studies have been conducted in countries outside of Africa and on a global scale to give policymakers evidence-based research to assist them in responding effectively to the current pandemic [52]. In Africa, the influence of environmental conditions on the transmission of COVID-19 has been the subject of few investigations.

According to the findings of the present study, the available data suggest that COVID-19 shares commonalities with other coronaviruses and the incidence of attacks decrease between the fall and winter. According to Phiri [29], the infection peaked between the months of April, May, June, and July before beginning to decline in August. This is comparable to what is seen in Figure 1. During the months of April, May, June, and July, the number of cases grew in three waves. August 2020 and August 2021 marked the beginning of the case's decline. The number of fatalities increased during April, May, June, and July in 2020 and 2021. The indication of these results requires that government prepares the safety policies during the cold season, in order to avoid massive infection of the COVID-19 virus [40].

It has been demonstrated that the rise in temperature is one of the reasons leading to the low number of COVID-19 transmissions across the majority of Africa [28,31,33,36,43,44]. Similar to other research conducted in Cyprus, it was determined that the rate of exponential growth of COVID-19-infected cases decreases with increasing temperature, reaching zero when the temperature reaches 30.1 ± 2.4 °C [53]. In addition, Chan et al.'s [19] research on previous SARS coronavirus epidemics demonstrated that the virus' viability was lost at high temperatures (e.g., 38 °C) and high specific humidity (>95%). This result explains why the frequency of cases in various African and Asian nations has decreased in recent months. However, even though this was the result, more research is still needed to figure out why the COVID-19 pandemic reacts differently to the weather conditions in different parts of Africa [32].

Other research findings released by the European Respiratory Society discussed the correlation between temperature and the dissemination of COVID-19 [54]. However, other studies have shown that temperature accounts for only approximately 18% of the variability in illness distribution during the pandemic, and other factors cannot be ignored [37]. The abundance of sunlight in Africa correlates with an increase in the availability of vitamin D, which is vital for protecting against COVID-19 infection by bolstering the immune system. The reported increase in UV light intensity closer to the equator increases the probability that populations closer to the equator have more appropriate endogenous vitamin D than populations farther away, hence decreasing the possibility of a deadly immunological malfunction in the presence of COVID-19 [38]. The majority of nations at risk for vitamin D deficiency are located in South Asia and the Middle East. The efficacy of vitamin D generation in the human body, particularly on the skin, is determined by the degree of sunlight to which the skin is exposed [55]. Africa's geographic location delivers sufficient UV light for the human body's health [46].

Air pollution has been identified as a further mechanism contributing to the spread of COVID-19 in highly industrialized nations. Long-term exposure to poor air quality in industrialized nations has increased the incidence of COVID-19 infection [56].

Air pollution is believed to be a further factor contributing to the high mortality rate associated with COVID-19 transmission. Research in Mozambique determined that the air quality is moderately hazardous, especially in Maputo, where the annual mean concentration of PM2.5 is 21 $g/m^3$, exceeding the WHO-recommended maximum of 10 $g/m^3$ [57]. The World Bank's estimate for PM2.5 pollution in the air in 2013 was found to be 40% lower than the records for 2019 [15]. This rise shows that the agency needs to put the sources of air pollution in Africa and the rest of the world at the top of its list in order to reduce the risks of COVID-19 and other related diseases spreading.

It has been reported that nations with greater levels of air pollution (PM2.5) and higher rates of obesity are more susceptible to the transmission of COVID-19 [46]. Moreover, the number of deaths from household air pollution in Africa is higher than the global average of 30 deaths per 100,000 people, which means that Africa has 30% of the world's disease burden from household air pollution [15]. People in Africa are at a high risk of getting sick and dying from long-term diseases like ischemic heart disease, lung cancer, chronic obstructive pulmonary disease (COPD), stroke, and type 2 diabetes. COVID-19 infection may make these diseases worse [15].

Since the first occurrence, the transmission and severity of the novel coronavirus pandemic have remained relatively low in sub-Saharan nations compared to other regions, such as Europe and the United States [4]. The countries of Sub-Saharan Africa share similar biological, meteorological, and cultural diversity [58]. In 2019, the average number of live births per woman will remain significantly higher than in Europe and North America [59]. The increase in human population mobility caused by international trade has a significant influence on the transmission of highly contagious infectious illnesses, such as COVID-19. Early instances of the pandemic demonstrated geographical diversity across sub-Saharan Africa and locations with a notably high prevalence [60,61]. With the rise of per-urban areas and packed trading areas in Africa, geographical location and land cover will play crucial roles in pandemic and epidemic development [62,63]. Therefore, it is important to ensure that urban planning plays an integral part in public health activity with the capacity to address health crises arising from infectious diseases, such as COVID-19, to improve sanitation and population density [50].

## 5. Conclusions

The information acquired about the impact of climatic and environmental factors on the transmission of COVID-19 in Africa indicates that climatic and environmental factors have an impact on the transmission of COVID-19. The annual epidemic curve illustrates that the number of illnesses increases exponentially with a reduction in temperature during the months of May, June, July, December, January, and February. During these months, the first, second, and third waves had the highest infection and mortality rates. In addition, climatic and environmental parameters, such as temperature, UV radiation, wind speed, humidity air quality, and land cover, have a substantial impact on the transmission of COVID-19. There is a need to ensure that public health interventions are planned to adapt effectively to the climatic and environmental variables that necessitate COVID-19 transmission. Additionally, it is crucial to ensure that proper preparations are made during seasons when the infection incidence is anticipated to be high. Due to the varying seasons encountered in the six regions of Africa, additional research is required to comprehend the climatic and environmental elements at the national level. On a national or regional level in Africa, the cost of the health problems caused by PM2.5 air pollution should be figured out. This includes how much it costs for people to die early or get sick because of air pollution. This will aid policymakers and implementors in the design of globally sustainable interventions. There is a need to enhance remote sensing in epidemiological studies to fully understand the distribution and transmission dynamics and how they correlate with climatic and environmental elements to increase the burden of disease.

**Author Contributions:** Conceptualization, A.M.M. and C.M.; methodology, A.M.M.; software, A.M.M.; validation, C.M.; formal analysis, A.M.M.; investigation, A.M.M. and M.S.; resources, C.M.; data curation, A.M.M. and M.S.; writing—original draft preparation, A.M.M. and M.S.; writing—review and editing, A.M.M., E.S., M.S., F.B. and C.M.; visualization, A.M.M.; supervision, C.M.; project administration, C.M. and A.M.M.; funding acquisition, A.M.M., F.B. and C.M. All authors have read and agreed to the published version of the manuscript.

**Funding:** National Science and Technology Council (NSTC) in Zambia funded this research. Project Number: 109370-NSTC-IDRCH-2-20.

**Institutional Review Board Statement:** Research and ethical clearance was obtained and granted by the Excellence in Research Ethics and Science (ERES) Converge, reference number 011-09-21.

**Informed Consent Statement:** Not applicable.

**Data Availability Statement:** All the data used are available under a creative commons license.

**Acknowledgments:** We wish to acknowledge the support from the National Science and Technology Council (NSTC) in Zambia for funding this research.

**Conflicts of Interest:** The authors declare no conflict of interest.

## Appendix A

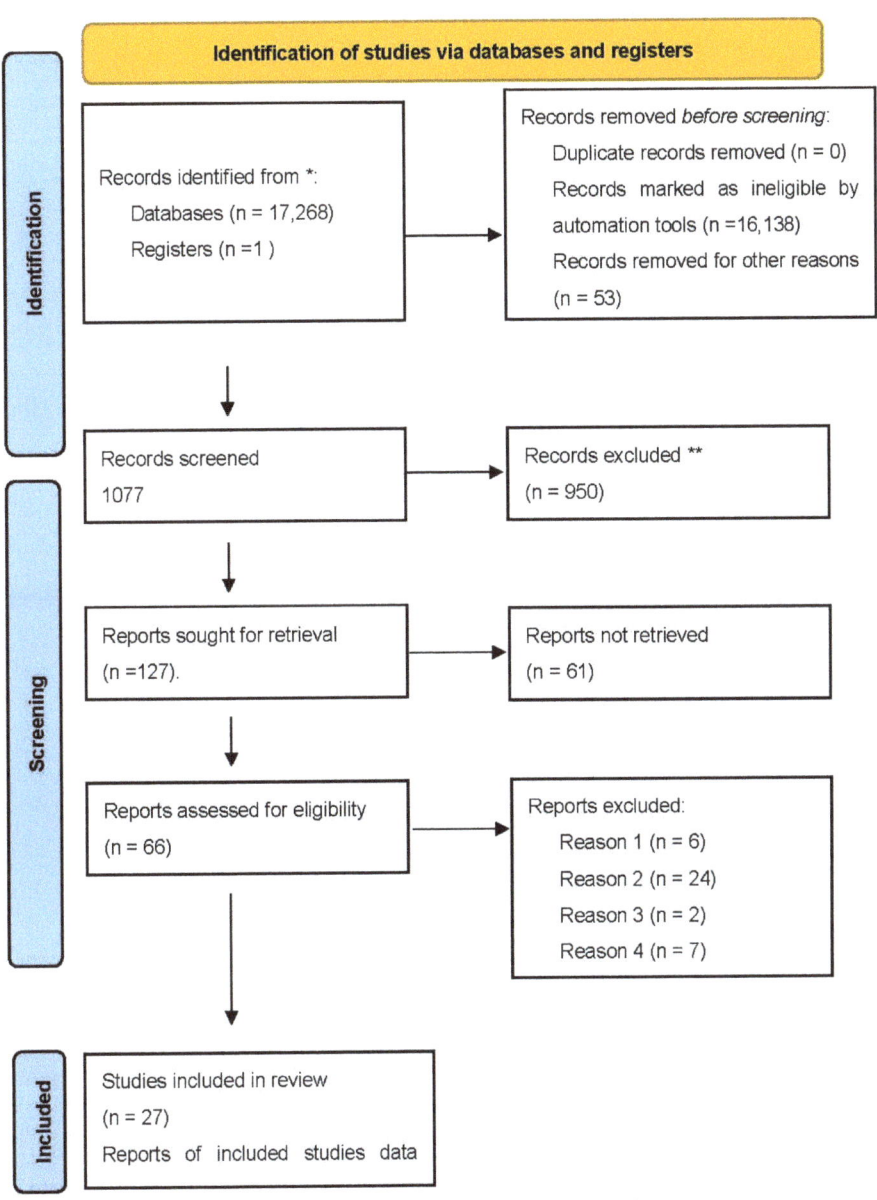

**Figure A1.** PRISMA Flow Diagram of Literature identification and selection. Literature identified * (database 17268, register 1), Records excluded ** 950. The final records from data bases 27 and 1 register.

## Appendix B

| Author and Year of Study | Study Aim | Study Design | Country | Study Findings | Needs Domain |
|---|---|---|---|---|---|
| Sumbana et al., 2020 [60]. | To examine the development and potential contributions of risk variables for COVID-19 severity based on Mozambique's data. | No method used, descriptive Statistics Used | Mozambique | The severity of COVID-19 increases significantly in the elderly and in people with underlying medical disorders, such as cancer, diabetes, obesity, and cardiovascular illness. Another contributing element to the high level of lethality is air pollution. | 1. However, there is little COVID-19 data available worldwide to analyze this association and still less in Mozambique. 2. Therefore, the need exists to increase laboratory diagnosis capacity and to monitor compliance of adhering to the intervention measures. |
| Fernandez et al., 2020 [52]. | Our study's objective is to evaluate the effects of those variables on COVID-19 mortality and geographic dissemination. | A retrospective, observational, longitudinal study | Global | According to the European Public Health Alliance, air pollution is also known to suppress the immune system and impair a person's capacity to fight against infection. 3.8 million fatalities have been attributed to household air pollution. Our research revealed a connection between COVID-19 and air pollution. However, not all nations experience the same effects because air pollution had a greater influence on HICs and UMICs. | The current COVID-19 pandemic can be associated with the global crises of biodiversity loss and environmental health. Thus, preservation and sustainable management of biodiversity might be necessary to mitigate climate disruption and prevent pandemics to protect health and well-being for the generations to come. Governments plan environmental and health policies as an alternative strategy to respond to new COVID-19 outbreaks and prevent future crises. |
| Yuan et al., 2020 [30]. | The importance of the climate and the environment function considered in transmission | Retrospective | Global | The mean temperature, wind speed, and relative humidity were adversely connected with daily new COVID-19 cases, although the diurnal temperature range was positively correlated. These relationships were more pronounced when the temperature and relative humidity were below normal (21.07 °C and 66.83%, respectively). The wind speed and diurnal temperature range were above average (3.07 m/s and 9.53 °C, respectively). The greatest RR of mean temperature was 1.30 below 23 °C at lag 10 days, the minimum RR of wind speed was 0.29 below 12 m/s at lag 24 days, the maximum RR of temperature range was 2.21 below 28 °C at lag 24 days, and the maximum RR of relative humidity was 1.35 below 4% at lag 0 days. Typically, meteorological influences have a delayed effect on human health. There was a nonlinear correlation between temperature and relative humidity and the number of daily cases. The correlation between humidity and the number of daily instances was negative. When the temperature is greater than 21 °C and the relative humidity is greater than 64%, a modest positive association is observed. | Active measures must be taken to control the source of infection, block transmission, and prevent further spread in all countries. There is relatively little information on the correlation between COVID-19 incidence and wind speed/diurnal temperature ranges globally. The results show that the world pandemic scenario in northern hemisphere countries may increase with the decrease in temperature in the next few seasons, so we should keep vigilant and take active measures. Although, COVID-19 is likely to be less prevalent in the Southern Hemisphere during the summer months, as COVID-19 transmission is influenced not only by meteorological factors, but the epidemic also still requires vigilance. We should take advantage of summer opportunities to prepare for better control of the disease in winter. |

| Author and Year of Study | Study Aim | Study Design | Country | Study Findings | Needs Domain |
|---|---|---|---|---|---|
| Francesco and Rubolini [26]. | While adjusting for a number of significant socioeconomic variables and airport links, we examined the effects of climatic conditions (temperature, humidity, and air pollution) on the dynamics of the early COVID-19 outbreak on a worldwide scale between January and May 2020. We demonstrated that COVID-19 growth rates were nonlinearly correlated with climate during the first stage of the global epidemic (January to March) with the quickest spread occurring in locations with a mean temperature of approximately 5 °C and in the most polluted regions. | Statistical analysis, Linear mixed models (LMMs) | Global | The environmental consequences of COVID-19, which spread during the 2020 global pandemic, were not long-lasting and vanished when aggressive containment measures were put in place. When outbreaks that began after mid-March were considered, the effects on the air quality were insignificant, but the effects on the climate lingered for a little longer (until mid-April) but finally vanished as well. Regions with high levels of pollution saw a quicker spread of disease. When later outbreaks were taken into account, the impacts of temperature and air pollution vanished entirely. First, high temperatures, somewhat high humidity, and sunlight reduce the persistence of COVID-19 and other coronaviruses outside the hosts. One of the largest societal challenges is without a doubt controlling COVID-19 outbreaks. Regardless of the climate, policy measures can effectively stop the spread of illness. | To improve the ability of epidemiological models to forecast the risk and time course of future outbreaks and to suggest adequate preventive or containment actions. Total environment ecological regression analyses have identified multiple complex relationships between COVID-19 spread and transmission patterns and diverse environmental features, providing a crucial stimulus to a rapidly evolving area of research. The correlative nature of these analyses should call for cautionary interpretations, as identifying the causal processes linking COVID-19 spread dynamics to environmental features remains challenging. |
| Salyer et al., 2021 [23]. | To assess reported COVID-19 epidemiology data in order to comprehend the spread of the pandemic in Africa. | A cross-sectional study | Africa | For wave analysis, the first wave's peak weekly incidence (97) with a mean of 18,273 new cases being reported per day for epidemiological week twenty-nine occurred in mid-July 2020. The second wave has not yet reached its apex on the African continent as of December 2020, but the weekly incidence reported for epidemiological week 53 was 129 and the mean number of new cases each day was 23,790. Of the 55 countries, 14 (25%) had only seen or were still seeing their first wave of cases, 40 (73%) had seen or were still seeing their second wave of cases, and four (7%) had seen or were still seeing their third wave of cases as of 31 December 2020. | Promoting efforts that help to better understand the true burden of COVID-19 and the outcomes associated with new circulating COVID-19 variants and their effect on vaccine efficacies are needed, along with campaigns to maintain population practices to prevent the spread of diseases. |

| Author and Year of Study | Study Aim | Study Design | Country | Study Findings | Needs Domain |
|---|---|---|---|---|---|
| Chabane and Arif [27]. | The fluctuations of the aerosol optical depth (AOD), black carbon, sulphate, and organic matter in the atmosphere in Blida City, Algeria, which was severely impacted by the COVID-19 pandemic, should be studied, estimated, and discussed. | Following the COVID-19 outbreak in Blida City, which was the most afflicted city in Algeria, we examined the effects of changes in the total AOD, black carbon, sulphate, and organic matter in the atmosphere (=550 nm) in the same period of 2019 and 2020. | Algeria | The quarantine that was implemented to stop the spread of COVID-19 had negative impacts that could be seen in the overall AOD as well as certain atmospheric components. When these factors were compared between 2019 and 2020 (during the quarantine months), it became clear that in April, the BCAOD values in 2020 were significantly lower than those in 2019. Low-level sulphur dioxide inhalation can make chronic respiratory conditions, such as asthma and emphysema, worse. Inhaling sulphur dioxide or consuming foods preserved with sulphates might trigger lung spasms in some asthmatics. | The variable related to aerosol optical depth (AOD) is sensitive to multiple pollutants in the atmosphere, including black carbon, sulphur, and organic materials. It is therefore an appropriate variable to study the transmission of viruses owing to pollution levels around the communities or geographical areas. |
| Sharif et al., 2020 [36]. | To assess the relationship between environmental variables and the COVID-19 pandemic and its epidemiology across nine nations and five continents. | Descriptive statistical analysis was conducted for the study regions. | Global | Environmental factors and COVID-19 survival were found to be statistically associated. Between 12 March 2020 and 30 June 2020, there were 61,172 cases and 1082 fatalities in South Africa's Western Cape, which is where the majority of cases in Africa were discovered. Daily average temperatures were 15 °C, relative humidity was 70%, UV index was 7 on average, and wind speed was 17 km/h. UV light destroyed microbes directly. The severity of the COVID-19 pandemic exacerbated in regions with lower UV indices. The average UV index for each day was calculated and displayed together with the number of cases and fatalities. In the Western Cape, 87% of cases and 93% of fatalities were found at 5.5 mean UV per day. | This study claims that, if necessary steps are not taken, the COVID-19 pandemic will become worse in the world during the winter days ahead with reduced temperature. |

| Author and Year of Study | Study Aim | Study Design | Country | Study Findings | Needs Domain |
|---|---|---|---|---|---|
| Yuan et al., 2020 [38]. | The effects of meteorological factors on daily new cases of COVID-19 in 127 countries as of 31 August 2020. | The log-linear generalized additive model (GAM) was used to analyze the effect of meteorological variables on daily new cases of COVID-19. | Global | In over 127 nations where temperature, relative humidity, and wind speed were below 20 °C, 70%, and 7 m/s, respectively, there may be a negative correlation between temperature, relative humidity, and wind speed and daily new COVID-19 cases. Daily new instances were strongly connected with temperature above 20 °C and relative humidity above 70%; however, the latter correlation was not strong. There was no statistically significant correlation between COVID-19 transmission and wind speed (above 7 m/s). | The basis of concluding about the effect of meteorological conditions on the transmission of COVID-19 is still controversial. To date, several studies examining the effects of meteorological variables on COVID-19 transmission have explored the role of temperature and other related climatic variables. |
| Yaro et al., 2020 [33]. | The effect of demographic and environmental variables on the transmission of severe acute respiratory syndrome coronavirus 2 (COVID-19) in Nigeria. | | Nigeria | The bioclimatic variables that had a significant impact on COVID-19 transmissibility in Nigeria included oscillation in day and night temperature (isothermally—BIO3), precipitation of the wettest month (BIO14), maximum temperature of the warmest month (BIO5), and mean temperature of the driest month (BIO10). The transmission rate of COVID-19 increases with increasing precipitation whereas it decreases with increasing temperature. | Therefore, there is a need for relevant stakeholders in the health sector to adopt a more collective and integrative approach to the control of the virus. |
| Adekunle et al., 2020 [34]. | To determine whether findings on the climatic circumstances of COVID-19 growth are regionally specific by looking at the impact of meteorological indicators on the development or not of coronavirus infections in Africa. | We rely on the generalized additive model (GAM). | Africa | The growth curve of COVID-19 in Africa is inversely correlated with both the mean temperature and the average wind speed. According to our research, there is no statistically significant correlation between relative humidity and the COVID-19 exposure-response curve in Africa. The crucial functions of wind speed and mean temperature in promoting and inhibiting COVID-19 growth in Africa, respectively, are explained by this study. In underdeveloped African nations with little access to clean water sources, social isolation and handwashing may be challenging; however, weather conditions that make COVID-19 less likely to survive may make up for these drawbacks. | The study is limited to the obtained findings permitted by the GAM model. Another pervasive limitation of this study could be traced to regional differences in testing rates, political interests to withhold information on COVID-19 cases and deaths, unavailability of data on non meteorological covariates, limited health system services and different travel patterns and contact rates with people from other continents. |

| Author and Year of Study | Study Aim | Study Design | Country | Study Findings | Needs Domain |
|---|---|---|---|---|---|
| Matthew et al., 2021 [35]. | | | | The spatial distribution of the illnesses revealed that the disease spread more quickly in the northern hemisphere (high latitudes, temperate or continental climate) with Europe and North America being the main destinations for the transmission. The findings showed that different climatic regions of the world saw varying effects of daily climatic fluctuations on the transmission of COVID-19 infection. In approximately 42 (68.85%) of the chosen nations, we discovered strong negative (0.510 r 0.967) and positive (0.519 r 0.9999) associations between climatic factors and confirmed COVID-19 instances. In 49.2% of the nations that were chosen, there were significant correlations between temperature and other variables (with 34.4% positive correlations and 14.6% negative correlations). | It should be seriously noted that climatic factors are not the only variables responsible for the observed variations in disease transmission. Further areas of research can look at the effects of climate on the spread of the disease while controlling for other factors that can affect transmissibility, such as adherence to COVID19 control measures, international travel, and population density |
| Notari et al., 2020 [40]. | In the month of the beginning epidemic growth, we look for a correlation between the rate and the average temperature T of each country. | | Global | Finally, additional environmental variables, including humidity, wind speed, air pressure, and pollution, may also be important. Since other coronaviruses have a similar decline at high temperatures, the drop is expected. The drop at low temperatures (less than 8 °C), which is included in the base dataset, is questionable though. | The limitation of the study is the use of average temperature, which is not very accurate for large countries, especially those that have a large spread in latitude and climatic conditions. |
| Lulbadda et al., 2020 [37]. | The main goal of this research is to better understand how COVID-19 dissemination relates to environmental factors including temperature, population density, median age, and healthcare facilities. | The relationships between the variables and COVID-19 cases during the study periods were determined using a negative binomial regression model. | Experiment | According to the findings, when considered separately in the model, population size, average temperature, and median age do not have a significant influence. They do, however, have a considerable impact on the number of instances when combined with other variables. | With the reported correlation between climatic and COVID-19 cases, it is difficult to explain precisely how the number of cases changes for a unit increase in each of the variables because that change depends on different values taken by other variables as well. |

| Author and Year of Study | Study Aim | Study Design | Country | Study Findings | Needs Domain |
|---|---|---|---|---|---|
| Mashrur F.R et al., 2021 [49]. | To enable policymakers to take proactive actions for the upcoming waves, it is important to identify the most important risk factors for spreading COVID-19. | Cross-section study | Global | Air pollution, PM2.5, the number of days to impose lockdown from the first case ($r = 0.38$, $p = 0.0424$), the total confirmed cases on the first lockdown ($r = 0.61$, $p = 0.0004$), and the number of days to impose lockdown from the first case were associated with outcome measures in the correlation analysis. The most important exposure variables for the spread of COVID-19 in the adjusted model were air pollution ($l = 4.5$, $p = 0.0127$, $|t| = 3.1$) and overweight prevalence ($l = 4.7$, $p = 0.0187$, $|t| = 2.9$). | The reported cases might not be the entire picture or representation of the COVID-19 situation in a country. Many affected patients remain undetected, making it too hard for them to get a sense of accurate total case information of a country. Second, the sample size used in the study was small. Future research should increase the number of countries. Third, we had only considered countries that crossed the peak of active cases from the curve until 10 June 2020. |
| Nguimkeu P and Tadadjeu S, 2020 [53]. | Intends to examine the influence of geographic and demographic (DG) characteristics in the SSA's lower level of epidemic severity than other regions. | Cross-section Study | Sub-Saharan African Countries | We discovered that while the average temperature around the first quarter of the year (January–March) is negatively associated with this epidemic outcome, the percentage of the population 65 years and older, population density, and urban population rate are all positively associated with the number of active cases. Sub-Saharan African nations are less impacted by these causes than other nations since they have higher levels of the latter and lower rates of the former. Therefore, compared to the rest of the globe, these characteristics are found to have smaller marginal effects on the number of active cases in sub-Saharan Africa. | The limitation of the analysis is the quality of the publicly available data that was used and the associated misreporting or underreporting in the outcome variable. Econometric approaches to deal with these issues such as the one employed may not fully mitigate it or fully identify some relevant components of the relationship, especially if the measurement errors are correlated with explanatory factors. It is worth noting another important limitation, which is the inability of the model to measure the endogenous behavioral responses of some of the key explanatory variables. |

| Author and Year of Study | Study Aim | Study Design | Country | Study Findings | Needs Domain |
|---|---|---|---|---|---|
| Phiri D et al., 2021 [29]. | Understanding the relationship between COVID-19 instances in Zambia, a sub-Saharan African nation, and environmental and socioeconomic aspects | The dataset was organized, extracted, and established using geospatial methods, and the factors connected to COVID-19 instances were examined using a classification tree (CT) technique. | Zambia | The findings demonstrated that socioeconomic variables as opposed to environmental ones significantly influenced the distribution of COVID-19 cases in Zambia. More specifically, the binary model revealed that the proximity to the airport, the density of the population, and the distance to the town centers were the factors that combined to have the greatest influence while the risk level analysis revealed that regions with higher rates of the human immunodeficiency virus (HIV) infection had a disproportionately higher likelihood of having a high number of COVID-19 cases than regions with lower HIV rates. Districts with lower COVID-19 case probabilities are those that are far from large urban centers and have hotter weather. | The data used was accessed at the district level, and hence some of the details might not have been captured because they need small mapping units. Furthermore, it was not possible for the data to include human behavior attributes, age group, and socioeconomic situation because of limited access to detailed information on COVID-19 patients. Second, the number of COVID-19 cases has continued to rise, especially during the cold season (July and August), and this is likely to affect the patterns and the distribution of COVID-19 cases. As such, these results might not be replicated or might vary if datasets for later dates are used, yet they remain relevant to use in controlling the surge of COVID-19 cases in similar situations. Third, the factors considered in this study do not represent all the potential factors that can be considered. Finally, due to the limitation in testing facilities and the logistics in fighting the COVID-19 pandemic, all the districts did not have the same testing facilities and opportunities. |
| Chen et al., 2021 [39]. | Multivariable regression analyses. | Visual examination of globe maps reveals that coronavirus disease 2019 (COVID-19), where heat and humidity are prone to be higher, is less common in nations closer to the equator. | Global | According to our findings, a nation that is 1000 km closer to the equator may anticipate 33% fewer cases per million people. Since the Earth's angular tilt changes by approximately 23.5° between the equinox and the solstice, one may anticipate a difference of 64% in cases per million people between two hypothetical nations whose climates vary by about as much as two nearby seasons. Our findings indicate that new COVID19 cases are predicted to decrease throughout the summer and increase during the winter in various nations. Our revised datasets contain larger numbers of observations. A 4.3% rise in COVID19 cases per million people is correlated with a 1° increase in absolute latitude. Summertime temperatures rising and prolonged exposure to sunlight may increase | It is worth noting that our findings are consistent with the generated hypothesis that higher temperatures and more intense UV radiation reduce COVID-19 transmission; the precise mechanisms for such an effect remain unclear and may indeed comprise not only biological but also behavioral factors which need to be accounted for. Thus, future research should aim at uncovering how the transmission of COVID-19 is affected by changes in (1) climatic factors, such as heat and humidity, (2) geographic factors, such as altitude and sunlight intensity, (3) factors related to human behavior, such as social interactions and pollution due to local economic activity at a more disaggregated level, and (4) the different potential of the human immune system to cope with diseases in summer as opposed to winter. Second, even though we included all countries worldwide for which data for this analysis were available, our final dataset included only 117 out of the world's countries, for reasons of data availability and for some countries not yet having surpassed the 100 COVID-19 case threshold. |

| Author and Year of Study | Study Aim | Study Design | Country | Study Findings | Needs Domain |
|---|---|---|---|---|---|
| Diouf et al., 2022 [32]. | Examining the possible impact of climate factors on COVID-19 transmission over sixteen carefully chosen nations in three different climate zones in Africa (the Sahel, the Maghreb, and the Gulf of Guinea). | Correlation | Africa | The findings show inverse associations between COVID-19 instances and temperature over the Maghreb and Gulf of Guinea regions that are statistically significant. Positive relationships, on the other hand, are discovered throughout the Sahel region, particularly in the central region, which includes Niger and Mali. The Sahelian and Gulf of Guinea countries show significant and positive values in correlations with certain humidity and water vapor parameters while the countries of the Maghreb show significant and negative values. The three climatic zones' respective influences on the COVID-19 pandemic transmission are (i) the cold and dry conditions over the Maghreb; (ii) the warm and humid conditions over the Sahel; and (iii) the cold and humid conditions over the Gulf of Guinea. | The findings of the study indicate the need for further studies to investigate why the COVID-19 pandemic has different sensitivities to the climate conditions observed across the three climatic regions. |
| Cambaza et al., 2020 [31]. | To analyze the relationships between weather and the frequency of confirmed COVID-19 cases in Mozambique, Southern Africa | Correlation | Africa | All areas showed negative correlations between temperature and the number of cases while Nampula Province and the Maputo region showed positive correlations. A bubble chart made it possible to visualize the relationship between the two weather variables and the overall number of cases, which suggests that the number of cases rises as pressure and temperature fall. In Mozambique, the number of confirmed cases of COVID-19 seems to be linked to the temperature and air pressure. | Decision makers should consider the weather as a predictor of the rate at which the pandemic is spreading in the country. |
| Aidoo et al., 2021 [43]. | The effect of some local weather variables (average temperature, average relative humidity, average wind speed and average atmospheric pressure) on the risk of Severe Respiratory Syndrome Coronavirus 2 (SARS-CoV-2) in Ghana | GAM, semi-parametric extension of generalized linear model (GLM) | Africa | Wind speed and pressure have a positive linear relationship with the spread risk of COVID-19 while temperature and humidity have a nonlinear relationship with the spread of COVID-19. | The need for policymakers to design effective countermeasures for controlling the spread as we are still within the low temperature season. |
| Mbandi M. A., 2020 [50]. | Air pollution in Africa in the time of COVID-19: the air we breathe indoors and outdoors | Commentary | Africa | With the reduction in air pollution due to lockdown measures in place during the COVID-19 pandemic, it seemed like indoor air quality was the major risk to African homes. | Despite the COVID-19 pandemic, there is still a lot of room for improvement in Africa when it comes to surveillance systems and hygiene. Moreover, as there is more evidence that COVID-19 is spreading in Africa, modeling must take into account environmental factors, such as air quality, trends in fuel use, and the link between disease outbreaks. |
| Reche et al., 2020 [45]. | To demonstrate that even in pristine environments, above the atmospheric boundary layer, the downward flux of viruses ranged from 0.26 × 10$^9$ to 7 × 10$^9$ m$^{-2}$ per day. | Experimental, MTX ARS 1010 automatic deposition collectors | Global | The daily deposition rates of viruses associated with aerosols < 0.7 μm in size explain observations that identical viral sequences occur at geographically distant locations and in very different environments. There is evidence that bacteria and viruses can still live after being carried by the air, which fits with the fact that microbes can be found in very different ecosystems. | The large amounts of bacteria and viruses that fall from the atmosphere may change the structure and function of ecosystems that they reach. These effects should be further investigated. |

| Author and Year of Study | Study Aim | Study Design | Country | Study Findings | Needs Domain |
|---|---|---|---|---|---|
| Meo et al., 2020 [28]. | To investigate the impact of weather conditions, heat, and humidity on the incidence and mortality of the COVID-19 pandemic in various regions of Africa | One-way ANOVA and correlation coefficient | Africa | In African countries, an increase in relative humidity and temperature was associated with a decrease in the number of daily cases and deaths due to the COVID-19 pandemic. Poisson regression results showed that with a 1% increase in humidity, the number of cases and deaths decreased ($=-0.037$, S.E. $= 0.0001$, $p < 0.001$) and deaths ($\beta = -0.035$, S.E. $= 0.0004$, $p = 0.001$) were significantly reduced by 3.6% and 3.7%, respectively. | Regional epidemiological trends and weather events related to the COVID-19 pandemic should be easier to predict. This will help the public be more aware and ready to take more appropriate steps and will help plan for the future to fight against pandemics. |
| Ogunjo et al., 2022 [42]. | Investigated the role of temperature, relative humidity, and particulate matter in the spread of COVID-19 cases within two densely populated cities of South Africa—Pretoria and Cape Town. | Linear and quantile regression and Granger Causality Test | South Africa | This study has shown that the effect of meteorological variables, especially temperature and relative humidity, is not the same everywhere. This suggests that other variables could be causing the causal relationships in places like Cape Town where they were seen. There was a significant relationship between particulate matter and COVID-19 in the two cities. Based on the significance of the causality test, particulate matter was found to be a good predictor of COVID-19 cases in Pretoria with a lag of seven days or more. | There is still a need for further studies, most importantly, when we have longer time series to unravel the role of meteorological data in COVID-19 transmission. Temperature and relative humidity are factors that should be given special attention, especially in the hinterlands. |
| Fisher et al., 2020 [48]. | To quantify how air pollution is affecting health, human capital, and the economy across Africa with a particular focus on Ethiopia, Ghana, and Rwanda. | Estimated economic output lost due to air pollution-related disease by country with use of labor income per worker, adjusted by the probability that a person (of a given age) was working | Africa | Air pollution was responsible for 1–1 million deaths across Africa in 2019. Household air pollution accounted for 697,000 deaths and ambient air pollution for 394,000. Ambient air pollution-related deaths increased from 361,000 in 2015 to 3,831,000 in 2019 with the greatest increases in the most highly developed countries. The majority of deaths due to ambient air pollution are caused by non-communicable diseases. The loss in economic output in 2019 due to air pollution-related morbidity and mortality was $3.02 billion in Ethiopia (1.16% of GDP), $1.63 billion in Ghana (0.95% of GDP), and $349 million in Rwanda (1.19% of GDP). PM25 pollution was estimated to be responsible for 196 billion lost IQ points in African children in 2019. | Courageous and visionary leaders who recognize the growing danger of ambient air pollution, engage civil society and the public, and take bold, evidence-based action to stop pollution at the source will be key to the prevention of air pollution in Africa. |

| Author and Year of Study | Study Aim | Study Design | Country | Study Findings | Needs Domain |
|---|---|---|---|---|---|
| Health Effect Institute, 2022 [15]. | Reports an overview of the state of air quality and its impact on health in Africa. | Compilation of disease project and from a recent global assessment of air pollution sources to discuss air pollution trends, sources, and associated disease burdens across this important region, with a particular focus on Egypt, Ghana, Democratic Republic of the Congo, Kenya, and South Africa. | Africa | In 2019, air pollution contributed to 1.1 million deaths in Africa. Of these, more than 63% were linked to exposure to household air pollution. In Africa, air pollution is the second-leading risk factor for deaths. Countries in Africa experience some of the highest PM2.5 exposures in the world. Although a lack of monitoring stations makes estimates uncertain, limited monitoring and modeled estimates indicate that most people in Africa breathe unhealthy levels of PM2.5 pollution. The burden of disease from household air pollution in Africa is among the highest in the world. | Most studies on the effects of air pollution on health in Africa have looked at respiratory health, but some have also looked at heart health or the health of mothers and children. Need for Comprehensive Air Pollution and Health Studies in Africa. |
| World Bank, 2022 [5]. | This publication aims to further contribute to the evidence base on air-quality management by providing up-to-date estimates of the global economic costs of air pollution. The analysis builds on previous estimates by the Bank and its partners and is based on cutting-edge scientific findings of the health effects of air pollution e comprehensive air-quality data from monitoring stations in a large number of cities across the world. | This report uses the GBD 2019 estimates of premature mortality and morbidity attributable to PM2.5 air pollution to value the economic cost in dollar terms. | Global and Region | There is no doubt that prolonged exposure to particulate matter pollution, particularly PM2.5, is linked to an increase in mortality from all causes, particularly cardiovascular causes, even at exposure levels below the 10 $g/m^3$ or PM2.5 annual exposure level that is currently recommended by the WHO (Chen and Hoek, 2020). There is strong evidence showing a robust, positive association between short-term exposure to PM10, PM2.5, NO$_2$, and O$_3$ and all-cause mortality, and between PM10 and PM2.5 and cardiovascular, respiratory, and cerebrovascular mortality (Orellano et al. 2020). Short-term exposure to sulfur dioxide (SO$_2$), ranging from increases in exposure from one hour to a 24 h average, is robustly associated with increased mortality (Orellano, Reynoso, and Quaranta, 2021). | As scientific research continues to evolve, there is a high probability that evidence will show that air pollution's health and economic burdens are even higher than in this report. Firstly, it indicates the importance of prioritising efforts to reduce air pollution emissions from coal-fired power plants and diesel-fueled vehicles because the particles in those emissions are more damaging to health than particles from most other air pollution sources (Thurston, Awe, Ostro, and Sánchez-Triana, 2021). Secondly, it demonstrated that particulate matter from dust should continue to be factored into global estimates of the burden of disease from air pollution given the substantial health impact of dust (Ostro, Awe, and Sánchez-Triana, 2021). Third, it makes a strong case for increasing efforts to set up ground-level networks to monitor air quality in low- and middle-income countries by showing that satellite-based estimates of air quality are not as accurate as data from the ground (World Bank, 2021). |

## References

1. Lu, H.; Stratton, C.W.; Tang, Y.-W. Outbreak of pneumonia of unknown etiology in Wuhan, China: The mystery and the miracle. *J. Med. Virol.* **2020**, *92*, 401–402. [CrossRef] [PubMed]
2. Adhikari, S.P.; Meng, S.; Wu, Y.-J.; Mao, Y.-P.; Ye, R.-X.; Wang, Q.-Z.; Sun, C.; Sylvia, S.; Rozelle, S.; Raat, H.; et al. Epidemiology, causes, clinical manifestation and diagnosis, prevention and control of coronavirus disease (COVID-19) during the early outbreak period: A scoping review. *Infect. Dis. Poverty* **2020**, *9*, 2019. [CrossRef] [PubMed]
3. Lone, A.S. Ahmad A COVID-19 pandemic—An African perspective. *Emerg. Microbes Infect.* **2020**, *395*, 1300–1308. [CrossRef]
4. Jiang, S.; Shi, Z.; Shu, Y.; Song, J.; Gao, F.G.; Tan, W.; Guo, D. A distinct name is needed for the new coronavirus. *Lancet* **2020**, *395*, 949. [CrossRef]
5. WHO. Novel Coronavirus—China. 2020. Available online: https://www.who.int/csr/don/12January-2020-novel-coronavirus-China/en/ (accessed on 1 February 2020).
6. WHO. WHO Coronavirus (COVID-19) Dashboard. Situation by Region, Country, Territory & Area. 2022. Available online: https://covid19.who.int/table (accessed on 11 November 2022).
7. Islam, A.; Sayeed, A.; Rahman, K.; Ferdous, J.; Shano, S.; Choudhury, S.D.; Hassan, M.M. Spatiotemporal patterns and trends of community transmission of the pandemic COVID-19 in South Asia: Bangladesh as a case study. *Biosaf. Health* **2021**, *3*, 39–49. [CrossRef]
8. Dzinamarira, T.; Dzobo, M.; Chitungo, I. COVID-19 A perspective of Africa's Capacity and Response. *J Med. Virol.* **2020**, *92*, 2465–2472. [CrossRef]
9. WHO. Coronavirus (COVID-19) Dash Bold 2021. Available online: https://covid19.who.int/table (accessed on 10 July 2022).
10. Mutombo, P.N.; Fallah, M.P.; Munodawafa, D.; Kabel, A.; Houeto, D.; Goronga, T.; Mweemba, O.; Balance, G.; Onya, H.; Kamba, R.S.; et al. COVID-19 vaccine hesitancy in Africa: A call to action. *Lancet Glob. Health* **2021**, *10*, e320–e321. [CrossRef] [PubMed]
11. OECD. Policy Responses to Coronavirus (COVID-19). The Territorial Impact of COVID Managing the Crisis across Levels of Government. 2019. Available online: http://www.oecd.org/coronavirus/policy-responses/the-territorial-impact-of-COVID-19-managing-the-crisis-across-levels-of-government-d3e314e1/ (accessed on 25 March 2021).
12. UN. Conference on Trade and Development Assessing the Impact of COVID-19 on Africa's Economic Development. UNCTAD/ALDC/MISC. 2020. Available online: https://unctad.org/system/files/official-document/aldcmisc2020d3_en.pdf (accessed on 22 September 2021).
13. Shao, L.; Ge, S.; Jones, T.; Santosh, M.; Silva, O.F.L.; Cao, Y.; Oliveira, S.L.M.; Zhang, M.; BéruBé, K. The role of airborne particles and environmental considerations in the transmission of SARS-CoV-2. *Geosci. Front.* **2021**, *12*, 101189. [CrossRef]
14. John Hopkins University. COVID-19. 2022. Available online: https://www.hopkinsmedicine.org/health/conditions-and-diseases/coronavirus/what-coronavirus-does-to-the-lungs (accessed on 15 November 2022).
15. Health Effects Institute. *The State of Air Quality and Health Impacts in Africa. A Report from the State of Global Air Initiative*; Health Effects Institute: Boston, MA, USA, 2022.
16. Vall, E.; Mburu, J.; Ndambi, A.; Sall, C.; Camara, A.D.; Sow, A.; Ba, K.; Corniaux, C.; Diaw, A.; Seck, D.; et al. Early effects of the COVID-19 outbreak on the African dairy industry: Cases of Burkina Faso, Kenya, Madagascar, and Senegal. *Cah. Agric.* **2021**, *30*, 14. [CrossRef]
17. Paraschivu, M.; Cotuna, O. Considerations on COVID 19 Impact on Agriculture and Food Security and Forward-Looking Statements. *Sci. Pap. Ser. Manag. Econ. Eng. Agric. Rural Dev.* **2021**, *21*, 573–581.
18. Mecenas, P.; Bastos, R.T.d.R.M.; Vallinoto, A.C.R.; Normando, D. Effects of temperature and humidity on the spread of COVID-19: A systematic review. *PLoS ONE* **2020**, *15*, e0238339. [CrossRef] [PubMed]
19. Chan, H.K.; Malik Peiris, S.J.; Lam, Y.S.; Poon, M.L.L.; Yuen, K.Y.; Seto, H.W. The Effects of Temperature and Relative Humidity on the Viability of the SARS Coronavirus. *Adv. Virol.* **2011**, *2011*, 734690. [CrossRef] [PubMed]
20. Goedel, W. Understanding Spatiotemporal Patterns in COVID-19 to Guide Local Public Health Action, Population Studies and Training Centre, Brown University. 2021. Available online: https://www.brown.edu/academics/populationstudies/event/ (accessed on 26 March 2021).
21. Ochani, R.; Asad, A.; Yasmin, F.; Shaikh, S.; Khalid, H.; Batra, S.; Sohail, M.R.; Mahmood, S.F.; Ochani, R.; Arshad, M.H.; et al. COVID-19 pandemic: From origins to outcomes. A comprehensive review of viral pathogenesis, clinical manifestations, diagnostic evaluation, and management. *Infez. Med.* **2021**, *29*, 20–36. [PubMed]
22. Eslami, H.; Jalili, M. The role of environmental factors to transmission of SARS-CoV-2 (COVID-19). *AMB Exp.* **2020**, *10*, 92. [CrossRef]
23. Salyer, S.J.; Maeda, J.; Sembuche, S.; Kebede, Y.; Tshangela, A.; Moussif, M.; Ihekweazu, C.; Mayet, N.; Abate, E.; Ouma, A.O.; et al. The first and second waves of the COVID-19 pandemic in Africa: A cross-sectional study. *Lancet* **2021**, *397*, 1265–1275. [CrossRef]
24. Franch-Pardo, I.; Napoletano, B.M.; Rosete-Verges, F.; Billa, L. Spatial analysis and GIS in the study of COVID-19. A review. *Sci. Total Environ.* **2020**, *739*, 140033. [CrossRef]
25. Hopkins, J. Our World in Data, COVID-19 Data Explorer. 2020. Available online: https://ourworldindata.org/explorers/coronavirus-data-explorer?zoomToSelection=true&time=earliest (accessed on 19 September 2022).
26. Francesco, F.G.; Rubolini, D. Containment measures limit environmental effects on COVID-19 early outbreak dynamics. *Sci. Total Environ.* **2021**, *761*, 144432. [CrossRef]

27. Chabane, F.; Arif, A. Determining the environmental and atmospheric effects of coronavirus disease 2019 (COVID-19) quarantining by studying the total aerosol optical depth, black carbon, organic matter, and sulphate in Blida City of Algeria. *Glob. Health J.* **2021**, *5*, 37–43. [CrossRef]
28. Meo, S.; Abukhalaf, A.; Alomar, A.; Aljudi, T.; Bajri, H.; Sami, W.; Shafi, K.M.; Meo, S.A.; Usmani, A.M.; Akram, J. Impact of weather conditions on incidence and mortality of COVID-19 pandemic in Africa. *Eur. Rev. Med. Pharmacol. Sci.* **2020**, *24*, 9753–9759.
29. Phiri, D.; Salekinb, S.; Nyirendac, R.V.; Simwandaa, M.; Ranagalage, M.; Murayama, Y. Spread of COVID-19 in Zambia: An assessment of environmental and socioeconomic factors using a classification tree approach. *Sci. Afr.* **2021**, *12*, e00827. [CrossRef]
30. Yuan, J.; Wu, Y.; Jing, W.; Liu, J.; Du, M.; Wang, Y.; Liu, M. Association between meteorological factors and daily new cases of COVID-19 in 188 countries: A time series analysis. *Sci. Total Environ.* **2021**, *780*, 146538. [CrossRef] [PubMed]
31. Cambaza, E.M.; Viegas, G.C.; Cambaza, C.M. Potential impact of temperature and atmospheric pressure on the number of cases of COVID-19 in Mozambique, Southern Africa. *J. Public Health Epidemiol.* **2020**, *12*, 246–260. [CrossRef]
32. Diouf, I.; Sy, S.; Senghor, H.; Fall, P.; Diouf, D.; Diakhaté, M.; Thiaw, W.M.; Gaye, A.T. Potential Contribution of Climate Conditions on COVID-19 Pandemic Transmission over West and North African Countries. *Atmosphere* **2022**, *13*, 34. [CrossRef]
33. Yaro, A.C.; Eneche, U.S.P.; Anyebe, A.D. Risk analysis and hot spots detection of SARS-CoV-2 in Nigeria using demographic and environmental variables: An early assessment of transmission dynamics. *Int. J. Environ. Health Res.* **2020**, *32*, 1111–1122. [CrossRef]
34. Adekunle, A.I.; Tella, A.S.; Oyesiku, K.O.; Oseni, O.I. Spatiotemporal analysis of meteorological factors in abating the spread of COVID-19 in Africa. *Heliyon* **2020**, *6*, e04749. [CrossRef]
35. Matthew, O.J.; Eludoyin, A.O.; Oluwadiya, K.S. Spatiotemporal variations in COVID-19 in relation to the global climate distribution and fluctuations. *Spat. Spatio-Temporal Epidemiol.* **2021**, *37*, 100417. [CrossRef]
36. Sharif, N.; Sarkar, M.K.; Ahmed, S.N.; Ferdous, R.N.; Nobel, N.U.; Parvez, A.K.; Talukder, A.A.; Dey, S.K. Environmental correlation and epidemiologic analysis of COVID-19 pandemic in ten regions in five continents. *Heliyon* **2021**, *7*, e06576. [CrossRef]
37. Lulbadda, K.T.; Kobbekaduwa, D.; Guruge, M.L. The impact of temperature, population size and median age on COVID-19 (SARS-CoV-2) outbreak. *Clin. Epidemiol. Glob. Health* **2021**, *9*, 231–236. [CrossRef]
38. Yuan, J.; Wu, Y.; Jing, W.; Liu, J.; Du, M.; Wang, Y.; Liu, M. Non-linear correlation between daily new cases of COVID-19 and meteorological factors in 127 countries. *Environ. Res.* **2021**, *193*, 110521. [CrossRef]
39. Chen, S.; Prettner, K.; Kuhn, M.; Geldsetzer, P.; Wang, C.; Bärnighausen, T.; Bloom, E.D. Climate and the spread of COVID-19. *Sci. Rep.* **2021**, *11*, 9042. [CrossRef]
40. Notari, A. Temperature dependence of COVID-19 transmission. *Sci. Total Environ.* **2020**, *763*, 144390. [CrossRef] [PubMed]
41. Whittemore, B.P. COVID-19 fatalities, latitude, sunlight, and vitamin D. *Am. J. Infect. Control* **2020**, *48*, P1042–P1044. [CrossRef] [PubMed]
42. Ogunjo, S.; Olusola, A.; Orimoloye, I. Association between weather parameters and SARS-CoV-2 confirmed cases in two South African cities. *GeoHealth* **2022**, *6*, e2021GH000520. [CrossRef] [PubMed]
43. Aidoo, E.N.; Adebanji, A.O.; Awashie, G.E.; Appiah, S.K. The effects of weather on the spread of COVID-19: Evidence from Ghana. *Bull. Natl. Res. Cent.* **2021**, *45*, 20. [CrossRef] [PubMed]
44. Osman, M. A COVID-19 transmission in Africa: Estimating the role of meteorological factors. *Heliyon* **2022**, *8*, e10901. [CrossRef] [PubMed]
45. Reche, I.; D'Orta, G.; Mladenov, N.; Winget, D.M.; Suttle, C.A. Deposition rates of viruses and bacteria above the atmospheric boundary layer. *ISME J.* **2018**, *12*, 1154–1162. [CrossRef]
46. Carleton, T.; Cornetet, J.; Huybers, P.; Meng, K.; Proctor, J. Global evidence for ultraviolet radiation decreasing COVID-19 growth rates. *Proc. Natl. Acad. Sci. USA* **2021**, *118*, e2012370118. [CrossRef]
47. Fisher, S.; Bellinger, C.D.; Cropper, L.M.; Kumar, P.; Binagwaho, A.; Koudenoukpo, B.J.; Park, Y.; Taghian, G.; Landrigan, J.P. Air pollution and development in Africa: Impacts on health, the economy, and human capital. *Lancet Planet. Health* **2021**, *5*, e681–e688. [CrossRef]
48. Mashrur, R.F.; Roy, D.A.; Chhoan, P.A.; Sarker, S.; Saha, A.S.M.; Hasan, N.; Saha, S. Impact of demographic, environmental, socioeconomic, and government intervention on the spreading of COVID-19. *Clin. Epidemiol. Glob. Health* **2021**, *12*, 100811. [CrossRef]
49. Mbandi, A. Air Pollution in Africa in the time of COVID-19: The air we breathe indoors and outdoors. *Clean Air J.* **2020**, *30*. [CrossRef]
50. World Bank. The Global Health Cost of PM2.5 Air Pollution: A Case for Action Beyond 2021. In *International Development in Focus*; World Bank: Washington, DC, USA, 2022.
51. Fernandez, D.; Gine-Vazquez, I.; Liu, I.; Yucel, R.; Nai Ruscone, M.; Morena, M.; García, V.G. Are environmental pollution and biodiversity levels associated with the spread and mortality of COVID-19? A four-month global analysis. *Environ. Pollut.* **2020**, *271*, 116326. [CrossRef]
52. Nguimkeu, P.; Tadadjeu, S. Why is the number of COVID-19 cases lower than expected in Sub-Saharan Africa? A cross-sectional analysis of the role of demographic and geographic factors. *World Dev.* **2020**, *138*, 105251. [CrossRef] [PubMed]

53. Livadiotis, G. Impact of environmental temperature on COVID-19 spread: Model and analysis of measurements recorded during the second pandemic in Cyprus. *medRxiv* **2021**. [CrossRef]
54. Cobbinah, B.P. Enabling Urban Planning Action in Africa: The Praxis and Oddity of COVID-19 Pandemic Response. *J. Plan. Lit.* **2022**, *37*, 83–87. [CrossRef] [PubMed]
55. Sharma, D.G.; Tiwari, K.A.; Jain, M.; Yadav, A.; Srivastava, M. COVID-19 and environmental concerns: A rapid review. *Renew. Sustain. Energy Rev.* **2021**, *148*, 111239. [CrossRef] [PubMed]
56. Laohavichien, P.; Boonchoo, T.; Cheunsaengaroon, N.; Kongprasertpong, C.; Poonnoy, V.; Rattanatamrong, P. Correlation Study of Global Weather Conditions and COVID-19 Transmission: A Clustering Approach. In Proceedings of the 19th International Conference on Electrical Engineering/Electronics, Computer, Telecommunications and Information Technology (ECTI-CON), Prachuap Khiri Khan, Thailand, 24–27 May 2022.
57. Edwards, M.H.; Cole, Z.A.; Harvey, N.C.; Cooper, C. The Global Epidemiology of Vitamin D Status. *J. Aging Res. Lifestyle* **2021**, *3*, 148–158. [CrossRef]
58. Travaglio, M.; Yu, Y.; Popovic, R.; Selley, L.; Leal, S.N.; Martins, M.L. Links between air pollution and COVID-19 in England. *Environ. Pollut.* **2020**, *268*, 115859. [CrossRef] [PubMed]
59. Sumbana, J.; Sacarlal, J.; Rubino, S. Air pollution and other risk factors might buffer COVID-19 severity in Mozambique. *J. Infect. Dev. Ctries.* **2020**, *14*, 994–1000. [CrossRef]
60. Serdeczny, O.; Adams, S.; Baarsch, F.; Coumou, D.; Robinson, A.; Hare, W.; Reinhardt, J. Climate Change Impacts in Sub-Saharan Africa: From Physical Changes to Their Social Repercussions. *Reg. Environ. Chang.* **2017**, *17*, 1585–1600. [CrossRef]
61. United Nations. How Certain Are the United Nations' Global Population, Department of Economic and Social Affairs, No. 2019/6. Available online: https://www.un.org/en/development/desa/population/publications/pdf/popfacts/PopFacts_2019-6.pdf (accessed on 10 June 2021).
62. Gayawan, E.; Awe, O.O.; Oseni, B.M.; Uzochukwu, I.C.; Adekunle, A.; Samuel, G.; Eisen, D.P.; Adegboye, O.A. The spatial-temporal epidemic dynamics of COVID-19 outbreak in Africa. *Epidemiol. Infect.* **2020**, *148*, e212. [CrossRef]
63. Siankwilimba, E.; Mwaanga, E.S.; Munkombwe, J.; Mumba, C.; Hang'ombe, B.M. Effective Extension Sustainability in the face of COVID-19 Pandemic in Smallholder Agricultural Markets. *Int. J. Res. Appl. Sci. Eng. Technol.* **2021**, *9*, 865–878. [CrossRef]

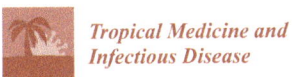 

*Systematic Review*

# Role of Arbovirus Infection in Arthritogenic Pain Manifestation—A Systematic Review

Rafaella de Carvalho Cardoso [1], Bismarck Rezende [2], Allan Kardec Nogueira Alencar [3], Fabrícia Lima Fontes-Dantas [2] and Guilherme Carneiro Montes [2,*]

[1] Healthy Sciences School, Brazilian Institute of Medicine and Rehabilitation (IBMR), Rio de Janeiro 22631-002, Brazil
[2] Department of Pharmacology and Psychobiology, Roberto Alcântara Gomes Institute Biology (IBRAG), Rio de Janeiro State University (UERJ), Rio de Janeiro 20551-030, Brazil
[3] Department of Biomedical Engineering, Tulane University, New Orleans, LA 70118, USA
* Correspondence: guilherme.montes@uerj.br

**Abstract:** The number of publications on the development of arthritic pain after CHIKV infection is increasing; however, there is still a gap in the pathophysiological mechanisms that explain these outcomes. In this review, we conducted a descriptive analysis of the findings of patients to understand their prognosis and to explore therapeutic options. Here, we searched the Cochrane, BVS, PubMed, and Scielo databases using the keywords "arthritis", "pain", "arbovirus", "disease", "arthritogenic", and "arthralgia" during the 2000 to 2022 period. Descriptive analyses were conducted to understand the association between CHIKV infection and arthritogenic pain. The present study shows the persistence of acute phase signals for months, making the chronic phase still marked by the presence of arthralgia, often disabling under stimuli, such as temperature variation. CHIKV infection appears to be remarkably similar to rheumatoid arthritis, since both diseases share common symptoms. Once diagnosed, patients are mostly treated with analgesics, nonsteroidal anti-inflammatory drugs (NSAIDs), corticosteroids, and disease modifying anti-rheumatic drugs (DMARD). As there are no prophylactic measures or specific treatments for arboviruses, this study gathered information on the development and manifestations of arthritogenic pain.

**Keywords:** arthritis; pain; arbovirus; disease; arthritogenic; arthralgia

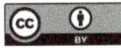

## 1. Introduction

Viral infections with unpredictable clinical outcomes occur frequently worldwide. To date, 87 countries have reported autochthonous transmission of arbovirus [1]. An example is the epidemics of arboviruses Zika (ZIKV) and Chikungunya (CHIKV) that occurred in Brazil in recent years, becoming endemic and causing irreparable damage to the population [2,3]. While more than 80% of cases of ZIKV infection are asymptomatic or have very mild symptoms, this relationship is practically reversed in relation to CHIKV infection, which is usually symptomatic [4–7]. In addition to the clinical manifestations that are central nervous system (CNS) and peripheral nervous system (PNS)-specific [8,9], nonspecific neurological and/or rheumatological symptoms, such as myalgia, hypogeusia, articular pain, and general malaise, have been reported in patients after CHIKV infection [3,10,11]. Interestingly, it has been observed that the main symptoms of CHIKV infection do not differ between sexes. Nevertheless, the symptomatologic profile might vary from case to case depending on the preexistence of comorbidities, such as diabetes mellitus and osteoarthritis, and advanced age [12–14]. Persistent joint pain is a common manifestation of arthropod-borne viral infections and can cause long-term disability, although the precise mechanisms of Chikungunya disease progression from acute fever to the chronic phase and its correlation with arthralgia remain poorly understood [8,15].

The immune process linked to articular pain is triggered, at least in part, by post-infectious inflammation [16]. Notably, acute symptomatic CHIKV disease resembles other common known arbovirus-induced diseases, such as dengue virus (DENV) and ZIKV disease, independent of strain [17]. In this context, physicians tend to identify similarities in the clinical onset of rheumatoid arthritis after infection by CHIKV, Dengue fever virus, Yellow Fever virus, and Zika virus, and it is believed that the mechanisms involved in the chronicity of both diseases are similar [18,19]. Indeed, the inflammation induced by the presence of the virus in the joints has been implicated as a key factor for the development of acute and chronic polyarthritis following alphavirus infection [15]; however, the severity of this manifestation is based not only on viral tissue tropism but also on a possible autoimmune response [20]. Vijayalakshmi et al., 2017, showed that molecular mimicry between viral protein E1 and host proteins contributes to the development of arthritic manifestations by CHIKV through increased immune and inflammatory responses [21]. Another important study identified conserved regions of the alphavirus structural polyprotein that are homologous to human proteins involved in rheumatoid arthritis, which can be recognized by B cells and the MHC class II receptor [22].

Furthermore, some studies have suggested a neuropathic component of arthritogenic pain [8,23–26]. Other lines of evidence concern the involvement of nociceptive and neuropathic mechanisms in arbovirus infection [27,28]. Neuropathic pain is usually caused by injuries that damage somatosensory pathways from peripheral nerves to central structures, including the spinal cord and brain [29]. Importantly, CHIKV infection might promote demyelination, the most typical injury that harms the entire structure of a peripheral nerve [26]. Given that there are no effective prevention methods or treatments for arboviral diseases, the aim of the present study was to conduct a systematic review of the literature to advance the understanding of the pathophysiological mechanisms of arboviruses-induced joint pain and to identify methods for diagnosis and treatment.

## 2. Materials and Methods

This systematic review was registered in the International Prospective Register of Systematic Reviews (PROSPERO) under the number protocol: CRD42022367576, https://www.crd.york.ac.uk/prospero/ (accessed on 1 November 2022). Additionally, this work was written in accordance with the Preferred Reporting Items for Systematic Reviews and Meta-Analyses (PRISMA) guidelines.

### 2.1. Search Strategy

A literature search was conducted using five databases to identify studies that examined the association between arbovirus infections and arthritic pain. The main terms and expressions used in this research were arthritis, pain, and arbovirus. The following databases were used to perform a search: PubMed, LILACS, SciELO, Cochrane (search tools strategies MeSH, PICO, and advanced search), and BVS, published between January 2000 and December 2020. For the systematization of the research question, the PICO strategy (PICO—patient, intervention, comparison, and outcomes) was used, where P (patient) was positive for arbovirus infections and arthritogenic pain; I (intervention) was drugs used in the treatment; C (comparison) was between patients who developed chronic pain and those who did not have persistent pain, and O (outcome) was relevant findings that could justify the appearance of signs and symptoms and the effectiveness of the methodology used for treatment. The GRADE approach was applied to assess the quality of evidence for the set of available evidence and important findings that corresponded to the research question. The data found and described were considered satisfactory and met the criteria for the GRADE approach. Two autonomous persons ran the survey in duplicate.

### 2.2. Inclusion and Exclusion Criteria

The object of interest this study was to collect research results that included studies of cohort, case–control, and clinical cases in human experimental models. Only files published in English were chosen for reading. Studies published in conferences, systematic and narrative reviews, or editorials were excluded. Duplicate quests were excluded from the study.

In addition, a considerable number of the selected studies presented as a primary patient outcome the manifestation of arthritogenic pain with increased levels of important pro-inflammatory molecules such interleukins (IL-6, IL-8, and IL-13), tumor necrose factor alpha (TNF-α), monocyte chemoattractant protein-1 (MCP-1), and macrophage inflammatory protein 1 (MIP-1) in the analysis of synovial fluid from pain-affected joints. It has been further observed that pain was not present in all patients. However, in cases of pain manifestation, it persisted for days or even years. The different diagnostic methodologies (clinical and symptomatic approaches, direct analyses such as the PCR technique, or indirect analyses such as serological tests for IgG and IgM detection), as well as different therapeutic interventions (anti-inflammatory and analgesic drugs), might be classified as secondary events and were not considered the focus of the current work.

*2.3. Study Selection and Data Extraction*

Two authors proceeded with the study selection and extracted the data independently by using the same predetermined data extraction patterns. After deleting duplicates and articles in languages other than English, two phases were completed. The first step was to appraise titles and abstracts for the selection of pertinent scientific articles that met the eligibility criteria. The second step consisted of a full-text reading of the articles approved in the first step to conduct a more complete judgment in compliance with the inclusion and exclusion survey criteria. A consensus was achieved in cases of disagreement between the authors. A third evaluator was not required. The following data were extracted and recorded: Table 1—author, year, country, ethnicity, study design, diagnosis, treatments, and relevant key findings. Quality control of eligible studies was assessed using the Critical Appraisal Skills Program tools [30] for cohort and case–control studies by two independent authors (F.L.F.D or G.M.).

Table 1. Characteristics of observational studies evaluating the association between arthritogenic pain and CHIKV infection.

| Author, Year | Country/Ethnicity | Study Design | Diagnoses | Treatments | Relevant Key Findings |
|---|---|---|---|---|---|
| F. Rosso et al., 2018 [31] | Colombia/Colombian | Case Report and Literature Review | Not mentioned | Corticosteroids in the management of inflammatory arthritis | Patients in this study underwent organ transplantation. Some of them developed leucopenia, neutropenia, and thrombocytopenia, and all of them developed lymphopenia. None developed graft rejection or died in process. |
| E. Bouquillard et al., 2017 [24] | France/French | Original article | Serological test and clinical symptoms | After the acute phase, joint pain is well-controlled with analgesics and NSAIDs; corticotherapy may be effective at moderate doses; and Chloroquine salt are sometimes prescribed, particularly in the case of chronic joints that are non-responsive to analgesics and NSAIDs. | Chronic joint pain was associated with synovitis of the patients, affecting primarily the wrists, the proximal interphalangeal joints of the fingers, and the ankles. Attempts to detect the viral genome in joint fluid and synovial tissue using the RT-PCR technique were repeatedly unsuccessful. |
| Ravindran et al., 2016 [32] | India/Indian | Original article | Clinical symptoms and serological test | DMARD combination to Chikungunya arthritis (CA); triple combination with methotrexate, sulfasalazine, and hydroxychloroquine; monotherapy with hydroxychloroquine. | Treatment with combination therapy leads to substantial improvement and reduces disability and pain in CA; levels of cytokines such as interleukin (IL)-6, IL-8 IL-13, and TNF; (MCP)-1; and (MIP)-1 also appear to play important roles in the pathogenesis of CA. Triple therapy is superior than monotherapy. |
| M. Blettery et al., 2019 [22] | France/French | Original article | Serological tests or PCR, then joints imaging studies by Doppler ultrasonography (DUS) | Not mentioned | DUS of painful joints revealed effusions in 92.8% of them (unilateral). Subcutaneous inflammatory infiltrations of the ankles were revealed at 29% of patients. Bone erosion was not observed. |
| A. Ribeiro et al., 2016 [25] | Brazil/Brazilian | Case Reports | Clinical symptoms. | Anti-inflammatory and analgesics drugs; in parallel, for local joints, applications include continuous ultrasound, infrared laser, and TENS-burst | The association of ultrasound, infrared laser, and TENS may accelerate the healing process by collaborating in different ways in cell recovery, speed of nerve conductions and collagen production, and extensibility. It could reduce inflammation, pain, and joints stiffness. |
| M.H. Pouriayevali, et al., 2019 [23] | Iran/Iranian | Original article | Serological test (ELISA and PCR tests) and clinical symptoms | Not mentioned | Correlation between abroad travel history and CHIKV infection; also, Iran-5300 strain showed a rare non-synonymous substitution T/C at nucleotide 10,560. |
| Y. Bedoui et al., 2021 [18] | France/French | Original article | Serological test, RT-PCR, immunohistochemistry, cytotoxicity assays | Methotrexate and dexamethasone | PIC and CHIKV enhanced mRNA expression of COX-2; PIC increased the mRNA levels of cPLA2α and mPGES-1, two other central enzymes in PGE2 production; IFNβ upregulated cPLA2α and COX-2 transcription levels; MTX failed to control the expression of all these enzymes, but dexamethasone was able to control the capacity of pro-inflammatory cytokines. |
| M. Agrawal et al., 2019 [33] | India/Indian | Original article | Not applicable | Not applicable | The modulation of AKT3 induces the TNF-α-mediated autophagy and cytokine secretion. Additionally, AKT3 has been reported to act via PI3K/AKT/mTOR pathway, which activates the antiapoptotic genes and sensitizes the fibroblasts to TNF-α and TRAIL-mediated apoptosis. Therefore, during CHIKV infection, suppression of the robust inflammatory response may be regulated by the induction of hsa-miR-4717-3p through AKT3 gene target. |
| J. J. Hoarau et al., 2010 [34] | France/French | Original article | RT-PCR, Mac-ELISA, Clinical examinations and biological symptoms; PFU evaluation, immunochemistry and Western blot analysis | Methotrexate | CHIKV (mRNA and proteins) persisting in synovial macrophages could contribute to tissue injuries, apoptosis in vitro, fibrosis, and a polarized inflammatory response reminiscent of rheumatoid arthritis. The expression of immunoregulatory cytokines, such as IL-10 and TGF-β1, was demonstrated at T0 (time 0, considered before symptoms appearance) and M6 (Month 6). |
| M.d.R.Q. Lima et al., 2021 [35] | Brazil/Brazilian | Original article | Mac-ELISA, RT-PCR | Not mentioned | The Euroimmun anti-CHIKV IgM ELISA test showed 100% sensitivity and 25.3% specificity due to cross reactivities observed with dengue. IgM positive and acute cases of dengue, the assay showed cross-reactivity of 46.7% and 31.6%, respectively, and so, molecular tests, such as RT-PCR, was used as an option to confirm cross-reactivity or not. |

## 3. Results

*Study Selection*

Eighteen articles were selected according to the search strategy. After applying the eligibility criteria, three articles were identified as duplicates, two were identified as systematic reviews, and four articles were written using languages other than English and were thus excluded of the final pool of studies (Figure 1). In total and based on data availability, we screened 18 studies by the title and abstracts and included 10 articles for a review of the observational analyses. There were 1036 patients in the total articles included, and most were female. The mean age of the patients was 50 years (6–87). Serum anti-CHIKV IgM and anti-CHIKV IgG levels were reported in 151 patients and were positive in only 19 and 28 patients, respectively, according to Pouriayevali et al., 2019 [23].

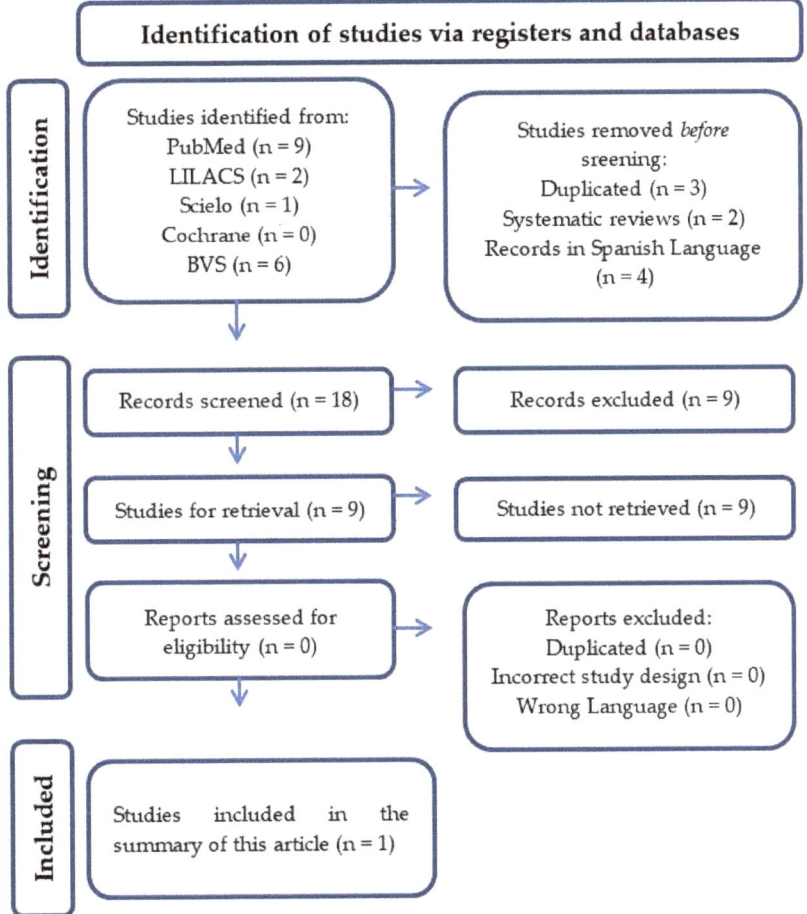

**Figure 1.** Illustrative flowchart of the rummage and article selection.

According to our search criteria, most records reporting CHIKV with joint signs/symptoms were from the European region (n = 387), followed by the Americas (n = 351) and the Asian continent (n = 289). Information about the symptomatologic profile of patients was documented in all studies, and the most frequently found symptoms were fever, rash, headache, myalgia, joint swelling, and pain due to a local inflammatory reaction.

Arthralgia and joint/articular pain were found in 98% (297 cases) of patients, according to Bouquillard et al., 2018. The most affected joints were the shoulders (168/300), elbows (37/300), wrists (216/300), hips (3/300), (161/300), ankles (212/300), and tarsus (152/300), according to the same author [24]. Patients diagnosed with rheumatoid arthritis were excluded from the study due to the similarity of symptoms with chronic pain after arbovirus infection. The duration of arthritis ranged from 2 days to 6 months among the nine cases who reported the time. The median treatment duration was approximately 10 days.

Different drug combinations were used as therapeutic strategies for mitigating signs and symptoms of infection. Corticosteroids in the management of inflammatory arthritis were effective at moderate doses and were used in the acute and chronic phases. In both the acute and chronic phases, joint pain was well-controlled with the administration of analgesics and NSAIDs. For patients unresponsive to this regular treatment, chloroquine proved to be a valid option, as evidenced by Bouquillard et al., 2018, and Ravindran et al., 2016 [24,32]. Ravindran et al., 2016, also demonstrated the efficacy of a triple combination of methotrexate, sulfasalazine, and hydroxychloroquine, which was superior to that of hydroxychloroquine monotherapy. According to the author, this drug combination led to a considerable reduction in pain levels by suppressing the expression of some pro-inflammatory cytokines, such as IL-6, IL-8, IL-13, TNF, MCP-1, and MIP-1, and for this reason, he considered triple therapy superior to monotherapy [32].

Bedoui et al., 2021, evaluated the expression levels of cPLA2α and mPGES-1 after therapy with methotrexate or dexamethasone. Methotrexate was not efficient in controlling the expression and activity of these enzymatic molecules; however, dexamethasone was shown to be able to normalize their levels [18].

An alternative method to drug treatment was pointed out by Ribeiro's study, which used anti-inflammatory drugs and analgesics in parallel with the continuous local application of infrared laser, ultrasound, and TENS-burst. This article argues that the association between focal treatments using stimuli of different wave frequencies accelerates the healing process by collaborating in different ways in cell recovery, speed of nerve conduction, and collagen production and extensibility, which may reduce inflammation and, consequently, pain and arthritic stiffness [25].

## 4. Discussion

Although global concern has focused on the COVID-19 pandemic since 2020, arthropod-borne viruses continue to cause outbreaks. It is already known that arboviruses induce self-limiting symptoms in adults [3,32,36], and the occurrence of short- and long-term pain syndromes has become increasingly common in patients infected by the CHIKV [3,32,36]. The most common viruses causing arthritis and/or arthralgias are parvoviruses; hepatitis B virus; hepatitis C virus; Epstein–Barr virus (EBV); and tropical viruses, such as Dengue, Zika, and CHIKV [37,38].

Arthritis is defined as swelling and tenderness of one or more joints and involves inflammation, whereas arthralgia is a joint pain with no inflammatory cause [39,40]. Although both may share many symptoms, each condition also has distinctive characteristics that make them different [41]. CHIKV-induced arthritis involves joints and a common pattern of leukocyte infiltration (innate and adaptive immune response cells, such as monocytes and T and B cells), cytokine production, and complement activation and is closely dependent on the possible virus persistence on hidden sides [42,43].

In joints, macrophages, synovial cells, and chondrocytes produce the eicosanoid named prostaglandin E2 (PGE2), which is an important pro-inflammatory molecule involved in bone erosion and pain [44]. Additional cytokines produced in this context are IL-1β and TNF-α, biomolecules that stimulate the synthesis of PGE2 and enhance its local concentration [8,16]. Since this inflammatory milieu is observed in the joints, NSAIDs are usually chosen as a therapeutic option. The general mechanism of action of NSAIDs is the inhibition of cyclooxygenases 1 and 2, enzymes involved in the synthesis of prostaglandins.

NSAIDs are commonly used to treat inflammatory diseases, such as rheumatic disorders, and aid in relieving pain and fever [45,46].

Serological tests, and clinical signs and symptoms have proven to be the basic and regular methods for diagnosing arboviruses. Furthermore, Zika and Chikungunya are infections with a very similar manifestation, and the clinical diagnosis may not be sufficient to differentiate them, requiring testing by other methods [4].

The most commonly used tests for differential diagnosis in the identification of serum levels of anti-antibodies (anti-IgM and anti-IgG) are ELISA (Mac-ELISA) and RT-PCR [47]. In addition, by performing immunohistochemistry, Bedoui et al., 2018, labeled a wide variety of primary antibodies used in cell cultures of synovial biopsy (hygroma), which originated from one of the patients in the study who had been in the chronic phase of the disease for at least 18 months, with persistent pain and relapsing arthralgia in more than one small joint. Moreover, RT-PCR from total RNA extracted from the same cell culture was performed. To verify the possible cytotoxic effects of the treatment, lactate dehydrogenase release was measured in the supernatants of HSF cell cultures 24 h post-treatment [18].

In addition, Blettery et al., 2019, combined serological tests and RT-PCR with joint imaging data acquired by Doppler ultrasonography. The Doppler ultrasound of painful joints revealed effusions in 92.8% of the examined joints (hands and wrists, ankles, and knees were involved, but shoulders and elbows were rarely affected). The majority (75.5%) of effusions were unilateral. No erosion was observed. Subcutaneous inflammatory infiltration (cellulitis) was observed in only a minor proportion of the participants [22]. In summary, RT-PCR was used in all studies that mentioned a diagnostic method, even in association with other alternative methodologies. This was the molecular technique of choice for the direct detection of viral RNA, which showed greater specificity and assertiveness. The Zika and Chikungunya epidemic in 2014–2016 in Brazil boosted the repositioning of drugs for the treatment of only acute symptoms; however, the identification of strategies for the management of persistent pain is still incipient [48]. The treatment is usually performed with common analgesics (e.g., acetaminophen) [49], NSAIDs (e.g., aspirin and ibuprofen) [50], dexamethasone [18], hydroxychloroquine, and DMARDs [32] such as methotrexate. Methotrexate acts by multiple mechanisms [51,52]. It decreases the nitric oxide production, stimulates adenosine release, activates the adenosine receptor $A_{2A}$ (a physiological receptor with anti-inflammatory properties [53]), inhibits purine and pyrimidine synthesis, participates in transmethylation reactions, promotes the translocation of the nuclear factor-κB to the nucleus, and reduces the signaling pathway of the Janus kinase signal transducer and the transcription factor STAT [52,54,55]. Furthermore, other therapies, such as local applications of continuous ultrasound, infrared laser, and TENS-burst alone or in combination might be used as alternative or additional treatments [56,57]. Nevertheless, these techniques are only partially effective. Finally, according to the studies reviewed in this work, the risk of bias was considered low; most groups were heterogeneous; and patients were mostly female, despite having a variable age according to each study. Most cases were between 41 and 69 years old, and treatment efficiency measures were used in different ways, including morphological assessments; HAQ score; ultrasound; DAS28 ESR; X-ray; serological, immunological, and biochemical tests.

## 5. Conclusions

Conflicting explanations were found in the reviewed studies regarding the origin and causes of chronic arthritogenic pain in arbovirus infections. The serological and clinical examination results support that pro-inflammatory cytokine, TNF-α, and PGE2 may infiltrate the joints and generate symptoms similar to rheumatic arthritis. Furthermore, leukopenia, lymphopenia, neutropenia, and thrombocytopenia are evidenced.

Antivirals such as ribavirin are cited as possible drugs to control the viral load in patients infected in the acute phase of the infection. Moreover, the use of aspirin and other NSAIDs has been suggested as symptomatic treatment for the chronic phase. There are no findings that clearly demonstrate the circumstances for the chronicity of arbovirus-induced arthritogenic pain. Therefore, research in this area is desperately needed for a better understanding and elucidation of the issues addressed in this systematic review.

**Author Contributions:** Conceptualization, R.d.C.C. and B.R.; methodology, R.d.C.C. and B.R.; validation, R.d.C.C., B.R., F.L.F.-D. and G.C.M.; formal analysis, F.L.F.-D. and G.C.M.; investigation, R.d.C.C.; resources, R.d.C.C. and B.R.; data curation, R.d.C.C. and B.R.; writing original draft preparation, R.d.C.C. and B.R.; writing review and editing, A.K.N.A., F.L.F.-D. and G.C.M.; visualization, R.d.C.C., B.R., A.K.N.A., F.L.F.-D. and G.C.M.; supervision, F.L.F.-D. and G.C.M.; project administration, F.L.F.-D. and G.C.M.; funding acquisition, G.C.M. All authors have read and agreed to the published version of the manuscript.

**Funding:** This research was funded by Fundação de Amparo à Pesquisa do Estado do Rio de Janeiro FAPERJ (E-26/211.795/2021). The funder had no role in the study design, data collection, analysis, decision to publish, or preparation of the manuscript.

**Acknowledgments:** We thank the Conselho Nacional de Desenvolvimento Científico e Tecnológico (CNPq) and the Coordenação de Aperfeiçoamento de Pessoal de Nível Superior (CAPES) for supporting.

**Conflicts of Interest:** The authors declare no conflict of interest.

# References

1. Wimalasiri-Yapa, B.; Yapa, H.E.; Huang, X.; Hafner, L.M.; Kenna, T.J.; Frentiu, F.D. Zika Virus and Arthritis/Arthralgia: A Systematic Review and Meta-Analysis. *Viruses* **2020**, *12*, 1137. [CrossRef] [PubMed]
2. Waggoner, J.J.; Gresh, L.; Vargas, M.J.; Ballesteros, G.; Tellez, Y.; Soda, K.J.; Sahoo, M.K.; Nunez, A.; Balmaseda, A.; Harris, E.; et al. Viremia and Clinical Presentation in Nicaraguan Patients Infected With Zika Virus, Chikungunya Virus, and Dengue Virus. *Clin. Infect. Dis.* **2016**, *63*, 1584–1590. [CrossRef] [PubMed]
3. Tritsch, S.R.; Encinales, L.; Pacheco, N.; Cadena, A.; Cure, C.; McMahon, E.; Watson, H.; Porras Ramirez, A.; Mendoza, A.R.; Li, G.; et al. Chronic Joint Pain 3 Years after Chikungunya Virus Infection Largely Characterized by Relapsing-remitting Symptoms. *J. Rheumatol.* **2020**, *47*, 1267–1274. [CrossRef]
4. Azeredo, E.L.; Dos Santos, F.B.; Barbosa, L.S.; Souza, T.M.A.; Badolato-Corrêa, J.; Sánchez-Arcila, J.C.; Nunes, P.C.G.; de-Oliveira-Pinto, L.M.; de Filippis, A.M.; Dal Fabbro, M.; et al. Clinical and Laboratory Profile of Zika and Dengue Infected Patients: Lessons Learned From the Co-circulation of Dengue, Zika and Chikungunya in Brazil. *PLoS Curr.* **2018**, *10*. [CrossRef] [PubMed]
5. Young, P.R. Arboviruses: A Family on the Move. *Adv. Exp. Med. Biol.* **2018**, *1062*, 1–10. [CrossRef]
6. Brito Ferreira, M.L.; Militão de Albuquerque, M.F.P.; de Brito, C.A.A.; de Oliveira França, R.F.; Porto Moreira, Á.J.; de Morais Machado, M.; da Paz Melo, R.; Medialdea-Carrera, R.; Dornelas Mesquita, S.; Lopes Santos, M.; et al. Neurological disease in adults with Zika and chikungunya virus infection in Northeast Brazil: A prospective observational study. *Lancet Neurol.* **2020**, *19*, 826–839. [CrossRef]
7. Burt, F.J.; Chen, W.; Miner, J.J.; Lenschow, D.J.; Merits, A.; Schnettler, E.; Kohl, A.; Rudd, P.A.; Taylor, A.; Herrero, L.J.; et al. Chikungunya virus: An update on the biology and pathogenesis of this emerging pathogen. *Lancet Infect. Dis.* **2017**, *17*, e107–e117. [CrossRef]
8. Burt, F.J.; Rolph, M.S.; Rulli, N.E.; Mahalingam, S.; Heise, M.T. Chikungunya: A re-emerging virus. *Lancet* **2012**, *379*, 662–671. [CrossRef]
9. Alves-Leon, S.V.; Ferreira, C.D.S.; Herlinger, A.L.; Fontes-Dantas, F.L.; Rueda-Lopes, F.C.; Francisco, R.D.S., Jr.; Goncalves, J.; de Araujo, A.D.; Rego, C.; Higa, L.M.; et al. Exome-Wide Search for Genes Associated With Central Nervous System Inflammatory Demyelinating Diseases Following CHIKV Infection: The Tip of the Iceberg. *Front. Genet.* **2021**, *12*, 639364. [CrossRef]
10. Rueda-Lopes, F.C.; da Cruz, L.C.H.; Fontes, F.L.; Herlinger, A.L.; da Costa Ferreira Junior, O.; de Aguiar, R.S.; Vasconcelos, C.C.F.; do Nascimento, O.J.M.; Alves-Leon, S.V. Clinical and magnetic resonance imaging patterns of extensive Chikungunya virus-associated myelitis. *J. Neurovirol.* **2021**, *27*, 616–625. [CrossRef]
11. Kumar, R.; Shrivastava, T.; Samal, S.; Ahmed, S.; Parray, H.A. Antibody-based therapeutic interventions: Possible strategy to counter chikungunya viral infection. *Appl. Microbiol. Biotechnol.* **2020**, *104*, 3209–3228. [CrossRef] [PubMed]
12. de Almeida Barreto, F.K.; Montenegro, R.M., Jr.; Fernandes, V.O.; Oliveira, R.; de Araujo Batista, L.A.; Hussain, A.; de Goes Cavalcanti, L.P. Chikungunya and diabetes, what do we know? *Diabetol. Metab. Syndr.* **2018**, *10*, 32. [CrossRef] [PubMed]
13. Kiely, P.D.W.; Lloyd, M.E. Ankle arthritis—An important signpost in rheumatologic practice. *Rheumatology* **2021**, *60*, 23–33. [CrossRef] [PubMed]
14. Benjamanukul, S.; Osiri, M.; Chansaenroj, J.; Chirathaworn, C.; Poovorawan, Y. Rheumatic manifestations of Chikungunya virus infection: Prevalence, patterns, and enthesitis. *PLoS ONE* **2021**, *16*, e0249867. [CrossRef] [PubMed]
15. Zaid, A.; Gerardin, P.; Taylor, A.; Mostafavi, H.; Malvy, D.; Mahalingam, S. Chikungunya Arthritis: Implications of Acute and Chronic Inflammation Mechanisms on Disease Management. *Arthritis Rheumatol.* **2018**, *70*, 484–495. [CrossRef]
16. Pathak, H.; Mohan, M.C.; Ravindran, V. Chikungunya arthritis. *Clin. Med.* **2019**, *19*, 381–385. [CrossRef]

17. de Lima Cavalcanti, T.Y.V.; Pereira, M.R.; de Paula, S.O.; Franca, R.F.O. A Review on Chikungunya Virus Epidemiology, Pathogenesis and Current Vaccine Development. *Viruses* **2022**, *14*, 969. [CrossRef]
18. Bedoui, Y.; Septembre-Malaterre, A.; Giry, C.; Jaffar-Bandjee, M.C.; Selambarom, J.; Guiraud, P.; Gasque, P. Robust COX-2-mediated prostaglandin response may drive arthralgia and bone destruction in patients with chronic inflammation post-chikungunya. *PLoS Negl. Trop. Dis.* **2021**, *15*, e0009115. [CrossRef]
19. Pineda, C.; Munoz-Louis, R.; Caballero-Uribe, C.V.; Viasus, D. Chikungunya in the region of the Americas. A challenge for rheumatologists and health care systems. *Clin. Rheumatol.* **2016**, *35*, 2381–2385. [CrossRef]
20. Venigalla, S.S.K.; Premakumar, S.; Janakiraman, V. A possible role for autoimmunity through molecular mimicry in alphavirus mediated arthritis. *Sci. Rep.* **2020**, *10*, 938. [CrossRef]
21. Reddy, V.; Desai, A.; Krishna, S.S.; Vasanthapuram, R. Molecular Mimicry between Chikungunya Virus and Host Components: A Possible Mechanism for the Arthritic Manifestations. *PLoS Negl. Trop. Dis.* **2017**, *11*, e0005238. [CrossRef] [PubMed]
22. Blettery, M.; Brunier, L.; Banydeen, R.; Derancourt, C.; de Bandt, M. Management of acute-stage chikungunya disease: Contribution of ultrasonographic joint examination. *Int. J. Infect. Dis. IJID Off. Publ. Int. Soc. Infect. Dis.* **2019**, *84*, 1–4. [CrossRef] [PubMed]
23. Pouriayevali, M.H.; Rezaei, F.; Jalali, T.; Baniasadi, V.; Fazlalipour, M.; Mostafavi, E.; Khakifirouz, S.; Mohammadi, T.; Fereydooni, Z.; Tavakoli, M.; et al. Imported cases of Chikungunya virus in Iran. *BMC Infect. Dis.* **2019**, *19*, 1004. [CrossRef]
24. Bouquillard, E.; Fianu, A.; Bangil, M.; Charlette, N.; Ribéra, A.; Michault, A.; Favier, F.; Simon, F.; Flipo, R.M. Rheumatic manifestations associated with Chikungunya virus infection: A study of 307 patients with 32-month follow-up (RHUMATOCHIK study). *Jt. Bone Spine* **2018**, *85*, 207–210. [CrossRef]
25. Ribeiro, A.M.B.M.; Pimentel, C.M.; Guerra, A.C.C.G.; Lima, M.R.D.O. Physiotherapeutic approach on the late phase of chikungunya: A case report. *Rev. Bras. Saúde Matern. Infant.* **2016**, *16*, S51–S56. [CrossRef]
26. Mostafavi, H.; Abeyratne, E.; Zaid, A.; Taylor, A. Arthritogenic Alphavirus-Induced Immunopathology and Targeting Host Inflammation as A Therapeutic Strategy for Alphaviral Disease. *Viruses* **2019**, *11*, 290. [CrossRef] [PubMed]
27. de Andrade, D.C.; Jean, S.; Clavelou, P.; Dallel, R.; Bouhassira, D. Chronic pain associated with the Chikungunya Fever: Long lasting burden of an acute illness. *BMC Infect. Dis.* **2010**, *10*, 31. [CrossRef] [PubMed]
28. Brito, C.A.; Sohsten, A.K.; Leitao, C.C.; Brito, R.C.; Valadares, L.D.; Fonte, C.A.; Mesquita, Z.B.; Cunha, R.V.; Luz, K.; Leao, H.M.; et al. Pharmacologic management of pain in patients with Chikungunya: A guideline. *Rev. Soc. Bras. Med. Trop.* **2016**, *49*, 668–679. [CrossRef]
29. Bouhassira, D. Neuropathic pain: Definition, assessment and epidemiology. *Rev. Neurol.* **2019**, *175*, 16–25. [CrossRef]
30. National Collaborating Centre for Methods and Tools. Critical Appraisal Skills Programme (CASP) Tools. Available online: https://casp-uk.net/glossary/systematic-review (accessed on 25 July 2022).
31. Rosso, F.; Rodriguez, S.; Cedano, J.A.; Mora, B.L.; Moncada, P.A.; Velez, J.D. Chikungunya in solid organ transplant recipients, a case series and literature review. *Transpl Infect Dis* **2018**, *20*, e12978. [CrossRef]
32. Ravindran, V.; Alias, G. Efficacy of combination DMARD therapy vs. hydroxychloroquine monotherapy in chronic persistent chikungunya arthritis: A 24-week randomized controlled open label study. *Clin. Rheumatol.* **2017**, *36*, 1335–1340. [CrossRef] [PubMed]
33. Agrawal, M.; Pandey, N.; Rastogi, M.; Dogra, S.; Singh, S.K. Chikungunya virus modulates the miRNA expression patterns in human synovial fibroblasts. *J. Med. Virol.* **2020**, *92*, 139–148. [CrossRef] [PubMed]
34. Hoarau, J.J.; Jaffar Bandjee, M.C.; Krejbich Trotot, P.; Das, T.; Li-Pat-Yuen, G.; Dassa, B.; Denizot, M.; Guichard, E.; Ribera, A.; Henni, T.; et al. Persistent chronic inflammation and infection by Chikungunya arthritogenic alphavirus in spite of a robust host immune response. *J. Immunol.* **2010**, *184*, 5914–5927. [CrossRef] [PubMed]
35. Lima, M.; de Lima, R.C.; de Azeredo, E.L.; Dos Santos, F.B. Analysis of a Routinely Used Commercial Anti-Chikungunya IgM ELISA Reveals Cross-Reactivities with Dengue in Brazil: A New Challenge for Differential Diagnosis? *Diagnostics* **2021**, *11*, 819. [CrossRef]
36. Hua, C.; Combe, B. Chikungunya Virus-Associated Disease. *Curr. Rheumatol. Rep.* **2017**, *19*, 69. [CrossRef]
37. Tiwari, V.; Bergman, M.J. Viral Arthritis. In *StatPearls*; StatPearls Publishing LLC.: Treasure Island, FL, USA, 2022.
38. Laine, M.; Luukkainen, R.; Toivanen, A. Sindbis viruses and other alphaviruses as cause of human arthritic disease. *J. Intern. Med.* **2004**, *256*, 457–471. [CrossRef]
39. Deane, K.D.; Holers, V.M. Rheumatoid Arthritis Pathogenesis, Prediction, and Prevention: An Emerging Paradigm Shift. *Arthritis Rheumatol.* **2021**, *73*, 181–193. [CrossRef]
40. van Steenbergen, H.W.; Aletaha, D.; Beaart-van de Voorde, L.J.; Brouwer, E.; Codreanu, C.; Combe, B.; Fonseca, J.E.; Hetland, M.L.; Humby, F.; Kvien, T.K.; et al. EULAR definition of arthralgia suspicious for progression to rheumatoid arthritis. *Ann. Rheum. Dis.* **2017**, *76*, 491–496. [CrossRef]
41. Ten Brinck, R.M.; van Steenbergen, H.W.; Mangnus, L.; Burgers, L.E.; Reijnierse, M.; Huizinga, T.W.; van der Helm-van Mil, A.H. Functional limitations in the phase of clinically suspect arthralgia are as serious as in early clinical arthritis; a longitudinal study. *RMD Open* **2017**, *3*, e000419. [CrossRef]
42. Amdekar, S.; Parashar, D.; Alagarasu, K. Chikungunya Virus-Induced Arthritis: Role of Host and Viral Factors in the Pathogenesis. *Viral Immunol.* **2017**, *30*, 691–702. [CrossRef]

43. Chirathaworn, C.; Chansaenroj, J.; Poovorawan, Y. Cytokines and Chemokines in Chikungunya Virus Infection: Protection or Induction of Pathology. *Pathogens* **2020**, *9*, 415. [CrossRef] [PubMed]
44. de Hair, M.J.; Leclerc, P.; Newsum, E.C.; Maijer, K.I.; van de Sande, M.G.; Ramwadhdoebe, T.H.; van Schaardenburg, D.; van Baarsen, L.G.; Korotkova, M.; Gerlag, D.M.; et al. Expression of Prostaglandin E2 Enzymes in the Synovium of Arthralgia Patients at Risk of Developing Rheumatoid Arthritis and in Early Arthritis Patients. *PLoS ONE* **2015**, *10*, e0133669. [CrossRef] [PubMed]
45. Crofford, L.J. Use of NSAIDs in treating patients with arthritis. *Arthritis Res. Ther.* **2013**, *15* (Suppl. 3), S2. [CrossRef] [PubMed]
46. Bindu, S.; Mazumder, S.; Bandyopadhyay, U. Non-steroidal anti-inflammatory drugs (NSAIDs) and organ damage: A current perspective. *Biochem. Pharmacol.* **2020**, *180*, 114147. [CrossRef]
47. Piantadosi, A.; Kanjilal, S. Diagnostic Approach for Arboviral Infections in the United States. *J. Clin. Microbiol.* **2020**, *58*. [CrossRef]
48. Kumar, R.; Ahmed, S.; Parray, H.A.; Das, S. Chikungunya and arthritis: An overview. *Travel Med. Infect. Dis.* **2021**, *44*, 102168. [CrossRef]
49. Kellstein, D.; Fernandes, L. Symptomatic treatment of dengue: Should the NSAID contraindication be reconsidered? *Postgrad. Med.* **2019**, *131*, 109–116. [CrossRef]
50. Pan, T.; Peng, Z.; Tan, L.; Zou, F.; Zhou, N.; Liu, B.; Liang, L.; Chen, C.; Liu, J.; Wu, L.; et al. Nonsteroidal Anti-inflammatory Drugs Potently Inhibit the Replication of Zika Viruses by Inducing the Degradation of AXL. *J. Virol.* **2018**, *92*. [CrossRef]
51. Marin, G.E.; Neag, M.A.; Burlacu, C.C.; Buzoianu, A.D. The Protective Effects of Nutraceutical Components in Methotrexate-Induced Toxicity Models-An Overview. *Microorganisms* **2022**, *10*, 2053. [CrossRef]
52. Alqarni, A.M.; Zeidler, M.P. How does methotrexate work? *Biochem. Soc. Trans.* **2020**, *48*, 559–567. [CrossRef]
53. Trevethick, M.A.; Mantell, S.J.; Stuart, E.F.; Barnard, A.; Wright, K.N.; Yeadon, M. Treating lung inflammation with agonists of the adenosine A2A receptor: Promises, problems and potential solutions. *Br. J. Pharmacol.* **2008**, *155*, 463–474. [CrossRef] [PubMed]
54. Cronstein, B.N.; Aune, T.M. Methotrexate and its mechanisms of action in inflammatory arthritis. *Nat. Rev. Rheumatol.* **2020**, *16*, 145–154. [CrossRef] [PubMed]
55. Harrington, R.; Al Nokhatha, S.A.; Conway, R. JAK Inhibitors in Rheumatoid Arthritis: An Evidence-Based Review on the Emerging Clinical Data. *J. Inflamm. Res.* **2020**, *13*, 519–531. [CrossRef] [PubMed]
56. Gibson, W.; Wand, B.M.; Meads, C.; Catley, M.J.; O'Connell, N.E. Transcutaneous electrical nerve stimulation (TENS) for chronic pain—An overview of Cochrane Reviews. *Cochrane Database Syst. Rev.* **2019**, *4*, CD011890. [CrossRef]
57. Macedo, L.B.; Josue, A.M.; Maia, P.H.; Camara, A.E.; Brasileiro, J.S. Effect of burst TENS and conventional TENS combined with cryotherapy on pressure pain threshold: Randomised, controlled, clinical trial. *Physiotherapy* **2015**, *101*, 155–160. [CrossRef]

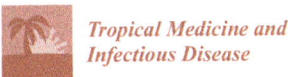 

*Tropical Medicine and Infectious Disease*

*Case Report*

# Putative Pathogenic Genes of *Leptospira interrogans* and *Leptospira weilii* Isolated from Patients with Acute Febrile Illness

Amira Wahida Mohamad Safiee [1], Mohammad Ridhuan Mohd Ali [2], Muhammad Zarul Hanifah Md Zoqratt [3], Tan Hock Siew [3], Chua Wei Chuan [4,5], Lee Lih Huey [4], Mohd Hashairi Fauzi [5,6], Alwi Muhd Besari [5,7], Chan Yean Yean [4,5] and Nabilah Ismail [4,5,*]

1. Microbiology Transfusion Unit, Department of Transfusion Medicine, Hospital Queen Elizabeth II, Lorong Bersatu Off Jalan Damai, Kota Kinabalu 88300, Sabah, Malaysia
2. Bacteriology Unit, Infectious Disease Research Center (IDRC), Institute for Medical Research, National Institutes of Health (NIH) Complex, Setia Alam, Shah Alam 40170, Selangor, Malaysia
3. School of Science, Monash University Malaysia, Bandar Sunway 47500, Selangor, Malaysia
4. Department of Medical Microbiology & Parasitology, School of Medical Sciences, Universiti Sains Malaysia, Health Campus, Kubang Kerian 16150, Kelantan, Malaysia
5. Hospital Universiti Sains Malaysia, Universiti Sains Malaysia, Health Campus, Kubang Kerian 16150, Kelantan, Malaysia
6. Department of Emergency Medicine, School of Medical Sciences, Universiti Sains Malaysia, Health Campus, Kubang Kerian 16150, Kelantan, Malaysia
7. Department of Medicine, School of Medical Sciences, Universiti Sains Malaysia, Health Campus, Kubang Kerian 16150, Kelantan, Malaysia
* Correspondence: drnabilah@usm.my

**Abstract:** Leptospirosis is an important worldwide tropical disease caused by pathogenic *Leptospira* spp. The determination of virulence genes is important, as it influences patients' clinical manifestations and clinical outcomes. This case report focused on detecting the pathogenic genes of *Leptospira* in association with the clinical manifestations of patients at the Hospital Universiti Sains Malaysia, Malaysia, who presented with acute febrile illness. Two cases were found and, to the best of our knowledge, these were the first two cases in Malaysia in which patients presented with febrile illness were associated with successful *Leptospira* isolation from clinical samples. Both clinical isolates were identified by 16S rRNA sequencing as *Leptospira weilii* and *Leptospira interrogans*, respectively, and they were classified as pathogenic *Leptospira* by the presence of different pathogenic genes, based on a polymerase chain reaction (PCR) amplification of targeted genes. This report emphasizes that different infecting *Leptospira* species and the presence of different virulence factors cause a slight difference in clinical manifestations and laboratory findings of leptospirosis. Genomic sequencing and annotation revealed the detection of classical leptospiral virulence factor genes that were otherwise missed using PCR for detection of *Leptospira weilii* genome B208.

**Keywords:** Leptospirosis; febrile illness; pathogenic genes; genomic sequencing

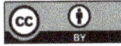

## 1. Introduction

Leptospirosis is recognized as a great mimicker because of its enormously wide variety of symptoms, ranging from subclinical diseases, such as a flu-like illness, to a severe syndrome of multi-organ infection with high mortality. The symptoms can imitate influenza, hepatitis, meningitis, viral hemorrhagic fever, and dengue fever. One study reported that 38% of the leptospirosis cases were misdiagnosed as hemorrhagic fever or dengue fever, due to similar clinical appearances [1]. The history of exposure and risk factors compatible with leptospirosis should alert clinicians to a possible diagnosis. Acute leptospirosis constantly presents with chills, headache, fever, conjunctival suffusion, vomiting, severe myalgia, nausea, anorexia, and malaise [2]. The vast majority of the infections are caused by pathogenic species, such as *L. interrogans*, *L. kirschneri*, *L. borgpetersenii*, *L. noguchii*, *L. santarosai*, *L. weilii*, and *L. alexanderi* [3]. The different species represent differences in DNA relatedness and possibly different geographical distributions, virulence, and clinical presentations.

The pathogenicity of *Leptospira* in humans are complex mechanisms that involve multi-protein interactions, including adhesion, that overcome host defense mechanisms followed by the expression of several virulence genes. Virulence genes are genes that code for factors, or for enzymes that produce factors, that are involved in interactions with the host; they are directly responsible for pathological damage during infection, and they are absent in nonpathogenic organisms [4].

This report focuses on detecting the pathogenic genes of *Leptospira* in association with the clinical manifestations of patients at the Hospital Universiti Sains Malaysia, Malaysia, who presented with acute febrile illness.

## 2. Description of the Cases

Here, we report two cases of leptospirosis patients in Malaysia who presented with febrile illness, in association with successful *Leptospira* isolation from clinical samples.

The first case (B208) was a 30-year-old man with no known medical illness who presented with febrile episodes for 3 days that were associated with myalgia, arthralgia, and headache. In addition, he had prominent gastrointestinal manifestations, presented with diarrhea for 5 days, and experienced poor oral intake. His further history revealed that he was involved with jungle trekking in a rural area, and that two of his companions developed similar symptoms. On admission to the medical ward, his vital signs were stable, with normal oxygenation and blood pressure. He was tachycardic and his body temperature was elevated. Physical examination was unremarkable, except for conjunctival suffusion. There was no hepatosplenomegaly and no palpable cervical lymphadenopathy. A laboratory investigation revealed slight leucocytosis at $12.5 \times 10^9$/L (the normal range is 4 to $11 \times 10^9$/L) and elevated C-reactive protein at >200 mg/L (the normal range is <10 mg/L), with otherwise normal blood cell counts. Liver and renal function tests were also normal. *Leptospira* IgM enzyme-linked immunosorbent assay (ELISA) and rapid *Leptospira* IgM Duo rapid test (ImmuneMed, Korea) were negative; however, an in-house real-time polymerase chain reaction (qPCR) was positive for *Leptospira* DNA and the isolation of *Leptospira* was also positive at day seven of cultivation. The patient was treated with intravenous ceftriaxone for 4 days, followed by 3 days of oral doxycycline, and he required intravenous hydration for 2 days. He subsequently became afebrile after 3 days of antimicrobial therapy and he was discharged 4 days after admission.

The second case (B004) was a 19-year-old man who was previously healthy and presented with a high-grade fever for 6 days. The febrile episodes were associated with nausea and persistent vomiting for 3 days, with epigastric pain and a poor appetite. On further questioning, the patient indicated that he had a history of swimming in a river about 10 days prior to the illness. As in the first case, the patient was tachycardic and had a raised body temperature on initial examination. Otherwise, the patient's blood pressure and oxygenation were normal. On abdominal examination, there was palpable tender liver at a two-finger breadth below the costal margin. The rest of the physical examination was unremarkable, with no jaundice or conjunctival suffusion noted. A laboratory investigation revealed that the patient had leukocytosis, with otherwise normal blood counts. His C-reactive protein was elevated at more than 200 mg/L (the normal range is <10 mg/L). There was also renal involvement with urea at 10.6 mmol/L (the normal range is 2.5 to 6.7 mmol/L), and creatinine at 182 μmol/L (the normal range is 70 to 100 μmol/L). The liver function test was normal. The *Leptospira* IgM Duo rapid test result (ImmuneMed, Korea) was intermediate; however, the microscopic agglutination test (MAT) result was negative. Then, *Leptospira* DNA was detected by in-house qPCR, and the isolation of *Leptospira* was positive on day 11 of cultivation. The patient initially required intravenous fluid and was treated with parenteral ceftriaxone for 4 days; subsequently, this was stepped down to 3 days of oral doxycycline. The condition improved and he was discharged 4 days after admission, with advice for an outpatient review of his renal profile.

## 3. Materials and Methods

Six ml of blood samples were collected from each patient prior to antibiotic administration and after obtaining their informed consent. The diagnosis of leptospirosis in both cases was confirmed by qPCR and positive isolation of *Leptospira* spp. Both clinical isolates, B208 and B004, were identified by 16S rRNA sequencing as *L. weilii* B208 (GenBank accession number JAMKEM000000000.1) and *L. interrogans* B004 (GenBank accession number JAMKEN000000000.1), respectively. Whole genomic sequencing for both isolates was performed and analyzed.

### 3.1. qPCR Detection of Leptospira

qPCR detection of *Leptospira* DNA was carried out, following a previous protocol [5]. Briefly, following DNA extraction, 8 µL of patient DNA was added to a PCR mix containing 1× Biorad SsoAdvanced™ Universal Probes Supermix, 200 nM forward and reverse primers, 100 nM probe, and PCR-grade water (adjusted to a total volume of 20 µL). The reactions were subjected to a thermal cycling condition, consisting of 95 °C (5 min) followed by 50 cycles of 95 °C for 30 s and 61.3 °C for 30 s.

### 3.2. Leptospira Isolation

The standard method to isolate *Leptospira* from the blood sample was by inoculating 1 to 5 drops (100 to 200 µL) of whole blood directly into EMJH media. The volume of the whole blood used for culturing was lower to avoid the inhibition of *Leptospira* growth by hemoglobin, antibiotics, antibodies, and other blood component factors [6,7]. The positive cultures from both patients were amplified and identified by PCR on the 16S rRNA gene by sequencing. In addition, the presence of the pathogenic genes was determined by using nine pathogenic genes: *lfb1*, *flaB*, *OmpL1*, *ligA*, *ligB*, *ligC*, *lipL21*, *lipL32*, and *lipL41*.

### 3.3. PCR Amplification of Virulence Genes

Amplification of the DNA was performed in a 25 µL reaction containing 1 mM of each primer, 12.5 µL of DreamTaq Green PCR Master Mix (Thermo Scientific, Malaysia), 2 µL of DNA template, and 8 µL of DNase-free water. The PCR cycling condition consisted of an initial denaturation step at 95 °C for 5 min, followed by 30 amplification cycles of denaturation at 95 °C for 30 s, annealing at a specified temperature for each primer for 30 s and extension at 72 °C for 30 s. A final extension step was performed at 72 °C for 5 min. The PCR cycles used in this study were based on the manufacturer's recommendations for PCR Master Mix (Thermo Scientific, Selangor, Malaysia).

### 3.4. Genome Sequencing, Assembly, and Quality Control

Genomic DNA was extracted from bacterial isolates using an MN NucleoSpin Tissue Genomic DNA Purification Kit (Apical Scientific, Selangor, Malaysia). The genomic DNA was quantitated using a Multiskan Sky Microplate Spectrophotometer (Thermo Fisher Scientific, Waltham, MA, USA) and a Qubit Fluorometer (Bio-Diagnostics, Selangor, Malaysia) before being shipped for library preparation at Bio3 Scientific Sdn Bhd company (Selangor, Malaysia). DNA fragmentation was carried out using Covaris S220 (Covaris, Woburn, MA, USA), followed by end repair, dA-tailing, adapter ligation, and purification using a VAHTS Universal DNA Library Prep Kit for Illumina (Nanjing Vazyme Biotech Co., Nanjing, China). The Agilent 2100 (Agilent, Santa Clara, CA, USA) and the Qubit Fluorometer (Thermo Fisher Scientific, Waltham, MA, USA) were used to determine library quality. Whole-genome sequencing was performed on a Novaseq 6000 platform (Illumina, San Diego, CA, USA). Upon completion, sequencing reads were quality-filtered using a FastQC (http://www.bioinformatics.babraham.ac.uk/projects/fastqc/; access date 10 February 2022) and adapter and were trimmed off using TrimGalore (https://www.bioinformatics.babraham.ac.uk/projects/trim_galore/; access date 10 February 2022) and CutAdapt (http://code.google.com/p/cutadapt/; access date 10 February 2022) [8] before genome assembly using SPAdes (http://bioinf.spbau.ru/spades; access date 10 February 2022) [9]. The quality of the genome assembly was assessed via EvalG (https://patricbrc.org/app/Annotation; access date 10 February 2022) [10].

### 3.5. Genomic Annotation

Genome annotation was carried out using Bakta version 1.3.3 (https://github.com/oschwengers/bakta; access date 10 February 2022) (database schema 3) [11]. The protein database included the UniRef protein sequence cluster universe. Then, reported *Leptospira* virulence genes were searched from the genome annotations [12], according to UniRef protein IDs (Table 1):

**Table 1.** Detection of *Leptospira* virulence factor genes by Bakta version 1.3.3.

| Gene | IDs | Note |
|---|---|---|
| lipL32 | UniRef90_Q6J0P4, UniRef50_Q6J0P4 | In *L. interrogans* genomes, the last three genomes have different versions. In *L. weilii* genomes, UniRef90_Q6J0P4 annotated as spirochaetales surface lipoprotein |
| lipL41 | UniRef90_A0A2M9XPR1, UniRef100_X5FKY1, UniRef90_A0A1D7V0C6 | |
| lipL21 | UniRef90_Q04WF0 | |
| ompL1 | UniRef90_Q6GXE0 | |
| lfb1 | UniRef90_E7DSE3, UniRef90_E7DSD4 | All *L. weilii* has only UniRef90_E7DSD4 form |
| ligA | UniRef90_Q72MA6, UniRef90_Q8EYU4 | |
| ligB | UniRef90_A0A540TD47, UniRef90_Q04UY1 | All *L. weilii* has only UniRef90_Q04UY1 form |
| ligC | UniRef_C0J1R0 | |
| secY | UniRef90_Q9XD16, UniRef90_M3CP76 | Housekeeping gene |
| flaB | UniRef90_O51941 | Housekeeping gene |

Annotation of antimicrobial resistance genes and virulence factor genes was conducted using Abricate (https://github.com/tseemann/abricate; access date 10 February 2022) against the comprehensive antibiotic resistance database (CARD) database and the virulence factor database (VFDB) database, respectively [13,14].

### 3.6. Taxonomic Assignment and Phylogenomic Tree Construction

Taxonomic assignment was carried out using GTDBtk (https://github.com/Ecogenomics/GTDBTk; access date 10 February 2022) against GTDB database release 202. An ANI value of over 95% in GTDBtk confirmed the assignment of the B004 genome as *L. interrogans* and the B208 genome as *L. weilii*.

The two genomes were analyzed against closely related *Leptospira* genomes that were accessible from the NCBI GenBank and RefSeq databases, based on SNPs. SNP calls were made against the sample genome, using snippy (https://github.com/tseemann/snippy; access date 10 February 2022). For sample B004 (*L. interrogans*), another 31 *L. interrogans* were used together for phylogenomic tree construction (gls454012v02 assembly as outgroup).

For genome B208 (*L. weilii*), another 18 *L. weilii* genomes were included, with assembly ASM200984v1 (*L. alexanderi* 56659) as the outgroup. Then, variant calls of respective *Leptospira* species were merged, using the snippy-core program.

The core SNP tree was constructed from merged variant calls using Gubbins v3.1.6 (https://github.com/nickjcroucher/gubbins; access date 10 February 2022) [15]. The phylogenetic tree was visualized using iTOL v6 (https://itol.embl.de/; access date 10 February 2022) [16].

### 3.7. Multi Locus Sequence Typing (MLST)

The MLST assignment was carried out against the pubMLST database, using the software MLST (https://github.com/tseemann/mlst; access date 10 February 2022) [17].

## 4. Results

### 4.1. Leptospirosis Investigation Results

The leptospirosis investigation results for both cases are summarized in Table 2.

**Table 2.** Summary of leptospirosis investigation results.

| Laboratory Test | Patient 1 (B208) | Patient 2 (B004) | Manufacturer |
|---|---|---|---|
| *Leptospira* IgM ELISA | Negative | - | Panbio, US |
| *Leptospira* IgM Duo Rapid | Intermediate | Negative | ImmuneMed, Korea |
| Microscopic agglutination test (MAT) | Negative | - | In-house |
| *Leptospira* in-house PCR | Positive | Positive | In-house |
| culture | Positive | Positive | In-house |
| 16S rRNA sequencing | *Leptospira weilii* | *Leptospira interrogans* | Apical, Malaysia |
| Genomic characteristics: | | | |
| Chromosome size (bp) | 4,298,595 | 4,858,647 | |
| Number of contigs | 220 | 169 | |
| N50 | 106460 | 83016 | |
| GC content (%) | 40.72 | 35.09 | |
| No. of coding sequences | 3854 | 3884 | |
| No. of RNAs rRNA | 3 | 3 | |
| tRNA | 36 | 37 | |
| tmRNA | 1 | 1 | |
| ncRNA | 4 | 4 | |
| CRISPR | 1 | 3 | |
| GenBank accession no. | JAMKEM000000000.1 | JAMKEN000000000.1 | |

### 4.2. Whole-Genome Sequencing

The taxonomy of *L. weilii* and *L. interrogans* was further confirmed based on whole-genome sequencing using GTDBtk (GTDB release 202). Both of the isolates were classified as pathogenic *Leptospira* and were determined by the presence of five and nine pathogenic genes, respectively, as shown in Table 3, based on the PCR amplification of the targeted genes. In this study, PCR products were amplified in all tested primers, suggesting that the second patient's isolate expressed all nine of the tested pathogenic genes, while the first patient's isolate only expressed *lfb1*, *flaB*, *ligB*, *ligC*, and *lipL32* genes.

MLST sequence type based on *Leptospira* scheme assigned genome B004 as sequence type 249, while there was no sequence type for genome B208. The raw output result from the MLST for *L. interrogans* and *L. weilii* are presented in Tables 4 and 5, respectively.

**Table 3.** Detection of pathogenic genes of the isolates from positive cultures, based on PCR amplification.

| Pathogenic Gene | Target Gene | Patient 1 (B208) | Patient 2 (B004) |
|---|---|---|---|
| *ligA* | *ligA* | - | + |
| *ligB* | *ligB* | + | + |
| *ligC* | *ligC* | + | + |
| *lipL21* | *lipL21* | - | + |
| *lipL32* | *lipL32* | + | + |
| *lipL41* | *lipL41* | - | + |
| *flaB* | *flaB* | + | + |
| *lfb1* | *lfb1* | + | + |
| *ompL1* | *ompL1* | - | + |

**Table 4.** Raw output result from the MLST software for *L. interrogans*.

| Genome | Scheme | ST | glmU_1 | pntA_1 | sucA_1 | tpiA_1 | pfkB_1 | mreA_1 | caiB_1 |
|---|---|---|---|---|---|---|---|---|---|
| gls454012v02 | Leptospira | 61 | 11 | 7 | 2 | 18 | 27 | 8 | 3 |
| gls454088v2.0 | Leptospira | 252 | 1 | 10 | 7 | 8 | 15 | 5 | 52 |
| ASM1028784v1 | Leptospira | 50 | 6 | 8 | 2 | 2 | 9 | 7 | 5 |
| gls454027v2.0 | Leptospira | 51 | 6 | 13 | 2 | 2 | 13 | 2 | 6 |
| Lint2002000621v2.0 | Leptospira | 51 | 6 | 13 | 2 | 2 | 13 | 2 | 6 |
| Lint2002000623v2.0 | Leptospira | 51 | 6 | 13 | 2 | 2 | 13 | 2 | 6 |
| gls454067v02 | Leptospira | 24 | 1 | 4 | 2 | 1 | 5 | 3 | 4 |
| LintsBulMalv1.0 | Leptospira | 112 | 1 | 1 | 1 | 2 | 2 | 1 | 2 |
| gls454077v2.0 | Leptospira | 49 | 5 | 1 | 1 | 1 | 3 | 2 | 7 |
| gls454092v02 | Leptospira | 49 | 5 | 1 | 1 | 1 | 3 | 2 | 7 |
| USM_B004 | Leptospira | 249 | 1 | 1 | 9 | 2 | 6 | 3 | 6 |
| ASM129261v1 | Leptospira | - | 1 | 1 | 2 | 2,2 | - | 4 | 8 |
| ASM168377v1 | Leptospira | - | 1 | 1 | 2 | 65 | 29 | 4 | - |
| IMG-taxon_2681812812_ annotated_assembly | Leptospira | 17 | 1 | 1 | 2 | 2 | 10 | 4 | 8 |
| LintFPW2026v1.0 | Leptospira | 47 | 4 | 18 | 2 | 2 | 3 | 3 | 5 |
| ASM237007v1 | Leptospira | 33 | 1 | 18 | 1 | 4 | 4 | 5 | 3 |
| gls454104v2.0 | Leptospira | 83 | 1 | 1 | 1 | 27 | 6 | 5 | 2 |
| gls454097v02 | Leptospira | 77 | 1 | 3 | 1 | 25 | 6 | 6 | 2 |
| gls454107v02 | Leptospira | 86 | 1 | 18 | 1 | 25 | 6 | 6 | 2 |
| gls454009v2.0 | Leptospira | 111 | 20 | 1 | 1 | 4 | 6 | 6 | 5 |
| gls454020v2.0 | Leptospira | 111 | 20 | 1 | 1 | 4 | 6 | 6 | 5 |
| gls454105v2.0 | Leptospira | 84 | 1 | 2 | 2 | 29 | 4 | 5 | 9 |
| gls454087v2.0 | Leptospira | 42 | 3 | 11 | 3 | 2 | 4 | 5 | 8 |
| LintL0996v0.2 | Leptospira | 46 | 4 | 1 | 1 | 4 | 4 | 6 | 6 |
| LintL0448v0.2 | Leptospira | 46 | 4 | 1 | 1 | 4 | 4 | 6 | 6 |
| gls454099v02 | Leptospira | 46 | 4 | 1 | 1 | 4 | 4 | 6 | 6 |
| gls454069v2.0 | Leptospira | 37 | 3 | 3 | 3 | 3 | 4 | 5 | 5 |
| gls454102v2.0 | Leptospira | 37 | 3 | 3 | 3 | 3 | 4 | 5 | 5 |
| gls454096v2.0 | Leptospira | 80 | 3 | 1 | 17 | 3 | 4 | 5 | 16 |
| gls454045v1.0 | Leptospira | 140 | 3 | 3 | 3 | 3 | 4 | 5 | 16 |
| gls454014v2.0 | Leptospira | 140 | 3 | 3 | 3 | 3 | 4 | 5 | 16 |
| ASM196907v1 | Leptospira | 140 | 3 | 3 | 3 | 3 | 4 | 5 | 16 |

**Table 5.** Raw output result from the MLST software for *L. weilii*.

| Genome | Scheme | ST | glmU_1 | pntA_1 | sucA_1 | tpiA_1 | pfkB_1 | mreA_1 | caiB_1 | Order |
|---|---|---|---|---|---|---|---|---|---|---|
| ASM200984v1 | Leptospira | 207 | 53 | 67 | 63 | 59 | 73 | 57 | 53 | 19 |
| gls454188v02 | Leptospira | 192 | 47 | 57 | 60 | 52 | 61 | 50 | 46 | 18 |
| ASM156937v1 | Leptospira | 191 | 50 | 62 | 58 | 54 | 65 | 53 | 48 | 17 |
| gls454043v02 | Leptospira | - | 48 | 63 | 59 | 51 | 69 | 52 | 45 | 16 |
| ASM156891v1 | Leptospira | 194 | 49 | 60 | 55 | 51 | 69 | 52 | 45 | 15 |
| ASM156840v1 | Leptospira | - | 48 | 63 | 59 | 53 | 69 | 49 | 45 | 14 |
| ASM156841v1 | Leptospira | - | 48 | 63 | 59 | 53 | 60 | 49 | 45 | 13 |
| ASM156938v1 | Leptospira | - | 49 | 63 | 55 | 51 | 69 | 49 | 45 | 12 |
| LweiUI13098v0.2 | Leptospira | 190 | 49 | 63 | 59 | 51 | 60 | 49 | 45 | 11 |
| ASM196993v1 | Leptospira | - | 49 | 63 | 55 | 51 | 80 | 49 | 45 | 10 |
| ASM156890v1 | Leptospira | 182 | 46 | 56 | 55 | 51 | 60 | 49 | 45 | 9 |
| gls454051v01 | Leptospira | - | 48 | 63 | 59 | 51 | 69 | 54 | 45 | 8 |
| gls454038v02 | Leptospira | - | 49 | 61 | 57 | 51 | 64 | 49 | 45 | 7 |
| USM_B208 | Leptospira | - | 49 | 61 | 57 | 53 | 63 | 52 | 45 | 6 |
| ASM156936v1 | Leptospira | - | 48 | 58 | 59 | 51 | 63 | 49 | 47 | 5 |
| gls454036v02 | Leptospira | - | 49 | 59 | 57 | 53 | 63 | 49 | 45 | 4 |
| ASM156952v1 | Leptospira | - | 46 | 59 | 57 | 53 | 63 | 55 | 47 | 3 |
| gls454086v02 | Leptospira | 183 | 46 | 59 | 57 | 53 | 63 | 49 | 45 | 2 |
| ASM687476v1 | Leptospira | 94 | 46 | 59 | 57 | 53 | 63 | 52 | 45 | 1 |
| ASM687474v1 | Leptospira | 94 | 46 | 59 | 57 | 53 | 63 | 52 | 45 | 0 |

*4.3. Phylogenomic Study*

The phylogenomic relationship of the B208 and B004 genomes conformed with the distribution of the virulence genes (Figures 1 and 2).

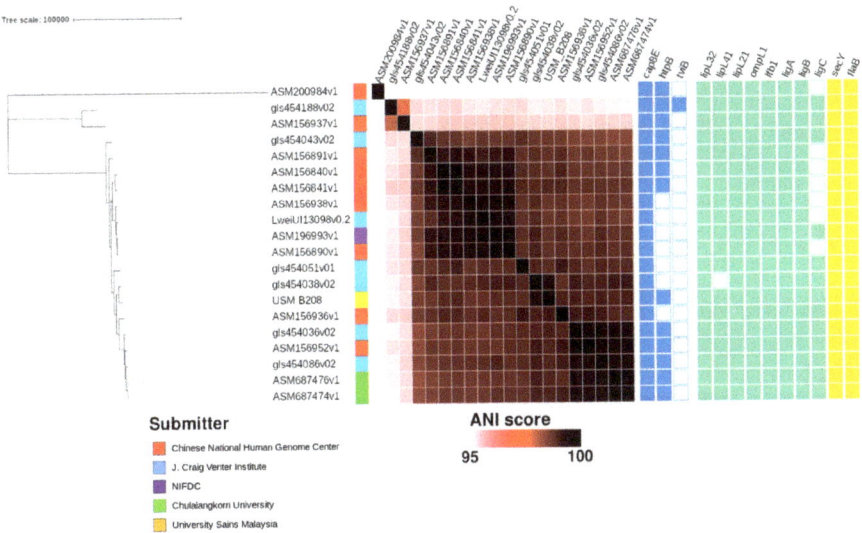

**Figure 1.** Phylogenomic tree of B208 genome against other *L. weilii* genomes. Metadata information provided in order are genome submitter, pairwise ANI score, predicted virulence genes in the virulence factor database (VFDB) and predicted virulence genes [12]. Assembly ASM200984v1 (*L. alexanderi*) acts as the outgroup.

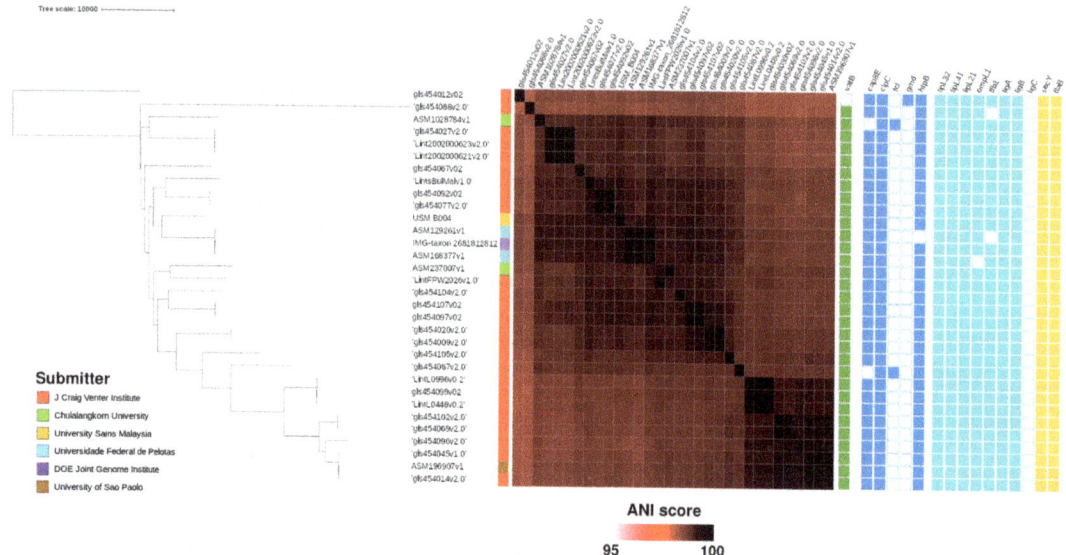

**Figure 2.** Phylogenomic tree of B004 genome against other L. interrogans genomes. Metadata information provided in order are genome submitter, pairwise ANI score, predicted antimicrobial resistance against the comprehensive antibiotic resistance database (CARD) and predicted virulence genes in VFDB, and predicted virulence genes [12].

## 5. Discussion

Leptospirosis is an endemic disease with global distribution, especially in Asia. In recent years, there have been increasing numbers of leptospirosis infection cases in Malaysia [18–20]. A case report showed that a real-time PCR assay was successfully used in a postmortem diagnosis of a woman whose death was caused by *L. interrogans* [21]. One study reported positively detected *Leptospira* cases and related risk factors in Sarawak, Malaysia [22]. Leptospirosis co-infected with other pathogens were normally seen in neighboring countries [23,24].

Advancements in molecular technology enable the expansion of the classical divisions of *L. interrogans* and *L. biflexa* into 64 species, based on DNA relatedness. These divisions are further classified into pathogenic species, non-pathogenic species, and species of indeterminate pathogenicity [25,26]. These classifications are quite different from the serologic classification, which may be of epidemiological value. The differences in genetic makeup among the pathogenic species may lead to the expression of different virulence factors, which may result in differences in clinical presentations [27].

Both of the clinical isolates in this study, *L. interrogans* and *L. weilii*, were pathogenic species. The slight difference in the presentations may be due to infection by different species of *Leptospira* with different virulence factors. *Leptospira interrogans* has a global distribution and there are some subgroups that are mostly isolated in the Asia–Pacific regions [28]. In comparison, *L. weilii* is a less commonly encountered species that has been previously reported in Australia [29]. In addition, the geographical distribution is related to the serovars [30]. However, a large number of patients infected by *Leptospira* have asymptomatic infections, particularly patients from endemic areas. Mild leptospirosis is the most common form of the disease, presenting in 90% of the cases [2] of patients who came from the endemic areas of leptospirosis.

Pathogenic *Leptospira* are responsible for human or animal infections. Although the pathogenic mechanisms of *Leptospira* are not clearly defined, potential virulence factors include lipopolysaccharide (LPS), OMPs, and adhesion molecule genes that are present in pathogenic *Leptospira* may help in understanding pathogenicity mechanisms. In animal cells, the pathways of Toll-like receptor 2 (TLR2) and Toll-like receptor 4 (TLR4) activate the host target, contrary to human cells that involve the activation of macrophage via TLR2 with the existence of CD14 [31]. The infection of *Leptospira* could result in problems with multiple organ systems or loss of life in unintentional hosts, such as humans, or merely moderate chronic or asymptomatic infections in reservoir hosts, including rodents [1]. All such primers were used to target the virulence factors and can be used to distinguish pathogenic from the saprophytic *Leptospira*. The differentiation of the pathogenic *Leptospira* is also crucial in classifying the pathogenic status for epidemiological and taxonomical study.

The role and contribution of individual virulence factors in the pathogenesis of leptospirosis are still not well defined. A combination of mechanisms, such as adhesions that allow adherence, immune-mediated responses, the ability of the host to recognize leptospiral LPS, toxin production, and surface proteins that result in immune evasion, may lead to a broad spectrum of clinical manifestation [32]. However, the spectrum and severity of clinical manifestations may also be influenced by several other factors, such as the duration of exposure to the pathogen, inoculum doses, and individual susceptibility.

Certain virulence factors found in pathogenic *Leptospira* can confer the ability to adhere to and enter mammalian host cells [12]. Several virulence factors, such as *lipL32* and leptospiral immunoglobulin-like genes *ligA*, *ligB*, and *ligC*, were only found in pathogenic *Leptospira* and not in their non-pathogenic counterparts [12,33]. The *lig* sequence is a virulence factor and plays a role in host cell attachment and invasion during *Leptospira* pathogenicity; *ligA* and *ligC* are present in a limited number of pathogenic serovar, while *ligB* is universally distributed among all of the pathogenic strains. Because *ligB* is present among all the pathogenic *Leptospira* strains, it may be useful in the identification and classification of *Leptospira* [34]. A drastic reduction in *L. interrogans* survival upon serum challenge was observed after experimenting with a concomitant and complete silencing of both LigA and LigB proteins by CRISPR-interference (CRISPRi) [35]. This process possibly signifies that *ligA* and *ligB* are virulence factors that enhance survival. In this study, we did not recover known *Leptospira* virulence factors from VFDB (Figures 1 and 2). Based on the detection of known *Leptospira* virulence factors of known *L. interrogans* and *L. weilii* genomes from genome annotation, we found that many of those virulence factors were broadly shared across all analyzed genomes. Genomic detection of a complete set of targeted virulence factors in the *L. weilii* genome B208 (Figure 1) contradicted PCR detection, as amplification for genes *ligA*, *lipL21*, *lipL41*, and *ompL1* on genome B208 were negative (Table 3). This suggests that the PCR amplification method is limited to protein sequences of *L. interrogans*, while possibly failing for other *Leptospira* species. This highlights the importance of reassessing conventional leptospiral diagnostic methods. For instance, PCR methods will fail to detect genes whenever mutations occur at the primer binding sites, which will consequentially lead to failure of primers to hybridizes to the target gene. Future PCR detection methods should account for the dissimilarity in sequences found in other *Leptospira* virulence genes and target more conserved genomic regions that are exclusive to pathogenic *Leptospira* genomes.

Another virulence factor, the outer membrane protein (OMP), plays an important role in pathogen virulence mechanisms, because this protein may evade the host's immune response [36]. OmpL1, LipL21, LipL32, and LipL41 have been used in this study to establish the pathogenicity of the isolate. All of the primers targeted a known gene sequence that was reported to be preserved among more than 200 of the pathogenic *Leptospira* serovars [34,36–39]. OmpL1 is a porin expressed in pathogenic *Leptospira* strains that allows the dispersion of hydrophilic solutes through the external membrane to the periplasm [40]. LipL32 is the most abundant protein in pathogenic *Leptospira*; it is absent in nonpathogenic organisms and expressed during human infection. It is mostly used in leptospirosis studies [36]. The sequence and expression of LipL32 are highly conserved among pathogenic *Leptospira* species. LipL41 is one of the immunogenic OMPs that is surface-exposed and it is expressed during infections [37,38]. In addition to those primers,

FlaB and Lfb were used to identify pathogenic *Leptospira*. The FlaB primer only amplifies a specific fragment from pathogenic *Leptospira*. A previous study reported that the FlaB PCR-based approach is an effective method for distinguishing and identifying the pathogenic *Leptospira* isolates [41,42].

The intake of doxycycline effectively cured leptospiral infection in both cases. Our results showed that the gene vatB was present in the majority of our *L. interrogans* genomes, but it was absent in *L. weillii* genomes, which suggest its role in *L. interrogans* survival, unlike its role with respect to *L. weillii*. If vatB is of no importance, the expression of vatB presents as a metabolic liability to *L. interrogans*. This indicates that, despite observations of horizontal gene transfer (HGT) in other pathogens, such as *Acinetobacter baumannii* [43], *Staphylococcus aureus* [44], and *Vibrio cholerae* [45], the conservation of the antimicrobial resistance (AMR) profile across *Leptospira* genomes suggests that HGT occurs minimally in *Leptospira*.

## 6. Conclusions

This report emphasized that different infecting *Leptospira* species and the presence of different virulence factors cause a slight difference in clinical manifestations and laboratory findings of leptospirosis. Genomic sequencing and annotation revealed the detection of classical leptospiral virulence factor genes that were otherwise missed using PCR for detecting *L. weilii* genome B208. Further large-scale investigation is needed to study the broad clinical manifestation of the disease in relation to species or serovar variation, antimicrobial susceptibility testing, virulence, and/or the pathogenicity of the *Leptospira* species.

**Author Contributions:** Conceptualization, N.I. and C.Y.Y.; methodology, N.I. and C.Y.Y.; formal analysis, A.W.M.S., M.R.M.A., M.Z.H.M.Z. and T.H.S.; investigation, A.W.M.S., M.R.M.A., M.Z.H.M.Z., T.H.S. and L.L.H.; resources, M.H.F., A.M.B., C.Y.Y. and N.I.; data curation, A.W.M.S., M.Z.H.M.Z., T.H.S. and C.W.C.; writing—original draft preparation, A.W.M.S. and C.W.C.; writing—review and editing, N.I., A.W.M.S., M.R.M.A., M.Z.H.M.Z., T.H.S. and L.L.H.; supervision, N.I and C.Y.Y.; project administration, N.I., M.H.F. and A.M.B.; funding acquisition, N.I., C.Y.Y. and M.R.M.A. All authors have read and agreed to the published version of the manuscript.

**Funding:** This study was funded by the Long-Term Research Grant Scheme (203/PPSP/6770004), a Research University Grant (1001/PPSP/812144), and a Bridging Grant (304/PPSP/6316187).

**Institutional Review Board Statement:** This study was approved by the Human Research Ethics Committee, Universiti Sains Malaysia (USM/JEPeM/16090300).

**Informed Consent Statement:** Written informed consent was obtained from all subjects involved in this study.

**Data Availability Statement:** The data presented in this study are available on request from the corresponding author.

**Acknowledgments:** We would like to give special thanks to the staff at the Department of Medical Microbiology and Parasitology, Health Campus, Universiti Sains Malaysia, for their direct and indirect contributions.

**Conflicts of Interest:** The authors declare no conflict of interest.

## References

1. Noor Rafizah, A.A.; Aziah, B.D.; Azwany, Y.N.; Kamarul Imran, M.; Mohamed Rusli, A.; Mohd Nazri, S.; Nabilah, I.; Siti Asma', H.; Zahiruddin, W.M.; Zaliha, I. Leptospirosis in Northeastern Malaysia: Misdiagnosed or coinfection? *Int. J. Collab. Res. Intern. Med. Public. Health* **2012**, *4*, 1419–1427.
2. Forbes, A.E.; Zochowski, W.J.; Dubrey, S.W.; Sivaprakasam, V. Leptospirosis and Weil's disease in the UK. *Q. J. Med.* **2012**, *105*, 1151–1162. [CrossRef] [PubMed]
3. Bulach, D.; Adler, B. Leptospiral genomics and pathogenesis. In *Current Topics in Microbiology and Immunology*; Adler, B., Ed.; Springer International Publishing: Cham, Switzerland, 2018; pp. 189–214.
4. Wassenaar, T.M.; Wim Gaastra, W. Bacterial virulence: Can we draw the line? *FEMS Microbiol. Lett.* **2001**, *201*, 1–7. [CrossRef] [PubMed]

5. Mohd Ali, M.R.; Mohd Safee, A.W.; Ismail, N.H.; Abu Sapian, R.; Mat Hussin, H.; Ismail, N.; Chan, Y.Y. Development and validation of pan-Leptospira Taqman qPCR for the detection of *Leptospira* spp. in clinical specimens. *Mol. Cell. Probes* **2018**, *38*, 1–6. [CrossRef]
6. Ellinghausen, H.C.; Mccullough, W.G. Nutrition of *Leptospira* Pomona and growth of 13 other Serotypes: A serum-free medium employing oleic albumin complex. *Am. J. Vet. Res.* **1965**, *26*, 39–44.
7. Faine, S.; Adler, B.; Bolin, C.; Perolat, P. *Leptospira and Leptospirosis*, 2nd ed.; Springer: Berlin/Heidelberg, Germany, 1999; 295p.
8. Martin, M. Cutadapt removes adapter sequences from high-throughput sequencing reads. *EMBnet. J.* **2011**, *17*, 10–12. [CrossRef]
9. Bankevich, A.; Nurk, S.; Antipov, D.; Gurevich, A.A.; Dvorkin, M.; Kulikov, A.S.; Lesin, V.M.; Nikolenko, S.I.; Pham, S.; Prjibelski, A.D.; et al. SPAdes: A new genome assembly algorithm and its applications to single-cell sequencing. *J. Comput. Biol.* **2012**, *19*, 455–477. [CrossRef] [PubMed]
10. Parrello, B.; Butler, R.; Chlenski, P.; Olson, R.; Overbeek, J.; Pusch, G.D.; Vonstein, V. and Overbeek, R. A machine learning-based service for estimating quality of genomes using PATRIC. *BMC BBioinform.* **2019**, *20*, 1–9.
11. Schwengers, O.; Jelonek, L.; Dieckmann, M.A.; Beyvers, S.; Blom, J.; Goesmann, A. Bakta: Rapid and standardized annotation of bacterial genomes via alignment-free sequence identification. *Microb. Genom.* **2021**, *7*, 000685. [CrossRef]
12. Ko, A.; Goarant, C.; Picardeau, M. *Leptospira*: The dawn of the molecular genetics era for an emerging zoonotic pathogen. *Nat. Rev. Microbiol.* **2009**, *7*, 736–747. [CrossRef]
13. Jia, B.F.; Raphenya, A.R.; Alcock, B.; Waglechner, N.; Guo, P.Y.; Tsang, K.K.; Lago, B.A.; Dave, B.M.; Pereira, S.; Sharma, A.N.; et al. CARD 2017: Expansion and model-centric curation of the comprehensive antibiotic resistance database. *Nucleic Acids Res.* **2017**, *45*, D566–D573. [CrossRef] [PubMed]
14. Chen, L.H.; Zheng, D.D.; Liu, B.; Yang, J.; Jin, Q. VFDB 2016: Hierarchical and refined dataset for big data analysis—10 years on. *Nucleic Acids Res.* **2016**, *44*, D694–D697. [CrossRef] [PubMed]
15. Croucher, N.J.; Page, A.J.; Connor, T.R.; Delaney, A.J.; Keane, J.A.; Bentley, S.D.; Parkhill, J.; Harris, S.R. Rapid phylogenetic analysis of large samples of recombinant bacterial whole genome sequences using Gubbins. *Nucleic Acids Res.* **2015**, *43*, e15. [CrossRef]
16. Letunic, I.; Bork, P. Interactive Tree of Life (iTOL) v5: An online tool for phylogenetic tree display and annotation. *Nucleic Acids Res.* **2021**, *49*, W293–W296. [CrossRef] [PubMed]
17. Jolley, K.A.; Maiden, M.C. BIGSdb: Scalable analysis of bacterial genome variation at the population level. *BMC Bioinform.* **2010**, *11*, 595. [CrossRef] [PubMed]
18. Garba, B.; Bahaman, A.R.; Khairani-Bejo, S.; Zakaria, Z.; Mutalib, A.R. Retrospective Study of Leptospirosis in Malaysia. *EcoHealth* **2017**, *14*, 389–398. [CrossRef]
19. Lim, J.K.; Murugaiyah, V.A.; Ramli, A.; Abdul Rahman, H.; Mohamed, N.; Shamsudin, N.; Tan, J.C. A Case Study: Leptospirosis In Malaysia. *Webmed Cent. Infect. Dis.* **2011**, *2*, WMC002764. [CrossRef]
20. Rao, M.; Amran, F.; Kamaruzaman, A.A.; Hakim Esa, H.A.; Hameed, A.A.; Mohamed Shabery, N.A. Case Report: Fatal Human Leptospirosis Caused by Leptospira interrogans Genotype ST149. *Am. J. Trop. Med. Hyg.* **2010**, *104*, 216–218. [CrossRef]
21. Hii, K.C.; Robie, E.R.; Saihidi, E.R.I.; Berita, A.; Alarja, N.A.; Xiu, L.S.; Merchant, J.A.; Binder, R.A.; Goh, J.K.T.; Guernier-Cambert, V.; et al. Leptospirosis infections among hospital patients, Sarawak, Malaysia. *Trop. Dis. Tra Vaccines* **2021**, *7*, 32. [CrossRef]
22. Mazhar, M.; Kao, J.J.; Bolger, D.T. A 23-year-old man with leptospirosis and acute abdominal pain. *Hawaii J. Med. Public Health* **2016**, *75*, 291–294.
23. Sachu, A.; Madhavan, A.; Vasudevan, A.; Vasudevapanicker, J. Prevalence of dengue and leptospirosis co-infection in a tertiary care hospital in South India. *Iran J. Microbiol.* **2018**, *10*, 227–232. [PubMed]
24. Sonthayanon, P.; Chierakul, W.; Wuthiekanun, V.; Limmathurotsakul, D.; Amornchai, P.; Smythe, L.D.; Day, N.P.; Peacock, S.J. Molecular confirmation of co-infection by pathogenic *Leptospira* spp. and Orientia tsutsugamushi in patients with acute febrile illness in Thailand. *Am. J. Trop. Med. Hyg.* **2013**, *89*, 797–799. [CrossRef] [PubMed]
25. Bratsch, N.; Fernandes, L.G.V.; Busch, J.D.; Pearson, T.; Rivera-Garcia, S.; Soltero, F.; Galloway, R.; Sahl, J.W.; Nally, J.E.; Wagner, D.M. Diverse lineages of pathogenic *Leptospira* species are widespread in the environment in Puerto Rico, USA. *PLoS Negl. Trop. Dis.* **2022**, *16*, e0009959. [CrossRef]
26. Vincent, A.T.; Schiettekatte, O.; Goarant, C.; Neela, V.K.; Bernet, E.; Thibeaux, R.; Ismail, N.; Mohd Khalid, M.K.N.; Amran, F.; Masuzawa, T.; et al. Revisiting the taxonomy and evolution of pathogenicity of the genus *Leptospira* through the prism of genomics. *PLoS Negl. Trop. Dis.* **2019**, *13*, e0007270. [CrossRef] [PubMed]
27. Bourhy, P.; Collet, L.; Brisse, S.; Picardeau, M. *Leptospira mayottensis* sp. nov., a pathogenic species of the genus *Leptospira* isolated from human. *Int. J. Syst. Evol. Microbiol.* **2014**, *64*, 4061–4067. [CrossRef] [PubMed]
28. Kumbhare, M.R.; Surana, A.R.; Arote, R.A.; Borse, G.D. Current status of Leptospirosis: A zoonotic tropical disease. *Int. J. Microbiol. Curr. Res.* **2019**, *1*, 14–19. [CrossRef]
29. Slack, A.T.; Symonds, M.L.; Dohnt, M.F.; Corney, B.G.; Smythe, L.D. Epidemiology of *Leptospira weilii* serovar Topaz infections in Australia. *Commun. Dis. Intell.* **2007**, *31*, 216–222.
30. Boonsilp, S.; Thaipadungpanit, J.; Amornchai, P.; Wuthiekanun, V.; Bailey, M.S.; Holden, M.T.G.; Zhang, C.C.; Jiang, X.G.; Koizumi, N.B.; Taylor, K.; et al. A single multilocus sequence typing (MLST) scheme for seven pathogenic *Leptospira* species. *PLoS Negl. Trop. Dis.* **2013**, *7*, e1954. [CrossRef]

31. Evangelista, K.V.; Coburn, J. Leptospira as an emerging pathogen: A review of its biology, pathogenesis and host immune responses. *Future Microbiol.* **2010**, *5*, 1413–1425. [CrossRef]
32. Nahori, M.A.; Fournié-Amazouz, E.; Que-Gewirth, N.S.; Balloy, V.; Chignard, M.; Raetz, C.R.; Saint Girons, I.; Werts, C. Differential TLR recognition of leptospiral lipid A and lipopolysaccharide in murine and human cells. *J. Immunol.* **2005**, *175*, 6022–6031. [CrossRef]
33. Samrot, A.V.; Sean, T.C.; Bhavya, K.S.; Sahithya, C.S.; Chan-Drasekaran, S.; Palanisamy, R.; Robinson, E.R.; Subbiah, S.K.; Mok, P.L. *Leptospiral* infection, pathogenesis and its diagnosis—A review. *Pathogens* **2021**, *10*, 145. [CrossRef] [PubMed]
34. Vieira, M.L.; Teixeira, A.F.; Pidde, G.; Ching, A.T.C.; Tambourgi, D.V.; Nascimento, A.L.T.O.; Herwald, H. *Leptospira interrogans* outer membrane protein LipL21 is a potent inhibitor of neutrophil myeloperoxidase. *Virulence* **2018**, *9*, 414–425. [CrossRef] [PubMed]
35. Fernandes, L.G.V.; Hornsby, R.L.; Nascimento, A.L.T.O.; Nally, J.E. Genetic manipulation of pathogenic Leptospira: CRISPR interference (CRISPRi)-mediated gene silencing and rapid mutant recovery at 37 °C. *Sci. Rep.* **2021**, *11*, 1768. [CrossRef] [PubMed]
36. Hsu, S.H.; Hung, C.C.; Chang, M.Y.; Ko, Y.C.; Yang, H.Y.; Hsu, H.H.; Tian, Y.C.; Chou, L.F.; Pan, R.L.; Tseng, F.G.; et al. Active components of *Leptospira* outer membrane protein LipL32 to toll-like receptor 2. *Sci. Rep.* **2017**, *7*, 8363. [CrossRef]
37. Takahashi, M.B.; Teixeira, A.F.; Nascimento, A.L.T.O. The leptospiral LipL21 and LipL41 proteins exhibit a broad spectrum of interactions with host cell components. *Virulence* **2021**, *12*, 2798–2813. [CrossRef]
38. Haake, D.A.; Zuckert, W.R. The leptospiral outer membrane. *Curr. Top. Microbiol. Immunol.* **2015**, *387*, 187–221. [CrossRef]
39. Dezhbord, M.; Esmaelizad, M.; Khaki, P.; Fotohi, F.; Moghaddam, A.Z. Molecular identification of the ompL1 gene within *Leptospira interrogans* standard serovars. *J. Infect. Dev. Ctries.* **2014**, *8*, 688–693. [CrossRef]
40. Yap, M.L.; Sekawi, Z.; Chee, H.Y.; Alan Ong, H.K.; Neela, V.K. Comparative analysis of current diagnostic PCR assays in detecting pathogenic *Leptospira* isolates from environmental samples. *Asian. Pac. J. Trop. Med.* **2019**, *12*, 472–478. [CrossRef]
41. Natarajaseenivasana, K.; Vijayacharib, P.; Sharmab, S.; Sugunanb, A.P.; Vedhagiria, K.; Selvina, J.; Sehgalb, S.C. FlaB PCR-based identification of pathogenic leptospiral isolates. *J. Microbiol. Immunol. Infect.* **2010**, *43*, 62–69. [CrossRef]
42. Chin, V.K.; Lee, T.Y.; Lim, W.F.; Wan Shahriman, Y.W.Y.; Syafinaz, A.N.; Zamberi, S.; Maha, A. Leptospirosis in human: Biomarkers in host immune responses. *Microbiol. Res.* **2018**, *207*, 108–115. [CrossRef]
43. Hernández-González, I.L.; Mateo-Estrada, V.; Castillo-Ramirez, S. The promiscuous and highly mobile resistome of *Acinetobacter baumannii*. *Microb. Genom.* **2022**, *8*, 000762. [CrossRef] [PubMed]
44. Lindsay, J.A. *Staphylococcus aureus* genomics and the impact of horizontal gene transfer. *Int. J. Med. Microbiol.* **2014**, *304*, 103–109. [CrossRef] [PubMed]
45. Verma, J.; Bag, S.; Saha, B.; Kumar, P.; Ghosh, T.S.; Dayal, M.; Senapati, T.; Mehra, S.; Dey, P.; Desigamani, A.; et al. Genomic plasticity associated with antimicrobial resistance in *Vibrio cholerae*. *Proc. Natl. Acad. Sci. USA* **2019**, *116*, 6226–6231. [CrossRef] [PubMed]

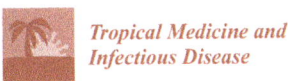 

*Brief Report*

# SARS-CoV-2 Infections in a High-Risk Migratory Population Arriving to a Migrant House along the US-Mexico Border

Nadia A. Fernández-Santos [1,2], Gabriel L. Hamer [2], Edith G. Garrido-Lozada [3] and Mario A. Rodríguez-Pérez [1,*]

1. Instituto Politécnico Nacional, Centro de Biotecnología Genómica, Reynosa 88710, Mexico
2. Department of Entomology, Texas A&M University, College Station, TX 77843, USA
3. Daughters of Charity of Saint Vincent de Paul (La Casa del Migrante), Reynosa 88520, Mexico
* Correspondence: mrodriguez@ipn.mx; Tel.: +52-899-9243627 (ext. 87719)

**Abstract:** Few reports exist on the COVID-19 epidemiology of migrant populations. We tested 370 migratory individuals from ten countries arriving at a migrant house along the US–Mexico border based on a rapid assay detecting SARS-CoV-2 antigen. Fifty-six were positive, for a prevalence of 15.1% (95%–CIs of 11.8–19.2%). Only 21 positive persons presented signs or symptoms associated with the infection (95%–CIs = 25–49%). Most (51.7%) positive migrants arrived in the previous two days before being tested, indicating that the virus infection was acquired during their transit. Out of the total of 56 positive individuals, 37.5% were from El Salvador, 33.9% from Honduras, and 21.4% from Guatemala. This study suggests that vulnerable populations traveling from countries in Latin America and seeking residence in the US are high-risk individuals for exposure to SARS-CoV-2. The rapid antigen COVID-19 testing on arrival at the migrant house, and subsequent 10-day quarantine, was a critical step to help minimize further transmission. Therefore, the present study demonstrates that public health services provided to migratory and vulnerable populations are necessary for pandemic control.

**Keywords:** COVID-19; SARS-CoV-2; México; migrants; infectious diseases; prevention

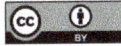

## 1. Introduction

The COVID-19 pandemic declared by the World Health Organization (WHO) on March 11, 2020, put the entire world in an unprecedented health crisis, which has led to a state of persistent uncertainty [1]. The groups most seriously affected by this health crisis are migrants and refugees, due to the increase in inequalities generated by the pandemic [2,3]. COVID-19 has emerged in a world closely connected with local and international population movements and with a greater number of people who move for work, education, family, tourism, and survival [4]. Migratory movements are dynamic and result from fundamental demographic, social, cultural, and economic phenomena that shape the local context where the pandemic, residents, and migrants co-exist [5]. Furthermore, geographic and geopolitical position, relative level of wealth, and international connections make some countries attractive destinations for migrant workers, international students, asylum seekers, and refugees [6]. The high number of migrants in these attractive countries underscores the specific need to include migrants in response and recovery efforts from the effects of COVID-19.

Organized caravans of persons from Central American countries traveling from southern to northern Mexico [7] results in many migrants being barred for months, and even years, at the borders of the different countries of origin and destination [8,9]. In this context of temporary housing, often in high densities, the transmission of SARS-CoV-2, the agent of COVID-19, can be high among resident and migrant populations. The COVID-19 problem is further exacerbated in migrant shelters, given the unsanitary conditions that prohibit basic preventive health measures. Migrants do not practice social distancing; there is absent or low coverage of face masks, no proper washing or regular hand washing, and little or no use of disinfectants, so the risk of exposure to SARS-CoV-2 is high in these populations [10,11]. In Mexico, as well as in other countries with a migrant population, support work for migrants is challenging; migrants often sleep in crowded closed dormitories with poor or no ventilation and sanitation, work illegally without decent conditions, or experience severe mobility restrictions, under different levels of scrutiny and/or facing public suspicion, even opprobrium, in a foreign country [10,12,13]. The Mexican Immigration Policy Unit (Registration and Identity of Persons) reported the delivery of 66,685 visitor cards for humanitarian reasons during 2020 at 2022 (March) [14]. Multiple entries are given through Tapachula city in Chiapas to migrants traveling mostly in caravans. From 2020 to March 2022, US Customs and Border Protection detected 3,488,674 undocumented immigrants on the border with Mexico [15]. In 2021, Mexico became the third country in the world to receive the largest number of new asylum applications [16]. People from various countries, including Haiti, countries in Central America, Venezuela, Cuba, the African continent, and elsewhere, submitted 562,549 asylum applications [16].

Those migrants, asylum seekers, and US deportees converge and concentrate mostly in 90 shelters run commonly by local government, religious, and non-governmental organizations (NGOs) located along nine northern Mexico cities: Ciudad Juarez, Mexicali, Reynosa, Nuevo Laredo, Rio Bravo, Matamoros, Nogales, Piedras Negras, and Tijuana [17], which are reference point areas of convergence and transit of the different demographic groups. Annually, Mexicans and ca. 50 other nationalities looking for temporary residence seek these destinations with the ultimate goal of reaching different cities in the US. Additionally, shelters in the Mexican territory are also receptor centers of US-expelled people (deportees) coming by land mainly from the nine processing offices of the US Southwest Customs and Border Protection Office of the Department of the Homeland Security [15]. These non-permanent people, which number in the thousands every year, are considered among the most vulnerable individuals in the social fabric of the border population, and this long interchange of people on both sides of the US-Mexico border creates a high risk for SARS-CoV-2 transmission.

The metropolitan city of Reynosa is the location of "The Migrant House" (TMH), which is run by the Daughters of Charity of Saint Vincent de Paul. This house offers a dignified and safe place to migrants who arrive in Reynosa, providing them with free basic services during their stay, such as food, clothing, personal hygiene items, telephone calls, medical attention, psychological attention, paperwork, and administration of personal documents. Within these facilities, a "Médecins Sans Frontières" (MSF) team provides medical and psychological consultations to this migrant population, but it also does so along its migratory route, prioritizing assistance to the most vulnerable groups. Likewise, other NGOs work for and with the migrants of this house. Due to the COVID-19 pandemic, they were forced to remain, indeterminately, in Reynosa. Migrants must cohabit in large groups of up to 20 people per dwelling; likewise, the temporary jobs to which they have access are of high risk for them and the local population. For example, cleaning the windshields of cars at traffic lights inso Reynosa is one form of income. This is in addition to the high-risk situation for COVID-19, since the Reynosa municipality officially presents the highest number of COVID-19 cases in Tamaulipas. As of 9 August 2022, the official figures in Reynosa were 24,388 confirmed cases of COVID-19 with 1628 deaths, which represents 14% and 20.4% of the total confirmed cases and deaths, respectively, for Tamaulipas [18]. During 2019–2022, TMH in Reynosa sheltered over 11,000 migrants; out of these, 10,548 were Mexicans, and 883 were from other countries. In total, 88% percent of the migrant population was male, and the remaining 12% was female and minors.

## 2. Materials and Methods

The study was carried out at "The Migrant House" (26°05′49.8″ N; 98°17′12.0″ W) in Reynosa, México. This was a cross-sectional study conducted from August to November, 2021 [19]. The inclusion criteria were all migrants, excluding newborns less than one year old. Eligible people arriving to TMH were continuously recruited to participate in the study and sampled until test supplies were exhausted (370 total migrants). A rapid lateral flow assay detecting SARS-CoV-2 antigen (PANBIO Covid-19 Ag rapid test; Abbott Laboratories de Mexico, S.A. de C.V. No. 41FK10) with nasopharyngeal swabs was used by health workers to test migrants. The specificity and sensitivity of this rapid test has been estimated by the manufacturer at 91.4 % (94.1 % for samples showing Ct-values = $\leq$33) and 99.8%, respectively (vs. nasopharyngeal PCR) [20]. However, the sensitivity may vary depending upon the time of testing and days from the onset of symptoms. Thus, a prevalence of 10.4% and sensitivity of 79.6% (95%–CIs = 67.0–88.8%) was reported when 412 symptomatic patients of healthcare centers in Spain were tested with the PANBIO rapid test [21].

We tested migrants on arrival to TMH; if the person tested positive, they were required to isolate for a 10-day quarantine period outside the communal environment per local health authorities. This strategy allowed TMH to continue to provide essential services to migrants while minimizing SARS-CoV-2 transmission, as migrants showed active and recent infections with SARS-CoV-2. The present study was conducted during the third COVID-19 "wave" in Mexico, when the incidence rate in Tamaulipas was 1.09% (maximum incidence of 3.39% in Mexico city) [19].

Statistical analysis. The 95% exact Bayes confidence intervals (95%–CIs) surrounding the point estimate of the COVID-19 prevalence was calculated as previously reported [22].

## 3. Results

We tested 370 migrants from ten countries, including 35.9% from Honduras, 26.4% from El Salvador, 18.3% from Guatemala, and 12.9% from Mexico (plus 1.6% from TMH staff). The other countries (Nicaragua, Venezuela, Haiti, United States, Colombia, and Ecuador) were less abundant, ranging from 0.2% to 1%. Of the 370 tested, 56 were positive to the antigen test (prevalence of 15.1%; 95%–CIs of 11.8–19.2%; Table 1). The refusal rate was 0.81%, as only three migrants were reluctant to participate and were, therefore, not admitted to enter the TMH.

Table 1. Percentages of migrants from 10 countries examined and tested positive for SARS-CoV-2.

| Country | No. Examined | % in Relation to Total Examined | No. Positives | % in Relation to Total Positives | % of No. Positives/Examined per Country |
|---|---|---|---|---|---|
| Colombia | 2 | 0.5 | 1 | 1.8 | 50.0 |
| Venezuela | 4 | 1.0 | 1 | 1.8 | 25.0 |
| El Salvador | 98 | 26.4 | 21 | 37.5 | 21.4 |
| Guatemala | 68 | 18.3 | 12 | 21.4 | 17.6 |
| Honduras | 133 | 35.9 | 19 | 33.9 | 14.2 |
| Mexico | 48 | 12.9 | 2 | 3.6 | 4.1 |
| Mexico (TMH *) | 6 | 1.6 | 0 | 0 | 0.0 |
| Nicaragua | 4 | 1.0 | 0 | 0 | 0.0 |
| Haití | 3 | 0.8 | 0 | 0 | 0.0 |
| USA | 3 | 0.8 | 0 | 0 | 0.0 |
| Ecuador | 1 | 0.2 | 0 | 0 | 0.0 |
| Total | 370 | 100 | 56 | 100 | 15.1 |

* TMH = The Migrant House staff.

The percent of migrants that tested positive by nationality ranged from 0% to 50%. By country of origin, we observed 50% prevalence (1 positive of 2 tested) of the individuals from Colombia, 25% from Venezuela (1 of 4), 21.4% from El Salvador (21 of 98), 17.6% from Guatemala (12 of 68), 14.2% from Honduras (19 of 133), and 4.17% from México (2 of 48). The other countries (Nicaragua, Haiti, United States, and Ecuador) and TMH staff had no positive cases of the people tested (Table 1). Thus, the top four positive for SARS-CoV-2 were: 21 people (37.5% of total positives) from El Salvador, 19 (33.9%) from Honduras, 12

(21.4%) from Guatemala, and 2 (3.6%) from Mexico. Only one person (1.8%) tested positive from the four and two people examined from Venezuela and Colombia, respectively.

Of the migrants positive for the SARS-CoV-2 antigen test, only 21 persons presented signs or symptoms associated with the infection (95%–CIs = 25–49%); the remaining 63% of positive persons were asymptomatic. The migrants testing positive by age group were as follows: children between 0 and 20 years old, 18.4% ($n$ = 163); followed by adults between 21 and 50 years old, 13.1% ($n$ = 199); and elderly people between 51 and 70, 0% ($n$ = 8). By gender, 135 and 235 men and female were examined, of which 25 and 31 were positive, respectively (Table 2).

**Table 2.** Testing results (no. of positives/no. of examined) for SARS-CoV-2 antigen in nasopharyngeal swabs of migrants arriving to "The Migrant House" in Reynosa, Mexico, according to country of origin, gender, and age group.

| Country | Males | Females | 0–20 Years Old | 21–50 Years Old | 51–70 Years Old |
|---|---|---|---|---|---|
| Honduras | 7/42 (31.1) | 12/91 (38.7) | 10/59 (16.9) | 9/72 (13) | 0/2 (0.0) |
| El Salvador | 7/30 (22.2) | 14/68 (28.9) | 14/48 (29.1) | 7/49 (14) | 0/1 (0.0) |
| Guatemala | 7/28 (20.7) | 5/40 (17) | 6/30 (20) | 6/37 (16) | 0/1 (0.0) |
| Mexico | 2/21 (15.6) | 0/27 (11.5) | 0/17 (0.0) | 2/28 (7.1) | 0/3 (0.0) |
| Venezuela | 1/4 (3) | ND | ND | 1/3 (33.3) | 0/1 (0.0) |
| Haití | 0/3 (2.2) | ND | ND | 0/3 (0.0) | ND |
| Mexico (TMH *) | 0/2 (1.5) | 0/4 (1.7) | 0/3 (0.0) | 0/3 (0.0) | ND |
| Colombia | 1/2 (1.5) | ND | ND | 1/2 (50) | ND |
| Ecuador | 0/1 (0.7) | ND | 0/1 (0.0) | ND | ND |
| Nicaragua | 0/1 (0.7) | 0/3 (1.3) | 0/2 (0.0) | 0/2 (0.0) | ND |
| USA | 0/1 (0.7) | 0/2 (0.9) | 0/3 (0.0) | ND | ND |

* TMH = The Migrant House staff. ND = no data (no individuals in this category).

Most (51.7%) positive migrants arrived to Reynosa within two days of being tested (Figure 1), suggesting that exposure to SARS-CoV-2 occurred during travel from their country of origin. The average amount of time for migrants to travel from southern to northern Mexico is 24 to 72 h according to the answers of 60 migrants, who responded to standardized questionnaires (unpublished data), which includes the incubation period for the delta variant, the most predominant variant of concern circulating in Mexico during this study [23,24].

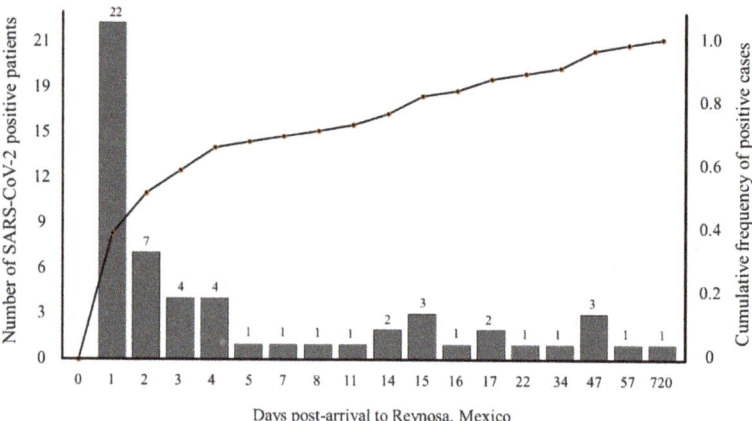

**Figure 1.** Cumulative frequency of the number of individual migrants arriving to "The Migrant House" in Reynosa, Mexico, that tested positive SARS-CoV-2 antigen at different days post-arrival.

Integrated health services supported by the network of TMH, MSF, and NGOs are paramount to improving access to rapid free tests in vulnerable populations [25], because testing for virus infection is critical to detecting COVID-19 cases for quarantine and contact tracing, as well as for providing medical care. Undoubtedly, migrants are a high-risk population for virus infection; it has been reported that migrants are disproportionately represented among COVID-19 cases and deaths. Risk factors for migrants include high-risk occupations, overcrowding, and barriers to healthcare, including imprecise information, languages, and limited human rights [26]. For example, in Saudi Arabia and Singapore, low-skilled migrant workers in crowded dormitories showed that 75 and 95%, respectively, of all newly confirmed cases were among migrants, and 93% of total cases were associated with migrants' dormitories in Singapore [27]. Although migrants depend heavily upon services of lodging, food, and medical care provided by the charitable network of TMH, MSF, and NGOs in Reynosa, this network lacks sufficient resources to provide all the needed services. The current scenario for migrants in northern border cities is worrisome, as expulsions from the US are ongoing. In addition, migrants seeking asylum in the US travel from Tapachula, a southern Mexico border city, to US–Mexico border cities. Here, the needs of migrants overwhelm the capacity of local health authorities and NGOs [28]. The emergence of new SARS-CoV-2 variants of concern will likely continue to result in epidemic waves. Thus, there is an urgent need to enhance medical care for this migrant population. Further studies are needed to confirm the role of migratory populations relative to resident populations in the spread of SARS-CoV-2 and similar emerging infectious diseases.

A limitation of the current study is that we were unable to confirm exactly when and where prior exposure to SARS-CoV-2 occurred for the migrants arriving to TMH in Reynosa. While we report variation among populations of migrants coming from different countries of origin, this prevalence does not necessarily reflect infection from the country of origin, and instead could reflect variation in the risk of exposure to SARS-CoV-2 during transport or staging in different locations along the route to the US.

## 4. Conclusions

Here, we tested 370 migrants from ten countries arriving at the US–Mexico border, and 56 tested positive for the SARS-CoV-2 antigen, which triggered a quarantine protocol to limit further spread. Thus, the present study documents a screening protocol of individuals arriving at TMH to guide actions for the prevention and control of SARS-CoV-2. Diagnostic rapid free testing for migratory populations is important for providing public health services to vulnerable populations that could contribute to SARS-CoV-2 spread [23].

**Author Contributions:** Conceptualization, N.A.F.-S. and M.A.R.-P.; methodology, N.A.F.-S. and E.G.G.-L.; validation, N.A.F.-S. and E.G.G.-L.; formal analysis, M.A.R.-P. and G.L.H.; investigation, N.A.F.-S.; resources, N.A.F.-S. and E.G.G.-L.; writing—original draft preparation, N.A.F.-S. and M.A.R.-P.; writing—review and editing, N.A.F.-S., M.A.R.-P. and G.L.H.; supervision, N.A.F.-S. and E.G.G.-L.; project administration, N.A.F.-S. and E.G.G.-L.; funding acquisition, N.A.F.-S., E.G.G.-L. and G.L.H. All authors have read and agreed to the published version of the manuscript.

**Funding:** This research was funded by Instituto Politécnico Nacional-Secretaría de Investigación y Posgrado, small-grant numbers 20210581, 20220163, and 20220299, and Texas A&M AgriLife Research.

**Institutional Review Board Statement:** The study was conducted in accordance with the Declaration of Helsinki and approved by the Ethics Committee of Escuela Nacional de Medicina y Homeopatía from Instituto Politécnico Nacional, Mexico (protocol code CBE/006/2020 and date of approval 21 December 2020), for studies involving humans.

**Informed Consent Statement:** Patient written consent was waived due to the SARS-CoV-2 test being compulsory for migrants to be admitted to The Migrant House. Instead, the Health Secretariat of México approved the use of oral consent, because the study was part of a routine public health national COVID-19 testing program conducted by the Mexican government. Meetings were held between TMN and Sanitary Jurisdiction No. IV of Reynosa to report that this testing activity was being carried out, and the information was provided to the jurisdiction.

**Acknowledgments:** We thank Francisco Gallardo, Father in Charge of Human Mobility in the Diocese, and Sor Maria Tello Claro, Director of The Migrant House, Daughters of Charity of Saint Vincent de Paul, for approval of the present study. We also thank Bernadita L. Reyes Berrones, Director of the State Laboratory of Public Health, Tamaulipas, Secretariate of Health, for advising on the test used here. We acknowledge Ariana Yaneth Fernández-Velázquez for designing the graphical abstract.

**Conflicts of Interest:** The authors declare no conflict of interest.

## References

1. World Health Organization (WHO). Coronavirus Disease (COVID-19) Pandemic. 2022. Available online: https://www.who.int (accessed on 19 September 2022).
2. Singh, A.K.; Gillies, C.L.; Singh, R.; Singh, A.; Chudasama, Y.; Coles, B.; Seidu, S.; Zaccardi, F.; Davies, M.J.; Khunti, K. Prevalence of co-morbidities and their association with mortality in patients with COVID-19: A systematic review and meta-analysis. *Diabetes Obes. Metab.* **2022**, *10*, 1915–1924. [CrossRef] [PubMed]
3. World Health Organization (WHO). Strengthening COVID-19 Vaccine Demand and Uptake in Refugees and Migrants: An Operational Guide to Support All Those Responsible for Planning and Implementing the Rollout of COVID-19 Vaccine to Refugees and Migrants at National and Local Levels. 14 March 2022. Available online: https://apps.who.int/iris/handle/10665/352415 (accessed on 19 September 2022).
4. Skeldon, R. *International migration, internal migration, mobility and urbanization: Towards more integrated approaches*; Migration Research Series No 53; International Organization for Migration (IOM); Geneva United Nations: New York, NY, USA, 2018.
5. International Organization for Migration (IOM). Migrants and the COVID-19 Pandemic: An Initial Analysis 2020. Available online: https://publications.iom.int/system/files/pdf/mrs-60.pdf (accessed on 19 September 2022).
6. IOM. World Migration Report. 2020. Available online: https://publications.iom.int/system/files/pdf/wmr_2020.pdf (accessed on 19 September 2022).
7. Milenio Digital (Milenio Diario, SA de CV) ¿Cuántas Caravanas Migrantes hay en México? Available online: https://www.milenio.com/estados/cuantas-caravanas-migrantes-hay-en-mexico-en-2021 (accessed on 19 September 2022).
8. Marschke, M.; Vandergeest, P.; Havice, E.; Kadfak, A.; Duker, P.; Isopescu, I.; MacDonnell, M. COVID-19, instability and migrant fish workers in Asia. *Marit. Stud.* **2021**, *20*, 87–99. [CrossRef] [PubMed]
9. Daniels, J.P. Venezuelan migrants "struggling to survive" amid COVID-19. *Lancet* **2020**, *395*, 1023. [CrossRef]
10. Bojorquez-Chapela, I.; Strathdee, S.A.; Garfein, R.S.; Benson, C.A.; Chaillon, A.; Ignacio, C.; Sepulveda, J. The impact of the COVID-19 pandemic among migrants in shelters in Tijuana, Baja California, Mexico. *BMJ Glob. Health* **2022**, *7*, e007202. [CrossRef] [PubMed]
11. Chander, M.; Rathod, P. Reorienting priorities of extension and advisory services in India during and post COVID-19 pandemic: A review. *Indian J. Ext. Educ.* **2020**, *56*, 1–9.
12. Suphanchaimat, R.; Pudpong, N.; Tangcharoensathien, V. Extreme exploitation in Southeast Asia waters: Challenges in progressing towards universal health coverage for migrant workers. *PLoS Med.* **2017**, *14*, e1002341. [CrossRef] [PubMed]
13. Platt, M.; Baey, G.; Yeoh, B.S.; Khoo, C.Y.; Lam, T. Debt, precarity and gender: Male and female temporary labour migrants in Singapore. *J. Ethn. Migr. Stud.* **2017**, *43*, 119–136. [CrossRef]
14. Gobierno de Mexico. Boletin Mensual de Estadisticas Migratorias 2022. Available online: http://portales.segob.gob.mx/es/PoliticaMigratoria/Boletines_Estadisticos (accessed on 19 September 2022).
15. U.S. Customs and Border Protection. Southwest Land Border Encounters. Available online: https://www.cbp.gov/newsroom/stats/southwest-land-border-encounters (accessed on 19 September 2022).
16. The UN Refugee Agency (UNHCR). Reporting Mexico 2021. Available online: https://reporting.unhcr.org/mexico (accessed on 19 September 2022).
17. El Colegio de la Frontera Norte (COLEF). Sedes Mexico 2020. Available online: https://www.colef.mx/sedes/ (accessed on 19 September 2022).
18. Gobierno del Estado de Tamaulipas. Situacion Geografica del Coronavirus 2022. Available online: https://coronavirus.tamaulipas.gob.mx/situacion-geografica-del-coronavirus/1 (accessed on 19 September 2022).
19. Gobierno de Mexico. Comprehensive Report on COVID-19 in Mexico, Numero 03-2022-9 de febrero 2022. Available online: https://coronavirus.gob.mx/wp-content/uploads/2022/02/Info-03-22-Int_COVID-19_16feb22.pdf (accessed on 19 September 2022).
20. PANBIO™ COVID-19 AG RAPID TEST DEVICE. Available online: https://www.globalpointofcare.abbott/es/product-details/panbio-covid-19-ag-antigen-test.html (accessed on 19 September 2022).
21. Albert, E.; Torres, I.; Bueno, F.; Huntley, D.; Molla, E.; Fernández-Fuentes, M.Á.; Martínez, M.; Poujois, S.; Forqué, L.; Valdivia, A.; et al. Field evaluation of a rapid antigen test (Panbio™ COVID-19 Ag Rapid Test Device) for COVID-19 diagnosis in primary healthcare centres. *Clin. Microbiol. Infect.* **2021**, *27*, 472.e7–472.e10. [CrossRef] [PubMed]

22. Armitage, P.; Berry, G. *Statistical Methods in Medical Research*, 3rd ed.; Blackwell Scientific Publications, Oxford: Boston, MA, USA, 1994.
23. Gobierno de Mexico. Genomic Surveillance Report of the SARS-CoV-2 Virus in Mexico National and State Distribution of Variants as of 30 August 2021. Available online: https://coronavirus.gob.mx/wp-content/uploads/2021/09/2021.08.30_ReporteVariantesCOVID-2.pdf (accessed on 19 September 2022).
24. Gobierno de Mexico. Genomic Surveillance Report of the SARS-CoV-2 Virus in Mexico National and State Distribution of Variants as of 18 October 2021. Available online: https://coronavirus.gob.mx/wp-content/uploads/2021/10/2021.10.18_ReporteVariantesCOVID_InDRE.pdf (accessed on 19 September 2022).
25. Yeager, S.; Abramovitz, D.; Harvey-Vera, A.Y.; Vera, C.F.; Algarin, A.B.; Smith, L.R.; Rangel, G.; Artamonova, I.; Patterson, T.L.; Bazzi, A.R.; et al. A cross-sectional study of factors associated with COVID-19 testing among people who inject drugs: Missed opportunities for reaching those most at risk. *BMC Public Health* **2022**, *22*, 842. [CrossRef]
26. Hayward, S.E.; Deal, A.; Cheng, C.; Crawshaw, A.; Orcutt, M.; Vandrevala, T.F.; Norredam, M.; Carballo, M.; Ciftci, Y.; Requena-Méndez, A.; et al. Clinical outcomes and risk factors for COVID-19 among migrant populations in high-income countries: A systematic review. *J. Migr. Health* **2021**, *3*, 100041. [CrossRef]
27. Migration Data Relevant for the COVID-19 Pandemic (Last Updated 1 April 2022). Available online: https://www.migrationdataportal.org/themes/migration-data-relevant-covid-19-pandemic#:~{}:text=Assuming%20zero%2Dgrowth%20in%20the,(UN%20DESA%2C%202020) (accessed on 19 September 2022).
28. Médecins Sans Frontières (Press Release 11 July 2022). Available online: https://www.msf.org/more-assistance-urgently-needed-people-arriving-mexico-northern-border-cities (accessed on 19 September 2022).

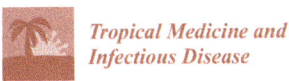

*Systematic Review*

# Prevalence and Characteristics of Malaria and Influenza Co-Infection in Febrile Patients: A Systematic Review and Meta-Analysis

Polrat Wilairatana [1,†], Wanida Mala [2,†], Kwuntida Uthaisar Kotepui [2] and Manas Kotepui [2,*]

1. Department of Clinical Tropical Medicine, Faculty of Tropical Medicine, Mahidol University, Bangkok 10400, Thailand
2. Medical Technology, School of Allied Health Sciences, Walailak University, Tha Sala, Nakhon Si Thammarat 80160, Thailand
* Correspondence: manas.ko@wu.ac.th; Tel.: +66-954392469
† These authors contributed equally to this work.

**Abstract:** Malaria and influenza are co-endemic in several geographical areas, and differentiation of their clinical features is difficult. The present study aimed to qualitatively and quantitatively analyze the prevalence and characteristics of malaria and influenza co-infection in febrile patients. The systematic review was registered at PROSPERO (CRD42021264525). Relevant literature that reported malaria and influenza co-infection in febrile patients were searched in PubMed, Web of Science, and Scopus from 20 June to 27 June 2021 and the risk of bias for each study was assessed. Quantitative analysis included pooled prevalence, and the odds of malaria and influenza virus co-infection among febrile patients were estimated using a random-effects model. Subgroup analyses were performed to summarize the effect estimate for each group. Funnel plot, Egger's test, and contour-enhanced funnel plot were used to demonstrate any publication bias among outcomes of included studies. Among 4253 studies retrieved, 10 studies that enrolled 22,066 febrile patients with 650 co-infected patients were included for qualitative and quantitative syntheses. The pooled prevalence of malaria and influenza virus co-infection among febrile patients was 31.0% in Nigeria, 1.0% in Tanzania, 1.0% in Uganda, 1.0% in Malawi, 1.0% in Ghana, 0% in Cambodia, 7.0% in the Central African Republic, and 7.0% in Kenya. Meta-analysis also showed co-infection occurrence by chance ($p = 0.097$, odds ratio 0.54, 95% CI 0.26–1.12, $I^2$ 94.9%). The prevalence of malaria and influenza virus co-infection among febrile patients was heterogeneous by country, characteristics of febrile participants, and diagnostic tests for influenza virus. Further studies should investigate severe clinical manifestations or differentiate clinical outcomes between mono-infected or co-infected individuals, whether the co-infection leads to severe disease outcome.

**Keywords:** malaria; *Plasmodium*; influenza; co-infection

## 1. Background

Malaria remains a major cause of death in children younger than 5 years old who live in Africa According to the World Health Organization (WHO), more than 241 million malaria cases and 558,000 deaths were reported, almost all (95%) in African countries, while 2% of malaria cases were reported in the WHO South-East Asia Region, and the remaining 3% from other regions [1]. The major cause of malaria in Africa was *Plasmodium falciparum*, although *P. vivax* malaria was also reported, albeit this is less endemic than *P. falciparum* owing to Duffy-negative populations in Africa. Nevertheless, recent evidence suggested that *P. vivax* can infect Duffy-negative individuals [2–4], and substantial epidemiological evidence suggests *P. vivax* as a cause of severe malaria [5–7]. In contrast to *P. falciparum* and *P. vivax*, a small number of patients develop severe complications derived from *Plasmodium* mixed infection [8], *Plasmodium ovale* [9], or *Plasmodium malariae* [10].

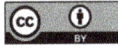

Influenza is an infectious respiratory disease caused by the influenza virus. In humans, severe disease and seasonal epidemics are mostly caused by influenza viruses A and B [11,12]. Previous studies reported the high incidence of influenza in Africa in Nigeria, Tanzania, Kenya, the Central African Republic, and Malawi [11,13,14]. At least 3 million severe influenza cases have been reported, with 290,000 to 650,000 deaths annually [15]. Transmission can occur by direct contact with aerosols and droplets through coughing and sneezing. The clinical symptoms of influenza range from mild respiratory tract infection to acute/chronic disease and are similar to those of other acute febrile illnesses (AFIs), such as pneumonia, typhoid fever, and malaria [11,14]. These overlapping symptoms include fever, chills, headache, and joint and muscle pain [13,16,17]. Children younger than 5 years old are the most vulnerable to morbidity and mortality caused by infection from malaria and influenza [14]. Pregnant women also constitute a risk group for complications from influenza, caused by pregnancy-specific immune changes arising from physiological and anatomical alterations, which lead to high morbidity and mortality especially in the second and third trimesters [11].

As malaria and influenza are co-endemic in several geographical areas, it is difficult to differentiate by the clinical features of the two diseases and other AFIs. To the best of our knowledge, few data regarding the prevalence and characteristics of their co-infection have been published. Therefore, the present study aimed to qualitatively and quantitatively analyze the prevalence and characteristics of malaria and influenza co-infection in febrile patients that have been reported in the literature. The results of this study should guide further investigations of febrile patients by clinicians in co-endemic areas.

## 2. Methods

### 2.1. Protocol and Registration

The systematic review was registered at PROSPERO with the registration number CRD42021264525. Reports of systematic reviews followed the Preferred Reporting Items for Systematic Reviews and Meta-Analyses (PRISMA) statement [18].

### 2.2. Search Strategy

Search terms were constructed and checked with Medical Subject Heading (MeSH). The potentially relevant search terms were combined as "(malaria OR plasmodium OR Paludism OR "Marsh Fever" OR "Remittent Fever") AND (influenza OR flu OR Influenzas OR Grippe)" (Table S1). The searches were performed in PubMed, Web of Science, and Scopus from 20 June to 27 June 2021 with restriction to the English language but with no restriction on year of publication.

We restricted the literatures in the English language because the articles in English language provided more flexibility for study selection and data extraction by review authors.

An additional search of reference lists of the included studies and another source, Google Scholar, was also performed to assure that potentially relevant studies were not overlooked during the searches.

### 2.3. Eligibility Criteria

The eligibility criteria followed the Participants/Outcome of interest/Context (PICo) principle. P represented febrile patients, I represented co-infection of malaria and influenza virus, and Co-represented the worldwide distribution of co-infection.

Therefore, the inclusion criteria of this study were prospective or retrospective observational studies that reported the concurrent infection of malaria and influenza virus among febrile participants who were suspected of malaria or other flu-like illnesses. The exclusion criteria were non-English articles, studies that reported co-infections but data of co-infections could not be extracted, case reports, case series, letters to editors, reviews, and systematic reviews.

*2.4. Study Selection and Data Extraction*

Potentially relevant studies were selected independently by two authors (M.K. and W.M.) on the basis of eligibility criteria. Disagreements between the two authors were consensualized by another author (P.W.). The flow of study selection after studies were retrieved from databases was as follows: (1) duplicates were removed; (2) title and abstract were screened and unrelated studies were excluded; (3) full texts of studies were examined and unrelated studies were excluded with reasons given; and (4) studies that met the eligibility criteria were included for syntheses. The following data were extracted: first author, publication year, study site, study design, participants and their characteristics, numbers of co-infections, numbers of malaria cases, numbers of influenza cases, diagnostic tests for malaria, and diagnostic tests for influenza. All information was extracted into a pilot standardized datasheet before further analysis. The data extraction was performed by two authors (M.K. and W.M.), and cross-checked by another author (P.W.).

*2.5. Risk of Bias*

The risk of bias for each study was assessed using the Joanna Briggs Institute (JBI) Critical Appraisal Tools for cross-sectional study [19]. The tool assessed the risk of bias for the following eight criteria: explanation of criteria for inclusion of participants, description of subjects and the setting, measurement of exposure validity and reliability, standard criteria used for measurement of the diseases, identification of confounding factors and identification of strategy to deal with them, measurement of outcome validity and reliability, and appropriateness of statistical analysis. A total score of 8 was given to a study that met all eight criteria. Studies with scores of 7–8 indicated a low risk of bias, scores of 5–6 indicated a moderate risk of bias, and scores of less than 5 indicated a high risk of bias.

*2.6. Data Syntheses*

Data syntheses comprise qualitative and quantitative syntheses. Qualitative synthesis is the narrative explanation of data from the included studies, while quantitative synthesis is the statistical analysis of the pooled evidence. The quantitative analysis included: (1) the pooled prevalence of malaria and influenza co-infection among febrile patients; (2) the pooled prevalence of influenza virus among patients with malaria; and (3) the odds of malaria and influenza virus co-infection among febrile patients. The effect estimates and 95% confidence interval (CI) including the pooled prevalence and the pooled odds were estimated using a random-effects model (DerSimonian and Laird). The point estimates and 95% CI of each study for one outcome were visualized in a forest plot. Subgroup analyses of participants, countries, and diagnostic tests for influenza virus were performed to summarize the pooled prevalence per group. Funnel plot, Egger's test, and contour-enhanced funnel plot were used to demonstrate any publication bias among the outcomes of the included studies. All analyses were performed using Stata version 14 (StataCorp, College Station, TX, USA).

**3. Results**

*3.1. Search Results*

Among 4253 studies that were retrieved from three databases (2459 from Scopus, 901 from Web of Science, and 893 from PubMed), 1232 duplicates were removed and 3021 studies were screened for titles and abstracts. Next, 2946 unrelated studies were removed, and 75 studies were examined for full texts. Sixty-five studies were then excluded with reasons as follows: (i) 25 in which no co-infection was reported, (ii) 13 in which only malaria was reported, (iii) 11 in which only influenza was reported, (iv) 6 reviews, (v) 4 with full text unavailable, (vi) 2 knowledge assessments, (vii) 2 with non-English language, (viii) 1 systematic review, and (ix) 1 co-infection study from which data could not be extracted. Additional searches from reference lists of the included studies and Google Scholar found no other relevant studies. Therefore, ultimately, 10 studies [11,13,14,20–26] were included for qualitative and quantitative syntheses (Figure 1).

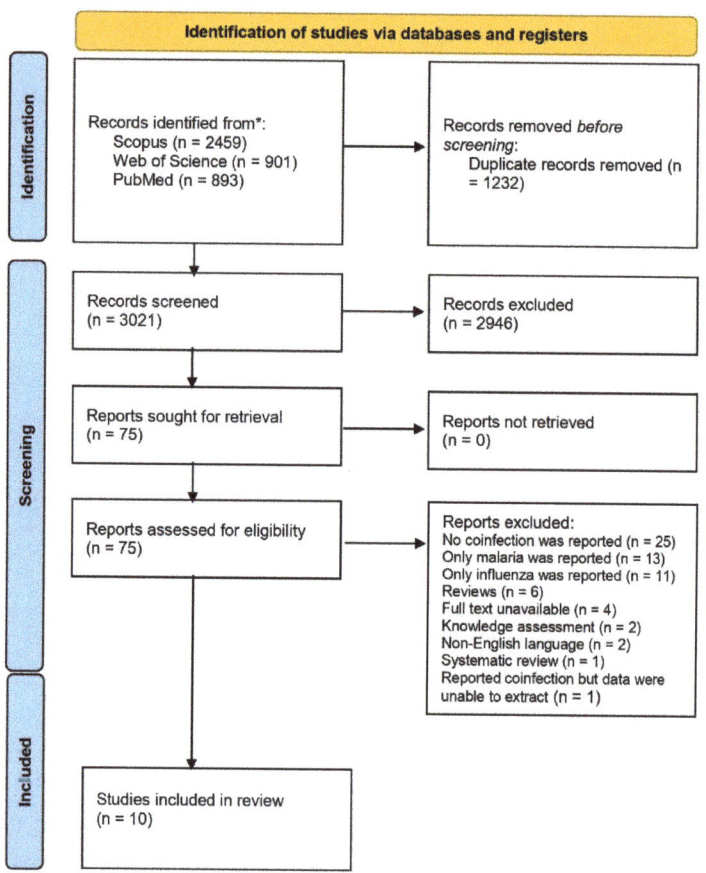

**Figure 1.** The PRISMA flow diagram showing study selection process. * mean from bibliographical databases.

*3.2. Characteristics of the Included Studies*

Characteristics of the included studies are shown in Table 1. All studies were conducted in the period 2006–2018 and published between 2012–2021. Eight studies were conducted in African countries, namely Nigeria [11], Tanzania [20,23], Uganda [21], Malawi [22], Ghana [24], the Central African Republic [13], and Kenya [14]. Two studies [25,26] were conducted in Cambodia (Figure 2). Eight studies [11,13,14,20,23–26] were observational, while two [21,22] were cohort studies. Two studies enrolled pregnant women [11,22], while other studies [14,20,24] enrolled febrile children, adults [21], and patients in all age groups [13,23,25,26]. For malaria diagnosis, five studies [14,20,22,24,25] used microscopy alone, two studies [13,21] used a rapid diagnostic test (RDT), one study [23] used RDT/microscopy, one study [26] used RDT/polymerase chain reaction (PCR), and one study [11] did not specify the diagnostic method. For influenza diagnosis, six studies [14,21,23–26] used PCR alone, one study [11] used enzyme-linked immunosorbent assay (ELISA) immunoglobulin M (IgM) alone, one study [20] used ELISA IgM/IgG/PCR, and two studies [13,22] did not specify the diagnostic method (Table 1).

Table 1. Characteristics of the included studies.

| Authors, Year | Study Site | Study Duration | Study Design | Participants | Age (Years) | Age Range (Years) | Co-Infections | Malaria Cases | Test for Malaria | Test for Influenza |
|---|---|---|---|---|---|---|---|---|---|---|
| Anjorin et al., 2020 | Nigeria | 2016–2018 | Observational study | 182 pregnant women with influenza-like illness | Median 29 | 18–45 | 56 | 56 | NS | ELISA IgM |
| Chipwaza et al., 2014 | Tanzania | 2013 | Observational study | 364 febrile children | NS | 2–13 | 1 | 83 | Microscopy | ELISA IgM, IgG, PCR |
| Cummings et al., 2021 | Uganda | 2017–2019 | Prospective cohort study | 431 febrile adults hospitalized with suspected sepsis | Median 32 | IQR: 26–42 | 3 | 58 | RDT | PCR |
| Divala et al., 2016 | Malawi | 2009–2010 | Prospective cohort study | 450 pregnant women | 20.2 ± 0.25 | ≥15 | 5 | 88 | Microscopy | NS |
| Hercik et al., 2017 | Tanzania | 2014–2015 | Prospective observational study | 997 febrile patients | Median 23 | 1–79 | 22 | 327 | RDT, Microscopy | PCR |
| Hogan et al., 2017 | Ghana | 2014–2015 | Prospective observational study | 1063 febrile children | Median 2 | IQR: 1–4 | 7 | NS | Microscopy | PCR |
| Kasper et al., 2012 | Cambodia | 2006–2009 | Prospective observational study | 9997 febrile patients | Median 13 | IQR: 6–28 | 8 | 716 | Microscopy | PCR |
| Mueller et al., 2014 | Cambodia | 2008–2010 | Prospective observational study | 1193 febrile patients | Mean 23.4 ± 10.6 | 7–49 | 32 | 644 | RDT, PCR | PCR |
| Nzoumbou-Boko et al., 2020 | The Central African Republic | 2015–2018 | Retrospective observational study | 5397 febrile patients | Median 11 | 2 months to 78 years | 367 | 3609 | RDT | NS |
| Thompson et al., 2012 | Kenya | 2009–2011 | Retrospective observational study | 1992 febrile patients | Mean 2.31 ± 1.34 | 0–5 | 149 | 1322 | Microscopy | PCR |

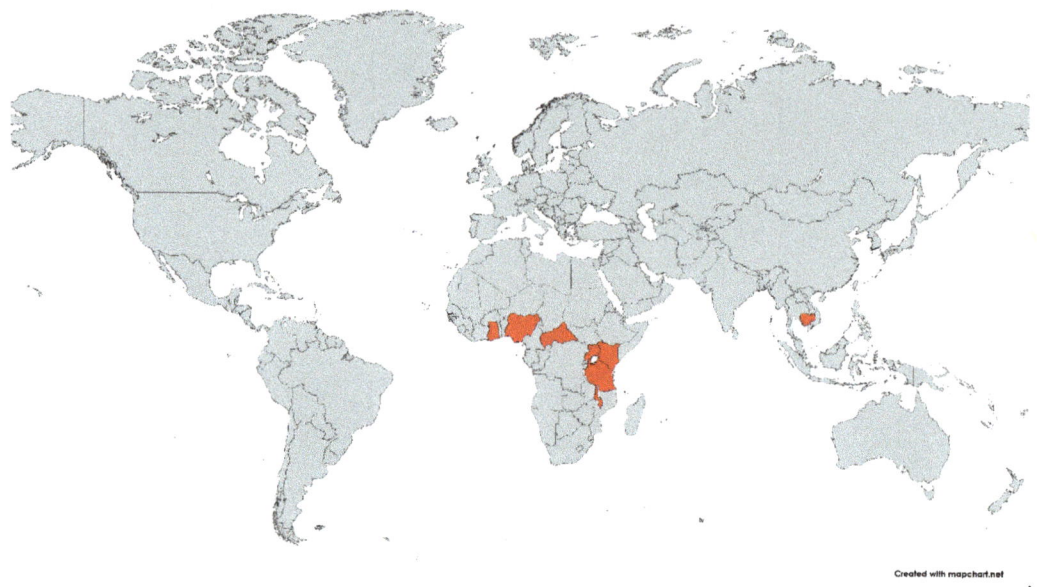

**Figure 2.** Malaria and influenza co-infection were documented in the following regions (marked in red). The map was made with the help of a map template found at https://mapchart.net/. By referencing mapchart.net, authors are permitted to use, alter, and modify any map made with it.

*3.3. Risk of Bias*

The risk of bias for each study was assessed using the JBI Critical Appraisal Tools for cross-sectional study. Six studies [14,20,23–26] were assessed as having a low risk of bias, while four studies [11,13,21,22] were assessed as having a moderate risk of bias (Table S2).

*3.4. Pooled Prevalence of Malaria and Influenza Virus Co-Infection*

The pooled prevalence of malaria and influenza virus co-infection (650 cases) among febrile patients (22,066 cases) was estimated using data from 10 studies [11,13,14,20–26]. On stratifying the prevalence by country, the pooled prevalence of malaria and influenza virus co-infection among febrile patients was 31.0% in Nigeria (95% CI: 25.0–38.0%), 1.0% in Tanzania (95% CI: 0–1.0%, $I^2$: 99.9%), 1.0% in Uganda (95% CI: 0–2.0%), 1.0% in Malawi (95% CI: 0–3.0%), 1.0% in Ghana (95% CI: 0–1.0%), 0% in Cambodia ($I^2$: 99.9%), 7.0% in the Central African Republic (95% CI: 6.0–8.0%), and 7.0% in Kenya (95% CI: 6.0–9.0%) (Figure 3).

For stratifying the prevalence by groups of participants, the pooled prevalence of malaria and influenza virus co-infection among febrile patients was 2.0% in pregnant women (95% CI: 1.0–3.0%, $I^2$: 99.9%), 3.0% in children (95% CI: 0–6.0%, $I^2$: 98.5%), 1.0% in adults (95% CI: 0–2.0%), and 4.0% in all age groups (95% CI: 1.0–7.0%, $I^2$: 97.6%) (Figure 4).

For stratifying the prevalence by diagnostic tests for influenza virus, the pooled prevalence of malaria and influenza virus co-infection among febrile patients was 31.0% in the study using ELISA IgM (95% CI: 25.0–38.0%), 0% in studies using ELISA IgM/IgG/PCR (95% CI: 0–2.0%), 2.0% in studies using PCR (95% CI: 1.0–4.0%, $I^2$: 97.7%), and 5.0% in studies that did not specify the diagnostic method for influenza virus (95% CI: 4.0–6.0%, $I^2$: 99.5%). Overall, the pooled prevalence of malaria and influenza virus co-infection among febrile patients was 3.0% (95% CI: 2.0–5.0%, $I^2$: 98.7%) (Figure 5).

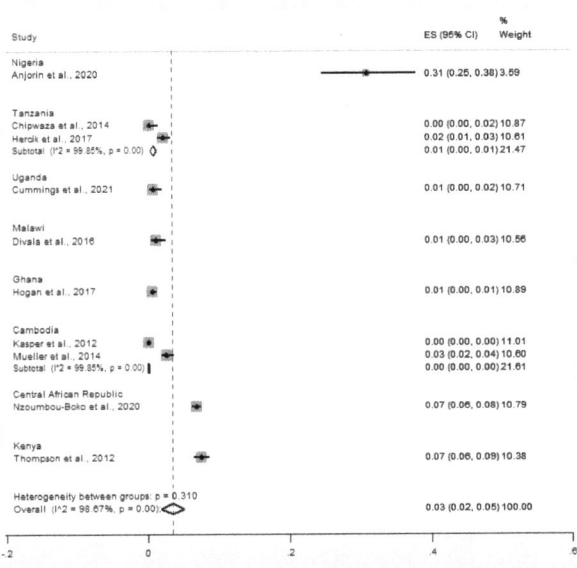

**Figure 3.** Countries with the highest rates of malaria and influenza co-infection among feverish patients. Percentage weight, each study's contribution to the pooled effect; black dot on black horizontal line, each study's point estimate; CI, confidence interval; white diamond, pooled prevalence; ES, effect size (prevalence).

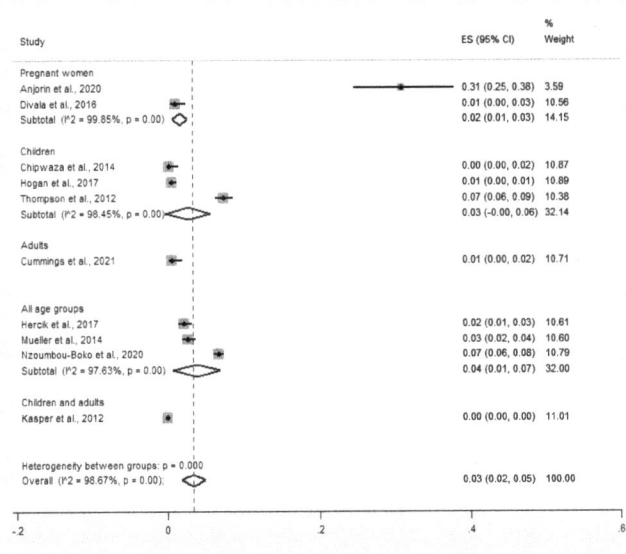

**Figure 4.** Malaria and influenza co-infection rates in febrile patients, broken down by participant groups. Percentage weight, the fraction of each study's impact on the pooled effect; black dot on black horizontal line, each study's point estimate; CI, confidence interval; white diamond, pooled prevalence; ES, effect size (prevalence).

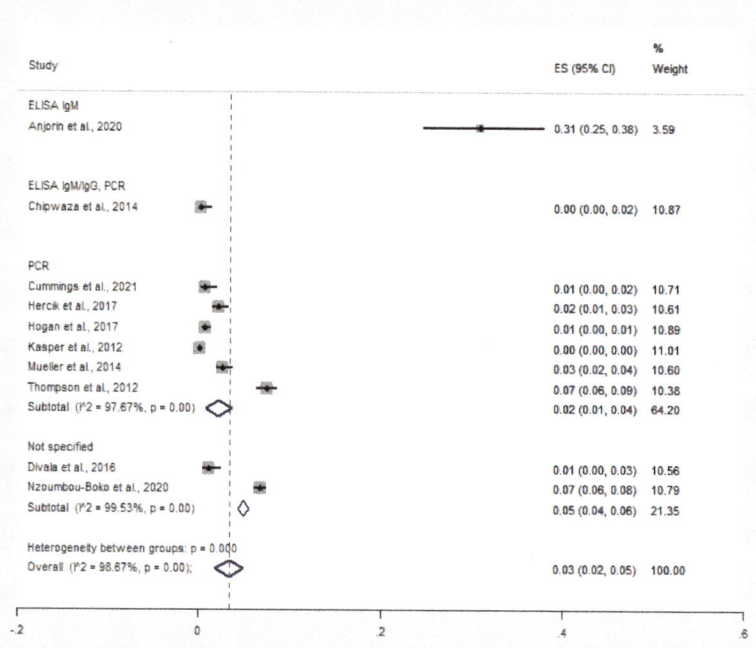

**Figure 5.** Diagnostic testing for influenza virus reveals the prevalence of malaria and influenza co-infection among feverish patients. Percentage weight, the fraction of each study's impact on the aggregated effect; black dot on black horizontal line, each study's point estimate; white diamond, pooled prevalence; CI, confidence interval; ES, effect size (prevalence).

*3.5. Pooled Prevalence of Influenza Virus Infection among Malaria-Positive Patients*

The pooled prevalence of influenza virus infection (587 cases) among malaria-positive patients (6847 cases) was estimated using data from eight studies [13,14,20–23,25,26]. On stratifying the prevalence by country, the pooled prevalence of influenza virus infection among malaria-positive patients was 4.0% in Tanzania (95% CI: 2.0–5.0%, $I^2$: 99.6%), 5.0% in Uganda (95% CI: 2.0–14.0%), 6.0% in Malawi (95% CI: 2.0–13.0%), 2.0% in Cambodia (95% CI: 1.0–2.0%, $I^2$: 99.6%), 10.0% in the Central African Republic (95% CI: 9.0–11.0%), and 11.0% in Kenya (95% CI: 10.0–13.0%) (Figure 6).

On stratifying the prevalence by groups of participants, the pooled prevalence of influenza virus infection among malaria-positive patients was 8.0% in children (95% CI: 6.0–9.0%, $I^2$: 99.6%), 5.0% in adults (95% CI: 2.0–14.0%), 6.0% in pregnant women (95% CI: 2.0–13.0%), and 7.0% in all age groups (95% CI: 4.0–11.0%, $I^2$: 93.2%) (Figure 7).

On stratifying the prevalence by diagnostic tests for influenza virus, the pooled prevalence of influenza virus infection among malaria patients was 1.0% in studies using ELISA IgM/IgG/PCR (95% CI: 0–7.0%), 6.0% in studies using PCR (95% CI: 1.0–10.0%, $I^2$: 96.8%), and 10.0% in studies that did not specify the diagnostic method for influenza virus (95% CI: 9.0–11.0%, $I^2$: 99.2%). Overall, the pooled prevalence of influenza virus infection among malaria patients was 6.0% (95% CI: 2.0–9.0%, $I^2$: 97.4%) (Figure 8).

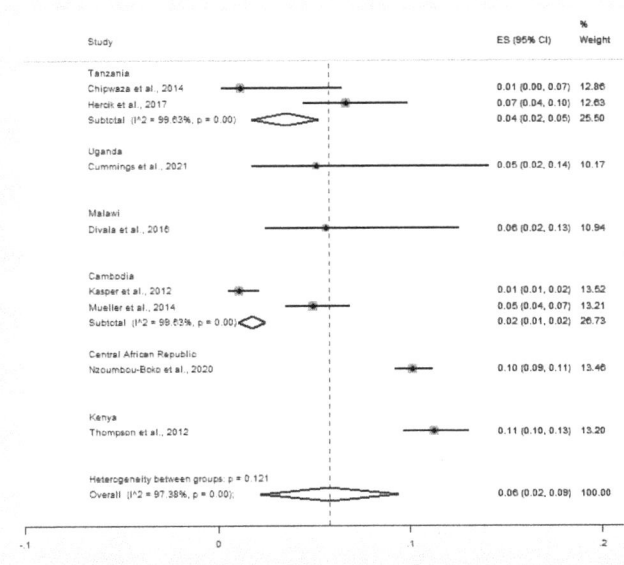

**Figure 6.** Countries with the highest rates of malaria and influenza co-infection among feverish patients. Percentage weight, the fraction of each study's impact on the pooled outcome; black dot on black horizontal line, each study's point estimate; white diamond, pooled prevalence; CI, confidence interval; ES, effect size (prevalence).

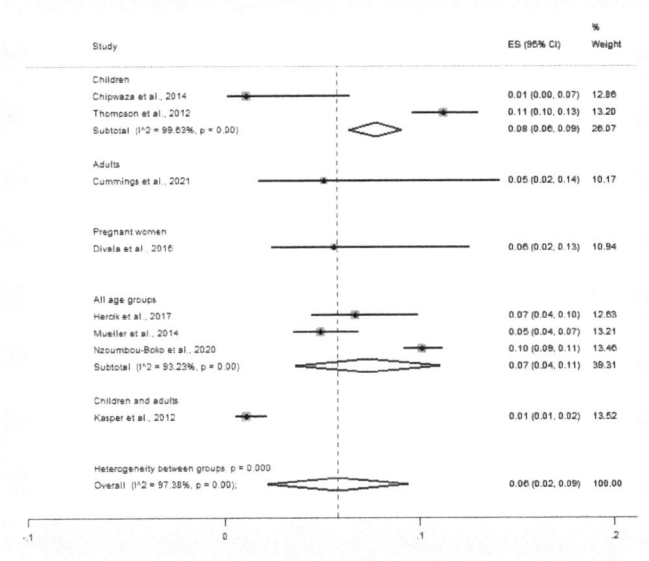

**Figure 7.** Influenza virus infection rates among malaria patients, broken down by participant groups. Percentage weight, the fraction of each study's impact on the pooled outcome; black dot on black horizontal line, each study's point estimate; white diamond, pooled prevalence; CI, confidence interval; ES, effect size (prevalence).

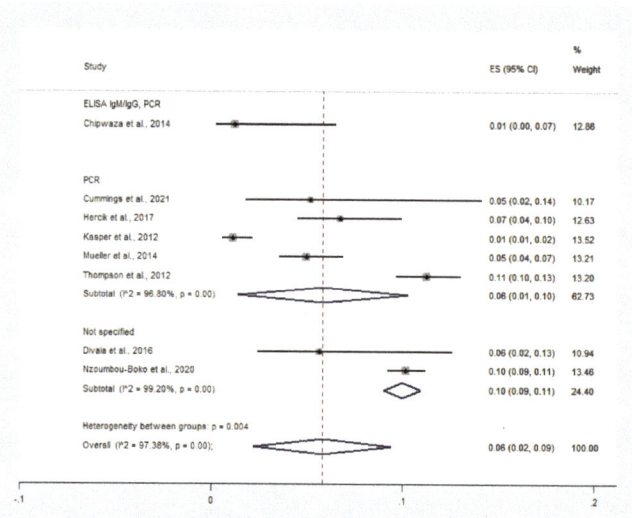

**Figure 8.** Diagnostic assays for influenza virus infection reveal the prevalence of influenza virus infection among malaria patients. Percentage weight, the fraction of each study's impact on the pooled outcome; black dot on black horizontal line, each study's point estimate; white diamond, pooled prevalence; CI, confidence interval; ES, effect size (prevalence).

### 3.6. Odds of Co-Infection

Odds of malaria and influenza virus co-infection were estimated using the data from seven studies [13,14,21–23,25,26]. Overall, the meta-analysis showed that co-infections occurred by chance ($p = 0.097$, odds ratio (OR): 0.54, 95% CI: 0.26–1.12, $I^2$: 94.9%). Results of individual studies showed that malaria and influenza virus co-infection occurred frequently in the study conducted in the Central African Republic during 2015–2018 [13], with less co-infection occurring in the study conducted in Cambodia during 2006–2009 [25] (Figure 9).

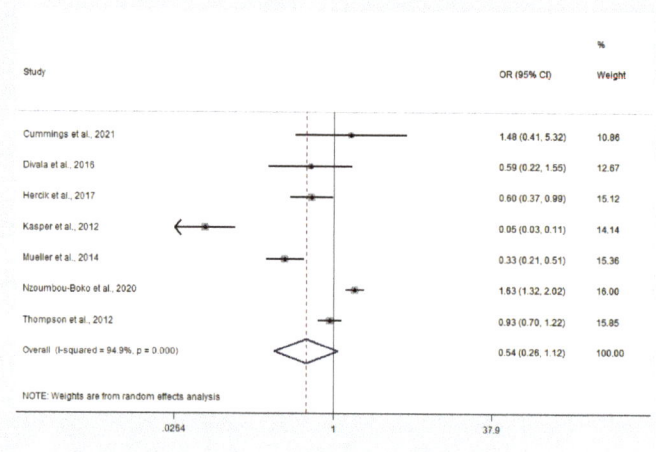

**Figure 9.** Malaria and influenza co-infections have a high chance of occurring. Percentage weight: each study's contribution to the pooled effect; black dot on black horizontal line, each study's point estimate.

## 3.7. Publication Bias

Publication bias was assessed by visualizing the funnel plot and analyzing by Egger's test. There was an asymmetrical distribution of the studies in the funnel plot, indicating the publication bias of the prevalence of co-infection among the included studies (Figure 10). Egger's test demonstrated that publication bias was caused by a small study effect ($p = 0.015$, co-efficient 6.97, standard error 2.26).

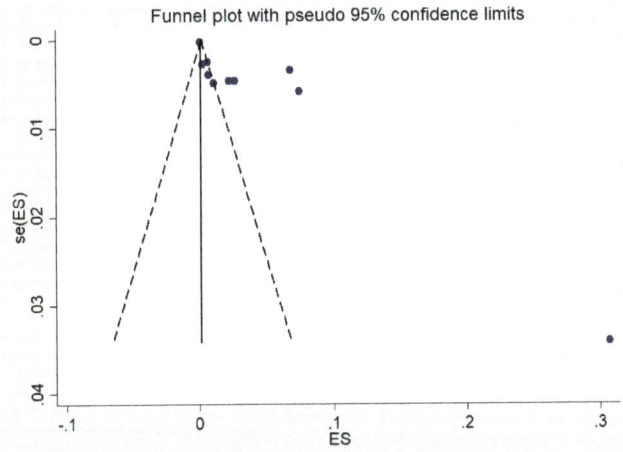

**Figure 10.** The asymmetrical distribution of the effect estimate (ES, prevalence of co-infection) and its standard error (se) is depicted in a funnel plot.

A contour-enhanced funnel plot was further created to demonstrate other possible causes of funnel-plot asymmetry. This showed that the effect estimates of the included studies were mostly located in the significant area ($p < 1.0\%$), indicating that the shape of the funnel plot was likely caused by publication bias (Figure 11).

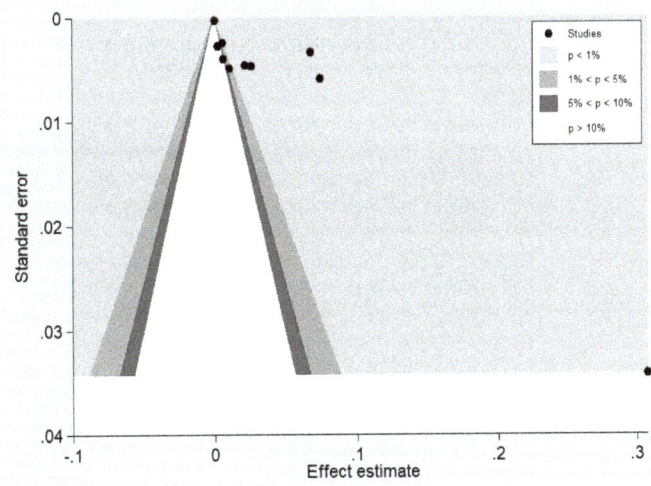

**Figure 11.** The distribution of the effect estimates of the included studies in the significant area ($p\ 1\%$) is shown in a contour-enhanced funnel plot.

## 4. Discussion

In this study, we found that the co-occurrence of malaria and influenza infections in febrile patients were published in the literatures between 2012 and 2021. The results of the meta-analysis showed that although the overall prevalence of malaria and influenza co-infection among febrile patients was low (3.0%), the causes of high heterogeneity among studies need to be considered. The difference in the prevalence of co-infections might due to the difference in countries, participants, and diagnostic tests for influenza virus in different studies. Interestingly, influenza virus infection among malaria patients was commonly found in Africa where falciparum malaria is endemic. These findings were consistent with those that previously reported a high prevalence of influenza A virus infection among malaria patients in Lagos State, Nigeria [11]. The incidence of malaria co-infection with influenza was also reported as approximately 6.8% in the Central African Republic between 2015 and 2018 [13]. In hyperendemic areas, where malaria is endemic in both urban and rural areas, the low prevalence of malaria and influenza virus co-infection in Africa might be caused by underdiagnosis by physicians in the absence of respiratory tract symptoms of influenza at presentation or misdiagnosis of co-infection. In hypoendemic areas such as South-East Asia, malaria is frequently found in rural populations; hence, the first differential diagnosis of patients who present with fever after spending time in the forest is malaria rather than influenza. Co-infection of malaria with other AFIs was reported in our previous studies [27–29]. Co-infections patients were less reported, perhaps because of under-reporting or underevaluation or misdiagnosis. Nevertheless, co-infection of malaria with leptospirosis or chikungunya tended to occur by chance [27,28]. Regarding malaria and influenza co-infection, the high prevalence of co-infection under poor living conditions might be associated with poor outcomes from influenza infection, especially in developing countries [30,31]. Given that several studies from Africa have reported a high prevalence of influenza virus infection associated with hospitalization [32,33], the relevant infection control strategies, including vaccination, warrant closer attention [32].

Subgroup analysis of study populations showed that the pooled prevalence of co-infection with influenza virus infection among malaria patients was highest in all age groups (4.0%) and children (8.0%). Lower prevalence was reported by studies that enrolled specific groups, such as pregnant women and adults. These results indicated that the co-infection of these two diseases could occur in all age groups, especially in children with influenza virus infection. This result was consistent with a report on the risk and severity of co-infection among children in Kenya [14,34], which showed that 45.0% of children < 5 years old with influenza virus infections were co-infected with malaria, while only 6.0% of malaria-positive patients were co-infected with influenza [14]. In addition, children aged 5–10 years (11.0%) were co-infected with malaria and influenza [34]. Longer hospitalization of children < 5 years old for co-infection with malaria and influenza was uncommon [14]. However, two studies [11,22] that recruited pregnant patients reported a low prevalence of co-infection in this group. Therefore, pregnant women who are infected by these two pathogens might not be the source of heterogeneity in the prevalence of co-infection in febrile illness. In Nigeria, pregnant women (56.6%) were IgM seropositive for influenza A virus and co-infection with malaria (54.0%) and typhoid fever (33.0%) [11]. Moreover, the most affected patients with co-infection had the highest seroprevalence estimated to occur among adults aged 21–30 years [11]. Possibly they were active working people and had risk to contact with other people including people with influenza.

Malaria and influenza share similar clinical symptoms with other febrile illnesses at the early stages of infection, which may leads to misdiagnosis and delays optimal treatment [35]. Influenza may be undiagnosed in febrile malaria patients if clinicians do not suspect influenza co-infection. In this study, the prevalence of co-infection was stratified by diagnostic tests for influenza virus infections, including ELISA (IgM), ELISA (IgM/IgG)/PCR, and PCR. The highest prevalence of co-infection and influenza virus infection among malaria patients was diagnosed using ELISA (IgM) and PCR. Moreover, the diagnostic tool for influenza diagnosis in the study in Nigeria was ELISA. Seropositivity by ELISA is used to detect IgM-specific antibodies to influenza A virus H1N1 and H3N2 [11]. The lowest prevalence of co-infection and chikungunya infection in malaria patients was diagnosed using ELISA (IgM/IgG)/PCR. In addition, two studies [13,22] did not specify the diagnostic method for the influenza virus. Currently there are several methods for the diagnosis of influenza infections, such as real-time reverse transcription-PCR assays, viral isolation in cell culture, immunofluorescence assays, and immunochromatography assays [36].

The meta-analysis showed that malaria and influenza virus co-infection occurred by chance. The rationale behind this occurrence might be the difference in vectors responsible for transmitting the diseases. While malaria is transmitted by female *Anopheles* mosquitoes, influenza is transmitted via direct contact with infected individuals or by inhalation of virus-laden aerosols. Nevertheless, a high probability of co-infection was demonstrated in the studies conducted in the Central African Republic during 2015–2018 [13]. The results of this study indicated that two diseases might enhance another infection. However, the low probability of co-infection was reported in the study conducted in Cambodia during 2006–2009 [25], which indicated that one infection might suppress another infection. Further studies are needed to investigate the interaction between these two diseases.

The present study had some limitations. First, the pooled prevalence of malaria and influenza virus co-infection in febrile patients or the pooled prevalence of influenza virus infection in malaria patients was heterogeneous. Therefore, the pooled prevalence must be interpreted with caution. Second, the number of publications that reported malaria and influenza co-infection was limited; hence, in the present study, the differences in clinical characteristics, laboratory data, and treatment outcome of co-infected patients could not be analyzed. Third, the prevalence of malaria and influenza virus co-infection was dependent on the diagnostic tests used for the influenza virus infection, which are not all confirmatory; therefore, the rate of co-infection might have been underestimated? in some of the included studies.

## 5. Conclusions

Prevalence of malaria and influenza virus co-infection among febrile patients was heterogeneous by country, characteristics of febrile participants, and diagnostic tests for influenza virus. Clinicians examining febrile patients in co-endemic areas such as Nigeria, Tanzania, Uganda, Malawi, Ghana, Cambodia, the Central African Republic, and Kenya should carefully examine patients for the possibility of co-infection. Influenza should also be suspected in febrile malaria patients in any country during influenza season. Moreover, further studies should investigate severe clinical manifestations or differentiate clinical outcomes between mono-infected or co-infected individuals, if the co-infection leads to severe disease outcomes.

**Supplementary Materials:** The following supporting information can be downloaded at: https://www.mdpi.com/article/10.3390/tropicalmed7080168/s1; Table S1: Search term; Table S2: Quality of the included studies.

**Author Contributions:** P.W., W.M. and M.K. carried out the study design, study selection, data extraction, and statistical analysis and drafted the manuscript; K.U.K. participated in the study selection and data extraction and drafted the manuscript. All authors have read and agreed to the published version of the manuscript.

**Funding:** This research received no external funding.

**Institutional Review Board Statement:** Not applicable.

**Informed Consent Statement:** Not applicable.

**Data Availability Statement:** All data related to the present study are available in this manuscript and supplementary files.

**Acknowledgments:** This research was financially supported by the new strategic research project (P2P) fiscal year 2022, Walailak University, Thailand.

**Conflicts of Interest:** The authors declare that there are no conflicts of interest regarding the publication of this article.

**Abbreviations**

AFIs: acute febrile illnesses; ELISA: enzyme-linked immunosorbent assay; JBI: Joanna Briggs Institute; MeSH: Medical Subject Heading; OR: odds ratio; WHO: World Health Organization.

## References

1. World Health Organization. *World Malaria Report 2021*; WHO: Geneva, Switzerland, 2021.
2. Gunalan, K.; Niangaly, A.; Thera, M.A.; Doumbo, O.K.; Miller, L.H. *Plasmodium vivax* infections of Duffy-negative erythrocytes: Historically undetected or a recent adaptation? *Trends Parasitol.* **2018**, *34*, 420–429. [CrossRef]
3. Mendes, C.; Dias, F.; Figueiredo, J.; Mora, V.G.; Cano, J.; de Sousa, B.; do Rosario, V.E.; Benito, A.; Berzosa, P.; Arez, A.P. Duffy negative antigen is no longer a barrier to *Plasmodium vivax*—Molecular evidences from the African West Coast (Angola and Equatorial Guinea). *PLoS Negl. Trop. Dis.* **2011**, *5*, e1192. [CrossRef] [PubMed]
4. Zimmerman, P.A. *Plasmodium vivax* infection in duffy-negative people in Africa. *Am. J. Trop. Med. Hyg.* **2017**, *97*, 636–638. [CrossRef] [PubMed]
5. Kotepui, M.; Kotepui, K.U.; Milanez, G.J.; Masangkay, F.R. Prevalence and risk factors related to poor outcome of patients with severe *Plasmodium vivax* infection: A systematic review, meta-analysis, and analysis of case reports. *BMC Infect. Dis.* **2020**, *20*, 363. [CrossRef] [PubMed]
6. Matlani, M.; Kojom, L.P.; Mishra, N.; Dogra, V.; Singh, V. Severe vivax malaria trends in the last two years: A study from a tertiary care centre, Delhi, India. *Ann. Clin. Microbiol. Antimicrob.* **2020**, *19*, 49. [CrossRef]
7. Geleta, G.; Ketema, T. Severe malaria associated with *Plasmodium falciparum* and *P. vivax* among children in Pawe hospital, Northwest Ethiopia. *Malar. Res. Treat.* **2016**, *2016*, 1240962. [CrossRef]
8. Kotepui, M.; Kotepui, K.U.; De Jesus Milanez, G.; Masangkay, F.R. *Plasmodium* spp. mixed infection leading to severe malaria: A systematic review and meta-analysis. *Sci. Rep.* **2020**, *10*, 11068. [CrossRef]
9. Kotepui, M.; Kotepui, K.U.; Milanez, G.D.; Masangkay, F.R. Severity and mortality of severe *Plasmodium ovale* infection: A systematic review and meta-analysis. *PLoS ONE* **2020**, *15*, e0235014. [CrossRef]
10. Kotepui, M.; Kotepui, K.U.; Milanez, G.D.; Masangkay, F.R. Global prevalence and mortality of severe *Plasmodium malariae* infection: A systematic review and meta-analysis. *Malar. J.* **2020**, *19*, 274. [CrossRef]
11. Anjorin, A.A.A.; Nwammadu, J.E. Seroepidemiology of seasonal influenza virus among unvaccinated pregnant women in Lagos, Nigeria. *Le Infez. Med.* **2020**, *28*, 407–415.
12. Ghebrehewet, S.; MacPherson, P.; Ho, A. Influenza. *BMJ* **2016**, *355*, i6258. [CrossRef] [PubMed]
13. Nzoumbou-Boko, R.; Yambiyo, B.M.; Ngoagouni, C.; Vickos, U.; Manirakiza, A.; Nakouné, E. Falciparum Malaria in febrile patients at sentinel sites for influenza surveillance in the Central African Republic from 2015 to 2018. *Interdiscip. Perspect. Infect. Dis.* **2020**, *2020*, 3938541. [CrossRef] [PubMed]
14. Thompson, M.G.; Breiman, R.F.; Hamel, M.J.; Desai, M.; Emukule, G.; Khagayi, S.; Shay, D.K.; Morales, K.; Kariuki, S.; Bigogo, G.M.; et al. Influenza and malaria coinfection among young children in western Kenya, 2009-2011. *J. Infect. Dis.* **2012**, *206*, 1674–1684. [CrossRef]
15. Iuliano, A.D.; Roguski, K.M.; Chang, H.H.; Muscatello, D.J.; Palekar, R.; Tempia, S.; Cohen, C.; Gran, J.M.; Schanzer, D.; Cowling, B.J.; et al. Estimates of global seasonal influenza-associated respiratory mortality: A modelling study. *Lancet* **2018**, *391*, 1285–1300. [CrossRef]
16. Grobusch, M.P.; Kremsner, P.G. Uncomplicated malaria. *Curr. Top. Microbiol. Immunol.* **2005**, *295*, 83–104.
17. Dalrymple, U.; Cameron, E.; Bhatt, S.; Weiss, D.J.; Gupta, S.; Gething, P.W. Quantifying the contribution of *Plasmodium falciparum* malaria to febrile illness amongst African children. *eLife* **2017**, *6*, e29198. [CrossRef] [PubMed]
18. Liberati, A.; Altman, D.G.; Tetzlaff, J.; Mulrow, C.; Gotzsche, P.C.; Ioannidis, J.P.; Clarke, M.; Devereaux, P.J.; Kleijnen, J.; Moher, D. The PRISMA statement for reporting systematic reviews and meta-analyses of studies that evaluate healthcare interventions: Explanation and elaboration. *BMJ* **2009**, *339*, b2700. [CrossRef]
19. Moola, S.M.Z.; Tufanaru, C.; Aromataris, E.; Sears, K.; Sfetcu, R.; Currie, M.; Qureshi, R.; Mattis, P.; Lisy, K.; Mu, P.-F. Chapter 7: Systematic reviews of etiology and risk. In *JBI Manual for Evidence Synthesis*; Aromataris, E.M.Z., Ed.; JBI: Adelaide, Australia, 2020.
20. Chipwaza, B.; Mugasa, J.P.; Selemani, M.; Amuri, M.; Mosha, F.; Ngatunga, S.D.; Gwakisa, P.S. Dengue and Chikungunya fever among viral diseases in outpatient febrile children in Kilosa district hospital, Tanzania. *PLoS Negl. Trop. Dis.* **2014**, *8*, e3335. [CrossRef]
21. Cummings, M.J.; Bakamutumaho, B.; Owor, N.; Kayiwa, J.; Namulondo, J.; Byaruhanga, T.; Muwanga, M.; Nsereko, C.; Baldwin, M.R.; Lutwama, J.J.; et al. Stratifying sepsis in Uganda using rapid pathogen diagnostics and clinical data: A prospective cohort study. *Am. J. Trop. Med. Hyg.* **2021**, *105*, 517–524. [CrossRef]
22. Divala, T.H.; Kalilani-Phiri, L.; Mawindo, P.; Nyirenda, O.; Kapito-Tembo, A.; Laufer, M.K. Incidence and seasonality of influenza-like illnesses among pregnant women in Blantyre, Malawi. *Am. J. Trop. Med. Hyg.* **2016**, *95*, 915–917. [CrossRef]

23. Hercik, C.; Cosmas, L.; Mogeni, O.D.; Wamola, N.; Kohi, W.; Omballa, V.; Ochieng, M.; Lidechi, S.; Bonventure, J.; Ochieng, C.; et al. A diagnostic and epidemiologic investigation of acute febrile illness (AFI) in Kilombero, Tanzania. *PLoS ONE* **2017**, *12*, e0189712. [CrossRef] [PubMed]
24. Hogan, B.; Ammer, L.; Zimmermann, M.; Binger, T.; Krumkamp, R.; Sarpong, N.; Rettig, T.; Dekker, D.; Kreuels, B.; Reigl, L.; et al. Burden of influenza among hospitalized febrile children in Ghana. *Influenza Other Respir. Viruses* **2017**, *11*, 497–501. [CrossRef] [PubMed]
25. Kasper, M.R.; Blair, P.J.; Touch, S.; Sokhal, B.; Yasuda, C.Y.; Williams, M.; Richards, A.L.; Burgess, T.H.; Wierzba, T.F.; Putnam, S.D. Infectious etiologies of acute febrile illness among patients seeking health care in south-central Cambodia. *Am. J. Trop. Med. Hyg.* **2012**, *86*, 246–253. [CrossRef] [PubMed]
26. Mueller, T.C.; Siv, S.; Khim, N.; Kim, S.; Fleischmann, E.; Ariey, F.; Buchy, P.; Guillard, B.; González, I.J.; Christophel, E.M.; et al. Acute undifferentiated febrile illness in rural Cambodia: A 3-year prospective observational study. *PLoS ONE* **2014**, *9*, e95868. [CrossRef]
27. Mala, W.; Wilairatana, P.; Kotepui, K.U.; Kotepui, M. Prevalence of malaria and chikungunya co-infection in febrile patients: A systematic review and meta-analysis. *Trop. Med. Infect. Dis.* **2021**, *6*, 119. [CrossRef]
28. Wilairatana, P.; Mala, W.; Rattaprasert, P.; Kotepui, K.U.; Kotepui, M. Prevalence of malaria and leptospirosis co-infection among febrile patients: A systematic review and meta-analysis. *Trop. Med. Infect. Dis.* **2021**, *6*, 122. [CrossRef]
29. Kotepui, M.; Kotepui, K.U. Prevalence and laboratory analysis of malaria and dengue co-infection: A systematic review and meta-analysis. *BMC Public Health* **2019**, *19*, 1148. [CrossRef]
30. Cohen, C.; Simonsen, L.; Kang, J.W.; Miller, M.; McAnerney, J.; Blumberg, L.; Schoub, B.; Madhi, S.A.; Viboud, C. Elevated influenza-related excess mortality in South African elderly individuals, 1998-2005. *Clin. Infect. Dis.* **2010**, *51*, 1362–1369. [CrossRef]
31. Phiri, M.; Gooding, K.; Peterson, I.; Mambule, I.; Nundwe, S.; McMorrow, M.; Desmond, N. Dust or disease? Perceptions of influenza in rural Southern Malawi. *PLoS ONE* **2019**, *14*, e0208155. [CrossRef]
32. McMorrow, M.L.; Wemakoy, E.O.; Tshilobo, J.K.; Emukule, G.O.; Mott, J.A.; Njuguna, H.; Waiboci, L.; Heraud, J.M.; Rajatonirina, S.; Razanajatovo, N.H.; et al. Severe acute respiratory illness deaths in sub-saharan Africa and the role of influenza: A case series from 8 countries. *J. Infect. Dis.* **2015**, *212*, 853–860. [CrossRef]
33. Nyamusore, J.; Rukelibuga, J.; Mutagoma, M.; Muhire, A.; Kabanda, A.; Williams, T.; Mutoni, A.; Kamwesiga, J.; Nyatanyi, T.; Omolo, J.; et al. The national burden of influenza-associated severe acute respiratory illness hospitalization in Rwanda, 2012-2014. *Influenza Other Respir. Viruses* **2018**, *12*, 38–45. [CrossRef] [PubMed]
34. Waitumbi, J.N.; Kuypers, J.; Anyona, S.B.; Koros, J.N.; Polhemus, M.E.; Gerlach, J.; Steele, M.; Englund, J.A.; Neuzil, K.M.; Domingo, G.J. Outpatient upper respiratory tract viral infections in children with malaria symptoms in Western Kenya. *Am. J. Trop. Med. Hyg.* **2010**, *83*, 1010–1013. [CrossRef] [PubMed]
35. Wang, H.; Zhao, J.; Xie, N.; Wang, W.; Qi, R.; Hao, X.; Liu, Y.; Sevalie, S.; Niu, G.; Zhang, Y.; et al. A prospective study of etiological agents among febrile patients in Sierra Leone. *Infect. Dis. Ther.* **2021**, *10*, 1645–1664. [CrossRef] [PubMed]
36. Vemula, S.V.; Zhao, J.; Liu, J.; Wang, X.; Biswas, S.; Hewlett, I. Current approaches for diagnosis of influenza virus infections in humans. *Viruses* **2016**, *8*, 96. [CrossRef] [PubMed]

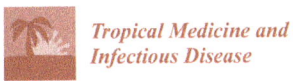

*Case Report*

# Post-Mortem Diagnosis of Pediatric Dengue Using Minimally Invasive Autopsy during the COVID-19 Pandemic in Brazil

Deborah N. Melo [1,2], Giovanna R. P. Lima [3], Carolina G. Fernandes [3], André C. Teixeira [1,3,4], Joel B. Filho [1], Fernanda M. C. Araújo [5], Lia C. Araújo [6], André M. Siqueira [7], Luís A. B. G. Farias [8], Renata A. A. Monteiro [9], Jaume Ordi [10,11], Miguel J. Martinez [11], Paulo H. N. Saldiva [9] and Luciano P. G. Cavalcanti [2,3,12,*]

[1] Serviço de Verificação de Óbitos Dr Rocha Furtado, Fortaleza 60842-395, Brazil; deborahnmb@gmail.com (D.N.M.); andrect3@hotmail.com (A.C.T.); joelpatologista@gmail.com (J.B.F.)
[2] Programa de Pós-graduação em Patologia, Universidade Federal do Ceará, Fortaleza 60020-181, Brazil
[3] Faculdade de Medicina, Centro Universitário Christus, Fortaleza 60190-180, Brazil; grolimlima@gmail.com (G.R.P.L.); carolfernandes.hp7@gmail.com (C.G.F.)
[4] Argos Laboratory, Fortaleza 60175-047, Brazil
[5] Fundação Oswaldo Cruz, Eusebio 61760-000, Brazil; fernandamontenegrocaraujo@gmail.com
[6] Programa de Residencia Medica em Patologia pela Universidade Federal do Ceará, 60, Fortaleza 60020-181, Brazil; araujolc@gmail.com
[7] Fundação Oswaldo Cruz, Rio de Janeiro 21040-360, Brazil; amsiqueira@gmail.com
[8] Hospital São José de Doenças Infecciosas, Fortaleza 60455-610, Brazil; luisarthurbrasilk@hotmail.com
[9] Departamento de Patologia, Faculdade de Medicina da Universidade de São Paulo, São Paulo 01246-903, Brazil; reacademic@gmail.com (R.A.A.M.); pepino@usp.br (P.H.N.S.)
[10] ISGlobal, Barcelona Institute for Global Health, Hospital Clínic, Universitat de Barcelona, 08036 Barcelona, Spain; jordi@clinic.cat
[11] ISGlobal, Hospital Clínic, University of Barcelona, 08007 Barcelona, Spain; myoldi@clinic.cat
[12] Programa de Pós-graduação em Saúde Coletiva, Universidade Federal do Ceará, Fortaleza 60020-181, Brazil
* Correspondence: luciano.pamplona@ufc.br; Tel.: +55-85-999878969

**Abstract:** We report the first pediatric disease in which the use of minimally invasive autopsy (MIA) confirmed severe dengue as the cause of death. During the COVID-19 pandemic, a previously healthy 10-year-old girl living in north-eastern Brazil presented fever, headache, diffuse abdominal pain, diarrhoea, and vomiting. On the fourth day, the clinical symptoms worsened and the patient died. An MIA was performed, and cores of brain, lungs, heart, liver, kidneys, and spleen were collected with 14G biopsy needles. Microscopic examination showed diffuse oedema and congestion, pulmonary intra-alveolar haemorrhage, small foci of midzonal necrosis in the liver, and tubular cell necrosis in the kidneys. Dengue virus RNA and NS1 antigen were detected in blood and cerebrospinal fluid samples. Clinical, pathological, and laboratory findings, in combination with the absence of other lesions and microorganisms, allowed concluding that the patient had died from complications of severe dengue.

**Keywords:** severe dengue; autopsy; minimally invasive autopsy; arbovirus; COVID-19

## 1. Introduction

Dengue is the most important arbovirus worldwide, causing epidemics with a high human health and economic impact. Severe symptoms mainly affect the pediatric population from endemic low- and middle-income countries [1,2].

In Brazil, dengue remains the most widespread disease caused by arbovirus, even after the introduction of Zika and chikungunya. In north-eastern Brazil, deaths from dengue are frequent, even in non-epidemic years, especially in socially vulnerable populations [1–3]. Clinically, most dengue infections are either asymptomatic or produce mild disease [1–3]. However, given the high number of infections, severe cases are often reported during epidemics and represent a challenge for diagnosis and clinical management. In fatal

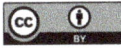

cases, most organs and systems are affected, particularly the heart, central nervous system, gastrointestinal tract, and kidneys.

After the establishment of Death Verification Services (DVS) in Brazil, the use of conventional autopsy (CA), the gold standard technique for the diagnosis of deaths caused by dengue, has contributed to the detection of patients clinically not diagnosed [4] and has significantly reduced neglected and underreported cases. However, the existence of few DVS in the cities, together with the low acceptability of CA among the relatives of the deceased and the lack of financial resources and specialised personnel, has resulted in limited implementation of this procedure [5]. Thus, the application of new strategies for post-mortem tissue collection is necessary, particularly for pediatric deaths, as rejection of CA by the relatives is very high in this population [5–10].

Minimally invasive autopsy (MIA) has been used as an alternative to CA with promising results [8,10–14]. This technique allows obtaining core biopsies of key organs by percutaneous puncture, with or without guidance with an imaging technique. MIA has been widely used in the context of the COVID-19 pandemic as a fast and non-disfiguring method with minimal biological risk for the personnel performing the procedure [8,9,15–17]. However, current knowledge of the performance of this technique for arboviral diseases in the paediatric population is very limited.

We report the first case of fatal dengue infection, which occurred in a previously healthy 10-year-old girl living in north-eastern Brazil during the COVID-19 pandemic. MIA sampling allowed correct diagnosis and showed complete agreement with the CA. We show that this acceptable, simplified, and non-disfiguring post-mortem technique can reliably diagnose death from severe dengue.

## 2. Case Report

A 10-year-old girl presented with fever, headache, diffuse abdominal pain, diarrhoea, and vomiting at the end of June 2021. She was previously healthy and had no comorbidities. A previously healthy 10-year-old girl with no comorbidities presented with fever, headache, diffuse abdominal pain, diarrhoea, and vomiting at the end of June 2021. The patient was initially treated with dipyrone. After 24 h, the patient presented dark stools. Two days later her clinical condition worsened and she was admitted to an emergency care unit (ECU), in which a blood count revealed thrombocytopenia ($57,000/mm^3$). Intravenous hydration, antipyretics, and antiemetics were administered. After 3 days, the abdominal pain worsened, and the patient developed cutaneous pallor, arterial hypotension, and drowsiness, and was transferred to a paediatric hospital, where she arrived pale, with cold skin, thin pulse, gasping, dehydrated, and with tense abdomen. Myocarditis was considered by the physician. A femoral central venous access allowed expansion with albumin. The blood count revealed mild anaemia (haemoglobin 11.9 g/dL, haematocrit 35.9%), lymphopenia ($92/mm^3$), and thrombocytopenia ($57,000/mm^3$ on admission, which dropped to $20,000/mm^3$ within a few hours). Liver enzymes were above reference levels during hospitalisation (aspartate aminotransferase 741.1 U/L; alanine aminotransferase 248.9 U/L). She also had altered renal function, hyperkalaemia (10 mmol/L), and severe metabolic acidosis (pH 6.7). Activated partial thromboplastin time and prothrombin time were prolonged (Table 1). The next day, the patient suffered cardiorespiratory arrest, unresponsive to resuscitation measures. There was profuse bleeding through the oropharynx, trachea, and stomach. The clinical diagnoses were severe acute hepatitis of unexplained cause, acute renal dysfunction, and shock.

The mother of the patient reported the presence of several neighbors with similar symptoms and the recent admission of an aunt who lived with her, who had been diagnosed with severe dengue. Neither respiratory symptoms nor recent contact with suspected or confirmed cases of COVID-19 were described. Remarkably, co-circulation of SARS-CoV-2 and dengue has recently been reported in the Americas [18].

Table 1. Results of laboratory tests.

| Exam | 27 June 2021 (3 Days of Symptom) | 28 June 2021 (4 Days of Symptom) | Reference Values |
|---|---|---|---|
| Red Cells | 4.29 million/mm$^3$ | 4.11 million/mm$^3$ | 4.1 to 5.3 million/mm$^3$ |
| Haemoglobin | 12.3 g/dL | 11.9 g/dL | 12 to 14.5 g/dL |
| Haematocrit | 35.9% | 35% | 36 to 43% |
| Leukocytes | 2300/mm$^3$ | 5600/mm$^3$ | 3400 to 10,800/mm$^3$ |
| Neutrophils | 1955/mm$^3$ | 4424/mm$^3$ | 1500 to 8500/mm$^3$ |
| Rod Neutrophils | 69/mm$^3$ | 224/mm$^3$ | 0 to 860/mm$^3$ |
| Segmented Neutrophils | 1886/mm$^3$ | 4200/mm$^3$ | 1500 to 8500/mm$^3$ |
| Eosinophils | 0/mm$^3$ | 56/mm$^3$ | 0 to 500/mm$^3$ |
| Lymphocytes | 92/mm$^3$ | 672/mm$^3$ | 1500 to 6500/mm$^3$ |
| Monocytes | 253/mm$^3$ | 336/mm$^3$ | 0 to 800/mm$^3$ |
| Basophils | 0/mm$^3$ | 0/mm$^3$ | 0 to 200/mm$^3$ |
| Platelets | 57,000/mm$^3$ | 20,000/mm$^3$ | 150 to 450 mil/mm$^3$ |
| Atypical Lymphocytes | - | 112/mm$^3$ | 0% |
| MPV | 8.3 fL | 7.5 fL | 9.2 to 12.6 fL |
| Ultrasensitive C-reactive protein | 2.96 mg/dL | 2.37 mg/dL | <0.10 mg/dL |
| Magnesium | - | 2.02 mg/dL | 2.02 to 2.75 mg/dL |
| Potassium | 4.0 mmol/L | 6.8 mmol/L | 3.5 to 5.1 mmol/L |
| Sodium | 136 mmol/L | 139 mmol/L | 136 to 145 mmol/L |
| AST | 83.3 U/L | 741.1 U/L | 17 to 33 U/L |
| ALT | 27.3 U/L | 248.9 U/L | 9 to 23 U/L |
| Urinary Urobilinogen | 3.0 mg/dL | - | < 1.0 mg/dL |
| Creatinine | - | 0.82 mg/dL | 0.32 to 0.61 mg/dL |
| Urea | - | 28.9 mg/dL | 19.2 to 46.2 mg/dL |
| TAP—prothrombin time | - | 16.8 s | 9.4 to 12.5 s |
| APTT- activated partial thromboplastin | - | 49.8 s | 25.1 to 36.5 s |
| | Laboratory tests performed after death | | |
| Blood culture | | | No microbial growth |
| RT-PCR for SARS-CoV-2 | | | Not Detectable |
| qRT-PCR for dengue | | | Positive |
| qRT-PCR for Zika | | | Negative |
| qRT-PCR for chikungunya | | | Negative |
| NS1 antigen | | | Positive |

Subtitle: MPV—mean platelet volume, AST—aspartate aminotransferase, ALT—alanine aminotransferase, TAP—prothrombin time, APTT—activated partial thromboplastin, RT-PCR—reverse transcriptase-polymerase chain reaction, qRT-PCR—quantitative reverse transcriptase-polymerase chain reaction.

The body was sent to the DVS Dr Rocha Furtado (DVS-RF), where an MIA followed by CA were performed, after consent provided by the mother. The post-mortem procedures were performed as part of a study approved by the Research Ethics Committee through protocol CAAE 27162619.1.0000.5049, number 3,851,684.

Nasopharyngeal swabs were routinely tested by quantitative reverse transcriptase-polymerase chain reaction (qRT-PCR) for SARS-CoV-2 in all DVS-RF autopsies performed during the COVID-19 pandemic. About 20 mL of blood and 2 mL of cerebrospinal fluid (CSF) were collected as part of the MIA procedure before the CA. The two post-mortem procedures were analysed by two different pathologists.

For the MIA, 20 cm, 14 Gauge percutaneous biopsy needles were used. Four brain cores (1.2 to 1.3 cm) were obtained by introducing the biopsy needle through the right and left nasal cavity, piercing the cribriform plate of the sphenoid bone. The right and the left lungs were punctured between the third and fourth intercostal spaces, and four cores from each lung (0.5 to 0.6 cm from the right lung; 1.2 to 1.4 cm from left lung) were collected. Four cores (0.8 to 0.9 cm) were obtained from the heart, after puncture in the fifth intercostal space. The liver was punctured in the right 11th intercostal space, in the anterior axillary line, and four tissue cores (0.7 to 1.0 cm) were obtained. Punctures directed to the kidneys were performed in the right and left subcostal spaces and four tissue fragments from each side were obtained (1.5 to 1.7 cm right, 1.0 to 1.2 cm left). Finally, four cores were collected from the splenic area (0.8 to 1.0 cm).

CA was performed following the DVS-RF protocol (4), after opening all cavities. The brain was swollen (weight 1310 g). Bilateral pleural effusion and ascites were observed. The lungs were oedematous and showed areas of haemorrhage (weight: 365 g left and 375 g right). The liver and the spleen showed congestion and weighed 1200 g and 415 g, respectively. One-hundred-and-fifty milliliters of fresh blood were identified in the stomach. The kidneys were pale and oedematous (weight: 110 g right and 100 g left). The adrenals showed no abnormalities.

Microscopic examination showed oedema and congestion in all organs, foci of intra-alveolar haemorrhage in the lungs, and foci of midzonal necrosis in the liver. Hypoplasia of the white pulp of the spleen was associated with abundant macrophages with large clear nuclei. There was extensive coagulative necrosis of the cortical tubules of the right kidney.

Samples of the left kidney and spleen of the MIA showed only skeletal muscle, connective tissue, vessels, and nerves under microscopy, with no cores of parenchyma.

The nasopharyngeal swab, blood, and CSF were sent to the Central Laboratory of Public Health of Ceará (LACEN-CE) for laboratory tests: qRT-PCR for respiratory viruses, arboviruses (dengue, Zika, and chikungunya), and detection of dengue NS1 antigen in blood and CSF [19]. A blood culture for bacterial research was also performed.

The following findings were of note: midzonal hepatocyte necrosis with rare acidophilic bodies seen only in the MIA samples, which were better preserved; enlargement of the alveolar septa by inflammatory cells (viral interstitial pneumonitis), edema and foci of intraalveolar hemorrhage seen in both MIA and CA; and acute tubular necrosis in the kidneys (Figure 1). Previous studies reporting histological findings in fatal cases of dengue have reported similar changes, including diffuse congestion and hemorrhage, alveolar edema, and liver cell necrosis [20].

The nasopharyngeal swab sample tested negative for SARS-CoV-2 RNA and there was no microbial growth in the blood culture. The qRT-PCR test for arboviruses identified the presence of DENV-2 RNA in the blood sample, and the NS1 antigen (kit J. Mitra & Co. Pvt. Ltd.) tests were positive for dengue in the blood and CSF samples [21] All tests performed for Zika and chikungunya viruses were negative (Table 1).

Clinical features, such as upper digestive and pulmonary hemorrhage, acute tubular necrosis, and shock causing death, in conjunction with the pathological and laboratory findings, were in keeping with the diagnosis of death due to complications of severe dengue. Remarkably, the samples collected by the MIA in this pediatric patient were sufficient to confirm the diagnosis of severe dengue and were completely in agreement with the samples collected by the CA (Figure 1).

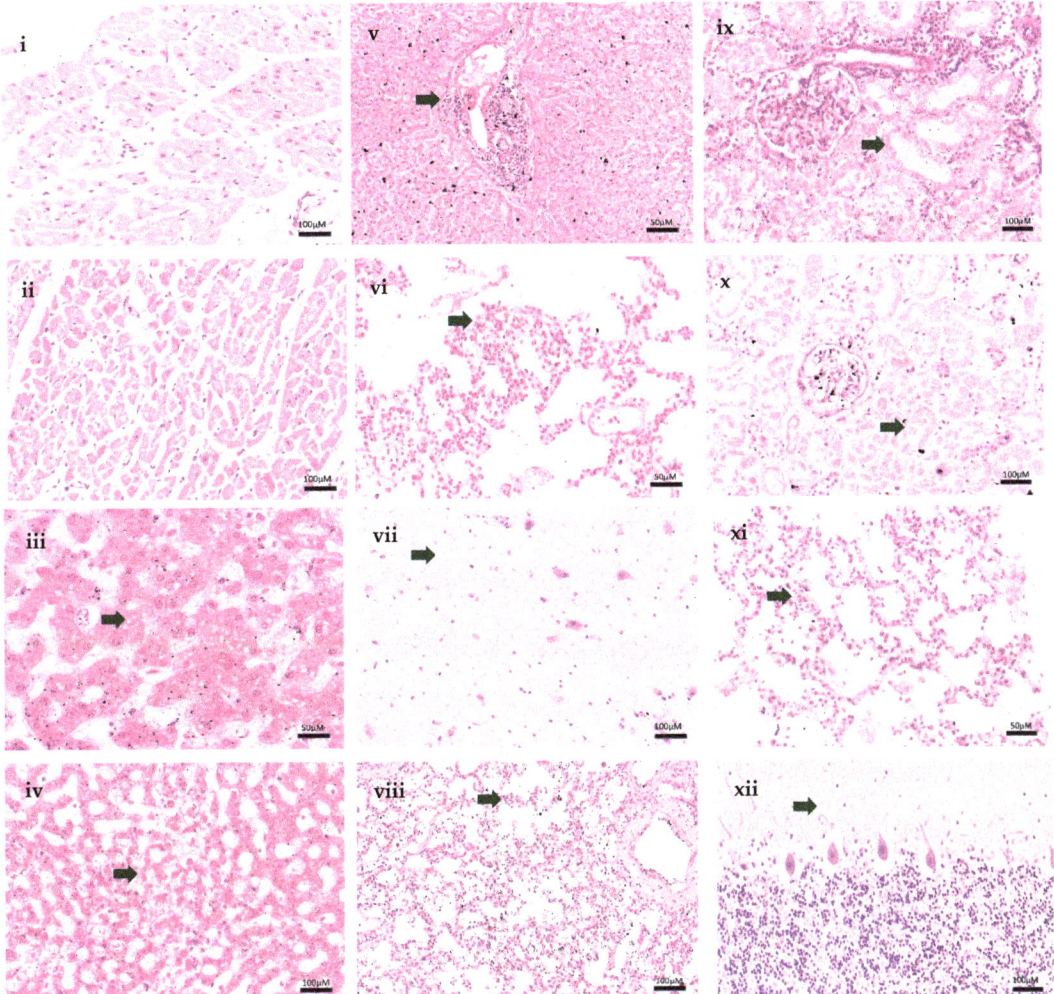

**Figure 1.** Images of MIA and CA samples of patient. (**i**)—Heart. Cardiac muscle fibres. (HE, 100X—MIA). (**ii**)—Heart. Cardiac muscle fibres. (HE, 100X—CA). (**iii**)—Liver. Mild microvesicular steatosis. (HE, 50X—MIA). (**iv**)—Liver. Midzonal necrosis of hepatocytes. (HE, 100X—MIA). (**v**)—Liver. Mononuclear portal infiltrate. Edema and congestion. (HE, 50X)—CA). (**vi**)—Lung. Interstitial pneumonitis. (HE, 50X—MIA). (**vii**)—Lung. Interstitial pneumonitis. (HE, 100X—CA). (**viii**)—Lung. Interstitial pneumonitis. Alveolar edema. (HE, 100X—CA). (**ix**)—Kidney R. Necrosis of renal tubules. (HE, 100X—MIA). (**x**)—Kidney Necrosis of renal tubules. (HE, 100X—CA). (**xi**)—Brain. Brain edema. (HE, 50X—MIA). (**xii**)—Cerebellum. Edema. (HE, 100X—CA). Legend: CA = conventional autopsy; MIA = minimally invasive autopsy.

## 3. Conclusions

Disease surveillance and patient healthcare requires adequate ascertainment of the cause of death, especially in the current context of circulation of multiple arboviruses and other pathogens with the potential of causing epidemics. In a scenario of reduced acceptability of CA, MIA is a promising tool, which has proven to be successful even during the COVID-19 pandemic, for diagnosing arboviral-related deaths.

**Author Contributions:** D.N.M., G.R.P.L., C.G.F., J.O., M.J.M., P.H.N.S. and L.P.G.C.—conceptualization; D.N.M., A.C.T., J.O., M.J.M. and P.H.N.S.—methodology; D.N.M., A.C.T., J.B.F. and L.P.G.C.—formal analysis; D.N.M., G.R.P.L., C.G.F., F.M.C.A., L.C.A. and L.P.G.C.—writing—original draft preparation; D.N.M., G.R.P.L., C.G.F., A.C.T., J.B.F., F.M.C.A., L.C.A., A.M.S., L.A.B.G.F., R.A.A.M., J.O., M.J.M., P.H.N.S. and L.P.G.C.—writing: review and editing. All authors have read and agreed to the published version of the manuscript.

**Funding:** This research was funded by REPLICK/DECIT/MS (process number 421724/2017-0 CNPQ) and SVS/MS (process number 707272/19-002).

**Institutional Review Board Statement:** The study was conducted in accordance with the Declaration of Helsinki and approved by the Institutional Review Board of Centro Universitario Christus, protocol code CAAE 27162619.1.0000.5049, number 3,851,684.

**Informed Consent Statement:** Informed consent was obtained from the family.

**Data Availability Statement:** Not applicable.

**Conflicts of Interest:** The authors declare no conflict of interest.

## References

1. Yang, X.; Quam, M.B.M.; Zhang, T.; Sang, S. Global burden for dengue and the evolving pattern in the past 30 years. *J. Travel Med.* **2021**, *28*, taab146. [CrossRef] [PubMed]
2. Du, M.; Jing, W.; Liu, M.; Liu, J. The Global Trends and Regional Differences in Incidence of Dengue Infection from 1990 to 2019: An Analysis from the Global Burden of Disease Study 2019. *Infect. Dis. Ther.* **2021**, *10*, 1625–1643. [CrossRef] [PubMed]
3. Martins, A.B.S.; Alencar, C.H. Ecoepidemiology of dengue in Brazil: From the virus to the environment. *One Health Implement. Res.* **2022**, *2*, 1–14. [CrossRef]
4. Cavalcanti, L.P.D.G.; Castiglioni, M.; da Silva, L.M.A.; Malta, D.L.; Pereira, R.A.D.C.; Silva-Junior, J.U.; Aguiar, M.G.; Pompeu, M.M.D.L.; Araújo, F.M.D.C.; Braga, D.N.D.M. Postmortem Diagnosis of Dengue as an Epidemiological Surveillance Tool. *Am. J. Trop. Med. Hyg.* **2016**, *94*, 187–192. [CrossRef]
5. Maixenchs, M.; Anselmo, R.; Sanz, A.; Castillo, P.; Macete, E.; Carrilho, C.; Ordi, J.; Menéndez, C.; Bassat, Q.; Munguambe, K. Healthcare providers' views and perceptions on post-mortem procedures for cause of death determination in Southern Mozambique. *PLoS ONE* **2018**, *13*, e0200058. [CrossRef]
6. Maixenchs, M.; Anselmo, R.; Zielinski Gutiérrez, E.; Odhiambo, F.O.; Akello, C.; Ondire, M.; Zaidi, S.S.H.; Soofi, S.B.; Bhutta, Z.A.; Diarra, K.; et al. Willingness to Know the Cause of Death and Hypothetical Acceptability of the Minimally Invasive Autopsy in Six Diverse African and Asian Settings: A Mixed Methods Socio-Behavioural Study. *PLoS Med.* **2016**, *13*, e1002172. [CrossRef]
7. Castillo, P.; Ussene, E.; Ismail, M.R.; Jordao, D.; Lovane, L.; Carrilho, C.; Lorenzoni, C.; Lacerda, M.V.; Palhares, A.E.M.; Rodríguez-Carunchio, L.; et al. Pathological Methods Applied to the Investigation of Causes of Death in Developing Countries: Minimally Invasive Autopsy Approach. *PLoS ONE* **2015**, *10*, e0132057. [CrossRef]
8. Bassat, Q.; Castillo, P.; Alonso, P.L.; Ordi, J.; Menéndez, C. Resuscitating the Dying Autopsy. *PLoS Med.* **2016**, *13*, e1001927. [CrossRef]
9. Bassat, Q.; Castillo, P.; Martinez, M.J.; Jordao, D.; Lovane, L.; Hurtado, J.C.; Nhampossa, T.; Ritchie, P.S.; Bandeira, S.; Sambo, C.; et al. Validity of a minimally invasive autopsy tool for cause of death determination in pediatric deaths in Mozambique: An observational study. *PLoS Med.* **2017**, *14*, e1002317. [CrossRef]
10. Menéndez, C.; Castillo, P.; Martinez, M.J.; Jordao, D.; Lovane, L.; Ismail, M.R.; Carrilho, C.; Lorenzoni, C.; Fernandes, F.; Nhampossa, T.; et al. Validity of a minimally invasive autopsy for cause of death determination in stillborn babies and neonates in Mozambique: An observational study. *PLoS Med.* **2017**, *14*, e1002318. [CrossRef]
11. Schwartz, D.A. Autopsy and Postmortem Studies Are Concordant: Pathology of Zika Virus Infection Is Neurotropic in Fetuses and Infants With Microcephaly Following Transplacental Transmission. *Arch. Pathol. Lab. Med.* **2016**, *141*, 68–72. [CrossRef] [PubMed]
12. Duarte-Neto, A.N.; Monteiro, R.; Johnsson, J.; Cunha, M.D.P.; POUR, S.Z.; Saraiva, A.C.; Ho, Y.-L.; Da Silva, L.F.F.; Mauad, T.; Zanotto, P.M.D.A.; et al. Ultrasound-guided minimally invasive autopsy as a tool for rapid post-mortem diagnosis in the 2018 Sao Paulo yellow fever epidemic: Correlation with conventional autopsy. *PLoS Negl. Trop. Dis.* **2019**, *13*, e0007625. [CrossRef] [PubMed]
13. Argueta, V. La importancia de la autopsia en epidemias. *Rev Me ´d (Col Me ´d Cir Guatem)* **2020**, *159*, 2–3. [CrossRef]
14. Martínez, M.J.; Massora, S.; Mandomando, I.; Ussene, E.; Jordao, D.; Lovane, L.; Muñoz-Almagro, C.; Castillo, P.; Mayor, A.; Rodriguez, C.; et al. Infectious cause of death determination using minimally invasive autopsies in developing countries. *Diagn. Microbiol. Infect. Dis.* **2016**, *84*, 80–86. [CrossRef]
15. Melo, D.N.; Coelho, T.M.; Lima, G.R.P.; Fernandes, C.G.; Alves, B.C.F.D.B.; Araújo, F.M.D.C.; Monteiro, R.A.D.A.; Ordi, J.; Saldiva, P.H.D.N.; Cavalcanti, L.P.D.G. Use of minimally invasive autopsy during the COVID-19 pandemic and its possibilities in the context of developing countries. *PLoS Negl. Trop. Dis.* **2021**, *15*, e0009729. [CrossRef]

16. Saldiva, P.H.N. Minimally invasive autopsies: A promise to revive the procedure. *Autops. Case Rep.* **2014**, *4*, 1–3. [CrossRef]
17. Rakislova, N.; Marimon, L.; Ismail, M.; Carrilho, C.; Fernandes, F.; Ferrando, M.; Castillo, P.; Rodrigo-Calvo, M.; Guerrero, J.; Ortiz, E.; et al. Minimally Invasive Autopsy Practice in COVID-19 Cases: Biosafety and Findings. *Pathogens* **2021**, *10*, 412. [CrossRef]
18. Reyes-Ruiz, J.M.; Campuzano-Vences, R.; Osuna-Ramos, J.F.; De Jesús-González, L.A.; Pérez-Méndez, M.J.; González-González, C.; Farfan-Morales, C.N.; Rivas-Tovar, L.; Dávila-González, E.; del Ángel, R.M.; et al. Case Report: Extrapulmonary Manifestations of COVID-19 and Dengue Coinfection. *Am. J. Trop. Med. Hyg.* **2021**, *105*, 363–367. [CrossRef]
19. Araújo, F.; Brilhante, R.; Cavalcanti, L.; Rocha, M.; Cordeiro, R.; Perdigão, A.; Miralles, I.; Araújo, L.; Lima, E.; Sidrim, J. Detection of the dengue non-structural 1 antigen in cerebral spinal fluid samples using a commercially available enzyme-linked immunosorbent assay. *J. Virol. Methods* **2011**, *177*, 128–131. [CrossRef]
20. Póvoa, T.F.; Alves, A.M.B.; Oliveira, C.A.B.; Nuovo, G.J.; Chagas, V.L.A.; Paes, M. The Pathology of Severe Dengue in Multiple Organs of Human Fatal Cases: Histopathology, Ultrastructure and Virus Replication. *PLoS ONE* **2014**, *9*, e83386. [CrossRef]
21. Araujo, F.M.C.; Araujo, M.S.; Nogueira, R.M.R.; Brilhante, R.S.N.; Oliveira, D.N.; Rocha, M.F.G.; Cordeiro, R.A.; Sidrim, J.J.C. Central nervous system involvement in dengue: A study in fatal cases from a dengue endemic area. *Neurology* **2012**, *78*, 736–742. [CrossRef] [PubMed]

MDPI
St. Alban-Anlage 66
4052 Basel
Switzerland
www.mdpi.com

*Tropical Medicine and Infectious Disease* Editorial Office
E-mail: tropicalmed@mdpi.com
www.mdpi.com/journal/tropicalmed

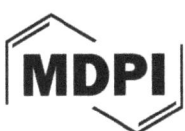

Disclaimer/Publisher's Note: The statements, opinions and data contained in all publications are solely those of the individual author(s) and contributor(s) and not of MDPI and/or the editor(s). MDPI and/or the editor(s) disclaim responsibility for any injury to people or property resulting from any ideas, methods, instructions or products referred to in the content.

www.ingramcontent.com/pod-product-compliance
Lightning Source LLC
LaVergne TN
LVHW070244100526
838202LV00015B/2173